Davidson's
Self-assessment in
Medicine

Davidson's
Self-assessment in
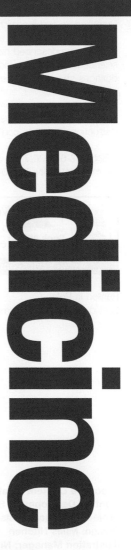

Edited by

Deborah Wake
MB ChB (Hons), BSc, PhD, Diploma Clin Ed, MRCPE
Clinical Reader, University of Edinburgh; Honorary Consultant
Physician, NHS Lothian, Edinburgh, UK

Patricia Cantley
MB ChB, FRCP, BSc Hons (Med Sci)
Consultant Physician, Midlothian Enhanced Rapid Response and
Intervention Team, Midlothian Health and Social Care Partnership
and also Royal Infirmary of Edinburgh and Midlothian Community
Hospital, Edinburgh, UK

ELSEVIER   Edinburgh   London   New York   Oxford   Philadelphia
St Louis   Sydney   2018

ELSEVIER

Notices

ISBN: 978-0-7020-7151-5
International ISBN: 978-0-7020-7145-4

  Working together to grow libraries in developing countries

www.elsevier.com • www.bookaid.org

Printed in Poland
Last digit is the print number: 9 8 7 6 5 4 3 2 1

Executive Content Strategist: Laurence Hunter
Content Development Specialist: Carole McMurray
Project Manager: Louisa Talbott
Design: Miles Hitchen
Illustration Manager: Nichole Beard
Illustrator: MPS North America LLC
Marketing Manager: Deborah Watkins

Contents

Preface

This is the first edition of *Davidson's Self-assessment in Medicine*, designed as an accompanying volume to the internationally renowned textbook *Davidson's Principles and Practice of Medicine*. Since the original *Davidson's* was first published in 1952, it has acquired a large following of medical students, doctors and health professionals. Alongside the success of the main textbook, a demand has emerged for a complementary self-assessment book covering a broad range of general medicine topics. Our new book uses typical clinical scenarios to test the reader. Each chapter is written by a specialty expert and the contents follow the style and chapter layout of *Davidson's*. This book can be used either independently or in conjunction with the main book.

This book has been built around modern educational principles and utilises a contemporary assessment style, in line with current undergraduate and postgraduate teaching. It is designed to help and support students in their final undergraduate years and in the early years after qualification. The style is compatible with that used in modern postgraduate examinations across the world.

The clinical scenarios have been chosen to be suitable for clinicians at any stage in their career, supporting ongoing professional development. Clinical reasoning and judgement are encouraged, with questions mirroring the situations and presentations that clinicians will meet in their everyday practice. The content is applicable to a global audience and is based on current evidence-based best practice.

The modern physician needs not only a sound knowledge base but also the ability to apply that understanding appropriately to individual patients. The vision of the editors is to create a resource that stimulates readers to build and apply their clinical knowledge to real-life scenarios, resulting in excellent patient-centred care.

Deborah Wake and Patricia Cantley
Edinburgh, 2018

Introduction

This book offers a broad education through formative self-assessment in general internal medicine. The majority of the questions have been designed around clinical scenarios, with a number of optional answers offered to the question posed. In general, the 'best fit' answer is sought unless otherwise stated. Full explanations are given as appropriate to assist the reader in their learning.

The questions aim to cover a wide range of topics, divided into specialist chapters in line with *Davidson's Principles and Practice of Medicine*. The questions have in general been based on UK clinical practice and pharmacology, but where appropriate generic drug names are used and the underlying principles are applicable internationally. Whilst the answers given are in line with best evidence-based clinical practice, patient choice and cultural factors should always be considered when applying the learning in individual patients and situations.

How to use this book

This self-assessment book can be used either independently or in conjunction with *Davidson's*. Readers may find it useful to read the relevant section of the main textbook in advance of tackling the self-assessment; or they can use it subsequently to explore the topic in greater detail.

The questions, followed by their corresponding answers, have been arranged in the same chapter order as *Davidson's*. The chapters are free-standing and can be read independently in any order.

Some of the questions are based on accompanying clinical images and radiology. Where it is appropriate to see the image in colour, it has also been reproduced in a colour photographic section at the back of the book.

Normal Reference Ranges for tests have not been used within the questions or explanations, but can be found in the laboratory reference range chapter, at the end of the book.

Standard abbreviations are found within the text and are generally explained at first use. A full list of abbreviations can be found at the front of the book.

Contributors

Anna Anderson MBChB, MRCP, PhD
Specialist Registrar Diabetes and Endocrinology,
Western General Hospital, Edinburgh, UK

**Brian J Angus BSc (Hons), DTM&H, FRCP,
MD, FFTM(Glas)**
Associate Professor, Nuffield Department of
Medicine, University of Oxford, UK

**Quentin M Anstee BSc (Hons), MBBS, PhD,
MRCP, FRCP**
Professor of Experimental Hepatology, Institute
of Cellular Medicine, Newcastle University,
Newcastle upon Tyne, UK; Honorary Consultant
Hepatologist, Freeman Hospital, Newcastle upon
Tyne NHS Hospitals Foundation Trust, Newcastle
upon Tyne, UK

Jennifer Bain MBChB, MRCP, FRCA, FFICM
Fellow in Vascular Anaesthesia, Scottish
Thoraco-abdominal & Aortic Aneurysm Service,
Royal Infirmary of Edinburgh, Edinburgh, UK

Leslie Burnett MBBS, PhD, FRCPA
Chief Medical Officer, Genome.One,
Garvan Institute of Medical Research,
Darlinghurst, Sydney; Honorary Professor,
University of Sydney, Sydney Medical School,
Sydney; Conjoint Professor, UNSW, St
Vincent's Medical School, Darlinghurst,
Sydney, Australia

**Mark Byers OBE, FRCGP, FFSEM, FIMC,
MRCEM**
Consultant in Pre-Hospital Emergency Medicine,
Institute of Pre-Hospital Care, London, UK

Harry Campbell MD, FRCPE, FFPH, FRSE
Professor of Genetic Epidemiology and Public
Health, Centre for Global Health Research, Usher
Institute of Population Health Sciences
and Informatics, University of Edinburgh,
Edinburgh, UK

**C Fiona Clegg BSc (MedSci), MBChB,
MRCP (UK)**
Clinical Lecturer in Gastroenterology, School of
Medicine, Medical Sciences and Nutrition,
University of Aberdeen, Aberdeen, UK

Gavin Clunie BSc, MBBS, MD, FRCP
Consultant Rheumatologist and Metabolic Bone
Physician, Cambridge University Hospitals NHS
Foundation Trust, Addenbrooke's Hospital,
Cambridge, UK

**Lesley A Colvin MBChB, BSc, FRCA, PhD,
FRCP (Edin), FFPMRCA**
Consultant/Honorary Professor in Anaesthesia
and Pain Medicine, Department of Anaesthesia,
Critical Care and Pain Medicine, University
of Edinburgh, Western General Hospital,
Edinburgh, UK

Bryan Conway MB, MRCP, PhD
Senior Lecturer, Centre for Cardiovascular
Science, University of Edinburgh; Honorary
Consultant Nephrologist, Royal Infirmary
Edinburgh, Edinburgh, UK

**Nicola Cooper MBChB, FAcadMEd, FRCPE,
FRACP**
Consultant Physician, Derby Teaching Hospitals
NHS Foundation Trust; Honorary Clinical
Associate Professor, Nottingham University,
Division of Medical Sciences and Graduate Entry
Medicine, Nottingham, UK

Dominic J Culligan BSc, MBBS, MD, FRCP, FRCPath
Consultant Haematologist and Honorary Senior Lecturer, Aberdeen Royal Infirmary, Aberdeen, UK

Ruth Darbyshire MB BChir, MA(Cantab)
Specialty Trainee in Ophthalmology, Yorkshire and Humber Deanery, Yorkshire, UK

Graham Dark MBBS, FRCP, FHEA
Senior Lecturer in Medical Oncology and Cancer Education, Newcastle University, Newcastle upon Tyne, UK

Richard J Davenport DM, FRCP (Edin), BM BS, BMedSci
Consultant Neurologist and Honorary Senior Lecturer, University of Edinburgh, Edinburgh, UK

David Dockrell MD, FRCPI, FRCP (Glas), FACP
Professor of Infection Medicine, MRC/University of Edinburgh Centre for Inflammation Research, University of Edinburgh, Edinburgh, UK

Emad El-Omar BSc (Hons), MBChB, MD (Hons), FRCP (Edin), FRSE
Professor of Medicine, St George and Sutherland Clinical School, University of New South Wales, Sydney, Australia

Sarah Fadden BA, MB BChir, FRCA
Senior Registrar in Anaesthesia, Royal Infirmary of Edinburgh, Edinburgh, UK

Catriona M Farrell MBChB, MRCP (UK)
Specialist Registrar Endocrinology and Diabetes, Ninewells Hospital, Dundee, UK

Amy Frost MA (Cantab), MBBS, MRCP
Clinical Genomics Educator, Affiliated to St George's University NHS Foundation Trust, London, UK

Neil Grubb MD, FRCP
Cardiology Consultant, Royal Infirmary of Edinburgh; Honorary Senior Lecturer, Cardiovascular Sciences, University of Edinburgh, Edinburgh, UK

Jyoti Hansi
Department of Gastroenterology, Royal Infirmary of Edinburgh, Edinburgh, UK

Sally H Ibbotson BSc (Hons), MBChB (Hons), MD, FRCP (Edin)
Professor of Photodermatology, Photobiology Unit, Dermatology Department, University of Dundee, Dundee, UK

Sara J Jenks Bsc (Hons), MRCP, FRCPath
Consultant in Metabolic Medicine, Department of Clinical Biochemistry, Royal Infirmary of Edinburgh, UK

Sarah Louise Johnston MB ChB, FCRP, FRCPath
Consultant in Immunology & HIV Medicine, Department of Immunology and Immunogenetics, North Bristol NHS Trust, Bristol, UK

David E J Jones MA, BM BCh, PhD, FRCP
Professor of Liver Immunology, Institute of Cellular Medicine, Newcastle University; Consultant Hepatologist, Freeman Hospital, Newcastle upon Tyne, UK

Peter Langhorne MBChB, PhD, FRCP (Glas), Hon FRCPI
Professor of Stroke Care, Institute of Cardiovascular and Medical Sciences, University of Glasgow, Glasgow, UK

Stephen Lawrie MD (Hons), FRCPsych, Hon FRCP (Edin)
Professor of Psychiatry, University of Edinburgh, Edinburgh, UK

John Paul Leach MD, FRCP
Consultant Neurologist, Institute of Neurological Sciences, Glasgow; Head of Undergraduate Medicine, University of Glasgow, Glasgow, UK

Andrew Leitch MBChB, BSc (Hons), PhD, MSc (Clin Ed), FRCPE (Respiratory)
Consultant Respiratory Physician, Western General Hospital; Honorary Senior Lecturer, University of Edinburgh, Edinburgh, UK

Gary Maartens MBChB, FCP(SA), MMed
Professor of Medicine, University of Cape Town, Cape Town, South Africa

Lucy Mackillop BM BCh, MA (Oxon), FRCP
Consultant Obstetric Physician, Oxford University Hospitals NHS Foundation Trust; Honorary Senior Clinical Lecturer, Nuffield Department of Obstetrics and Gynaecology, University of Oxford, Oxford, UK

Michael MacMahon MBChB, FRCA, FICM, EDIC
Consultant in Anaesthesia and Intensive Care, Victoria Hospital, Kirkcaldy, Fife, UK

Rebecca Mann BMedSci, BMBS, MRCP, FRCPCh
Consultant Paediatrician, Taunton and Somerset NHS Foundation Trust, Taunton, UK

Lynn Manson MBChB, MD, FRCP, FRCPath
Consultant Haematologist, Scottish National Blood Transfusion Service, Department of Transfusion Medicine, Royal Infirmary of Edinburgh, Edinburgh, UK

Amanda Mather MBBS, FRACP, PhD
Consultant Nephrologist, Department of Renal Medicine, Royal North Shore Hospital; Conjoint Senior Lecturer, Faculty of Medicine, University of Sydney, Sydney, Australia

Simon R Maxwell BSc, MBChB, MD, PhD, FRCP, FRCPE, FHEA
Professor of Student Learning/Clinical Pharmacology & Prescribing, Clinical Pharmacology Unit, University of Edinburgh, Edinburgh, UK

David McAllister MBChB, MD, MPH, MRCP, MFPH
Wellcome Trust Intermediate Clinical Fellow and Beit Fellow, Senior Clinical Lecturer in Epidemiology and Honorary Consultant in Public Health Medicine, University of Glasgow, Glasgow, UK

Mairi H McLean BSc (Hons), MBChB (Hons), PhD, MRCP
Senior Clinical Lecturer in Gastroenterology, School of Medicine, Medical Sciences and Nutrition, University of Aberdeen; Honorary Consultant Gastroenterologist, Digestive Disorders Department, Aberdeen Royal Infirmary, Aberdeen, UK

Francesca E M Neuberger MBChB, MRCP (UK)
Consultant Physician in Acute Medicine and Obstetric Medicine, Southmead Hospital, Bristol, UK

David E Newby BA, BSc (Hons), PhD, BM, DM, DSc, FMedSci, FRSE, FESC, FACC
British Heart Foundation John Wheatley Chair of Cardiology, British Heart Foundation Centre for Cardiovascular Science, University of Edinburgh, Edinburgh, UK

John Olson MD, FRPCE, FRCOphth
Consultant Ophthalmic Physician, Aberdeen Royal Infirmary; Honorary Reader, University of Aberdeen, UK

Paul J Phelan MBBCh, MD, FRCP (Edin)
Consultant Nephrologist and Renal Transplant Physician, Honorary Senior Lecturer, University of Edinburgh, Royal Infirmary of Edinburgh, Edinburgh, UK

Eric M Przybyszewski BS, MD
Resident Physician, Department of Medicine, Massachusetts General Hospital, Boston, USA

Stuart H Ralston MBChB, MRCP, FMedSci, FRSE
Professor of Rheumatology, Rheumatic Diseases Unit, University of Edinburgh, Edinburgh, UK

Jonathan Sandoe MBChB, PhD, FRCPath
Associate Clinical Professor, University of Leeds, UK

Gordon Scott BSc, FRCP
Consultant in Genitourinary Medicine, Chalmers Sexual Health Centre, Edinburgh, UK

Alan G Shand MD, FRCP (Ed)
Consultant Gastroenterologist, Gastrointestinal Unit, Western General Hospital, Edinburgh, UK

Robby Steel MA, MD, FRCPsych
Department of Psychological Medicine, Royal Infirmary of Edinburgh; Honorary (Clinical) Senior Lecturer, Department of Psychiatry, University of Edinburgh, Edinburgh, UK

Grant D Stewart BSc (Hons), FRCSEd (Urol), MBChB, PhD
University Lecturer in Urological Surgery, Department of Surgery, University of Cambridge; Honorary Consultant Urological Surgeon, Department of Urology, Addenbrooke's Hospital, Cambridge; Honorary Senior Clinical Lecturer, University of Edinburgh, Edinburgh, UK

David R. Sullivan MBBS, FRACP, FRCPA
Clinical Associate Professor, Clinical Biochemistry, Royal Prince Alfred Hospital, Camperdown, NSW, Australia

Victoria Ruth Tallentire BSc (Hons), MD, FRCP (Edin)
Consultant Physician, Western General Hospital; Honorary Clinical Senior Lecturer, University of Edinburgh, Edinburgh, UK

Simon H Thomas MD, FRCP
Professor of Clinical Pharmacoloy and Therapeutics, Medical Toxicology Centre, Newcastle University, Newcastle upon Tyne, UK

Craig Thurtell BMedSci (Hons), MBChB MRCP
Specialty Registrar, Department of Diabetes & Endocrinology, Ninewells Hospital, Dundee, UK

Henry Watson MBChB, MD
Consultant Haematologist, Aberdeen Royal Infirmary, Aberdeen, UK

Julian White MBBS, MD
Professor and Department Head, Toxinology Department, Women's & Children's Hospital, North Adelaide, Australia

Miles D Witham BM BCh, PhD, FRCP (Ed)
Clinical Reader in Ageing and Health, Department of Ageing and Health, University of Dundee, Dundee, UK

Abbreviations

11β-HSD	11β-Hydroxysteroid dehydrogenase	**APL**	Acute promyelocytic leukaemia
^{131}I	Radioisotope iodine-131	**APS**	Antiphospholipid syndrome
2,3-DPG	2,3-Diphosphoglycerate	**APTT**	Activated partial thromboplastin time
20WBCT	20-Minute whole-blood clotting test	**ARDS**	Acute respiratory distress syndrome
5-ASA	5-Aminosalicylic acid	**ART**	Antiretroviral therapy
5-HIAA	5-Hydroxyindoleacetic acid	**AS**	Ankylosing spondylitis
AAV	ANCA-associated vasculitis	**AST**	Aspartate aminotransferase
ACE	Angiotensin-converting enzyme	**ATCG**	Adenine, thymine, cytosine, guanine
AChR	Acetylcholine receptor	**ATG**	Anti-thymocyte globulin
ACPA	Anti-citrullinated peptide antibody	**ATN**	Acute tubular necrosis
ACR	Albumin : creatinine ratio	**AVNRT**	Atrioventricular nodal re-entrant tachycardia
ACTH	Adrenocorticotrophic hormone		
ADH	Antidiuretic hormone, vasopressin	**AVP**	Arginine vasopressin
ADP	Adenosine diphosphate	**AVRT**	Atrioventricular re-entrant tachycardia
ADR	Adverse drug reaction		
AED	Antiepileptic drug	**axSpA**	Axial spondyloarthritis
AFLP	Acute fatty liver of pregnancy	**BAL**	Bronchoalveolar lavage
AFP	Alpha-fetoprotein	**BCC**	Basal cell carcinoma
AICTD	Autoimmune connective tissue disease	**BCG**	Bacille Calmette–Guérin
		BD	Behçet's disease
AIDS	Acquired immune deficiency syndrome	**BiPAP**	Bi-level positive airway pressure
		BMD	Bone mineral density
AIH	Autoimmune hepatitis	**BMI**	Body mass index
AK	Actinic keratosis	**BNP**	Brain natriuretic peptide
AKI	Acute kidney injury	**BP**	Blood pressure
ALL	Acute lymphoblastic leukaemia	**BPH**	Benign prostatic hypertrophy
ALP	Alkaline phosphatase	**BPPV**	Benign paroxysmal positional vertigo
ALT	Alanine transaminase		
AMA	Antimitochondrial antibody	**BRCA1**	BReast CAncer genes 1
AMD	Age-related macular degeneration	**BRCA2**	BReast CAncer genes 2
AML	Acute myeloid leukaemia	**Ca^{2+}**	Calcium
ANA	Antinuclear antibody	**CA-MRSA**	Community-acquired meticillin-resistant *Staphylococcus aureus*
ANCA	Antineutrophil cytoplasmic antibody		
anti-EMA	Anti-endomysial antibody	**CAH**	Congenital adrenal hyperplasia
anti-tTG	Anti-tissue transglutaminase	**cAMP**	Cyclic adenosine monophosphate
APC	Argon plasma coagulation	**CAP**	Community-acquired pneumonia
APKD	Autosomal dominant polycystic kidney disease	**CBT**	Cognitive behavioural therapy
		CCF	Congestive cardiac failure

CD4	Cluster of differentiation 4	**DIPJ**	Distal interphalangeal joints
CDC	Centers for Disease Control and Prevention	**DIT**	Diiodotyrosine
		DKA	Diabetic ketoacidosis
CF	Cystic fibrosis	**DLBL**	Diffuse large B-cell lymphoma
CFTR	Cystic fibrosis transmembrane conductance regulator	**DLQI**	Dermatology Life Quality Index
		DM1	Myotonic dystrophy type 1
CGA	Comprehensive Geriatric Assessment	**DMARD**	Disease-modifying antirheumatic drug
CGH	Comparative genomic hybridisation	**DMSA**	Dimercaptosuccinic acid
		DNA	Deoxyribonucleic acid
CGRP	Calcitonin gene-related peptide	**DOAC**	Direct oral anticoagulant
CIDP	Chronic inflammatory demyelinating polyneuropathy	**DPP-4**	Dipeptidyl peptidase 4
		DRE	Digital rectal examination
CIM	Critical illness myopathy	**DRESS**	Drug reaction and eosinophilia with systemic symptoms
CJD	Creutzfeldt–Jakob disease		
CK	Creatine kinase	**DVT**	Deep vein thrombosis
CKD	Chronic kidney disease	**DXA**	Dual X-ray absorptiometry
CLL	Chronic lymphocytic leukaemia	**E, V, M**	Eye, verbal, motor (in Glasgow Coma Scale)
CML	Chronic myeloid leukaemia		
CMV	Cytomegalovirus	**EBUS-FNA**	Endobronchial ultrasound-guided fine needle aspiration
CN	Cranial nerve		
CNS	Central nervous system	**EBV**	Epstein–Barr virus
CNV	Copy number variant	**ECF**	Extracellular fluid
CO₂	Carbon dioxide	**ECF**	Epirubicin, cisplatin and fluorouracil (cancer chemotherapy combination)
COL4A5	Collagen type IV alpha 5 chain		
COPD	Chronic obstructive pulmonary disease		
		ECG	Electrocardiography
COX	Cyclo-oxygenase	**ECMO**	Extracorporeal membrane oxygenation
CPAP	Continuous positive airway pressure		
CPE	Carbapenemase-producing Enterobacteriaceae	**ECT**	Electroconvulsive therapy
		ED	Erectile dysfunction
CPPD	Calcium pyrophosphate disease	**ED₅₀**	Median effective dose: the dose that produces a quantal effect (all or nothing) in 50% of the population that takes it
CPR	Cardiopulmonary resuscitation		
CRP	C-reactive protein		
CRPS	Complex regional pain syndrome		
CSF	Cerebrospinal fluid	**EEG**	Electroencephalography
CT	Computed tomography	**eGFR**	Estimated glomerular filtration rate
CT-PET	CT positron emission tomography	**EGFR**	Epidermal growth factor receptor
CTKUB	CT scan of kidneys, ureters and bladder	**EIA**	Enzyme immunoassay
		ELISA	Enzyme-linked immunosorbent assay
CTPA	CT pulmonary angiogram		
CTS	Carpal tunnel syndrome	**EMG**	Electromyography
CVC	Central venous catheter	**ENA**	Extractable nuclear antigens
CVD	Cardiovascular disease	**ENT**	Ear, nose and throat
CVP	Central venous pressure	**EPO**	Erythropoietin
CXR	Chest X-ray	**ERCP**	Endoscopic retrograde cholangiopancreatography
CYP	Cytochrome P		
DBS	Deep brain stimulation	**ESR**	Erythrocyte sedimentation rate
DDAVP	Desmopressin	**ESRD**	End-stage renal disease
DGI	Disseminated gonococcal infection	**ESWL**	Extracorporeal shockwave lithotripsy
DILI	Drug-induced liver injury	**ET**	Essential tremor
DILS	Diffuse inflammatory lymphocytosis syndrome	**EUS**	Endoscopic ultrasound
		FAP	Familial adenomatous polyposis

FAST HUG	Feeding, analgesia, sedation, thromboprophylaxis, head of bed elevation, ulcer prophylaxis, glucose control (mnemonic to help prevent intensive care complications)	**HBeAg**	Hepatitis B e antigen
		HBsAg	Hepatitis B surface antigen
		HBV	Hepatitis B virus
		HCC	Hepatocellular carcinoma
		hCG	Human chorionic gonadotrophin
FDG	Fludeoxyglucose	**HCO$_3^-$**	Bicarbonate
FEV$_1$	Forced expiratory volume in 1 second	**HCV**	Hepatitis C virus
		HDL	High-density lipoprotein
FFP	Fresh frozen plasma	**HDV**	Hepatitis D virus
FHH	Familial hypocalciuric hypercalcaemia	**HELLP**	Haemolysis, elevated liver enzymes, low platelet count
FiO$_2$	Fraction of inspired oxygen	**HER**	Human epidermal growth factor receptor
FODMAP	Fermentable oligosaccharides, disaccharides, monosaccharides and polyols	**HEV**	Hepatitis E virus
		HG	Hyperemesis gravidarum
FSGS	Focal segmental glomerulosclerosis	**HHS**	Hyperosmolar hyperglycaemic state
FSH	Follicle-stimulating hormone	**HIT**	Heparin-induced thrombocytopenia
FVC	Forced vital capacity		
FXR	Farnesoid X receptor	**HIV**	Human immunodeficiency virus
G-CSF	Granulocyte colony-stimulating factor	**HIVAN**	HIV-associated nephropathy
		HL	Hodgkin lymphoma
G6PD	Glucose-6-phosphate dehydrogenase	**HLA**	Human leucocyte antigen
		HLH	Haemophagocytic lymphohistiocytosis
GABA	γ-Aminobutyric acid		
GAD	Glutamic acid decarboxylase	**HMS**	Hypermobility syndrome
GBD	Global Burden of Disease	**HNF**	Hepatocyte nuclear factor
GBL	Gamma butyrolactone	**HPOA**	Hypertrophic pulmonary osteoarthropathy
GBM	Glomerular basement membrane		
GBS	Guillain–Barré syndrome	**HPV**	Human papilloma virus
GCA	Giant cell arteritis	**HRCT**	High-resolution CT
GCS	Glasgow Coma Scale	**HSV**	Herpes simplex virus
GFR	Glomerular filtration rate	**HTLV**	Human T-cell lymphotropic virus
GGE	Genetic generalised epilepsies	**HUS**	Haemolytic uraemic syndrome
GGT	γ-Glutamyl transferase	**IA-2**	Islet antigen 2
GH	Growth hormone	**IABP**	Intra-aortic balloon pump
GHB	Gamma hydroxybutyrate	**IARC**	International Agency for Research on Cancer
GI	Gastrointestinal		
GIP	Gastric inhibitory polypeptide	**IBD**	Inflammatory bowel disease
GIST	Gastrointestinal stromal cell tumour	**IBS**	Irritable bowel syndrome
		ICD	Implantable cardiac defibrillator
GLP-1	Glucagon-like peptide-1	**ICD**	International Classification of Diseases
GLUTs	Glucose transporters		
GnRH	Gonadotrophin-releasing hormone	**ICF**	Intracellular fluid
GORD	Gastro-oesophageal reflux disease	**ICP**	Intracranial pressure
GPA	Granulomatosis with polyangiitis	**ICS**	Inhaled corticosteroid
GVHD	Graft-versus-host disease	**ICU**	Intensive care unit
H$^+$	Hydrogen ion	**IDU**	Intravenous drug user
HACE	High-altitude cerebral oedema	**Ig**	Immunoglobulin
HAP	Hospital-acquired pneumonia	**IgA**	Immunoglobulin A
HAPE	High-altitude pulmonary oedema	**IgE**	Immunoglobulin E
HAV	Hepatitis A virus	**IGF**	Insulin-like growth factor
HbA$_{1c}$	Glycated haemoglobin	**IgG**	Immunoglobulin G
HBc	Hepatitis B core antigen	**IgM**	Immunoglobulin M

IGRA	Interferon-gamma release assay	**MERS-CoV**	Middle East respiratory syndrome coronavirus
IIH	Idiopathic intracranial hypertension		
ILD	Interstitial lung disease	**Mg²⁺**	Magnesium
IM	Intramuscular	**MGUS**	Monoclonal gammopathy of uncertain significance
INN	International non-proprietary name		
INR	International normalised ratio	**MHC**	Major histocompatibility complex
IPF	Idiopathic pulmonary fibrosis	**MI**	Myocardial infarction
IPSS	International Prostate Symptom Score	**MIT**	Monoiodotyrosine
		MM	Multiple myeloma
IRIS	Immune reconstitution inflammatory syndrome	**MMF**	Mycophenolate mofetil
		MODY	Maturity-onset diabetes of the young
ITP	Immune thrombocytopenia		
IV	Intravenous	**MPA**	Microscopic polyangiitis
IVIg	Intravenous immunoglobulins	**MRCP**	Magnetic resonance cholangiopancreatography
JC virus	John Cunningham virus		
JIA	Juvenile idiopathic arthritis	**MRD**	Minimal residual disease
JVP	Jugular venous pressure	**MRI**	Magnetic resonance imaging
K⁺	Potassium	**mRNA**	Messenger ribonucleic acid
K$_{CO}$	Carbon monoxide transfer coefficient	**MRSA**	Meticillin-resistant *Staphylococcus aureus*
LABA	Long-acting β₂-agonist	**MS**	Multiple sclerosis
LADA	Latent autoimmune diabetes of adulthood	**MSE**	Mental state examination
		MSM	Man who has sex with men
LAMA	Long-acting muscarinic antagonist	**MSU**	Mid-stream urine
LDH	Lactate dehydrogenase	**MTP**	Metatarsophalangeal
LDL	Low-density lipoprotein	**MuSK**	Muscle-specific kinase
LEMS	Lambert–Eaton myasthenic syndrome	**MVA**	Mosaic variegated aneuploidy
		Na⁺	Sodium
LFTs	Liver function tests	**NAD**	Nicotinamide adenine dinucleotide
LH	Luteinising hormone	**NAFLD**	Non-alcoholic fatty liver disease
LMWH	Low-molecular-weight heparin	**NASH**	Non-alcoholic steatohepatitis
LR	Likelihood ratio	**NFFC**	Non-front-fanged colubrid (snake)
LSD	Lysosomal storage disease	**NGS**	Next-generation sequencing
LUL	Left upper lobe	**NHL**	Non-Hodgkin lymphoma
LUTS	Lower urinary tract symptoms	**NICE**	National Institute for Health and Care Excellence
MALT	Mucosa-associated lymphoid tissue		
		NIV	Non-invasive ventilation
MAP	Mean arterial pressure	**NMDA**	*N*-methyl-D-aspartate
MCI	Minimal cognitive impairment	**NMO**	Neuromyelitis optica
MCP	Metacarpophalangeal	**NNRTI**	Non-nucleoside reverse transcriptase inhibitor
MCPJ	Metacarpophalangeal joint		
MCTD	Mixed connective tissue disease	**NNT**	Number needed to treat
MCV	Mean corpuscular volume	**NR**	Normalised ratio
MDP	Methylene diphosphonate	**NRTI**	Nucleoside reverse transcriptase inhibitor
MDRD	Modification of Diet in Renal Disease		
		NSAID	Non-steroidal anti-inflammatory drug
MDS	Myelodysplastic syndromes		
MEGX	Monoethylglycinexylidide	**NSIP**	Non-specific interstitial pneumonia
MELAS	Mitochondrial encephalopathy, lactic acidosis and stroke-like episodes	**O₂**	Oxygen
		OA	Osteoarthritis
		OBMT	Omeprazole, bismuth subcitrate, metronidazole and tetracycline
MELD	Model for End-Stage Liver Disease		
		OCD	Obsessive–compulsive disorder
MEN	Multiple endocrine neoplasia	**OCP**	Oral contraceptive pill
MERS	Middle East respiratory syndrome	**OGD**	Oesophago-gastroduodenoscopy

OGTT	Oral glucose tolerance test	PTE	Pulmonary thromboembolism
OPIDN	Organophosphate-induced delayed polyneuropathy	PTH	Parathyroid hormone
		PTLD	Post-transplant lymphoproliferative disorder
OSA	Obstructive sleep apnoea		
$PaCO_2$	Partial pressure of carbon dioxide in arterial blood	PTSD	Post-traumatic stress disorder
		PUO	Pyrexia of unknown origin
pANCA	Perinuclear antineutrophil cytoplasmic antibody	PVD	Posterior vitreous detachment
		RA	Rheumatoid arthritis
PaO_2	Partial pressure of oxygen in arterial blood	RAAS	Renin–angiotensin–aldosterone system
PARP	Poly-ADP ribose polymerase	RAPD	Relative afferent pupillary defect
PASI	Psoriasis Area and Severity Index	RBILD	Respiratory bronchiolitis–interstitial lung disease
PBC	Primary biliary cirrhosis	RFA	Radiofrequency ablation
PBI	Pressure bandage and immobilisation	RIC	Reduced-intensity conditioning
		RNA	Ribonucleic acid
PCI	Percutaneous coronary intervention	ROSC	Return of spontaneous circulation
PCNL	Percutaneous nephrolithotomy	ROSIER	Rule Out Stroke In the Emergency Room (clinical stroke tool)
PCOS	Polycystic ovary syndrome		
PCP	*Pneumocystis* pneumonia	RPR	Rapid plasma reagin
PCR	Polymerase chain reaction	rt-PA	Recombinant tissue plasminogen activator
PD	Parkinson's disease		
PDB	Paget's disease of bone	RTA	Renal tubular acidosis
PDT	Photodynamic therapy	RV	Residual volume
PEA	Pulseless electrical activity	SAAG	Serum–ascites albumin gradient
PEEP	Positive end-expiratory pressure	SABA	Short-acting β_2-agonist
PEFR	Peak expiratory flow rate	SaO_2	Arterial oxygen saturation
PEP	Post-exposure prophylaxis	SARS	Severe acute respiratory syndrome
PET	Positron emission tomography		
PHT	Pulmonary hypertension	SBP	Spontaneous bacterial peritonitis
PIP	Proximal interphalangeal	SCC	Squamous cell carcinoma
PIPJ	Proximal interphalangeal joints	SCLC	Small cell lung cancer
PI	Protease inhibitor	SCRA	Synthetic cannabinoid receptor agonist
PKD	Polycystic kidney disease		
PLE	Polymorphic light eruption	SeHCAT	^{75}Se-homocholic acid taurine
PMF	Progressive massive fibrosis	SGLT2	Sodium and glucose co-transporter 2
PMR	Polymyalgia rheumatica		
PO_2	Partial pressure of oxygen	SHBG	Sex hormone-binding globulin
POCT	Point-of-care test	SIADH	Syndrome of inappropriate antidiuretic hormone (vasopressin) secretion
POEM	Peroral endoscopic myotomy		
POMC	Pro-opiomelanocortin		
PPARγ	Peroxisome proliferator-activated receptor gamma	SIJ	Sacroiliac joint
		SLE	Systemic lupus erythematosus
PPCI	Primary percutaneous coronary intervention	SO_2	Saturation of haemoglobin with oxygen
PPI	Proton pump inhibitor	SOFA	Sequential Organ Failure Assessment
PRV	Polycythaemia rubra vera		
PSA	Prostate-specific antigen	SpA	Spondyloarthritis
PsA	Psoriatic arthritis	SPC	Summary of product characteristics
PSC	Primary sclerosing cholangitis		
PSP	Primary spontaneous pneumothorax	SPECT	Single-photon emission computed tomography
PSS	Primary Sjögren's syndrome	SpO_2	Peripheral capillary oxygen saturation
PT	Prothrombin time		

SScl	Systemic sclerosis	**TPPA**	*Treponema pallidum* particle agglutination assay
SSRI	Selective serotonin re-uptake inhibitor	**TRAbs**	TSH receptor antibodies
STI	Sexually transmitted infection	**TRM**	Treatment-related mortality
SVR	Sustained viral response	**tRNA**	Transfer ribonucleic acid
T₃	Triiodothyronine	**TSH**	Thyroid-stimulating hormone
T₄	Thyroxine	**TTP**	Thrombotic thrombocytopenic purpura
TAC	Trigeminal autonomic cephalalgia	**UDCA**	Ursodeoxycholic acid
TACE	Transarterial chemoembolisation	**UFH**	Unfractionated heparin
TB	Tuberculosis	**UMOD**	Uromodulin
TBG	Thyroxine-binding globulin	**USS**	Ultrasound scan
T$_{co}$	Transfer factor for carbon monoxide	**UVB**	Ultraviolet B
TEN	Toxic epidermal necrolysis	**V̇/Q̇**	Ventilation–perfusion
TFTs	Thyroid function tests	**V2**	Vasopressin 2
TGA	Transient global amnesia	**VAP**	Ventilator-associated pneumonia
TGF	Transforming growth factor	**V$_d$**	Volume of distribution
TIA	Transient ischaemic attack	**VEGF**	Vascular endothelial growth factor
TIPSS	Transjugular intrahepatic portosystemic stent shunt	**VGCC**	Voltage-gated calcium channel
TKI	Tyrosine kinase inhibitor	**VIP**	Vasoactive intestinal peptide
TKR	Total knee replacement	**VLDL**	Very low-density lipoprotein
TNF	Tumour necrosis factor	**VSD**	Ventricular septal defect
TNM	System used in cancer staging: T = size and extent of the main/ primary tumour; N = number of nearby lymph nodes involved; M = metastasis	**VTE**	Venous thromboembolism
		vWD	von Willebrand disease
		vWF	von Willebrand factor
		vWF:Ag	von Willebrand factor antigen
		VZV	Varicella zoster virus
		WCC	White cell count
		WHO	World Health Organization
TPOs	Thyroid peroxidise antibodies	**ZnT8**	Zinc transporter 8

N Cooper

Clinical decision-making

1.1. In the specialty of internal medicine, diagnostic error occurs in approximately what percentage of cases?

A. 0–5%
B. 6–10%
C. 11–15%
D. 16–20%
E. 21–25%

1.2. A doctor is considering whether a patient presenting with headache, fever and nuchal rigidity may have meningitis. Regarding likelihood ratios (LRs) for each clinical finding, which of the following statements is true?

A. An LR greater than 1 decreases the probability of disease
B. An LR greater than 1 increases the probability of disease
C. An LR is the probability of the finding in patients with the disease
D. An LR of 0 means the diagnosis is unlikely
E. An LR of 1 means the diagnosis is certain

1.3. A test is performed to detect the presence of a disease. The results of the test can be summarised in the table below.

	Disease	No disease
Positive test	A	B
Negative test	C	D

Which of the following describes the sensitivity of the test?

A. A/(A+B) × 100
B. A/(A+C) × 100
C. A/(A+D) × 100
D. D/(D+B) × 100
E. D/(D+C) × 100

1.4. A test is performed to detect the presence of a disease in a specific population. The results of the test can be summarised in the table below.

	Disease	No disease
Positive test	A	B
Negative test	C	D

Which of the following describes the positive predictive value of the test?

A. A/(A+B) × 100
B. A/(A+C) × 100
C. A/(A+D) × 100
D. D/(D+B) × 100
E. D/(D+C) × 100

1.5. An elderly woman fell and hurt her left hip. On examination the left hip was extremely painful to move and she was unable to stand. The pre-test probability of a hip fracture was deemed to be high. Plain X-rays of the pelvis and left hip were requested.

Which of the following statements best describes 'post-test probability'?

A. The adjustment of probability after taking individual patient factors in to account
B. The chance that a test will detect true positives
C. The prevalence of disease in the population to which the patient belongs
D. The probability of a disease after taking new information from a test result into account
E. The proportion of patients with a test result who have the disease

1.6. A doctor is considering whether to treat a patient with antibiotics for a urinary tract infection. The term 'treatment threshold' describes a situation in which various factors are evenly weighted. What is the best description of the factors involved?

A. The cost of the treatment, and whether the treatment is likely to succeed
B. The quality of life of the patient, and risks and benefits of treatment
C. The risk and benefits of treatment
D. The risks of the test, and risk and benefits of treatment
E. The wishes of the patient, and whether the treatment is likely to succeed

1.7. Dual process theory describes two distinct processes of human decision-making. What is the accepted estimate of the proportion of time we spend engaged in type 2 (analytical) thinking?

A. 5%
B. 25%
C. 50%
D. 75%
E. 95%

1.8. In terms of human thinking and decision-making, what tendency does confirmation bias describe?

A. To look for supporting evidence to confirm a theory and ignore evidence that contradicts it
B. To rely too much on the first piece of information offered
C. To stop searching because we have found something that fits
D. To subconsciously see what we expect to see
E. To want to confirm our diagnoses with others before making a decision

1.9. Which of these factors is most likely to lead to an increased incidence of errors in clinical decision-making?

A. Age
B. Fatigue
C. Gender
D. Use of checklists
E. Working alone

1.10. In a case of suspected pulmonary embolism in an ambulatory care setting, which of the following individual signs on physical examination carries the most diagnostic weight in either a positive or negative direction?

A. Blood pressure greater than 120/80 mmHg
B. Heart rate less than 90 beats/min
C. Oxygen saturations greater than 94% on air
D. Respiratory rate less than 20 breaths/min
E. Temperature less than 37.5°C

1.11. Which of the following statements best describes 'patient-centred evidence-based medicine'?

A. The application of best available evidence taking individual patient factors into account
B. The application of best available evidence to patient care
C. The application of clinical decision aids in decision-making
D. The implementation of a management plan based on patient wishes
E. The use of evidence-based care bundles

1.12. According to research, under what circumstances are patients more likely to comply with recommended treatment and less likely to re-attend?

A. If relative risk instead of absolute risk is used in explanations
B. If the consultation is longer
C. If the patient is male
D. If they feel that they have been listened to and understand the treatment plan
E. If visual aids have been used instead of text to explain the treatment plan

1.13. Which of the following statements best describes what is meant by the term 'human factors'?

A. An understanding of diagnostic error
B. How equipment is designed to take human behaviour into account
C. How fatigue affects human thinking and decision-making
D. How healthcare professionals communicate in a team
E. The science of the limitations of human performance

1.14. In terms of human thinking and decision-making, anchoring describes what tendency?

A. To look for supporting evidence to confirm a theory and ignore evidence that contradicts it

1

B. To rely too much on the first piece of information offered

C. To stop searching because we have found something that fits

D. To subconsciously see what we expect to see

E. To want to confirm our diagnoses with others before making a decision

1.15. The D-dimer test has a sensitivity of at least 95% in detecting acute venous thromboembolism (VTE). However, it has a low specificity of around 40%. Which of the

following statements is true regarding the interpretation of a D-dimer result?

A. A negative D-dimer result in a high clinical probability patient excludes acute VTE

B. A positive D-dimer result means that acute VTE is present

C. D-dimer is a useful screening test in patients presenting with breathlessness

D. D-dimer testing in suspected acute VTE results in lots of false negatives

E. D-dimer testing in suspected acute VTE results in lots of false positives

Answers

1.1. Answer: C.
It is estimated that diagnosis is wrong 11–15% of the time in the undifferentiated specialties of internal medicine, emergency medicine and general practice. Diagnostic error is associated with greater morbidity than other types of medical error, and the majority of diagnostic errors are considered to be preventable.

1.2. Answer: B.
Likelihood ratios (LRs) are clinical diagnostic weights.

$$LR = \frac{\text{probability of finding in patients } \textbf{with} \text{ disease}}{\text{probability of finding in patients } \textbf{without} \text{ disease}}$$

An LR greater than 1 increases the probability of disease (the greater the value, the greater the probability). An LR less than 1 decreases the probability of disease. LRs are developed against a diagnostic standard (in the case of meningitis, lumbar puncture results) so do not exist for all clinical findings. LRs illustrate how a probability changes – *but do not determine the prior probability of disease*. If the starting probability is high to begin with, an LR of around 1 does not affect this.

1.3. Answer: B.

$$\text{Sensitivity} = A/(A + C) \times 100$$

Sensitivity is the ability to detect true positives; specificity is the ability to detect true negatives. There is no test that can 100% of the time detect people with a disease and

exclude those without it. Even a very good test, with 95% sensitivity, will miss 1 in 20 people with the disease. Every test therefore has 'false positives' and 'false negatives'.

A very sensitive test will detect most disease but may generate abnormal findings in healthy people. A negative result will therefore reliably exclude the disease, but a positive test is likely to require further evaluation. On the other hand, a very specific test may miss significant pathology but is likely to establish the diagnosis beyond doubt when the result is positive.

1.4. Answer: A.

$$\text{Positive predictive value} = A/(A + B) \times 100$$

Predictive values combine sensitivity, specificity and prevalence. Sensitivity and specificity are characteristics of the test; the population does not change this. However, as doctors, we are interested in the question, 'What is the probability that a person with a positive test actually has the disease?' The positive predictive value is the proportion of patients with a test result who have the disease and is calculated from a table of results in a specific population. It is not possible to transfer this value to a different population.

1.5. Answer: D.
Post-test probability is the probability of a disease after taking new information from a test result into account. The pre-test probability of disease is decided by the doctor – it is an *opinion* based on gathered evidence prior to ordering the test. Bayes' Theorem can be used

to calculate post-test probability for a patient in any population. It is a mathematical way to describe the post-test probability of a disease by incorporating pre-test probability, sensitivity and specificity.

1.6. Answer: D.
The treatment threshold combines factors such as the risks of the test, and the risks versus benefits of treatment. The point at which the factors are all evenly weighted is the threshold. If a test or treatment for a disease is effective and low risk, then one would have a lower threshold for going ahead. On the other hand, if a test or treatment is less effective or high risk, one requires greater confidence in the clinical diagnosis and potential benefits of treatment first. In principle, if a diagnostic test will not change the management of the patient, then it should not be requested, unless there are other compelling reasons to do so.

1.7. Answer: A.
Psychologists believe we spend 95% of our daily lives engaged in type 1 thinking – the intuitive, fast, subconscious mode of decision-making. In everyday life we spend little time (5%) engaged in type 2 thinking. Imagine driving a car; it would be impossible to function efficiently if every decision and movement was as deliberate, conscious, slow and effortful as in our first driving lesson. With experience, complex procedures become automatic, fast and effortless. The same applies to medical practice.

1.8. Answer: A.
Cognitive biases are *subconscious* errors that lead to inaccurate judgement and illogical interpretation of information. In evolutionary terms, it is thought that cognitive biases developed because speed was often more important than accuracy. This property of human thinking is highly relevant to clinical decision-making. Confirmation bias is the tendency to look for confirming evidence to support a theory rather than looking for contradictory evidence to refute it, even if the latter is clearly present. Confirmation bias is common when a patient has been seen first by another doctor.

1.9. Answer: B.
Cognition is affected by things like fatigue, illness, emotions, interruptions, cognitive overload and time pressure. Poor team communication and poorly designed equipment or clinical processes also increase the likelihood of error. Age, gender and working alone are not factors that affect cognition. Use of checklists has been shown to improve decision-making in clinical settings.

1.10. Answer: B.
Suspected pulmonary embolism is a common problem referred to UK ambulatory emergency care centres. Unexplained pleuritic chest pain and/or a history of breathlessness are the most common symptoms. Vital signs at rest and the physical examination may be normal. The only feature presented with a negative likelihood ratio in the diagnosis of pulmonary embolism is a heart rate of less than 90 beats/min. In other words, the other normal physical examination findings (including normal oxygen saturations) carry little diagnostic weight.

1.11. Answer: A.
'Patient-centred evidence-based medicine' refers to the application of best available research evidence *while taking individual patient factors into account* – these include clinical factors (e.g. bleeding risk when considering anticoagulation) and non-clinical factors (e.g. the patient's inability to attend for regular blood tests if started on warfarin).

1.12. Answer: D.
Many studies demonstrate a correlation between effective clinician–patient communication and improved health outcomes. If patients feel they have been listened to and understand the problem and proposed treatment plan, they are more likely to adhere to their medication and less likely to re-attend. Whenever possible, doctors should quote numerical information using consistent denominators (e.g. '90 out of 100 patients who have this operation feel much better, 1 will die during the operation and 2 will suffer a stroke'). Visual aids can be used to present complex statistical information.

Relative risk exaggerates small effects that distort people's understanding of true probability. Longer consultations and the use of visual aids are tools to facilitate good communication but in themselves do not guarantee this is the case. Gender by itself is not a factor.

1.13. Answer: E.
Human factors is *the science of the limitations of human performance* and how technology, our work environment and team communication can adapt for this to reduce diagnostic and other types of error. Analysis of serious adverse events in health care show that human factors and poor team communication play a significant role when things go wrong. Human factors training is being introduced into undergraduate and postgraduate medical curricula and multi-professional team training in many countries.

1.14. Answer: B.
Cognitive biases are *subconscious* errors that lead to inaccurate judgement and illogical interpretation of information. In evolutionary terms, it is thought that cognitive biases developed because speed was often more important than accuracy. This property of human thinking is highly relevant to clinical decision-making. Anchoring describes the common human tendency to rely too heavily on the first piece of information offered (the 'anchor') when making decisions.

1.15. Answer: E.
A very sensitive test will detect most disease but generate abnormal findings in healthy people. A negative result therefore means the disease is unlikely, but a positive result is likely to require further evaluation. As with all diagnostic tests, a low pre-test probability plus a negative D-dimer virtually excludes acute VTE. However, if the pre-test probability is very high, a negative D-dimer still leaves a small but significant chance that acute VTE is present.

D-dimer is commonly raised in conditions that have nothing to do with acute VTE: for example, old age, pregnancy, heart failure, sepsis and cancer. This is the reason for its low specificity. It should be used only when the history and physical examination are consistent with acute VTE.

2

Clinical therapeutics and good prescribing

Multiple Choice Questions

2.1. Which of the following drugs exerts its action directly at an enzyme target?

A. Aspirin
B. Hydrocortisone
C. Insulin
D. Lidocaine
E. Morphine

2.2. Which of the following statements best describes the term 'potency'?

A. A less potent drug will always have a lower efficacy than a more potent drug
B. More potent drugs have a lower ED_{50}
C. The potency of a drug has no bearing on recommended dose ranges
D. The potency of a drug is the extent to which the drug can produce a response when all of the available receptors are occupied
E. The potency of a drug is unrelated to its affinity for a receptor

2.3. Which of the following statements best describes how a non-competitive antagonist drug affects the pharmacodynamic actions of an agonist?

A. Binding irreversibly with the receptor to remove receptors as potential binding sites for the agonist
B. Binding to a different population of receptors that produce a response antagonistic to that of the agonist
C. Causing cell death so that it cannot function
D. Increasing the total number of receptors for the agonist, thereby reducing the proportion that it can occupy

E. Reacting chemically with the agonist to reduce the agonist concentration available to bind to receptors

2.4. Which of the following drugs induce the hepatic cytochrome P450 enzymes that are responsible for drug metabolism?

A. Cimetidine
B. Ciprofloxacin
C. Erythromycin
D. Rifampicin
E. Valproate

2.5. Which of the following drugs may exhibit zero-order drug kinetics at therapeutic drug concentrations?

A. Carbamazepine
B. Ciprofloxacin
C. Lamotrigine
D. Phenytoin
E. Vancomycin

2.6. Which of the following statements about the estimated volume of distribution (V_d) of a drug is true?

A. Drugs that are highly bound to albumin have a lower V_d
B. Drugs with a large V_d are eliminated more rapidly after discontinuation
C. Larger V_d is associated with a shorter half-life
D. V_d cannot be greater than the volume of the body
E. V_d of lipid-soluble drugs is larger in males than females (of equivalent mass)

2.7. Which of the following factors might be expected to favour increased bioavailability of a drug that is given by mouth?

A. Enterohepatic circulation of the active drug
B. Gastroenteritis
C. Hypoalbuminaemia
D. Impaired renal function
E. Solid rather than liquid formulations

2.8. For which of the following drugs do pharmacogenetic differences commonly influence the clinical effect in Western populations?

A. Amlodipine
B. Codeine
C. Gliclazide
D. Omeprazole
E. Simvastatin

2.9. Which of the following features is most characteristic of hypersensitivity adverse drug reactions?

A. They are associated with human leucocyte antigen (HLA) class haplotypes
B. They are discovered early in the drug development process
C. They are dose related
D. They manifest several months after initial exposure
E. They occur at the higher part of the therapeutic dose range

2.10. Which of the following is an advantage of the spontaneous voluntary reporting methods of pharmacovigilance?

A. It captures the majority of adverse drug reactions
B. It is able to quantify the risk of an adverse drug reaction (ADR) after exposure to a drug
C. It is specific for events that really are caused by the drug
D. It provides early signal generation after marketing of a new drug
E. Its information is generated by highly qualified professionals

2.11. A 23 year old woman is taking a combined oral contraceptive preparation. She has developed an infection sensitive to a number of common antibiotics. Which of the following antibiotic choices is most likely to interact with the contraceptive preparation to cause contraceptive failure?

A. Amoxicillin
B. Ciprofloxacin
C. Doxycycline
D. Erythromycin
E. Rifampicin

2.12. A 71 year old woman with ischaemic heart disease recently started taking amiodarone 200 mg orally daily for control of her atrial fibrillation. She has now been admitted to hospital 3 months later with episodes of dizziness and bradycardia (heart rate 48 beats/min). The electrocardiogram shows a prolonged QT interval (530 ms).
   Which of her current regular medicines below is most likely to interact with amiodarone to cause the QT prolongation?

A. Clopidogrel
B. Moxifloxacin
C. Nicorandil
D. Simvastatin
E. Thyroxine

2.13. Which of the following is the commonest cause of prescribing errors in hospital practice?

A. Calculation errors
B. Duplicated prescribing
C. Failed medicines reconciliation
D. Prescribing without indication
E. Unintentional prescribing

2.14. Which of the following is NOT information required as part of the regulatory process leading to the granting of a marketing authorisation ('license')?

A. Cost-effectiveness compared to standard treatment
B. Efficacy in the licensed indication
C. Product information literature
D. Quality of the manufacturing process
E. Toxicology studies

2.15. A trial of 5000 hypertensive patients randomised them to treatment with a new oral anticoagulant or a matched placebo. After a follow-up period of 5 years, 150 patients in the active treatment arm and 250 patients in the placebo arm had suffered a stroke.
   What is the number of patients that need to be treated (NNT) with the new treatment over 5 years to prevent one stroke?

A. 10
B. 15

C. 20
D. 25
E. 30

2.16. An 82 year old man has a routine medication review with his family physician. He has a history of a transient ischaemic attack, hypertension and attacks of gout.

Which of the following prescriptions should probably be discontinued?

A. Allopurinol 100 mg orally daily
B. Amlodipine 5 mg orally daily
C. Aspirin 75 mg orally daily
D. Diclofenac 25 mg orally 3 times daily
E. Ramipril 5 mg orally daily

2.17. Which of the following drugs would pose the greatest risk of teratogenic effects if prescribed during the first trimester of pregnancy?

A. Amoxicillin
B. Mebeverine hydrochloride
C. Rifampicin
D. Sodium valproate
E. Sulfasalazine

2.18. A 63 year old woman has progressively deteriorating renal function presumed to be due to the effects of renal scarring secondary to chronic reflux nephropathy in childhood. Her most recent estimated glomerular filtration rate (eGFR) is 26 mL/min/1.73 m^2.

Which of the patient's prescriptions below would need to be amended?

A. Clopidogrel 75 mg orally daily
B. Doxazosin 8 mg orally daily
C. Metformin hydrochloride 1 g orally twice daily
D. Pregabalin 50 mg orally twice daily
E. Tamoxifen 20 mg orally daily

2.19. A 44 year old man with alcoholic cirrhosis of the liver is admitted to hospital with delirium, irritability and painful distension of the abdomen as a result of ascites. His investigations show that he is anaemic (haemoglobin 82 g/L), jaundiced (bilirubin 65 µmol/L (3.8 mg/dL)), hypoalbuminaemic (albumin 20 g/L) and has a mild coagulopathy (international normalised ratio (INR) 1.6).

His initial prescription chart contains the five prescriptions below. Which of the prescriptions should be discontinued?

A. Codeine phosphate 60 mg orally 4 times daily
B. Lactulose 20 g 3 times daily
C. Pabrinex (vitamins B and C) intravenous high-potency solution for injection 2 pairs of 5 mL ampoules 3 times daily
D. Spironolactone 100 mg orally daily
E. Terlipressin acetate 1.5 mg intravenously 4 times daily

2.20. The following dose expressions have been found on a hospital inpatient chart.

Which dose expression violates acceptable prescribing practice?

A. 1 sachet
B. 1.4 g
C. 20 mL
D. 26 units
E. 100 µg

2.21. Which of the following drugs should be prescribed by its proprietary (brand) name in preference to the generic international non-proprietary name (INN)?

A. Atorvastatin
B. Ciclosporin
C. Ciprofloxacin
D. Irbesartan
E. Methyldopa

2.22. A 76 year old woman has been treated successfully with digoxin 187.5 µg orally daily over a number of months to control the ventricular response rate to her atrial fibrillation. She has recently complained of some nausea and so the plasma digoxin concentration has been measured to investigate the possibility of digoxin toxicity as an explanation. On examination, the radial pulse rate is irregularly irregular and 64 beats/min. The plasma digoxin concentration is 1.8 µg/L (target 0.8–2.0 µg/L).

What is the most appropriate course of action with regard to her digoxin prescription?

A. Change digoxin dosage to 187.5 µg orally on alternate days
B. Maintain the digoxin dosage at 187.5 µg orally daily
C. Reduce the digoxin dosage to 62.5 µg orally daily
D. Reduce the digoxin dosage to 125 µg orally daily
E. Stop digoxin and start bisoprolol 2.5 mg orally daily

2.23. A 56 year old man is being treated with intravenous gentamicin for Gram-negative septicaemia that is presumed to be of urinary tract origin. He is well hydrated and his renal function is normal. He has had two previous doses of gentamicin 360 mg as a 30-minute intravenous infusion at 1000 hrs on Wednesday and Thursday. Both previous plasma gentamicin concentrations have been checked by the senior doctor in charge of the ward and the third dose of gentamicin has been prescribed and is now due (Friday morning at 1000 hrs).

When should the next plasma gentamicin concentration be taken?

A. 0400 hrs (Saturday)
B. 1400 hrs (Friday)
C. 1800 hrs (Friday)
D. Immediately after the infusion is completed
E. Immediately before the third dose

2.24. A 78 year old woman is reviewed in the emergency department of a hospital with bruising. She is taking warfarin 3 mg and 4 mg orally on alternate days as prophylaxis against recurrent pulmonary emboli. Her last 3-monthly INR measurement was 2.7. She has been otherwise well with no other new symptoms and she has not been put on any new medicines. Her investigations reveal a normal full blood count but an INR of 6.7.

What is the appropriate course of action?

A. Stop warfarin and give phytomenadione (vitamin K₁) 1–3 mg by slow intravenous injection
B. Stop warfarin and give phytomenadione (vitamin K₁) 1–5 mg by mouth
C. Stop warfarin and start apixaban
D. Stop warfarin and start low-molecular-weight heparin injections
E. Stop warfarin for 2 days only

Answers

2.1. Answer: A.
Aspirin acts on the enzyme cyclo-oxygenase and is a non-selective and irreversible inhibitor. Hydrocortisone is a corticosteroid and acts on a DNA-linked receptor. Insulin acts on a kinase-linked receptor. Lidocaine blocks a voltage-sensitive Na^+ channel. Morphine acts on a G-protein-coupled receptor.

2.2. Answer: B.
The potency of a drug is related to its affinity for a receptor. Less potent drugs are given in higher doses. The lower potency of a drug can be overcome by increasing the dose. Option D refers to the 'efficacy' of a drug.

2.3. Answer: A.
The term 'non-competitive antagonist' is used to describe two distinct situations where an antagonist binds to a receptor, or its associated signal transduction mechanism, to prevent the agonist activating the receptor. The common feature is that increasing the concentration of agonist cannot outcompete the antagonist. The receptor is rendered inactive and so the maximal response of which the cell or tissue is capable is reduced. This can occur in three ways: (i) the antagonist binds to an allosteric site of the receptor, (ii) the antagonist binds to

the same active site as the agonist but does so irreversibly, or (iii) the antagonist interferes with the signal transduction mechanism preventing receptor–agonist binding resulting in a pharmacological effect.

2.4. Answer: D.
Rifampicin is a very potent enzyme inducer. All of the other options are well recognised as enzyme inhibitors.

2.5. Answer: D.
The clearance rate of most drugs increases progressively as their plasma concentration increases ('first-order metabolism'). For a small number of common medicines, their metabolism is 'saturable', meaning that the rate of clearance cannot increase further ('zero-order kinetics'). For those drugs, further dose increases can cause disproportionate increases in exposure and the likelihood of toxicity.

2.6. Answer: A.
The apparent volume of distribution (V_d) is the volume into which a drug appears to have distributed following intravenous injection. It is calculated from the equation $V_d = D/C_0$, where D is the amount of drug given and C_0 is the

initial plasma concentration. Drugs that are highly bound to plasma proteins may have a V_d below 10 L (e.g. warfarin, aspirin), while those that diffuse into the interstitial fluid but do not enter cells because they have low lipid solubility may have a V_d between 10 and 30 L (e.g. gentamicin, amoxicillin). It is an 'apparent' volume because those drugs that are lipid soluble and highly tissue-bound may have a V_d of greater than 100 L (e.g. digoxin, amitriptyline). Drugs with a larger V_d have longer half-lives, take longer to reach steady state on repeated administration and are eliminated more slowly from the body following discontinuation. Females have a greater proportionate content of fat in their bodies and so the volume of distribution of lipid-soluble drugs is increased.

2.7. Answer: A.

Drugs that enter the enterohepatic circulation are reabsorbed into the body after excretion in the bile. This occurs because intestinal flora split the water-soluble conjugated drug, allowing the free drug to be reabsorbed into the body and thus increasing its bioavailability. Gastroenteritis favours more rapid transit through the small intestinal absorptive region of the bowel and reduces oral bioavailability. Hypoalbuminaemia may alter the proportion of the drug retained in plasma after absorption but does not alter the overall bioavailability in the body. Impaired renal function may influence clearance of a drug but does not influence bioavailability. Aqueous solutions, syrups, elixirs, and emulsions do not present a dissolution problem and generally result in fast and often complete absorption as compared to solid dosage forms. Due to their generally good systemic availability, solutions are frequently used as bioavailability standards against which other dosage forms are compared.

2.8. Answer: B.

Codeine is an opioid analgesic drug that is licensed for the treatment of mild to moderately severe pain, and it belongs to the drug class of opioid analgesics. Codeine is metabolised by the hepatic cytochrome P450 2D6 (CYP2D6) enzyme, which also metabolises many other prescribed drugs. CYP2D6 converts codeine to its active metabolite, morphine, which is responsible for the analgesic effect. The analgesic effect of codeine is attenuated in individuals who carry two inactive copies of

CYP2D6 ('poor metabolisers'), and are less able to deliver sufficient morphine levels. Some individuals carry more than two functional copies of the *CYP2D6* gene ('ultra-rapid metabolisers') and are able to metabolise codeine to morphine more rapidly and completely. They may develop symptoms of morphine toxicity (e.g. drowsiness, delirium and shallow breathing) even at low doses.

2.9. Answer: A.

Drug hypersensitivity is typically immune mediated. Some drugs (especially large molecules) may themselves stimulate immune reaction but many others (or their metabolites) act as 'haptens' that bind covalently to serum or cell-bound proteins, including peptides embedded in major histocompatibility complex (MHC) molecules. This makes the protein immunogenic, stimulating antibody production targeted at the drug or T-cell responses against the drug. The reaction can produce a variety of reactions ranging from mild rashes through to life-threatening anaphylaxis. These reactions are often rare and discovered later in the drug development process. The susceptibility to hypersensitivity reactions is, in many cases, strongly related to genetics. Those who are susceptible will often react immediately to minimal exposure to the drug, making it very difficult to identify a dose–response relationship.

2.10. Answer: D.

Voluntary reporting is a continuously operating and effective early warning system for previously unrecognised rare ADRs. It is better suited than most other methods to early detection of previously unknown reactions, especially for medicines that are prescribed in high volume. Although doctors were initially the main source of reporting, most other healthcare professional groups, and patients, are now able to report in the UK. Their reports have been shown to be of equivalent value to those produced by the medical reporters. Its weaknesses include low reporting rates (only 3% of all ADRs and 10% of serious ADRs are ever reported), an inability to quantify risk (because the ratio of ADRs to prescriptions is unknown) and the influence of prescriber awareness on likelihood of reporting (reporting rates rise rapidly following publicity about potential ADRs).

2.11. Answer: E.
Although there have been past suggestions that broad-spectrum penicillins might interfere with gut flora to alter the enterohepatic recycling of oestrogens (reducing their bioavailability in the body), it is now thought that the only types of antibiotic that interact with hormonal contraception and make it less effective are rifampicin-like antibiotics. The metabolism of oestrogens is accelerated by rifamycins, leading to a reduced contraceptive effect with combined oral contraceptives, contraceptive patches and vaginal rings. Erythromycin is a well-recognised inhibitor of the hepatic metabolism of many drugs (including oestrogens) but this will not result in contraceptive failure.

2.12. Answer: B.
Moxifloxacin is a quinolone antibiotic that can be used to treat sinusitis, community-acquired pneumonia, exacerbations of chronic bronchitis, mild to moderate pelvic inflammatory disease, or complicated skin and soft tissue infections. Along with other quinolones, it may block cardiac potassium channels and delay the repolarisation phase of the action potential to prolong QT interval. This may potentiate the similar actions of amiodarone. Patients with a prolonged QT interval are at risk of suffering episodes of torsades de pointes, which may progress to cause cardiac arrest.

2.13. Answer: C.
Medication reconciliation is the process of creating the most appropriate list of medications for the patient – including drug name, dosage, frequency and route – at a transition of care from one provider to another. Failure to take an adequate medication history from the patient (or relative), obtain information from another professional or another source increases the chance that important medicines will be inadvertently omitted. Medicines reconciliation is also about considering that information in the light of the clinical circumstances and altering or discontinuing prescriptions as necessary. The medicines reconciliation process is particularly important at the admission, transfer and/or discharge from hospital. Omission of medicines on admission or discharge from hospital may account for a third of all recorded errors in some studies.

2.14. Answer: A.
New drugs are given a 'market authorisation' based on the evidence of quality, safety and efficacy presented by the manufacturer. The regulator will not only approve the drug but will also take great care to ensure that the accompanying information reflects the evidence that has been presented. The summary of product characteristics (SPC), or 'label', provides detailed information about indications, dosage, adverse effects, warnings, monitoring, etc.

2.15. Answer: D.
The calculation of NNT can be undertaken in two ways. First, the number of patients prevented from suffering a stroke in the active treatment compared to control arm was 100 out of a total number at risk of 2500. Therefore, the numbers treated for each one who benefitted was 2500/100 = 25. An alternative approach that works easily in less rounded numbers is to consider the difference in the percentage of patients in each group who had a stroke, i.e. active treatment $150/2500 \times 100$ = 6% and placebo $250/2500 \times 100$ = 10%. The difference is 4%, meaning that if a single at-risk group of just 100 patients were considered, then 4 would benefit and so the NNT is 100/4 = 25.

2.16. Answer: D.
Diclofenac sodium is a non-steroidal anti-inflammatory drug (NSAID) that is indicated for the treatment of inflammatory arthritis and other musculoskeletal conditions. NSAIDs are contraindicated in elderly patients because of their increased risk of adverse effects, notably on the gastrointestinal mucosa and renal function. The likelihood of each of these outcomes is increased by co-prescription of aspirin and ramipril, respectively. All of the other medicines appear to have a clear indication for use. Best practice will be to discuss the medications involved with the patient himself.

2.17. Answer: D.
Sodium valproate is associated with a risk of major and minor congenital malformations (in particular neural tube defects) as well as long-term neurodevelopmental effects. It should be avoided during pregnancy unless there is no safer alternative and only after a carefully discussing the risks with the patient.

2.18. Answer: C.
The UK National Institute for Health and Care Excellence (NICE) recommends that the dose of metformin should be reviewed if the eGFR is less than 45 mL/min/1.73 m^2 and that it should be avoided if the eGFR is less than 30 mL/min/1.73 m^2. (Type 2 diabetes in adults: management. NICE guideline [NG28]. Published December 2015.)

2.19. Answer: A.
This patient has severe liver disease demonstrated by the failure to synthesise clotting factors and albumin, and is showing features of hepatic encephalopathy. In severe liver disease many drugs can further impair cerebral function and may precipitate hepatic encephalopathy. These include all sedative drugs, opioid analgesics (e.g. codeine phosphate), those diuretics that produce hypokalaemia and drugs that cause constipation (e.g. codeine phosphate). Patients with hepatic encephalopathy must avoid constipation, and lactulose is a preferred laxative. Spironolactone is indicated in the management of ascites. B vitamins are important in avoiding Wernicke's encephalopathy in chronically malnourished patients. Terlipressin acetate is a vasoconstrictor that helps to reduce bleeding from oesophageal varices.

2.20. Answer: E.
The only acceptable abbreviations of mass to be used on a written prescription chart are 'mg' and 'g'. 'Micrograms' should be written out in full to avoid the risk that the Greek symbol mu (μ) is mistaken for an 'm'. This would run the risk of a serious dosing error.

2.21. Answer: B.
Where non-proprietary ('generic') titles are given, they should be used by prescribers. This allows a pharmacist to dispense any suitable product, which avoids delay to the patient and sometimes expense to the health service. The only exception to this preference for generic prescribing is where there is a demonstrable difference in clinical effect between each manufacturer's version of the formulation, making it important that the patient should always receive the same brand. Ciclosporin is available in the UK as Neoral, Capimune, Deximune and ciclosporin. Other examples of

such medicines include diltiazem, lithium, theophylline, phenytoin and insulin. Non-proprietary names are also preferred in the case of many compound and modified-release preparations.

2.22. Answer: D.
The patient has excellent control of her ventricular rate and so digoxin appears to be very effective. However, she is complaining of nausea, which is a very common toxic effect of digoxin although there could be numerous other explanations. The plasma digoxin concentration is at the top end of the normal 'target' range. Although within that range it is perfectly possible (and likely) that, because of natural inter-patient variation, this patient's nausea is indeed caused by digoxin. Given that the rate control is so good, the optimal course of action is to keep this patient on digoxin but reduce the dosage in the hope of relieving the symptoms but maintaining the therapeutic effect. In other words, be guided by the beneficial and adverse effects of the medicine for your specific patient rather than the published reference ranges alone.

2.23. Answer: C.
Gentamicin can cause significant toxic effects if it accumulates in the body (especially nephrotoxicity and ototoxicity). It is almost exclusively cleared by the kidney so the risk of accumulation is increased in patients with impaired renal function. Whatever the baseline renal function, all patients should have the serum gentamicin concentration monitored after each dose as a guide to the next dose and the dose interval. This patient has had two doses administered already and each has been followed by a serum concentration that has indicated it is appropriate to maintain the same dose and dose interval. The issue now is when to take the next serum concentration. The normal recommended window is between 6 and 14 hours post-dose: measurements taken before or after this interval are less likely to reflect the gentamicin exposure produced by the previous dosage. Most hospitals have a nomogram (based on the original Hartford nomogram) that helps clinicians to respond appropriately to the serum concentration.

2.24. Answer: E.
The patient is taking warfarin as prophylaxis against future recurrent pulmonary emboli. The

target INR should be 2.5. She now presents with the INR out of control and this can be caused by several different factors (e.g. erratic tablet taking, altered liver function, dietary change, interacting drug). The loss of control puts her at increased risk of bleeding although there are no symptoms suggestive of a serious bleeding episode. The appropriate course of action at this point is to withhold the warfarin for 2 days and then resume (at a lower dose) before re-measuring the INR. In the absence of bleeding or an INR greater than 8.0, there is no indication to give vitamin K, which will largely reverse the action of warfarin and put the patient at risk of thromboembolic events until it can be restarted or replaced with an alternative anticoagulant.

3

Clinical genetics

Multiple Choice Questions

3.1. Deoxyribonucleic acid (DNA) repair mechanisms exist to repair damage that may arise spontaneously or as a result of environmental exposures. Failure to repair DNA damage prior to replication results in mutations. Spontaneous deamination of a cytosine results in its conversion to a uracil. If this were not repaired prior to replication, what would be the result?

A. Conversion of a GA pair to a CT pair
B. Conversion of a GC pair to an AT pair
C. Conversion of a GT pair to an AC pair
D. Conversion of an AC pair to a GT pair
E. Conversion of an AT pair to a GC pair

3.2. The central dogma of molecular biology describes the steps by which information encoded by the DNA determines protein production. One of these steps is transcription. Which of the following elements are all essential components in transcription?

A. Promoter sequence, deoxynucleotides, DNA polymerase
B. Promoter sequence, DNA template, DNA polymerase
C. Promoter sequence, DNA template, ribonucleic acid (RNA) polymerase
D. Ribosomes, DNA template, RNA polymerase
E. Ribosomes, messenger RNA (mRNA) template, transfer RNAs (tRNAs)

3.3. In thyroid C cells, the calcitonin gene encodes the osteoclast inhibitor calcitonin, whereas in neurons, the same gene encodes calcitonin-gene-related peptide. Which of the mechanisms of controlling gene expression listed below is responsible for this multi-functionality?

A. Acetylation of histone protein
B. Alternative splicing
C. Epigenetic modification
D. Gene silencing by microRNA species
E. Post-translational glycosylation

3.4. You receive a genetic test result for a 3 year old boy with a history of Wilms' tumour and microcephaly, confirming a diagnosis of mosaic variegated aneuploidy (MVA), a rare inherited predisposition to chromosomal non-dysjunction. The genetic test has identified a mutation in *BUB1B*, a key component of the mitotic spindle checkpoint. You now need to explain these results to his parents. Non-dysjunction occurs during cell division when the sister chromatids attach to the mitotic spindle and are pulled apart to separate poles of the cell. What is this phase of the cell cycle called?

A. Anaphase
B. Interphase
C. Metaphase
D. Prophase
E. Telophase

3.5. You receive a referral to see a 32 year old woman who has recently been diagnosed with triple-negative breast cancer. Triple-negative breast cancer is defined by the absence of oestrogen receptors, progesterone receptors and human epidermal growth factor receptor 2 (HER2) expression, and this tumour type is particularly common in *BRCA1* mutation carriers. Genetic testing of the *BRCA1* and *BRCA2* genes reveals a heterozygous *BRCA1* mutation (*BRCA1* c.3748G>T). This mutation substitutes a G for a T, resulting in the creation of a premature stop codon and a truncated protein, a so-called 'stop-gain mutation'. What other name is commonly used for this type of mutation?

A. Deletion
B. Frameshift mutation
C. Missense mutation
D. Nonsense mutation
E. Synonymous mutation

3.6. A 37 year old woman with type 1 myotonic dystrophy (DM1) attends your clinic for genetic counselling. She is 8 weeks pregnant. Which of the following pieces of advice is correct?

A. A baby inheriting the condition is at risk of being more severely affected than her
B. Her chance of having a baby affected by this condition is 1 in 4
C. Her partner should be referred for genetic testing
D. Only a male baby will be affected with this condition
E. The mutation causing her condition is likely to have arisen post-zygotically

3.7. A 16 year old girl is referred to your clinic with primary amenorrhoea. On examination she is on 0.4th centile for height. You request a karyotype, the result of which is shown below. What is your diagnosis?

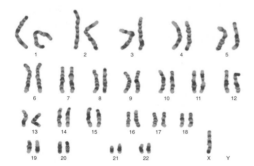

A. Edward's syndrome
B. Klinefelter's syndrome
C. Lynch's syndrome
D. Patau's syndrome
E. Turner's syndrome

3.8. You receive a referral to review an 18 month old girl with developmental delay. She is the first child of unrelated parents and there is no significant family history. On examination she has microcephaly (occipitofrontal circumference 0.4th centile), some subtle dysmorphic features and global developmental delay. Which of the investigations listed below is the most appropriate first-line investigation?

A. Array comparative genomic hybridisation (CGH)
B. Exome sequencing
C. Fragile X testing
D. Karyotype
E. Whole-genome sequencing

3.9. Random double-stranded breaks in DNA are a necessary feature of meiotic recombination. The frequency of these breaks is dramatically increased by exposure to ionising radiation. These breaks are usually repaired accurately by DNA repair mechanisms within the cell; however, some will instead undergo non-homologous end-joining. Which of the following is a possible outcome of non-homologous end-joining between fragments from different chromosomes?

A. Deletion
B. Duplication
C. Paracentric inversion
D. Pericentric inversion
E. Translocation

3.10. Osteogenesis imperfecta type II is a lethal condition causing severe bone deformity and respiratory failure. It is caused by mutations in type I collagen genes, resulting in the production of an abnormal protein that interferes with the normal functioning of the wild-type protein. What is the name for this type of mutation?

A. Dominant negative mutation
B. Gain-of-function mutation
C. Loss-of-function mutation
D. Protein-truncating mutation
E. Stop-gain mutation

3.11. You are asked to review a 17 year old boy with a diagnosis of Becker muscular dystrophy. He has two siblings, an unaffected brother and a sister whose status is unknown. His parents are fit and well; however, his maternal grandfather also had Becker muscular dystrophy. You need to construct an appropriate pedigree for your notes. What symbol would you conventionally use to represent his mother in this case?

A. A diamond
B. A half-shaded circle
C. A shaded circle
D. An open circle
E. An open circle with a central dot

3.12. You meet a family affected by Lynch syndrome, an autosomal dominant condition causing increased predisposition to cancer, mainly of the colon and endometrium. You need to explain the concept of autosomal dominant inheritance to the family. Which of the following is a typical feature of autosomal dominant inheritance?

A. 25% recurrence risk for a couple with an affected child
B. 50% chance of an unaffected child with an affected sibling being a carrier
C. Affected individuals occurring in a single generation
D. Males more commonly affected than females
E. Variable penetrance

3.13. You receive a referral to review a 12 year old girl with a 2-year history of worsening muscle weakness and pain, recurrent migraines and vomiting. Her neurologist requested a genetic test, which confirmed the diagnosis of MELAS (mitochondrial encephalopathy, lactic acidosis and stroke-like episodes), a rare mitochondrial disorder. She and her parents wish to discuss the inheritance of this condition and its implications for their family. Which of the following statements is true in relation to her condition?

A. Affected males cannot transmit the condition to their daughters
B. Affected males cannot transmit the condition to their sons but all their daughters would be carriers
C. Female carriers may be variably affected due to X-inactivation
D. Females are affected more often than males
E. The condition has arisen de novo and her siblings do not require genetic testing

3.14. You are asked to provide genetic counselling for a couple who are expecting their third child. They have two older children, a normally developing 9 year old daughter and a son who, at age 5, has significant learning difficulties. There is a family history of learning difficulties in the maternal grandfather and a maternal uncle, and his daughter, in turn, has a degree of developmental delay. You construct a pedigree (Fig. 3.14) with the affected family members represented by the filled symbols.

The couple has just found out that they are expecting a boy, and are concerned that, since in their family it is boys more than girls that seem to be affected, he may be at risk. They have heard that learning difficulties are commonly X-linked conditions, and want to know whether you think this could be the case in their family and, if so, whether they could have genetic testing of the X chromosome.

When reviewing a pedigree, which of these features is NOT consistent with X-linked inheritance?

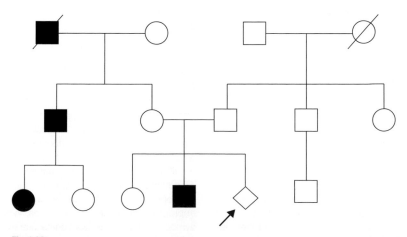

Fig. 3.14

A. Affected father and affected son
B. Affected members in each generation
C. Affected son and affected maternal uncle
D. The presence of an affected female
E. Variable expressivity

3.15. You review a 39 year old woman with advanced breast cancer. She has been referred to you for genetic testing because of her young age at diagnosis. You undertake diagnostic genetic testing but are unable to identify a pathogenic mutation in either *BRCA1* or *BRCA2*. Which of the following mechanisms could be a contributing mechanism in her tumour formation?

A. Apoptosis
B. Autocrine stimulation
C. Gain-of-function mutation in a tumour suppressor gene
D. Loss-of-function mutation in an oncogene
E. Passenger mutation

3.16. You receive an array comparative genomic hybridisation (array CGH) report for a patient with developmental delay and autism. The report is normal and has not identified a cause for the patient's difficulties. Which of the following statements is true about what array CGH is able to reliably detect?

A. It will reliably detect aneuploidy
B. It will reliably detect balanced translocations
C. It will reliably detect intragenic deletions
D. It will reliably detect mosaicism at the 1% level
E. It will reliably detect triploidy

3.17. A 2 year old boy with global developmental delay and facial dysmorphism attends with his parents for the results of his array CGH testing. His parents are healthy and there is no family history of note. The test has identified a 446-kB deletion at 18p23, which has been reported as a copy number variant (CNV) of uncertain significance. What would be your next step in his management?

A. Exome sequencing of the boy and his parents
B. Intellectual disability gene panel testing
C. Parental array CGH testing
D. Repeat the array using more closely spaced probes to give a higher resolution
E. Request a karyotype to exclude a balanced translocation

3.18. A 27 year old woman is referred to your clinic by her family physician for advice. She was worried about her family history of breast cancer and decided to undergo genetic testing through a private company offering a next-generation sequencing (NGS) breast cancer susceptibility gene panel test. They sent her the report but she is having trouble understanding some of the terminology used and needs some clarification. In NGS, what does the term 'capture' refer to?

A. Binding of the library fragments as they are washed over the flow cell
B. Downloading the relevant read data into the analysis software
C. Identifying the differences between the reads and the reference genome
D. Pulling out the part of the genome to be sequenced
E. Successfully identifying a disease-causing variant

3.19. You review a family, several members of whom have the same, rare condition, for which no genetic cause has yet been identified. You are considering a clinical research project with the aim of identifying the disease-causing mutation in this family. You are trying to decide whether whole-exome sequencing or whole-genome sequencing would be a better approach. Which of the following is an advantage of whole-genome sequencing over whole-exome sequencing?

A. Increased detection of gene dosage abnormalities
B. Increased detection of mosaicism
C. Increased likelihood that a variant detected will be pathogenic
D. Less expensive
E. Lower risk of identifying incidental findings

3.20. You are asked to review a 39 year old woman who has had a positive result for trisomy 21 during non-invasive prenatal testing for aneuploidy screening. She is very upset and is asking you if there is any chance that the test could be wrong. Which of the following is a possible cause of a false-positive result in this circumstance?

A. Confined placental mosaicism
B. High maternal body mass index (BMI)
C. Maternal smoking
D. Previous miscarriage of aneuploid fetus
E. Test done too early in gestation

3.21. You are reviewing a 35 year old woman with triple-negative breast cancer, in whom you have identified an underlying *BRCA1* mutation. Her oncologist has recommended that she enters a trial of treatment with a poly ADP ribose polymerase (PARP) inhibitor. She wants to know more about how they work. Which of the following statements about the mechanism of PARP inhibitors is true?

A. They block the double-stranded DNA break-repair pathway

B. They block the double-stranded DNA break-repair pathway and up-regulate the single-stranded DNA break-repair pathway

C. They block the single-stranded DNA break-repair pathway

D. They repair the double-stranded DNA break-repair pathway

E. They repair the single-stranded DNA break-repair pathway

3.22. You review a 42 year old woman who developed breast cancer at the age of 27 that was successfully treated, and has now developed an osteosarcoma in her right femur. On discussion of her family history she tells you that her mother died when she was very young of brain cancer (glioblastoma) and that her brother is currently receiving treatment for a rhabdomyosarcoma. Apart from evidence of a previous mastectomy, there are no additional phenotypic features on physical examination. You suspect a familial cancer predisposition syndrome. Which of the following cancer predisposition syndromes would be the best fit for this tumour spectrum?

A. Birt–Hogg–Dubé syndrome

B. Cowden's syndrome

C. Gorlin's syndrome

D. Li–Fraumeni syndrome

E. Lynch's syndrome

Answers

3.1. Answer: B.
In DNA, bases are paired as follows: adenine (A) with thymine (T) and guanine (G) with cytosine (C). In RNA, the pairing is the same except that adenine (A) pairs with uracil (U). If unrepaired prior to replication, deamination of a cytosine (C) to a uracil (U) will result in pairing with adenine (A), ultimately replacing the original GC pair with an AT pair.

3.2. Answer: C.
Transcription describes the production of RNA from the DNA template. RNA polymerase binds to the promoter sequence on the DNA template strand, then moves along the strand producing a complementary mRNA molecule. DNA polymerase is not required for transcription but is an essential component of DNA replication. Translation (production of the protein encoded by the mRNA) occurs on the ribosome, and requires an mRNA template and tRNAs.

3.3. Answer: B.
Transcription produces a nascent transcript, which then undergoes splicing to generate the shorter 'mature' mRNA molecule that provides the template for protein production. Splicing removes the intronic regions and joins together the exons. Different combinations of exons may

be joined together (alternative splicing) to produce more than one form of mRNA, which may be tissue specific, as in this example.

3.4. Answer: A.
Whilst the other answers are all stages of the cell cycle, it is during anaphase that the spindle fibres attach to the sister chromatids and pull them apart.

3.5. Answer: D.
A stop-gain (or nonsense) mutation introduces a premature stop codon, resulting in a truncated protein. A synonymous mutation is a base substitution that does not result in a change in the amino acid (because more than one codon may encode a particular amino acid). A missense (or non-synonymous) mutation is a base substitution that results in a change in the encoded amino acid. A deletion is the loss of one or more nucleotides. If the number of nucleotides deleted from within a coding region is not a multiple of three, this results in a frameshift mutation, with a typically severe effect.

3.6. Answer: A.
Myotonic dystrophy type 1 (DM1) is a triplet-repeat disorder, caused by pathological

3

expansion of a run of CTG repeats within the *DMPK* gene, located on chromosome 19. It shows autosomal dominant inheritance so there is a 50% chance that the patient's baby will be affected, regardless of gender. Expanded repeats are unstable and may expand further during meiosis, so that offspring inheriting the condition are often more severely affected than the affected parent – a phenomenon known as anticipation. Anticipation most commonly occurs during the transmission of the condition from mother to child. The vast majority of individuals with DM1 have inherited their expanded CTG allele from a parent; new expansions of a normal allele are rare.

3.7. Answer: E.
Turner's syndrome is a sex chromosome aneuploidy where there is monosomy of the X chromosome (note the single X chromosome and absence of Y chromosome in the karyotype). Girls with Turner's syndrome are typically shorter than average and have underdeveloped ovaries, resulting in delayed or arrested development of secondary sexual characteristics, delayed or absent menstruation and commonly infertility.

3.8. Answer: A.
The initial management step here is to exclude a chromosomal cause for her difficulties. Array CGH would be the most appropriate first-line investigation as it provides a genome-wide screen for chromosomal abnormalities. It has superseded the use of karyotyping in this context as it provides a much higher-resolution screen. Fragile X is a recognised cause of developmental delay but is unlikely here in the context of the microcephaly. If the array CGH is normal, then you may wish to proceed to exome sequencing, or a developmental delay gene panel.

3.9. Answer: E.
Translocation is the result of joining of two segments of DNA from different chromosomes. All the other answers describe structural rearrangements that may be found within a single chromosome.

3.10. Answer: A.
A dominant negative mutation interferes with the function of the wild-type protein. A protein-truncating (or stop-gain) mutation

produces a shorter, non-functional protein and is therefore an example of a loss-of-function mutation. A gain-of-function mutation results in activation or alteration of a protein's normal function.

3.11. Answer: E.
Becker muscular dystrophy is an X-linked disorder. Since his grandfather was also affected, the condition cannot have arisen in your patient de novo and his mother is an obligate carrier. In genetic pedigrees, females are represented by circles, and unaffected female carriers of X-linked conditions are represented by an open circle with a central dot. Female carriers of autosomal recessive conditions are represented by a half-shaded circle. Fully shaded symbols represent affected family members. Diamonds are used to represent ongoing pregnancies.

3.12. Answer: E.
Autosomal dominant conditions typically show variable penetrance – not all people who inherit a mutation will develop the disease. Affected individuals typically occur in each generation (unless the mutation has arisen de novo in an affected individual). Males and females are equally affected.

The recurrence risk for a couple with an affected child will depend on whether the mutation has arisen de novo in the affected child (in which case it is low, typically < 1%), or has been inherited from a parent, in which case it is 50%.

3.13. Answer: A.
In mitochondrial inheritance, the mutation is in the mitochondrial DNA and, since mitochondria are contributed by the oocyte and not by the sperm, inheritance is exclusively via the maternal line. Males and females are equally affected. Variable penetrance and expressivity is common in mitochondrial disorders due to the degree of mitochondrial heteroplasmy (not due to X-inactivation, as in X-linked disorders). Whilst it is possible that the condition has arisen in the proband de novo, it is more likely that it was inherited from her mother. If her mother is indeed a carrier, she will have transmitted the condition to all her offspring. Both the mother and siblings should therefore be offered genetic testing, regardless of clinical symptoms.

3.14. Answer: A.
X-linked conditions are not passed from father to son, as the mutation is on the X chromosome. Whilst X-linked conditions are mostly restricted to males, occasionally female carriers may exhibit signs of an X-linked disease due to skewed X-inactivation. Also, when considering a pedigree, beware of the possible presence of phenocopies (i.e. individuals with a similar phenotype who do not carry the mutation); with a phenotype as common and multifactorial as developmental delay/learning difficulties, this could be a confounding factor in your analysis.

3.15. Answer: B.
If a mutation results in activation of a growth factor gene or receptor, then that cell will replicate more frequently as a result of autocrine stimulation. Tumour formation is promoted by gain-of-function mutations in oncogenes and loss-of-function mutations in tumour suppressor genes, not the other way around. Passenger mutations accumulate within cancer cells but do not in themselves promote growth (unlike 'driver' mutations). Apoptosis is programmed cell death and does not have a role in tumour formation. (The *BRCA* test result is not relevant here – the question is simply testing knowledge of mechanisms promoting tumourigenesis.)

3.16. Answer: A.
Array CGH provides a high-resolution genome-wide screen for chromosomal abnormalities. Mosaicism down to a 10% level can often be detected. Since it relies on analysis of comparative dosage across the genome, triploidy (all chromosomes present in an extra copy) may be missed. Similarly, because with balanced translocations dosage is unaffected, these may not be picked up and, if suspected, karyotyping should be undertaken. Even with the most powerful modern arrays, the resolution is limited to around 10 kB. This would therefore miss many smaller intragenic deletions. Larger deletions and duplications (or indeed aneuploidy) would, however, be reliably detected.

3.17. Answer: C.
The next step would be to test his parents to see whether either of them carried the same CNV. Since they are both phenotypically normal with no history of developmental problems, if either of them also carried the CNV it would be unlikely that it was contributing significantly to his phenotype. It is not uncommon to identify benign inherited CNVs during array CGH testing. If the CNV is not inherited from an unaffected parent it is harder to assess its significance. You would need to carefully consider any genes that could be potentially disrupted. If you remain unconvinced that the CNV provides an explanation for his difficulties you may wish to proceed to further genetic testing, and consider an intellectual disability gene panel or exome sequencing.

3.18. Answer: D.
In NGS, 'capture' refers to the 'pull-down' of a targeted region of the genome for sequencing. This may constitute a single gene, a number of genes associated with a given phenotype or condition (a gene panel), the exons of all coding genes known to be associated with disease (a clinical exome) or the exons of all known coding genes (an exome).

3.19. Answer: A.
Whole-genome sequencing enables more even coverage of genes, allowing better identification of gene dosage anomalies than whole-exome sequencing. (Gene dosage refers to the number of copies of a gene that are present in a genome, and anomalies may be caused by CNVs such as deletions or duplications.) Whole-exome sequencing is, however, less expensive, and allows deeper sequencing and consequently better detection of mosaicism. Whole-genome sequencing will detect many more variants, so it is associated with a greater risk of incidental findings, and the likelihood of any given variant detected being pathogenic is reduced.

3.20. Answer: A.
Confined placental mosaicism (the aneuploidy being present in placental tissue but not in the fetus) is the most well-recognised cause of false-positive results during non-invasive aneuploidy screening. Results should be viewed in the context of ultrasound findings, and positive results need confirmation with invasive testing. High maternal BMI and early gestation are recognised causes of false-negative results. A previous pregnancy will have no effect on these results as cell-free fetal DNA is cleared from the maternal circulation within 30 minutes of delivery.

3.21. Answer: C.

PARP inhibitors work by blocking the single-stranded DNA break-repair pathway. In a *BRCA1/2* mutation-positive tumour with an already compromised double-stranded DNA break-repair pathway, the additional loss of the single-stranded break-repair pathway will drive the tumour cell towards apoptosis (programmed cell death).

3.22. Answer: D.

Mutations in the *TP53* gene cause Li–Fraumeni syndrome, a hereditary predisposition to sarcoma, breast carcinoma, brain cancer (especially glioblastoma) and adrenocortical carcinoma. There are no additional clinical features other than the cancer susceptibility in this syndrome. The other answers are also examples of other rare cancer predisposition syndromes, with different spectrums of tumour susceptibility, and in some cases additional phenotypic clinical features.

3

4

Clinical immunology

Multiple Choice Questions

4.1. Which of the following statements best describes a key feature of innate immunity?

A. It improves with repeated exposure to a given antigen

B. It includes interaction between pattern recognition receptors on phagocytes and pathogen-associated molecular patterns

C. It is not associated with primary immune deficiency

D. It requires antigen processing for activation

E. Memory and specificity are characteristic features

4.2. Which of the following statements best describes a key feature of phagocytes?

A. They are derived from thymic progenitors

B. They are involved in intra- and extracellular killing of microorganisms

C. They do not damage host tissue

D. They have a long half-life

E. They include monocytes, macrophages, neutrophils and natural killer (NK) cells

4.3. Which of the following statements describes a key function of cytokines?

A. They are routinely measured in clinical practice

B. They are small molecules that act as intercellular messengers

C. They do not require receptor interaction

D. They have distinct and non-overlapping biological functions

E. They have not been shown to have a role in disease pathogenesis

4.4. Which of the following statements is correct with regard to adaptive immunity?

A. Each component is able to function independently

B. It is ready to act immediately on pathogen exposure

C. Primary lymphoid tissues include the spleen and mucosa-associated lymphoid tissue

D. T- and B-cell receptors are antigen specific

E. Vaccination efficacy does not require functional adaptive immunity

4.5. Which of the following statements is correct regarding primary immune deficiency?

A. A number of X-linked conditions are recognised

B. Bone marrow transplantation is required for B-cell immune deficiency

C. Gene therapy has not yet been applied to primary immune deficiencies

D. Primary immune deficiency is invariably fatal without treatment

E. Primary immune deficiency only presents in childhood

4.6. Which of the following statements is correct in relation to immunoglobulins?

A. They are constructed of two identical heavy chains and two identical light chains

B. They are derived from thymic precursors

C. They are limited to the intravascular compartment

D. They include six isotypes

E. They protect predominantly against intracellular infection

4.7. Which of the following statements is most consistent with immunoglobulin deficiency?

A. It commonly presents with opportunistic infection
B. It has no association with autoimmune disease
C. It is not associated with end-organ damage
D. It is unlikely in myeloma
E. It may require immunoglobulin replacement therapy

4.8. Which of the following statements most accurately describes the complement system?

A. Complement proteins are reduced as part of the acute phase response
B. It can be activated by one of two pathways – the classical or alternative pathway
C. It does not contribute to local inflammation
D. It ends with a final common pathway leading to bacterial lysis
E. It refers to a series of immune proteins produced by the primary lymphoid tissues

4.9. Which of the following statements best describes complement deficiency?

A. C1 inhibitor deficiency leads to a low C3, even between attacks of angioedema
B. It can be routinely treated with complement replacement therapy
C. It is associated with connective tissue disease
D. It is not associated with recurrent infection
E. It is not influenced by complement control proteins

4.10. Which of the following statements best describes secondary immune deficiency?

A. It can be drug induced
B. It is generally not associated with opportunistic infection
C. It is less common than primary immune deficiency
D. It is rarely life-threatening
E. It is reversible with management of the underlying cause

4.11. Which of the following statements is correct regarding hypersensitivity reactions?

A. The predominant cell type involved in type IV hypersensitivity is the basophil
B. Type I hypersensitivity is IgG mediated
C. Type II hypersensitivity results in circulating immune complexes
D. Type III hypersensitivity results in complement activation

E. Type IV hypersensitivity is typically immediate in onset

4.12. Which of the following clinic features would be UNUSUAL in acute systemic type I hypersensitivity?

A. Bronchospasm
B. Eczematous rash
C. Hypotension
D. Urticarial rash
E. Vomiting

4.13. Which of the following statements is correct regarding mast cell tryptase measurement?

A. It has a half-life of 24 hours
B. It is a less reliable marker of mast cell activation than plasma histamine
C. It is elevated in all cases of anaphylaxis
D. Mast cell tryptase is unstable in serum
E. Serial measurement following appropriate acute patient management can be helpful in confirming a mast cell-activating event

4.14. Which of these statements most accurately describes anaphylaxis?

A. Desensitisation therapy is recommended for nut-induced anaphylaxis
B. It is rarely fatal
C. It leads to increased vascular permeability
D. It results from cross-linking of pre-formed, allergen-specific IgG on the surface of mast cells with subsequent mast cell activation
E. Onset from allergen exposure is typically delayed by 24 hours

4.15. Which of these statements most accurately describes autoimmune disease?

A. It can affect multiple organ systems
B. It is not influenced by environmental factors
C. It is typically life-threatening
D. It is typically monogenic
E. It requires immunosuppressive therapy

4.16. Which one of the following statements is true regarding disease-modifying therapy in autoimmune disease?

A. Anti-tumour necrosis factor (TNF) therapy has been shown to alter the course of disease progression in rheumatoid arthritis
B. Biological agents are generally now considered first-line therapy for inflammatory bowel disease

C. Inhibition of integrins has no proven efficacy
D. Mononclonal antibodies used in autoimmune disease have not been associated with serious side-effects
E. Small-molecule inhibitors targeting intracellular signalling pathways have yet to be developed

4.17. Which of the following statements is true regarding organ transplantation?

A. Acute rejection typically occurs within the first week post-transplant
B. Chronic rejection is immune mediated
C. Co-stimulatory blockade has not been shown to improve outcomes
D. Hyperacute rejection occurs as a result of recipient pre-formed antibody
E. Post-transplant immunosuppression is only required for the first 6 months

4.18. A 57 year old woman with a 20-year history of rheumatoid arthritis presents to the emergency department with a right basal pneumonia. She has received a number of disease-modifying drugs for the arthritis, including methotrexate, and has most recently been on rituximab, an anti-CD20 monoclonal antibody targeting B cells. Which of the following statements is correct?

A. Immunoglobulin measurement is unlikely to be informative
B. Immunoglobulin measurement should include paraprotein assessment for appropriate interpretation
C. Methotrexate is not a risk factor for secondary immune deficiency
D. Opportunistic infection does not need to be considered
E. The patient is at low risk of secondary immune deficiency

4.19. A 5 year old boy presents to the paediatric team with right upper quadrant pain and fever. He has a temperature of 38.5°C, tenderness over a mildly enlarged liver and is noted to have gingivitis. At the age of 3 years he developed a cutaneous abscess following minor trauma. His younger brother died at 2 years of age of sepsis; further details are not known. On imaging he is found to have a 5×6 cm hepatic abscess, aspiration confirming *Staphylococcus aureus* infection. On the post-take ward round you are asked to consider the differential diagnosis and

diagnostic tests. Which of the following statements best fits the clinical scenario?

A. A defect in T-cell immunity is most likely
B. A periodic fever syndrome is most likely
C. An X-linked immune deficiency is most likely
D. Primary immune deficiency is ruled out by the patient's age
E. The diagnostic test would be lymphocyte immunophenotyping

4.20. A 70 year old man presents to his family physician with recurrent lower respiratory tract infection. Sputum culture has confirmed *Streptococcus pneumoniae* and *Moraxella catarrhalis* on multiple occasions. Which of the following tests would have the lowest yield (i.e. would be LEAST helpful) in this context?

A. Full blood count with white cell differential
B. Lymphocyte immunophenotyping
C. Neutrophil function tests
D. Serum immunoglobulins and electrophoresis
E. Thoracic computed tomography (CT) imaging

4.21. A 35 year old woman presents to the allergy clinic for investigation of venom hypersensitivity. She reports rapid onset of localised swelling at the site of a wasp sting on her forearm, with subsequent dyspnoea and altered vision prior to collapsing. She was treated at the scene by the paramedics prior to transfer to her local hospital. She lives in a rural area, is a keen cyclist and often cycles in remote areas. Which of the following statements is correct?

A. Component-resolved diagnostics should be the first-line test
B. From the clinical history given, an adrenaline (epinephrine) auto-injector is not indicated
C. The clinical history is not suggestive of anaphylaxis
D. The patient's regular drug history is not relevant
E. Venom immunotherapy should be considered for this patient

4.22. Which of the following clinical scenarios is correctly paired with the underlying immune deficiency?

A. A 26 year old man presenting with oesophageal candidiasis = primary antibody deficiency
B. A 40 year old woman presenting with increasing delirium; cerebral imaging and biopsy confirm central nervous system (CNS)

lymphoma = human immunodeficiency virus (HIV)

C. A 54 year old man presenting with cerebral toxoplasmosis = complement deficiency

D. A 6 year old boy presenting with osteomyelitis and fungal pneumonia = severe combined immune deficiency

E. A previously well 9 year old boy presenting with *Haemophilus influenzae* otitis media = secondary immune deficiency

4.23. A 54 year old man with chronic hepatitis C presents with lower limb palpable purpura, arthralgia and neuropathy. His alanine aminotransferase (ALT) is 80 U/L (10–60 U/L), albumin 32 g/L (35–50 g/L), C-reactive protein 18 mg/L (<6 mg/L), platelets 90×10^9/L (150–400×10^9/L), complement C4 0.08 g/L (0.15–0.5 g/L); urinalysis confirms proteinuria and microscopic haematuria. Which one of the following statements is true?

A. Diagnostic serum analysis can be reliably undertaken on routine blood sampling

B. Systemic lupus erythematosus (SLE) is most likely

C. Type I cryoglobulinaemia is most likely

D. Type II cryoglobulinaemia is most likely

E. With a normal C3, genetic C4 deficiency is most likely

4.24. A 35 year old woman presents with cough 3 months after a live related donor renal transplantation for end-stage renal disease secondary to IgA nephropathy. She is prescribed prednisolone, tacrolimus and mycophenolate immunosuppression. She also received additional immunosuppression as an early post-transplant biopsy confirmed acute rejection. Her chest X-ray confirms bilateral airspace shadowing, predominantly in the mid-zones. Which of the following statements is correct?

A. At such an early stage, post-transplant opportunistic infection is unlikely

B. Early bronchoscopy with bronchoalveolar lavage needs to be considered

C. Immunosuppression needs to be immediately withdrawn

D. Tuberculosis is the most likely diagnosis

E. The white cell differential is unlikely to be helpful

Answers

4.1. Answer: B.
Pathogen-associated molecular patterns, found on invading pathogens, are recognised by pattern recognition receptors on phagocytic cells, allowing phagocytosis and subsequent pathogen destruction. Memory, specificity and the need for antigen processing are features of adaptive immunity. Primary immune deficiencies affecting innate immunity are well recognised.

4.2. Answer: B.
Phagocytic cells are derived from bone marrow precursors. They include monocytes, macrophages and neutrophils, and are involved in intra- and extracellular killing of microorganisms. They may cause damage to host tissue and have a short half-life.

4.3. Answer: B.
Cytokines are small molecules that act as intercellular messengers via interaction with specific cytokine receptors. They have overlapping biological functions. Many

cytokines have a role in disease pathogenesis. They are not currently routinely measured in clinical practice.

4.4. Answer: D.
T and B lymphocytes carry unique antigen-specific receptors, conferring specificity of the adaptive immune response. Antigen processing is required by T cells, such that the adaptive response requires time to develop. Components of the adaptive immune response work in concert rather than functioning independently. Primary lymphoid tissues are the bone marrow and thymus.

4.5. Answer: A.
Primary immune deficiency often presents in childhood but can present later. A number of X-linked conditions are recognised. Immunoglobulin replacement therapy is standard treatment for primary B-cell immune deficiency. Gene therapy has been applied to a number of specific primary immune deficiencies. There is a spectrum of immune

deficiency disorders; not all are invariably fatal without treatment.

4.6. Answer: A.
Immunoglobulins (Ig) are constructed of two identical heavy chains and two identical light chains. IgG, IgA, IgM, IgE and IgD isotypes are recognised. IgM is the isotype limited to the intravascular compartment. They are produced by B cells and predominantly protect against extracellular infection.

4.7. Answer: E.
Symptomatic immunoglobulin deficiency may require immunoglobulin replacement therapy. Secondary immunoglobulin deficiency can occur with myeloma. Opportunistic infection is not commonly seen without additional T-cell deficiency. End-organ damage such as bronchiectasis can occur, as can autoimmune disease.

4.8. Answer: D.
Complement proteins are produced by the liver as part of the acute phase response and can be activated by three pathways, the classical, alternate and lectin pathways. All three pathways end in the membrane attack complex, leading to bacterial lysis. Local inflammation is induced by complement breakdown products.

4.9. Answer: C.
Complement deficiency is associated with connective tissue disease and recurrent infection, late complement protein deficiency being particularly associated with recurrent neisserial infection. Complement deficiency is not routinely treated with complement replacement therapy. C1 inhibitor deficiency can, however, be treated with C1 inhibitor concentrate. Patients with this condition have a low C4, even between attacks of angioedema. Complement control proteins have an important role in controlling complement activity.

4.10. Answer: A.
Secondary immune deficiency can be drug induced, for example with immunosuppressive agents. It is much more common than primary immune deficiency, can be associated with opportunistic infection and can be life-threatening. Secondary immune deficiency may not be reversible with management of the underlying condition.

4.11. Answer: D.
Type III hypersensitivity results in circulating immune complexes, immune complex deposition and subsequent complement activation. The basophil is not the predominant cell type in type IV hypersensitivity. Type I hypersensitivity is IgE mediated.

4.12. Answer: B.
Bronchospasm, urticarial rash, vomiting and hypotension are well-recognised features of type I hypersensitivity. Eczematous rash is more consistent with type IV hypersensitivity.

4.13. Answer: E.
Mast cell tryptase is stable in serum at room temperature and is a more reliable marker of mast cell activation than plasma histamine. It has a half-life of 2.5 hours. Serial measurement can be helpful in confirming a mast cell-activating event but a negative result does not exclude anaphylaxis.

4.14. Answer: C.
Anaphylaxis leads to increased vascular permeability, is typically rapid in onset following allergen exposure and can be fatal. It results from cross-linking of allergen-specific IgE on mast cells. Desensitisation therapy is currently not routinely recommended for food allergy.

4.15. Answer: A.
Autoimmune disease is generally not monogenic and is influenced by environmental factors. Many autoimmune conditions are not life-threatening, e.g. vitiligo or hypothyroidism. Not all conditions require immunosuppression: e.g. coeliac disease, where gluten withdrawal is required. It can affect multiple organs.

4.16. Answer: A.
Anti-TNF therapy has been shown to alter the course of disease progression in rheumatoid arthritis. Small-molecule inhibitors targeting intracellular signalling pathways are in development. Natalizumab, an integrin inhibitor, has proven efficacy in multiple sclerosis. Monoclonal therapy is not without potentially serious side-effects (e.g. natalizumab and progressive multifocal leucoencephalopathy). Biological agents are generally second line.

4.17. Answer: D.
Hyperacute rejection occurs as a result of recipient pre-formed antibody. Acute rejection

typically occurs at 5–30 days post-transplant. Chronic rejection is multifactorial. Co-stimulatory blockade has been shown to improve outcome. Post-transplant immunosuppression is required for more than 6 months.

4.18. Answer: B.
In this case, secondary immune deficiency has to be considered. Rituximab can lead to B-cell depletion, usually transient, and can be associated with antibody deficiency. Paraprotein assessment should be undertaken for appropriate interpretation of immunoglobulin results.

4.19. Answer: C.
An immune deficiency is likely; the patient's age does not rule this out. With the family history, an X-linked condition should be considered. With the organisms identified, X-linked chronic granulomatous disease, a disorder of phagocytes, rather than a T-cell defect, is most likely, in which case neutrophil function testing would be diagnostic.

4.20. Answer: C.
The clinical history is most consistent with symptomatic antibody deficiency. This may be primary or secondary, for example with chronic lymphocytic leukaemia, and may be associated with end-organ damage. Neutrophil function testing is indicated in the investigation of chronic granulamotous disease rather than antibody deficiency. Chronic granulomatous disease presents at a much younger age usually, with staphylococcal and fungal infection, abscess formation and granulomas; the clinical history does not suggest this.

4.21. Answer: E.
The clinical history is suggestive of anaphylaxis, in which case venom immunotherapy should be considered. Component-resolved diagnostics is not the first-line test. The patient may be on medication that could influence future anaphylaxis management, e.g. angiotensin-converting enzyme inhibitor or β-blocker.

4.22. Answer: B.
CNS lymphoma, driven by Epstein–Barr virus infection, is seen in immune deficiency, typically late-stage HIV infection or following systemic immunosuppressive therapy. A previously well 9 year old is unlikely to have a secondary immune deficiency. *Candida* oesophagitis is more consistent with T-cell immune deficiency, as is toxoplasmosis. Severe combined immune deficiency is likely to have presented before the age of 6 years and the clinical findings described are more consistent with a primary phagocyte deficiency.

4.23. Answer: D.
A type II cryoglobulinaemia in the context of hepatitis C is most likely, from the clinical history, raised ALT, elevated inflammatory markers and low C4. SLE is on the differential diagnosis but crypglobulinaemia typically presents with rash, arthralgia and neuropathy. Warm separated serum is required for appropriate investigation. Genetic deficiency of C4 is less likely in this context.

4.24. Answer: B.
Early bronchoscopy should be considered. Opportunistic infection could occur at 3 months. The white cell differential will help to determine the risk of opportunistic infection. Immunosuppression needs to be carefully considered rather than immediately withdrawn; withdrawal would compromise the transplanted organ. *Pneumocystis* pneumonia is the most likely diagnosis.

D McAllister, H Campbell

5

Population health and epidemiology

Multiple Choice Questions

5.1. Which of the following diseases was among the top 15 ranked causes of global premature mortality (measured by years of life lost) in 2013 as part of the Global Burden of Disease (GBD) Exercise?

A. Alzheimer's disease
B. Asthma
C. Colorectal cancer
D. Congenital anomalies
E. Protein energy malnutrition

5.2. Global premature mortality is measured by years of life lost, with higher ranking meaning higher number of premature deaths. Between 1990 and 2013, which of the following rose in the rankings of conditions causing global premature mortality?

A. Human immunodeficiency virus (HIV)/ acquired immune deficiency syndrome (AIDS)
B. Iron deficiency anaemia
C. Maternal disorders
D. Measles
E. Meningitis

5.3. Which one of the following diseases is among the top 15 ranked causes of global disability (measured by years of life lived with disability; YLD) in 2013?

A. Alcohol use disorders
B. Epilepsy
C. Lens cataract
D. Neural tube defects
E. Schizophrenia

5.4. Which of the following diseases is among the top 10 ranked risk factors underlying GBD in 2013 (ranked in terms of the proportion of GBD that they cause)?

A. Alcohol use
B. Low-fibre diet
C. Low physical activity
D. Suboptimal breastfeeding
E. Vitamin A deficiency

5.5. Patients who respond positively to an invitation for screening tend to be less socioeconomically deprived than those who do not. In view of this, what needs to be considered when evaluating such a programme?

A. Incomplete follow-up
B. Lead-time bias
C. Length bias
D. Recall bias
E. Self-selection bias

5.6. Which of the following is one of Wilson and Jungner's criteria for the evaluation of a national screening programme?

A. The case-finding should be a once-and-for-all project
B. The condition sought should be an important health problem
C. The condition sought should be self-limiting
D. The condition sought should have a low mortality
E. The condition sought should only be treatable if detected at screening

5.7. In a clinical trial where participants are randomly allocated to a treatment or control group, which one of the following statements is true?

A. In randomisation, the doctor generally knows which treatment the patient will be allocated to before they are enrolled in the trial
B. In randomisation, the patient generally knows which treatment they will be allocated to before they are enrolled in the trial
C. Randomisation is performed so that the number of patients in the treatment and control groups are the same
D. Randomisation is primarily used to reduce bias
E. Randomisation is primarily used to reduce confounding

5.8. In a case–control study examining the effect of coffee consumption on lung cancer, which one of the following might lead to confounding?

A. People with lung cancer are more likely to over-report smoking
B. People with lung cancer are more likely to under-report coffee consumption
C. Smokers with lung cancer drink more coffee than smokers without lung cancer
D. Smoking is commoner in coffee drinkers
E. There is a lot of variation in the amount of caffeine in different coffees

5.9. Which of the following is a true description of a cohort study, as used in epidemiological research?

A. Cohort studies generally enrol people without disease
B. Odds ratios cannot be calculated
C. Participants are randomly assigned to different exposures
D. People with the disease of interest are selected along with similar people without the disease of interest
E. Risk ratios cannot be calculated

5.10. Which of the following is true of the number needed to treat (NNT), calculated from a randomised controlled trial?

A. The more effective a treatment, the larger the NNT

B. The NNT is one minus the absolute risk reduction
C. The NNT is the number of patients who will benefit from a treatment if 100 typical patients are treated
D. The NNT is the reciprocal (inverse) of the difference in risk between different treatment groups
E. The NNT is the reciprocal (inverse) of the risk ratio

5.11. In a clinical trial, 2000 patients were randomly allocated on a 1-to-1 basis to either a placebo or 'Novotreat', a new drug. After 1-year of follow-up, 130 patients in the placebo group and 100 in the treatment group had died. What was the absolute risk reduction?

A. 3%
B. 23%
C. 0.77
D. 1.30
E. 33.33

5.12. A city has a population of 100 000. Each year 10 000 people are diagnosed with heart disease for the first time after presenting to their doctor and 5000 people die of heart disease. Of the latter, 1000 are not found to have heart disease until after they died. Assuming that there are no other ways that new cases are identified, which of the following is true of heart disease in this city?

A. The case fatality is 20%
B. The incidence is 10 per 100 person-years
C. The incidence is 11 per 100 person-years
D. The incidence is 5 per 100 person-years
E. The prevalence is 10%

5.13. Which of the following is true of national health information systems?

A. Definitions of non-psychiatric illnesses are agreed nationally
B. Few countries produce national mortality statistics
C. Incidence rates can generally be easily compared across countries
D. Most countries record attendances at primary care facilities by cause
E. Most countries use an international standard classification system for recording cause of death

Answers

5.1. Answer: D.

Congenital anomalies were ranked 10 in 2013 in the GBD Exercise initiated by the World Bank. Asthma is a major cause of burden of disease but not of premature deaths. Protein energy malnutrition has been declining as an important cause of death due to economic development globally. Alzheimer's disease and colorectal cancer are both important causes of premature death but are both outside the top 20 (rank 29 and 27, respectively).

5.2. Answer: A.

HIV/AIDS rose from rank 27 in 1990 to rank 6 in 2013 due to the global epidemic. Most other infections, including meningitis, measles and maternal infections, fell due to increased implementation of successful control measures. Iron deficiency anaemia ranking fell from 35 to 45.

5.3. Answer: E.

Schizophrenia was ranked 11 as a cause of YLD in 2013. Epilepsy is an important cause of YLD but outside the top 20 (rank 23). Cataract, neural tube defects and alcohol use disorders are causes of disability but are all well below the top 15 ranked causes.

5.4. Answer: A.

Alcohol use was ranked 6 as a cause of GBD in 2013. Suboptimal breastfeeding is ranked 19 in 2013, down from rank 11 in 1990, and vitamin A deficiency is ranked 23, down from rank 36. Low-fibre diet (25) and low physical activity (17) are also of lower rank.

5.5. Answer: E.

Self-selection bias, lead-time bias and length bias are all classic sources of bias in evaluation of screening trials. Incomplete follow-up is also an important problem in all trials. Screening evaluations normally are based on recorded events for their primary evaluations and do not depend on recall of past events, so recall bias is not one of the most important problems.

5.6. Answer: B.

The important question is how common is the condition in the specific population in whom the screening will be implemented. It is possible for a disease to be important globally, e.g. malaria or primary liver cancer, but not important in a specific country. The test should be whether it is an important public health problem in the specific country or region.

5.7. Answer: E.

Randomisation is performed primarily to ensure that, on average, different treatment (or intervention) groups are similar, apart from the intervention being studied. It is only true to say that the groups are the same on average, however, as differences can arise by chance. Randomisation only works if the treatment allocation is masked until after the decision is taken to enrol a participant. In some trials, the treatment allocation continues to be concealed after enrolment, but this is done for a separate reason, to reduce bias.

5.8. Answer: D.

Confounding is where a cause of the disease (or a marker of such a cause) is commoner in the exposure group of interest, and is not itself a consequence of that exposure. If coffee per se, caused smoking, it would not be confounding but a causal chain.

5.9. Answer: A.

Cohort studies are observational studies where participants are selected to reflect some population, characterised according to their baseline characteristics and followed up over time to observe occurrences of one or more diseases of interest. The relationship between an exposure and outcome of interest can then be studied. Risk ratios, odds ratios and rate ratios can all be calculated in cohort studies. Studies that enrol people with disease and then follow up these people over time are better called case series with follow-up.

5.10. Answer: D.

Developed by David Sackett, the number needed to treat (NNT) aims to provide doctors and patients with a more intuitive statistic for quantifying treatment effects than the standard ratios and differences. It is calculated as the inverse of the absolute risk reduction (or risk difference) between treatment groups. Like absolute risk reductions, NNTs are only comparable if the risks being reported are the same, including the time over which the risk applied, e.g. 1-year absolute risk reductions and 5-year absolute risk reductions are not comparable.

5.11. Answer: A.

There are many ways to represent the effect of drug treatments. The other measures are, in order, (1) the number needed to treat, (2) the risk ratio of the placebo versus the treatment group, (3) the risk ratio of the treatment versus the placebo group and the (4) relative risk reduction.

5.12. Answer: C.

The incidence rate is the number of new events per unit of person-time. As 1000 of the people who died with heart disease were not previously diagnosed, these also represent new events. You do not have sufficient information to estimate the case-fatality as you do not know the proportion of the people with heart disease who die from any cause. Additional assumptions would also be needed to estimate the prevalence of heart disease.

5.13. Answer: E.

Globally, the vast majority of countries use the World Health Organization International Classification of Diseases (ICD) system. For psychiatric illnesses, the disease is also defined. In most countries (the most notable exception being the USA where the Diagnostic and Statistical Manual of Mental Disorders is used), ICD criteria are also used to define psychiatric illnesses. For non-psychiatric illnesses, definitions are not included as part of the ICD system, although there are some separate definitions of certain conditions such as diabetes which have been adopted widely (http://www.who.int/diabetes/publications/diagnosis_diabetes2006/en/).

5

JAT Sandoe, DH Dockrell

6

Principles of infectious disease

Multiple Choice Questions

6.1. A 53 year old lawyer from South Africa who is human immunodeficiency virus (HIV)-seropositive has a medical review, which reveals a positive interferon-gamma release assay (IGRA), showing T cells reactive to *Mycobacterium tuberculosis* antigens. He is asymptomatic and a chest X-ray is reported as negative. Which of these most accurately describes his mycobacterial status?

A. Active pulmonary disease
B. Commensal flora
C. Extrapulmonary infection
D. Latent infection
E. Opportunistic infection

6.2. A 9 month old infant has a temperature of 39.5°C and is not feeding. The parents attend the local clinic where the doctor can find no abnormalities on physical examination other than erythema of the right tympanic membrane. Treatment with which of the following is appropriate as a simple and safe intervention that may decrease the body temperature?

A. Anti-tumour necrosis factor (TNF) antibody
B. Aspirin
C. Erythromycin
D. Paracetamol
E. Penicillin

6.3. A 44 year old woman is diagnosed with HIV infection and a low CD4 T-cell count. She starts antiretroviral therapy to treat her infection and is seen at clinic 3 months later when she has an undetectable HIV viral load and a significant increase in her CD4 T-cell counts.

She complains of severe headaches, slurred speech and right arm weakness, and a computed tomography (CT) head scan shows multiple space-occupying lesions in her brain. What are her symptoms most likely due to?

A. Antiretroviral drug-related side-effect
B. HIV-related damage to brain
C. Immune reconstitution inflammatory syndrome (IRIS)
D. Metastatic carcinoma
E. Syphilitic gumma

6.4. A 59 year old woman presents with a pelvic tumour and is found to have cervical carcinoma. The use of which vaccine in childhood would have reduced the chance of this cancer developing?

A. Hepatitis B virus vaccine
B. Human papilloma virus (HPV) vaccine
C. Measles vaccine
D. Pneumococcal conjugate vaccine
E. Rubella vaccine

6.5. A 33 year old Nigerian man who has had a haematopoeitic stem cell transplant for aplastic anaemia six months previously returns to visit his family in Nigeria once a year. He attends your vaccine clinic. Which of the following vaccines should be avoided?

A. Hepatitis B virus vaccine
B. Influenza inactivated vaccine
C. Pneumococcal protein conjugate vaccine
D. Tetanus toxoid
E. Yellow fever virus vaccine

6.6. A 45 year old man is admitted to the intensive care unit with a short history of respiratory symptoms and shortness of breath. He arrived in the country 2 days ago. Initial polymerase chain reaction (PCR) for routine respiratory viruses is negative but a sample sent to the national laboratory detects a specific geographically restricted coronavirus. Travel to which of the following countries is most likely to be associated with this virus?

A. Brazil
B. China
C. Saudi Arabia
D. United States of America
E. Zambia

6.7. A 63 year old retired international aid worker who last worked abroad 15 months ago presents with fever and fatigue. He had worked in many African countries but particularly in Sudan and West Africa. On examination he is found to have splenomegaly and his full blood count reveals anaemia and thrombocytopenia. Which of the following tropical infections is most consistent with the clinical scenario?

A. Dengue
B. Leishmaniasis
C. *Plasmodium falciparum*
D. *Trypanosoma brucei gambiense*
E. Typhoid fever

6.8. Your hospital has had three cases of severe community-acquired pneumonia in the last 3 weeks that have had positive tests for urinary *Legionella* antigen. You typically have one to two cases per year. The cases were cared for in different units and there was no direct contact between the cases while hospitalised. All three cases have the same postal code. You contact the public health doctors to discuss these cases. How would you best describe the clustering of these cases?

A. Common source outbreak
B. Epidemic
C. Nosocomial linked cluster
D. Pandemic
E. Person-to-person community spread

6.9. A 56 year old patient has had multiple orthopaedic operations to deal with complications of a road traffic accident. These have involved plates and screws for several fractures. Three weeks after the last operation

there is purulent drainage from a wound in the right hip and a CT scan reveals a collection, which is aspirated. The microbiologists identify Gram-positive cocci in clusters that they identify as *Staphylococcus aureus*. The presence of which genetic element will influence therapy decisions for this patient?

A. *ampC* extended-spectrum β-lactamase
B. *mecA* penicillin-binding protein
C. NDM-1 carbapenemase
D. TEM-12 β-lactamase
E. *vanA* gene cluster

6.10. A 73 year old patient develops *Staphylococcus aureus* bacteraemia with a meticillin-sensitive strain that remains persistent despite flucloxacillin therapy. All prosthetic material and collections of infection have been removed or drained. Which intervention may enhance the success of the therapy?

A. Administering therapy as an infusion
B. High-dose once-a-day therapy
C. Increasing the dose frequency
D. Prolonging treatment duration
E. Switching to glycopeptide therapy

6.11. A 60 year old man with acute myeloid leukaemia develops pulmonary aspergillosis. He is placed on treatment with voriconazole. Which of the following is a recognised adverse effect of voriconazole therapy that the patient should be counselled about?

A. Aplastic anaemia
B. Dermatitis
C. Oesophageal ulcer
D. Proximal renal tubular injury
E. Tendon rupture

6.12. A 33 year old man develops chicken pox with pulmonary involvement. He is previously fit and well and has had no prior therapy for viral infections. He is hypoxic and has tachypnoea. His chest X-ray reveals widespread nodules. In addition to oxygen, which antiviral agent should he receive?

A. Aciclovir
B. Amantadine
C. Cidofovir
D. Foscarnet
E. Valaciclovir

6.13. A 35 year old wildlife photographer plans a trip to Kenya and asks for advice about antimalarial treatment. She has a long history of depression but is currently not on any treatment. The medical history is otherwise unremarkable. Which is the best choice of malaria prophylaxis in this case?

A. Atovaquone plus proguanil
B. Chloroquine
C. Doxycycline
D. Ivermectin
E. Mefloquine

6.14. A 50 year old tourist returns from a trip in Kenya where she visited game parks and remembers receiving some tick bites. She has a necrotic eschar at the site of one bite a maculopapular rash and fever plus headache. A diagnosis of boutonneuse fever due to *Rickettsia conorii* is made and she is prescribed doxycycline. She has diabetes mellitus and hypertension as well as osteoporosis. Which medication that she currently takes should not be taken at the same time as doxycycline?

A. Calcium
B. Metformin
C. Paracetamol
D. Ramipril
E. Simvastatin

6.15. A 63 year old patient develops bowel perforation after abdominal surgery and is admitted to the intensive care unit where he requires pressors and ventilation. Microbiology shows a mixed infection including coliforms, enterococci and *Candida* spp. He requires a range of antimicrobials initially including teiocoplanin, meropenem and caspofungin, but subsequently develops a nosocomial *Acinetobacter baumannii* infection and receives colistin and tigecycline. He makes steady progress but when weaned from the ventilator is found to have encephalopathy. Which of the antimicrobials he has received is associated with development of encephalopathy?

A. Caspofungin
B. Colistin
C. Meropenem
D. Teicoplanin
E. Tigecycline

Answers

6.1. Answer: D.
The test result with a positive IGRA but no symptoms or signs on chest X-ray suggesting infection and no evidence of active disease point to latent infection. Active pulmonary and extrapulmonary disease would have signs and/or symptoms and *M. tuberculosis* would not be found as commensal flora.

6.2. Answer: D.
Temperature elevation involves generation of cytokines and prostaglandins. Paracetamol is a simple intervention that can inhibit generation of prostaglandins and act as antipyretic. Although aspirin would do the same, it is not recommended routinely for children due to the risk of Reye's syndrome. Anti-TNF therapy has other medical indications and antimicrobials would not be appropriate for what appears to be a viral illness.

6.3. Answer: C.
The symptoms in this case have come on after therapy was commenced, which raises

suspicion of a drug-related side-effect, but the nature of the lesions on brain scan are not consistent. They have occurred at a time when the immunodeficiency associated with HIV has been reversed, which raises suspicion of IRIS. HIV itself can cause chronic loss of brain volume but not space-occupying lesions, and syphilitic gumma or metastatic carcinoma (although differential diagnoses) are not associated with therapy and immune reconstitution.

6.4. Answer: B.
The HPV vaccine is now part of the vaccine schedule for girls in many countries and decreases the risk of cervical carcinoma. The hepatitis B vaccine also reduces the incidence of a cancer, in this case hepatocellular carcinoma, but the other vaccines do not have an obvious link to reduction of cancer incidence.

6.5. Answer: E.
Live vaccines should, in general, be avoided in immunocompromised patients or only given

after careful risk–benefit analysis in exceptional cases. Yellow fever virus vaccine is a live virus vaccine. The other vaccines are not live vaccines.

6.6. Answer: C.
The symptoms of severe respiratory syndrome and presence of a geographically restricted coronavirus raise the possibility of Middle East respiratory syndrome (MERS) coronavirus. Travel-related cases have been seen in many countries but the majority of cases have initially been associated with travel to countries in the Middle East.

6.7. Answer: B.
The clinical scenario with fever, splenomegaly and abnormalities on the full blood count could be seen with most of these travel-associated infections, although at this late stage *Trypanosoma brucei* would generally present with encephalopathy. The key feature here is the incubation period. Of these infections, only leishmaniasis and sleeping sickness would present with such a long incubation period. The clinical scenario suggests visceral leishmaniasis not sleeping sickness.

6.8. Answer: A.
The cases are most consistent with a common source outbreak that is linked to some common environmental source. Since the patients were cared for in different units, there is no evidence of hospital transmission. Person-to-person transmission in the community would be a less likely scenario for this organism. The numbers are not consistent with a pandemic or epidemic.

6.9. Answer: B.
The *mecA* gene encodes a penicillin-binding protein with low affinity for penicillins, including antistaphylococcal penicillins, and is the usual basis of resistance in meticillin-resistant *Staph. aureus* (MRSA). Presence of this genetic element, which is often screened for in *Staph. aureus* strains, necessitates use of an antimicrobial other than an antistaphylococcal penicillin (e.g. flucloxacillin). *vanA* encodes a penicillin-binding protein that has low affinity for glycopeptides and is found in enterococci. The other options are β-lactamase or carbapenemase enzymes that mediate resistance in Gram-negative bacteria.

6.10. Answer: A.
Persistent bacteraemia increases the risk of complications. When the strain is sensitive to antistaphylococcal penicillins (e.g. flucloxacillin) these should be prescribed in preference to other agents. Penicillins work by time-dependent killing so the efficacy is, in theory, improved by continuous infusion. Increasing the dose would be appropriate only for antimicrobials that kill by dose-dependent killing (e.g. aminoglycosides).

6.11. Answer: B.
Voriconazole can cause photosensitive dermatitis and patients should be advised to avoid sun exposure or to use a high-level sunblock on light-exposed areas. The other side-effects are associated with other antimicrobials.

6.12. Answer: A.
All the listed choices except amantadine are active against herpes virus infections but for someone with an end-organ complication such as pneumonia, high-dose intravenous therapy aciclovir would be indicated. Valaciclovir would be appropriate for milder disease and foscarnet for someone who has an infection with resistance to aciclovir as may occur in an immunocompromised patient with frequent exposure.

6.13. Answer: A.
Atovaquone when combined with proguanil is active against *Plasmodium falciparum*. This is a good choice as it is well tolerated. Mefloquine is associated with neurocognitive side-effects and can worsen symptoms of pre-existing psychiatric conditions. Doxycycline is another option but can cause photosensitive dermatitis and may not be a good choice for someone who will be working out of doors. Resistance means chloroquine is no longer a suitable option in most malaria-endemic areas. Ivermectin is used against helminths not malaria.

6.14. Answer: A.
Tetracyclines absorption is limited by cations such as calcium, iron and antacids that contain aluminium or magnesium. The other medications will not alter absorption. Tetracyclines should be taken at a different time, several hours separate from the cation-containing medicine.

6.15. Answer: B.

Although there are a range of potential causes of encephalopathy in a patient who has received ventilation for critical illness including infection, medication-related causes should always be considered. Of the antimicrobials listed, colistin is associated, in particular, with neurotoxicity including encephalopathy.

7

SHL Thomas

Poisoning

Multiple Choice Questions

7.1. Which one of the following is most likely to produce significant toxicity if ingested accidentally by a child?

A. A 1 cm length of pencil lead
B. One combined oral contraceptive tablet
C. One liquid laundry detergent capsule
D. One mouthful of emulsion paint
E. One prednisolone 5 mg tablet

7.2. A patient develops prolonged and recurrent episodes of torsades de pointes associated with no palpable cardiac output after an overdose of sotalol. All of these interventions may be useful except one. Which one is NOT likely to be helpful in the management of this situation?

A. Cardiac pacing
B. Correction of hypokalaemia
C. Intravenous bolus dose of magnesium sulphate
D. Intravenous infusion of isoproterenol
E. Intravenous bolus dose of procainamide

7.3. A 33 year old male attends the emergency department with breathlessness and chest pain after using a recreational substance/street drug. On examination he looks cyanosed and has a tachycardia (120 beats/min). On supplemental oxygen, his arterial blood gases show H$^+$ 52.5 nmol/L (pH 7.28), $PaCO_2$ 2.7 kPa (20.3 mmHg), PaO_2 17.3 kPa (129.8 mmHg) and 35% methaemoglobinaemia. Which of the following is the most likely causative agent?

A. Cocaine
B. Gamma hydroxybutyrate
C. Isopropyl nitrite

D. Isosorbide mononitrate
E. Paracetamol

7.4. A family of four people living in Jamaica develop vomiting, diarrhoea and abdominal pain a few hours after eating a well-cooked meal of snapper fish in a seafood restaurant. This subsequently progresses to unsteadiness of gait, blurred vision and tingling in the hands and feet. Which of the following is the most likely diagnosis?

A. Aconite poisoning
B. Ciguatera poisoning
C. Paralytic shellfish poisoning
D. *Salmonella* poisoning
E. Scombrotoxic fish poisoning

7.5. Which of the following is the most likely explanation for the following clinical features in an adult patient after drug overdose: tachycardia, delirium, hallucinations, fever, diarrhoea, shivering, inducible prolonged clonus, seizures, raised creatine kinase?

A. Anticholinergic toxidrome
B. Intercurrent infection
C. Recent use of gamma hydroxybutyrate
D. Serotonin syndrome
E. Stimulant toxidrome

7.6. A 54 year old man presents unconscious. His pulse is 88 and blood pressure 142/78. Initial investigations reveal normal urea and electrolytes, creatinine of 101 μmol/L (1.14 mg/dL) and glucose 7.3 mmol/L (131.4 mg/dL). Arterial blood gases results include H$^+$ 81.3 nmol/L (pH 7.09), $PaCO_2$ 1.8 kPa (13.5 mmHg), base excess of –13 mmol/L, carboxyhaemoglobin of 2% and lactate of 17.3 mmol/L (155.9 mg/dL). Paracetamol and salicylate are not detected. A computed tomography (CT) scan of the head is normal. Which of the following is the most likely diagnosis?

A. Carbon monoxide poisoning
B. Cyanide poisoning
C. Diabetic ketoacidosis
D. Ethylene glycol poisoning
E. Salicylate poisoning

7.7. A 34 year old painter/decorator presents with fatigue and anaemia after spending several weeks thermally stripping lead-based paint without using adequate personal protective equipment. His blood lead concentration is substantially elevated. Which of the following chelating agents is the most appropriate antidote for treatment of chronic lead poisoning?

A. Desferrioxamine
B. Dicobalt edetate
C. Dimercaprol
D. Dimercaptosuccinic acid (DMSA)
E. Hydroxocobalamin

7.8. Which of the following results indicates the largest anion gap (all results are in mmol/L)?

A. Sodium 119, potassium 2.6, chloride 90, bicarbonate 27
B. Sodium 131, potassium 4.3, chloride 96, bicarbonate 18
C. Sodium 135, potassium 5.6, chloride 101, bicarbonate 24
D. Sodium 136, potassium 4.1, chloride 102, bicarbonate 25
E. Sodium 149, potassium 3.9, chloride 94, bicarbonate 21

7.9. A 24 year old man presents to hospital after smoking a herbal mixture. Which of the following features are characteristic of exposure to synthetic cannabinoid receptor agonists (SCRAs) but are not usually associated with use of herbal cannabis?

A. Ataxia
B. Conjunctival irritation
C. Psychosis
D. Seizures
E. Tachycardia

7.10. A 23 year old female develops muscle cramps and numbness about 3 weeks after an intentional ingestion of an insecticide product used on the farm where she lives. Her features progress to flaccid paralysis of lower and upper limbs with reduced tendon reflexes. A diagnosis of organophosphate-induced delayed polyneuropathy (OPIDN) is made. Which of the following is the most likely causative agent?

A. Bendiocarb
B. Dichlorvos
C. Methomyl
D. Sarin
E. Tabun

7.11. A 21 year old man presents to hospital after snorting a white powder purchased as a 'research chemical' via the internet. He develops tachycardia and hypertension. Which of the following compounds is most likely to have been in the powder used?

A. Cannabis
B. Gamma hydroxybutyrate
C. Heroin
D. Isobutyl nitrite
E. Mephedrone

7.12. Two adult males present to hospital after they both used the same unidentified recreational substance. Both have a Glasgow Coma Scale score <9 and bradycardia. Pupils are mid-sized. One has been incontinent for urine and both display myoclonus. Blood gases show a mixed respiratory and metabolic acidosis in both. What substance is most likely to be responsible?

A. Diazepam
B. Ethanol
C. Gamma hydroxybutyrate
D. Heroin
E. Ketamine

7.13. In relation to ingestion of a toxic substance, which of the following characteristics make a substance less appropriate for removal by haemodialysis?

A. Large volume of distribution
B. Long half-life
C. Low molecular weight
D. Non-polar molecule
E. Not bound to activated charcoal

7.14. An 18 year old male presented to hospital after a deliberate overdose involving unknown substances. At presentation there was a high concentration of paracetamol in the blood. Over the subsequent 3 days he developed worsening abnormalities of liver function (elevated bilirubin and alanine transaminase), clotting (raised international normalised ratio) and renal function (elevated creatinine) and episodes of hypoglycaemia. All the features below are consistent with paracetamol overdose, except one. Which feature is most likely to be caused by another substance?

A. Acute kidney injury
B. Early unconsciousness
C. Elevated international normalised ratio
D. Hypoglycaemia
E. Liver failure

7.15. A 23 year old man develops toxicity after deliberately ingesting a carbamate insecticide. Clinical features include headache, vomiting, diarrhoea, hypersalivation, abdominal pain, tachycardia, muscle weakness, fasciculation and reduced ventilation due to respiratory muscle involvement. Which one of the following is an example of a cholinergic (muscarinic) effect?

A. Fasciculation
B. Mydriasis
C. Respiratory muscle paralysis
D. Salivation
E. Tachycardia

7.16. A 2 year old child develops tachycardia, delirium, fever associated with a flushed face, mydriasis and seizures after eating part of a plant. Which of the following is most likely to be responsible?

A. Autumn crocus (*Colchicum autumnale*)
B. Deadly nightshade (*Atropa belladonna*)
C. Jequirity bean (*Abrus precatorius*)
D. Laburnum (*Laburnum anagyroides*)
E. Wolf's bane (*Aconitum napellus*)

7.17. A 17 year old female patient presents unconscious having had a witnessed seizure after an intentional drug overdose. Following the seizure she is drowsy but vital signs are otherwise satisfactory. Which of the following is most likely to be responsible?

A. Amlodipine
B. Diazepam
C. Digoxin
D. Mefenamic acid
E. Paracetamol

7.18. Deliberate release of a chemical warfare agent is suspected when 12 people develop similar symptoms after an explosion on an underground train. Initially these include anxiety, breathlessness, vomiting and headache, but five cases have also developed convulsions. Three patients have become unconscious and two have died. Survivors have dilated pupils and no respiratory tract or skin abnormalities are found. Investigations show raised plasma lactate but plasma acetylcholinesterase activity is normal. This clinical picture is most characteristic of exposure to which of the following?

A. Cyanide
B. Lewisite
C. Phosgene
D. Sarin
E. Sulphur mustard

Answers

7.1. Answer: C.
These are all substances of low toxicity (Box 7.1) with the exception of liquid laundry detergent capsules, which can cause CNS depression in children and are also corrosive, sometimes causing stridor, pulmonary aspiration and airway burns, as well as ocular damage if the liquid gets into the eyes.

7.2. Answer: E.
These are all useful interventions for torsades de pointes except procainamide. Magnesium sulphate reduces the risk of torsades without

---

i 7.1 Substances of very low toxicity

Writing/educational materials, e.g. pencil lead, crayons, chalk

Decorating products, e.g. emulsion paint, wallpaper paste

Cleaning/bathroom products (except dishwasher tablets and liquid laundry detergent capsules, which can be corrosive)

Pharmaceuticals: oral contraceptives, most antibiotics (but not tetracyclines or antituberculous drugs), vitamins B, C and E, prednisolone, emollients and other skin creams, baby lotion

Miscellaneous: plasticine, silica gel, most household plants, plant food, pet food, soil

i	7.2 Complications of poisoning and their management	
Complication	**Examples of causative agents**	**Management**
Coma	Sedative agents	Appropriate airway protection and ventilatory support Oxygen saturation and blood gas monitoring Pressure area and bladder care Identification and treatment of aspiration pneumonia

Seizures	NSAIDs
	Anticonvulsants
	TCAs
	Theophylline
		Appropriate airway and ventilatory support
		IV benzodiazepine (e.g. diazepam 10–20 mg,
		  lorazepam 2–4 mg)
		Correction of hypoxia, acid–base and metabolic
		  abnormalities

Acute dystonias	Typical antipsychotics Metoclopramide	Procyclidine, benzatropine or diazepam
Hypotension		
Due to vasodilatation	Vasodilator antihypertensives Anticholinergic agents TCAs	IV fluids Vasopressors (rarely indicated)
Due to myocardial suppression	β-blockers Calcium channel blockers TCAs	Optimisation of volume status Inotropic agents
Ventricular tachycardia		

Monomorphic, associated with
  QRS prolongation
	Sodium channel blockers	Correction of electrolyte and acid–base abnormalities
		  and hypoxia
		Sodium bicarbonate (e.g. 50 mL 8.4% solution,
		  repeated if necessary)

Torsades de pointes,
  associated with QT$_c$
  prolongation
	Anti-arrhythmic drugs (quinidine,
	  amiodarone, sotalol)
	Antimalarials
	Organophosphate insecticides
	Antipsychotic agents
	Antidepressants
	Antibiotics (erythromycin)
		Correction of electrolyte and acid–base abnormalities
		  and hypoxia
		Magnesium sulphate, 2 g IV over 1–2 mins, repeated
		  if necessary

(NSAID = non-steroidal anti-inflammatory drug; TCA = tricyclic antidepressant)

affecting the QT interval and is first-line treatment (Box 7.2). Isoproterenol and pacing increase the underlying ventricular rate and reduce the risk of recurrence, as torsades is a bradycardia-dependent arrhythmia, although they are infrequently needed. Hypokalaemia worsens the risk of torsades, so correction is beneficial. Procainamide is a class Ia anti-dysrhythmic drug that further prolongs ventricular repolarisation and would worsen the risk of torsades.

7.3. Answer: C.
Methaemoglobinaemia is commonly caused by organic nitrites, such as isopropyl nitrite, which oxidise haemoglobin. Other causes are shown in Fig. 7.3. The other substances listed in the question do not have this effect directly. Note, however, that occasionally cocaine is contaminated with oxidising adulterants such as benzocaine or phenacetin, which may occasionally produce unexpected methaemoglobinaemia.

7.4. Answer: B.
The clinical features could be consistent with options B or C but the association with eating predator fish suggests ciguatera, which is prevalent in the Caribbean. These neurological features are not found with *Salmonella* poisoning. Scombrotoxic fish poisoning causes symptoms associated with histamine release, which may include gastrointestinal disturbance, but neurological features are not characteristic. Aconite can also cause gastrointestinal disturbances and paraesthesia but a plant is less likely to be involved in this episode.

7.5. Answer: D
These are all characteristic features of serotonin syndrome (Box 7.5A). Inducible clonus and shivering are not characteristic of the anticholinergic or stimulant toxidromes or gamma hydroxybutyrate (GHB) toxicity (although myoclonus may be seen after GHB; Box 7.5B). Clonus would not suggest intercurrent infection.

Causes	Consequences	Treatment
Non-toxic • Congenital methaemoglobinaemias *Toxic (Oxidising agents)* • Organic nitrites • Nitrates • Benzocaine • Dapsone • Chloroquine • Aniline dyes • Chlorobenzene • Naphthalene • Copper sulphate	• Haemoglobin–oxygen dissociation curve is shifted to the left • Oxygen delivery to tissues is reduced • There is apparent 'cyanosis' • Breathlessness, fatigue, headache and chest pain occur • Delirium, impaired consciousness and seizures may occur in severe cases	• Methylthioninium chloride ('methylene blue') 1–2 mg/kg (intravenous) is given • Reduces methaemoglobin (see below) • Used for symptomatic patients with severe methaemoglobinaemia (e.g. >30%) • Patients with anaemia or other comorbidities may need treatment at lower concentrations

7

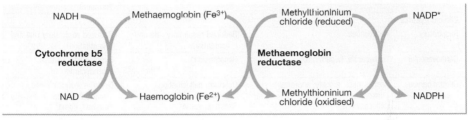

Fig. 7.3

	7.5A Anticholinergic and serotonergic feature clusters	
	Anticholinergic	**Serotonin syndrome**
Common causes	Benzodiazepines Antipsychotics TCAs Antihistamines Scopolamine Benzatropine Belladonna Some plants and mushrooms (see Box 7.16B)	SSRIs MAOIs TCAs Amphetamines Tryptamines Buspirone Bupropion (especially in combination)
Clinical features		
Cardiovascular	Tachycardia, hypertension	Tachycardia, hyper- or hypotension
Central nervous system	Delirium, hallucinations, sedation	Delirium, hallucinations, sedation, coma
Muscle	Myoclonus	Shivering, tremor, myoclonus, raised creatine kinase
Temperature	Fever	Fever
Eyes	Diplopia, mydriasis	Normal pupil size
Abdomen	Ileus, palpable bladder	Diarrhoea, vomiting
Mouth	Dry	
Skin	Flushing, hot, dry	Flushing, sweating
Complications	Seizures	Seizures Rhabdomyolysis Renal failure Metabolic acidosis Coagulopathies

(MAOI = monoamine oxidase inhibitor; SSRI = selective serotonin re-uptake inhibitor; TCA = tricyclic antidepressant)

7.6. Answer: B.
This patient has marked metabolic acidosis with greatly elevated lactic acid. While all of these diagnoses may cause metabolic acidosis, only cyanide and carbon monoxide are associated with elevated lactic acid in the absence of cardiovascular shock. Carbon monoxide poisoning has probably been excluded by the normal carboxyhaemoglobin result, unless exposure was many hours earlier. Diabetic ketoacidosis and salicylate poisoning are also excluded by the normal blood glucose and salicylate concentration, respectively.

7.7. Answer: D.
Lead poisoning can be treated with oral DMSA (also called succimer) or parenteral sodium calcium edetate (Box 7.7). Indications for the other listed chelating agents include poisoning with cyanide (hydroxocobalamin, dicobalt edetate) or iron (desferrioxamine). Dimercaprol has been used for heavy metal poisoning, including mercury, but has now been largely superseded by other chelating agents, because these are better tolerated.

7.8. Answer: E.
The anion gap measures the difference between measured cations (sodium and potassium) and anions (chloride and bicarbonate) and is usually calculated as [Na$^+$ + K$^+$] – [Cl$^-$ + HCO$_3^-$]. The 'gap' reflects the

i   7.5B Stimulant, sedative and opioid feature clusters

	Stimulant	Sedative hypnotic	Opioid
Common causes	Amphetamines MDMA ('ecstasy') Ephedrine Pseudoephedrine Cocaine Cannabis Phencyclidine Cathinones (e.g. mephedrone) Benzylpiperazine	Benzodiazepines Barbiturates Ethanol GHB	Heroin Morphine Methadone Oxycodone Dihydrocodeine Codeine Pethidine Dipipanone Buprenorphine Dextropropoxyphene Tramadol
Clinical features			
Respiratory	Tachypnoea	Reduced respiratory rate and ventilation*	Reduced respiratory rate and ventilation
Cardiovascular	Tachycardia, hypertension	Hypotension*	Hypotension, relative bradycardia
Central nervous system	Restlessness, anxiety, anorexia, insomnia Hallucinations	Delirium, hallucinations, slurred speech Sedation, coma*	Delirium, hallucinations, slurred speech Sedation, coma†
Muscle	Tremor	Ataxia, reduced muscle tone	Ataxia, reduced muscle tone
Temperature	Fever	Hypothermia	Hypothermia
Eyes	Mydriasis	Diplopia, strabismus, nystagmus Normal pupil size	Miosis
Abdomen	Abdominal pain, diarrhoea	–	Ileus
Mouth	Dry	–	–
Skin	Piloerection	Blisters, pressure sores	Needle tracks†
Complications	Seizures Myocardial infarction Dysrhythmias Rhabdomyolysis Renal failure Intracerebral haemorrhage or infarction	Respiratory failure* Aspiration	Respiratory failure† Non-cardiogenic pulmonary oedema Aspiration

Especially barbiturates.
†*IV use.*
(GHB = gamma hydroxybutyrate; MDMA = 3,4-methylene-dioxymethamphetamine)

i   7.7 Specific antidotes used to treat poisoning

Mechanism of action	Examples of antidote	Poisoning treated
Glutathione repleters	Acetylcysteine Methionine	Paracetamol
Receptor antagonists	Naloxone Flumazenil Atropine	Opioids Benzodiazepines Organophosphorus compounds Carbamates
Alcohol dehydrogenase inhibitors	Fomepizole Ethanol	Ethylene glycol Methanol
Chelating agents	Desferrioxamine Hydroxocobalamin Dicobalt edetate DMSA Sodium calcium edetate	Iron Cyanide Lead
Reducing agents	Methylthioninium chloride	Organic nitrites
Cholinesterase reactivators	Pralidoxime	Organophosphorus compounds
Antibody fragments	Digoxin Fab fragments	Digoxin

(DMSA = dimercaptosuccinic acid)

7.8 Anion and osmolar gaps in poisoning		
	Anion gap	Osmolar gap
Calculation	[Na$^+$ + K$^+$] − [Cl$^-$ + HCO$_3^-$]	[Measured osmolality] − [(2 × Na) + Urea + Glucose]*
Reference range	12–16 mmol/L	< 10
Common toxic causes of elevation	Ethanol Ethylene glycol Methanol Salicylates Iron Cyanide	Ethanol Ethylene glycol Methanol

All units should be in mmol/L. For non-SI units, the corresponding formula is [Osm (measured)] − [(2 × Na (mEq/L)) + Urea/2.8 (mg/dL) + Glucose/18 (mg/dL)].

concentrations of unmeasured anions such as albumin and phosphate and the normal range is 12–16 mmol/L. Anion gap is increased by the presence of toxic anions such as the metabolites of ethylene glycol or methanol.

In these examples, the calculated values are: (A) 4.6; (B) 21.3; (C) 15.6; (D) 13.1; and (E) 37.9 mmol/L. For more information see Box 7.8.

N.B. for simplicity some recommend ignoring potassium in the calculation of anion gap (anion gap = Na$^+$ − [Cl$^-$ + HCO$_3^-$]), as potassium makes a limited contribution. Using this calculation, the normal range is 8–12 mmol/L. Use of this method gives the same answer for this question.

7.9. Answer: D.

Tachycardia, ataxia, conjunctival irritation and psychosis can all be characteristic of exposure to both cannabis and synthetic cannabinoid receptor agonists. Seizures, however, are often reported after use of SCRAs but rarely after use of cannabis. Unlike cannabis, SCRAs have also been reported to cause hypokalaemia, acute kidney injury and coma with respiratory acidosis.

7.10. Answer: B.

Dichlorvos is an organophosphate insecticide that can sometimes cause OPIDN, but this complication is rare with nerve agents (e.g. sarin, tabun) and non-organophosphate carbamate insecticides (e.g. methomyl, bendiocarb). Nerve agents would not be found on farms.

7.11. Answer: E.

Mephedrone is a white powder commonly taken by nasal insufflation ('snorting'), and

tachycardia and hypertension would be typical stimulant effects. Cannabis is not a white powder. While pure heroin (diamorphine) is white, street heroin is usually discoloured brown and smoked or injected rather than snorted. GHB and isobutyl nitrite are liquids. None of these others are likely to cause tachycardia and hypertension.

7.12. Answer: C.

These features (especially myoclonus and incontinence) are characteristic of poisoning with GHB and the related substances gamma butyrolactone (GBL) and 1,4 butanediol. The other four substances can all cause coma but bradycardia and incontinence are not typical. Small pupils would be seen with heroin toxicity.

7.13. Answer: A.

Characteristics associated with efficacy for haemodialysis as a treatment for poisoning include small volume of distribution (high proportion of body load in the blood/plasma), low molecular weight, lipid soluble/non-polar at physiological pH (can cross dialysis membrane) and a long half-life after overdose. Binding to activated charcoal is not relevant for haemodialysis (only haemoperfusion).

7.14. Answer: B.

Paracetamol toxicity is characteristically associated with liver failure (including hypoglycaemia and abnormal clotting) and renal failure. Paracetamol does not generally cause unconsciousness, although this can be a feature of late-stage liver failure. It may also be caused by co-ingestants.

7.15. Answer: D.

These could all be cholinergic effects, but tachycardia, reduced ventilation, mydriasis and fasciculation are all cholinergic *nicotinic* (rather than muscarinic) effects (Box 7.15).

7.16. Answer: B.

The child has features consistent with an anticholinergic toxidrome (Box 7.16A). Plants with this effect include *Atropa belladonna* (deadly nightshade), *Datura stramonium* (jimson weed, thorn apple) and *Brugmansia* spp. (angel's trumpet). While ingestion of jequirity beans, wolf's bane and laburnum could potentially also cause convulsions, anticholinergic effects would not be expected. Autumn crocus causes gastrointestinal effects,

7

i 7.15 Cholinergic features in poisoning*	Muscarinic	Nicotinic
Respiratory	Bronchorrhoea, bronchoconstriction	Reduced ventilation
Circulation	Bradycardia, hypotension	Tachycardia, hypertension
Higher mental function	Anxiety, delirium, psychosis	
Muscle	–	Fasciculation, paralysis
Temperature	Fever	–
Eyes	Diplopia, miosis, lacrimation	Mydriasis
Abdomen	Vomiting, profuse diarrhoea	–
Mouth	Salivation	–
Skin	Sweating	–
Complications	Coma, seizures, respiratory depression	

Both muscarinic and nicotinic features occur in organophosphorus poisoning. Nicotinic features occur in nicotine poisoning and black widow spider bites. Cholinergic features are sometimes seen with some mushrooms.

i 7.16A Anticholinergic and serotonergic feature clusters	Anticholinergic	Serotonin syndrome
Common causes	Benzodiazepines Antipsychotics TCAs Antihistamines Scopolamine Benzatropine Belladonna Some plants and mushrooms (see Box 7.16B)	SSRIs MAOIs TCAs Amphetamines Tryptamines Buspirone Bupropion (especially in combination)
Clinical features		
Cardiovascular	Tachycardia, hypertension	Tachycardia, hyper- or hypotension
Central nervous system	Delirium, hallucinations, sedation	Delirium, hallucinations, sedation, coma
Muscle	Myoclonus	Shivering, tremor, myoclonus, raised creatine kinase
Temperature	Fever	Fever
Eyes	Diplopia, mydriasis	Normal pupil size
Abdomen	Ileus, palpable bladder	Diarrhoea, vomiting
Mouth	Dry	
Skin	Flushing, hot, dry	Flushing, sweating
Complications	Seizures	Seizures Rhabdomyolysis Renal failure Metabolic acidosis Coagulopathies

(MAOI = monoamine oxidase inhibitor; SSRI = selective serotonin re-uptake inhibitor; TCA = tricyclic antidepressant)

hypotension and cardiogenic shock (Box 7.16B).

7.17. Answer: D.

Mefenamic acid is a non-steroidal anti-inflammatory drug (NSAID) with a very high propensity to cause seizures. Other common causes of seizures in the context of drug overdose include tricyclic antidepressants, antipsychotic drugs, antiepileptic drugs, other NSAIDs (although much less commonly than with mefenamic acid), anticonvulsants and theophylline (Box 7.17). Paracetamol, diazepam and digoxin do not cause seizures. Seizures have been reported with severe amlodipine

poisoning but are uncommon and likely to be associated with severe cardiovascular effects.

7.18. Answer: A.

These are typical features of cyanide poisoning. Sarin can also cause vomiting, breathlessness (associated with bronchospasm and bronchorrhoea) and convulsions, but small pupils, abnormalities on respiratory examination and reduced plasma or red cell acetylcholinesterase activity would be expected. Sulphur mustard, lewisite and phosgene can cause respiratory effects but convulsions and coma would not be expected.

i 7.16B Some poisonous plants and their clinical effects

Species (common name)	Toxins	Important features of toxicity
Plants		
Abrus precatorius (jequirity bean)	Abrin	Gastrointestinal effects, drowsiness, delirium, convulsions, multi-organ failure
Ricinus communis (castor oil plant)	Ricin	
Aconitum napellus (aconite, wolf's bane, monkshood)	Aconite	Gastrointestinal effects, paraesthesiae, convulsions, ventricular tachycardia
Aconitum ferox (Indian aconite, bikh)		
Atropa belladonna (deadly nightshade)	Atropine, scopolamine, hyocyamine	Anticholinergic toxidrome (see Box 7.16A)
Datura stramonium (Jimson weed, thorn apple)		
Brugmansia spp. (angel's trumpet)		
Colchicum autumnale (autumn crocus)	Colchicine	Gastrointestinal effects, hypotension, cardiogenic shock
Conium maculatum (hemlock)	Toxic nicotinic alkaloids	Hypersalivation, gastrointestinal effects, followed by muscular paralysis
Digitalis purpurea (foxglove)	Cardiac glycosides	Cardiac glycoside toxicity
Nerium oleander (pink oleander)		
Thevetia peruviana (yellow oleander)		
Laburnum anagyroides (laburnum)	Cytosine	Gastrointestinal effects; convulsions in severe cases
Taxus baccata (yew)	Taxane alkaloids	Hypotension, bradycardia, respiratory depression, convulsions, coma, arrhythmias
Fungi		
Amanita phalloides (death cap mushroom)	Amatoxins	Gastrointestinal effects, progressing to liver failure
Cortinarius spp.	Orellanine	Gastrointestinal effects, fever, progressing to renal failure
Psilocybe semilanceata ('magic mushrooms')	Psilocybin, psilocin	Hallucinations

i 7.17 Complications of poisoning and their management

Complication	Examples of causative agents	Management
Coma	Sedative agents	Appropriate airway protection and ventilatory support Oxygen saturation and blood gas monitoring Pressure area and bladder care Identification and treatment of aspiration pneumonia
Seizures	NSAIDs Anticonvulsants TCAs Theophylline	Appropriate airway and ventilatory support IV benzodiazepine (e.g. diazepam 10–20 mg, lorazepam 2–4 mg) Correction of hypoxia, acid–base and metabolic abnormalities
Acute dystonias	Typical antipsychotics Metoclopramide	Procyclidine, benzatropine or diazepam
Hypotension		
Due to vasodilatation	Vasodilator antihypertensives Anticholinergic agents TCAs	IV fluids Vasopressors (rarely indicated)
Due to myocardial suppression	β-blockers Calcium channel blockers TCAs	Optimisation of volume status Inotropic agents
Ventricular tachycardia		
Monomorphic, associated with QRS prolongation	Sodium channel blockers	Correction of electrolyte and acid–base abnormalities and hypoxia Sodium bicarbonate (e.g. 50 mL 8.4% solution, repeated if necessary)
Torsades de pointes, associated with QT_c prolongation	Anti-arrhythmic drugs (quinidine, amiodarone, sotalol) Antimalarials Organophosphate insecticides Antipsychotic agents Antidepressants Antibiotics (erythromycin)	Correction of electrolyte and acid–base abnormalities and hypoxia Magnesium sulphate, 2 g IV over 1–2 mins, repeated if necessary

(NSAID = non-steroidal anti-inflammatory drug; TCA = tricyclic antidepressant)

J White

8

Envenomation

Multiple Choice Questions

8.1. A patient presenting with suspected envenoming requires a rapid but careful and targeted assessment to determine if envenoming is present and what urgent responses are required. Which is the most important first response in ensuring a good outcome?

A. Check for breathing and circulatory problems and institute cardiopulmonary resuscitation (CPR) if indicated

B. Give antivenom

C. If the animal that caused the bite/sting is available, try and identify it, so that likely risks can be determined and targeted treatment provided

D. Insert an intravenous (IV) line and consider an early IV fluid load

E. Urgently examine for signs of developing neurotoxic flaccid paralysis and bleeding tendency secondary to coagulopathy

8.2. A 32 year old man presents to your hospital with a history of working in a rice paddy and being bitten by something, not seen. He appears unwell and has swelling around the bite on his foot, with two bite marks that are bleeding. What is a key test that might help you determine the type of snake and need for antivenom?

A. 20-Minute whole-blood clotting test (20WBCT)

B. Arterial blood gas

C. Blood pressure

D. Extended coagulation studies

E. Serum electrolytes

8.3. Considering the patient in Question 8.2, above, if we knew he came from somewhere in India or Sri Lanka, given the particular circumstances of this bite, and that testing showed a coagulopathy, which of the following venomous animals would be most likely as a cause for his bite?

A. Cobra

B. Indian red scorpion

C. Krait

D. Russell's viper

E. Saw-scaled viper

8.4. Our patient in Questions 8.2 and 8.3 is clearly envenomed and needs antivenom urgently. In giving him antivenom, which is the most important drug to have available?

A. Adrenaline (epinephrine)

B. Antihistamine

C. Dopamine

D. Hydrocortisone

E. Prazosin

8.5. The patient in Questions 8.2 to 8.4 has now developed a low urine output, despite adequate IV fluids. In this small rural hospital setting, what test might best help in deciding that acute kidney injury and renal failure is occurring?

A. Dipstick test for proteinuria

B. Measure serum creatinine level

C. None of the above

D. Renal biopsy

E. Renal ultrasound

8.6. A patient presents at a small rural hospital you are working in, with a history of snakebite and on investigation she has local bruising and swelling around the bite site with oozing of blood, a coagulopathy, renal failure and developing flaccid neurotoxic paralysis. In which country is this hospital likely to be?

A. Bangladesh
B. Burma
C. India
D. South Africa
E. Sri Lanka

8.7. You are working in a hospital in Brazil and you are asked to assess a young man with a history of snakebite, occurring at around dusk. He did not see the snake properly, so cannot provide a description. The bite site is not showing much swelling or local pain, but there are obvious fang marks and he has bilateral ptosis and a positive 20WBCT. Which snake is the most likely cause?

A. Coral snake (*Micrurus frontalis*)
B. Green racer (*Philodryas olfersii*)
C. Jararaca (*Bothrops jararaca*)
D. Neotropical rattlesnake or cascabel (*Crotalus durissus terrificus*)
E. Tiger snake (*Notechis scutatus*)

8.8. You are working in a hospital in rural Nigeria. A patient presents with a snakebite and already has local swelling and bruising around the bite site. A 20WBCT is positive (blood not clotted at 20 minutes). Which of the following snakes is most likely involved?

A. Black-necked spitting cobra (*Naja nigricollis*)
B. Forest cobra (*Naja melanoleuca*)
C. Green mamba (*Dendroaspis jamesoni*)
D. Puff adder (*Bitis arietans*)
E. Saw-scaled (carpet) viper (*Echis ocellatus*)

8.9. For a forest cobra bite (*Naja melanoleuca*), which of the following is likely to be the most useful and effective first aid, if applied correctly?

A. Electric shock
B. Pressure bandage and immobilisation (PBI)
C. None of these listed
D. Scarification of the bite site
E. Tourniquet

8.10. Snakebite is variously claimed to be either an important or quite unimportant medical problem. Which of the following epidemiological data is considered, by experts, to be a reliable figure indicating the impact of snakebite?

A. Snakebite causes about 3000 deaths per year in India
B. Snakebite causes about 45000 deaths per year in India
C. Snakebite causes more than 200000 deaths per year worldwide
D. Snakebite causes only about 20000 deaths per year worldwide
E. Snakebite is less important than land mines in causing injuries requiring an amputation

8.11. You are working in a hospital in northern England, near areas of national parks, when a 10 year old boy is presented with a history of stepping on and being bitten by a snake while playing in his garden, near natural parkland. The boy's father, who was not present when the bite occurred, describes the snake as grey in colour, with indistinct darker markings along the sides of the body and a pale narrow band, like a collar, behind the head. What type of snake might this be?

A. A European adder (*Vipera berus*)
B. A form of legless lizard ('slow worm', *Anguis fragilis*)
C. A grass snake (*Natrix natrix*)
D. A smooth snake (*Coronella austriaca*)
E. An escaped exotic snake, most likely a small mamba

8.12. With regard to the patient in Question 8.11, this boy has now developed significant local swelling and bruising around the bite site, which is painful and swelling extends to much of the bitten limb. He appears shocked, has poor urine output and the preliminary report from the laboratory indicates he may have a coagulation abnormality. Questioning also reveals that the father's description of the snake may not be accurate. What do you now think is most likely to have bitten this boy?

A. A European adder (*Vipera berus*)
B. A form of legless lizard ('slow worm', *Anguis fragilis*)
C. A grass snake (*Natrix natrix*)
D. A smooth snake (*Coronella austriaca*)
E. An escaped exotic snake, most likely a small mamba

8.13. A young man presents to the emergency department of the London hospital you are

8

working in, claiming he has been bitten by a large spider that he was keeping as a pet. The bite occurred 6 hours ago, has been very painful locally and his attempts to control the pain with oral analgesia have failed. He was given the spider by a friend who worked for an importer of fruit such as bananas. He does not know what type of spider it is. What sort of spider would you be concerned about?

A. Australian funnel web spider
B. Black widow spider
C. Brazilian wandering spider
D. Brown recluse spider
E. Mexican orange-kneed tarantula

Answers

8.1. Answer: A.

Options C, D and E are all necessary urgent requirements in managing a patient with suspected envenoming, but ensuring there is no problem with the classic 'ABC' of airway, breathing and circulation, and treating any problems found, is the most urgent action. Snakebite patients, particularly in Asia, still die unnecessarily because bystanders and health professionals forget about the ABC and fail to provide airway protection and external respiratory support, when required, following envenoming by neurotoxic snakes such as kraits and some cobras.

Option B might seem like an obvious answer, but not every patient bitten/stung by a venomous animal will develop medically significant envenoming, therefore not every patient needs antivenom. The other issue is choosing which antivenom to use, and what dose to administer, particularly in countries with several different antivenoms. In countries such as India, where only a polyvalent antivenom is available, there is no requirement to delay while choosing the right antivenom, but that does not imply every patient should be given antivenom, so CPR, if indicated, takes precedence.

8.2. Answer: A.

A number of snakes may cause rapid envenoming with development of a coagulopathy that can present as prolonged bleeding from the bite site, any other recent wound, or the gums. The 20WBCT is a rapid and simple test that can provide a useful guide to the presence of snakebite coagulopathy. That, in turn, can help in determining what type of snake may be involved and, if there are several different antivenoms available, which one to consider using.

Blood pressure is certainly an important test, but an abnormal result is not a specific marker for envenoming. Serum electrolytes may be useful, but not critical to initial assessment, and may be hard to obtain in a rural hospital setting, as may extended coagulation studies. The latter will take far more time to provide an answer than will the 20WBCT. Arterial blood gas is not a critical test in initial assessment of snakebite and if there is a coagulopathy, insertion of the needle or a line may pose significant risks for the patient.

8.3. Answer: D.

The history tells us he was bitten in a paddy field, so likely a wetlands agricultural area, a classic setting for a Russell's viper (*Daboia russelii* and *Daboia siamensis*) and this snake causes coagulopathy, plus other effects. In some areas, such as Myanmar, Russell's vipers also commonly cause acute renal failure.

Saw-scaled vipers (*Echis* spp.) also cause coagulopathy, but tend to inhabit dry areas rather than paddy fields. However, there are sometimes exceptions, so knowing precisely where the bite occurred and matching that to the known local venomous fauna might assist in deciding if a saw-scaled viper might be the cause. Cobras (*Naja* spp.) do not cause coagulopathy, neither do kraits (*Bungarus* spp.) nor Indian red scorpions (*Hottentotta tamulus*).

8.4. Answer: A.

The greatest risk when giving antivenom is an anaphylactic reaction, which, if not correctly managed, may prove fatal. Managing anaphylaxis requires a multifaceted approach, but the key drug is adrenaline (epinephrine), in most instances administered intramuscularly. Adrenaline should always be immediately available, in an appropriate dose, prior to giving any antivenom.

Adrenaline, as a dilute subcutaneous injection, has also been suggested as a pre-medication prior to giving antivenom, in certain situations and countries, a practice now supported by clinical trials in Sri Lanka, where its use was associated with a reduced incidence of anaphylactic reactions to antivenom.

Hydrocortisone and antihistamines have also been suggested as pre-medication prior to giving antivenom, but clinical trial evidence does not support their use. Prazosin has, in the past, been the recommended treatment for envenoming by the Indian red scorpion, but more recent clinical trial evidence indicates that specific antivenom is more effective. Dopamine might be required in managing intractable hypotension, but is not an alternative to adrenaline as the drug of first choice in treating anaphylaxis.

8.5. Answer: A.

In this setting it is likely that a simple urine dipstick test will be available and if this shows proteinuria, in this clinical scenario, it is very likely the patient is developing renal failure.

A serum creatinine level may certainly help, but even if available, may take time to gain an answer. Renal ultrasound is unlikely to be available and may not assist in diagnosis. Renal biopsy is inappropriate given the active coagulopathy.

8.6. Answer: E.

The combination of coagulopathy, renal failure and neurotoxic flaccid paralysis is classic for Sri Lankan Russell's viper envenoming. It is rarely seen elsewhere within the range of this snake, although there are a few reports from part of southern India. If the hospital was in south eastern Australia (not an option listed), then a tiger snake (*Notechis scutatus*) bite should be considered.

8.7. Answer: D.

Because of the likely snake fauna in Brazil, early development of paralysis (as evidenced by ptosis) plus coagulopathy is typical of a significant South American rattlesnake bite, quite different to rattlesnake bites in North America.

The jararaca and related *Bothrops* spp. are the most common cause of significant snakebites in Brazil and often cause coagulopathy plus significant local bite site injury, but not paralysis. Coral snakes mostly cause only minor local bite effects and

classically cause paralysis, but not coagulopathy. The green racer may, in some cases, cause coagulopathy, but not paralysis, though like most non-front-fanged colubrid (NFFC) snakes, the clinical picture is not well defined.

8.8. Answer: E.

The saw-scaled vipers routinely cause both significant tissue damage around the bite site and a severe coagulopathy.

Forest cobras cause only minor local bite site effects, major flaccid paralysis and do not cause coagulopathy. Black-necked spitting cobras can cause severe local tissue injury, but not coagulopathy. Puff adders cause severe local tissue injury, but not a clear coagulopathy, although there may be bruising and oozing of blood around the bite site. Green mambas cause local and paralytic effects, not coagulopathy.

8.9. Answer: B.

The forest cobra causes principally flaccid neurotoxic paralysis, without major local tissue damage around the bite site. Therefore, the most important consideration is slowing venom movement from the bite site to the rest of the body, a process that initially occurs particularly via the lymphatic system. The Australian-developed PBI first aid is the most effective safe way of achieving this. Because the pressure is applied to the bite area and bitten limb, it has the potential, for bites by snakes causing extensive bite site tissue injury, to worsen that injury. Therefore, the PBI method is not recommended for bites by snakes likely to cause such local tissue injury; for these snakes, simple immobilisation of the bitten limb is recommended instead.

Tourniquets, while effective in the short term in preventing venom movement, are painful and have a well-established reputation for causing major ischaemic limb injury, often necessitating amputation; therefore, tourniquets are not recommended first aid for any snakebite. Electric shock treatment for snakebite has been proven to cause injury and provides no benefit; it should never be used as first aid for any envenoming. Scarification of the bite site, although commonly used as first aid for snakebite, has no benefit, causes significant harm and should never be used for snakebite.

8

8.10. Answer: B.

The 'Million Death Study' in India provided the best available data on the impact of snakebite in that country and estimated at least 45 000 Indians die from snakebite every year, far higher than official Indian Government data, which uses only hospital data.

The precise number of snakebite deaths each year worldwide is unknown, with estimates varying from a low of about 25 000 (almost certainly far too low), to >100 000, with some experts speculating that up to 200 000 deaths may occur, although this latter figure is not yet supported by definitive data.

Snakebite causes nearly 100 times more limb injuries requiring amputation, each year, than land mines. Fortunately most of those injuries caused by snakebites require only amputation of digits or parts of a limb – less commonly whole-limb amputation.

8.11. Answer: C.

The grass snake is a non-dangerous snake, arguably the most common native snake in the UK. The pale band or collar behind the head is a useful diagnostic feature present in many specimens, although not all.

There are legless lizards ('slow worms') in the UK, but they generally do not have this pattern of coloration. The European northern adder (*Vipera berus*) is the only venomous snake native to the UK. It is often grey in colour, with darker blotchy markings on the body. Mambas are tree-dwelling snakes and do not accord with the description given. Consider the possibility of an escaped exotic venomous snake (depending on the setting) if the patient develops envenoming inconsistent with a European adder bite.

8.12. Answer: A.

The European northern adder does cause snakebites in the UK, maybe as many as 70–100 cases per year and, particularly in children, it can cause severe, even life-threatening envenoming, characterised by local pain, swelling, bruising and sometimes shock and a coagulopathy. Kidney injury can occur, although is rare.

Legless lizards are harmless, non-venomous, as are grass snakes. Mambas (*Dendroaspis* spp.) cause a quite different clinical picture of envenoming.

8.13. Answer: C.

The severe local pain following a bite from a large spider could be caused by a number of exotic species, but is a particular feature of bites by the Brazilian wandering spider (*Phoneutria nigriventer*), otherwise known as the banana spider because it is sometimes accidentally imported in containers of fruit, notably bananas.

The Australian funnel web spiders (there are a number of genera and species; the best known is the Sydney funnel web spider, *Atrax robustus*) can cause local severe pain, but the major risk is systemic envenoming causing a catecholamine-storm-like clinical picture and this develops quickly within minutes to an hour or so after the bite. Your patient does not have this clinical picture, so even if it was a funnel web spider, he is out of the danger period. Black widow spiders (*Latrodectus* spp.) are not large and, while they can cause local pain, it progresses to more regional, then generalised pain, plus features of neuroexcitation, so your patient does not really fit this picture. Brown recluse spiders (*Loxosceles* spp.) generally cause little or no pain initially and it is only many hours to days after people are bitten that local necrosis and sometimes a significant systemic envenoming can develop; they are not large spiders, so do not fit the picture presented by your patient. The Mexican orange-kneed tarantula (*Brachypelma smithi*) may cause locally painful bites, but more commonly causes skin or eye irritation from shed abdominal hairs.

M Byers

9

Environmental medicine

Multiple Choice Questions

9.1. Research on individuals exposed to radiation from the atomic bombs in Hiroshima and Nagasaki has shown an increased relative risk of developing malignancy (leukaemia, oral cavity, oesophagus, stomach, colon, lung, breast, ovary, urinary bladder, thyroid, liver, non-melanoma skin and nervous system) as a result of radiation exposure. Which of these statements best describes this observation?

A. The Japanese have higher rates of cancer than the world average
B. This is a deterministic effect of radiation
C. This is a stochastic (random) effect of radiation
D. This is an observational effect unrelated to the atomic bomb
E. This is because of background radiation in Japan

9.2. Radiation can be divided into ionising and non-ionising forms. Ionising radiation carries enough energy to free electrons from atoms or molecules, thereby ionising them, and this can damage tissues and cells. Which of these forms of therapy is most likely to cause long-term radiation injury through high levels of ionising radiation exposure to patients?

A. Chest X-ray to diagnose a spontaneous pneumothorax
B. Radiofrequency ablation for cardiac arrhythmias
C. Serial whole-body computed tomography (CT) for cancer screening
D. Transurethral microwave therapy for prostatic hypertrophy
E. Ultraviolet therapy for psoriasis

9.3. A 67 year old patient is brought to the emergency department having been found unwell in an unheated apartment during the winter in Northern Europe. Severe reversible hypothermia is best characterised by which of the following?

A. A core temperature below 32°C
B. Bradycardia, a J wave on the electrocardiogram and loss of consciousness
C. Chest and abdomen rigidity with a core temperature below 13°C and serum potassium > 12 mmol/L.
D. Shivering, white peripheries and irritability
E. Tachycardia, tachypnoea and slight delirium

9.4. A family consult their family physician for advice regarding a forthcoming holiday in the tropics. Heat illness is a spectrum of disease affecting both the young and old. Which of these statements is most correct?

A. Complications of heat stroke include hypovolaemic shock, lactic acidosis, rhabdomyolysis, hepatic failure and pulmonary oedema
B. Exertional heat illness is more common in the elderly than in younger people
C. Heat acclimatisation is characterised by decreased sweat volume, reduced sweat sodium content and secondary hyperaldosteronism to maintain body sodium balance
D. Heat stroke commonly occurs above 39°C
E. Heat syncope is another term for heat stroke

9.5. Acclimatisation is the process of the body adjusting to the decreased availability of oxygen at high altitudes. This becomes noticeable above 2500 m. Which of these changes occurs in healthy individuals?

A. A shift in the oxygen dissociation curve to the left after 2–3 days
B. Deep prolonged sleep with vivid dreams
C. Deep, slow breathing to maximise oxygen uptake
D. Erythropoiesis and haemoconcentration mediated through the endocrine system
E. Fluid retention to counteract the raised haematocrit due to hypoxia

9.6. A 36 year old mountaineer ascends to 3800 m. He complains of feeling tired and unwell. His companions notice that he is staggering and delirious. Which of the following statements is true regarding illness at altitude?

A. Acetazolamide is the treatment of choice for high-altitude cerebral oedema (HACE)
B. Altitude sickness usually occurs between 1500 m and 2500 m, is characterised by vomiting and resolves spontaneously after a few days
C. High-altitude pulmonary oedema (HAPE) is a life-threatening condition that initially presents with symptoms of dry cough, exertional dyspnoea and extreme fatigue
D. Monge's disease (chronic mountain sickness) is characterised by polycythemia and hypoxia that does not improve if the patient moves to lower altitudes to live
E. The cardinal signs of HACE are headache, unilateral pupillary dilatation and dizziness

9.7. A 5 year old boy is brought to the emergency department following a drowning incident. Which of the following statements is true with regard to a drowned patient?

A. Fresh water is hypotonic and impairs surfactant function, causing alveolar collapse and left-to-right shunting of unoxygenated blood

B. In about 10% of cases, no water enters the lungs and death follows intense laryngospasm ('dry' drowning)
C. Long-term outcome depends on the severity of the cerebral hypoxic injury and is predicted by the duration of immersion and delay in resuscitation, but is independent of the presence of cardiac arrest
D. Salt water is hypertonic and inhalation provokes alveolar oedema, producing a distinct clinical picture from freshwater drowning
E. Those rescued alive (near-drowning) are often unconscious and not breathing. Hypoxaemia and metabolic alkalosis are common features during resuscitation

9.8. A 48 year old woman is planning to do some diving on her forthcoming holiday to the Caribbean. She is reading about the possible risks involved. Which of the following statements is true?

A. Ambient pressure under water increases by 101 kPa (1 atmosphere, 1 ata) for every 10 m of seawater depth, with the nitrogen in air causing narcosis below 30 m of seawater and oxygen becoming toxic at inspired pressures above 40 kPa (0.4 ata)
B. As divers descend, the partial pressures of the gases they are breathing decrease and the blood and tissue concentrations of dissolved gases change accordingly
C. She can be confident that she will be able to undertake a final dive on the morning of her return flight home provided she has taken enough time on her final ascent
D. She should hold her breath on ascent to avoid arterial embolisation through a patent foramen ovale
E. The bends are caused by bubbles of carbon dioxide being released into the body tissues whilst a diver ascends; this can be treated with recompression therapy

Answers

9.1. Answer: C.
Stochastic (chance) effects occur with increasing probability as the dose of radiation increases. Carcinogenesis represents a stochastic effect, with not all exposed individuals being affected. With acute exposures, leukaemias may arise after an

interval of around 2–5 years and solid tumours after an interval of about 10–20 years.

9.2. Answer: C.
CT scans result in relatively high-radiation exposure and whole-body CT screening has not been demonstrated to meet generally

accepted criteria for screening. The risks associated are outweighed by the benefits of diagnostic CT and there is a small increase in lifetime risk of developing cancer. Options B, D and E are non-ionising radiations and the radiation dose from one chest X-ray is negligible.

9.3. Answer: B.

Hypothermia occurs when the core temperature drops below 35°C. Severe hypothermia is characterised by a temperature below 28°C, bradycardia, bradypnoea, arrhythmias and loss of consciousness. A rigid chest and abdomen with a core temperature below 13°C and serum potassium >12 mmol/L is probably incompatible with life.

Body temperature is controlled in the hypothalamus, which is directly sensitive to changes in core temperature and indirectly responds to temperature-sensitive neurons in the skin. The normal 'set-point' of core temperature is tightly regulated within 37±0.5°C.

9.4. Answer: A.

Exertional heat illness is more common in athletes and sweat volumes increase with acclimatisation. Heat stroke is rare below 40°C and heat syncope is a distinct condition and far less serious than heat stroke.

9.5. Answer: D.

Hyperventilation is caused by hypoxia sensed through the carotid bodies and a diuresis occurs secondary to haemoconcentration. After 2–3 days the oxygen dissociation curve moves to the right, making it easier for haemoglobin to release oxygen to the tissues. Sleep and nocturnal breathing patterns are frequently disturbed at altitude.

9.6. Answer: C.

Above 2500 m, high-altitude illnesses may occur in previously healthy people, and above 3500 m these become common. Acute mountain sickness (AMS) symptoms develop a few hours after ascent and include dizziness, fatigue and headache.

The cardinal signs of HACE are ataxia and altered consciousness. It is rare, life-threatening and usually preceded by AMS. In addition to features of AMS, the patient suffers confusion, disorientation, visual disturbance, lethargy and ultimately loss of consciousness. Monge's disease improves if the patient moves to lower altitudes to live.

9.7. Answer: B.

Drowning remains a common cause of accidental death throughout the world and is relatively common in young children. Fresh water causes alveolar collapse and right-to-left shunting of unoxygenated blood. Saltwater and freshwater drowning produce a similar clinical picture. In near-drowning, metabolic acidosis is almost universal and cardiac arrest is a poor prognostic indicator in recovery from drowning. It is true that in about 10% of cases, no water enters the lungs and death follows intense laryngospasm ('dry' drowning).

9.8. Answer: A.

The underwater environment is extremely hostile. Other than drowning, most diving illness is related to changes in barometric pressure and its effect on gas behaviour. Partial pressures of gases increase with descent and the bends are caused by the nitrogen bubbles on ascending again. Arterial embolisation may occur if the gas load in the venous system exceeds the lungs' abilities to excrete nitrogen, or when bubbles pass through a patent foramen ovale. A patent foramen ovale occurs in 25–30% of asymptomatic individuals. A diver must ascend slowly and breathe regularly during ascent to avoid barotrauma.

Recompression is the definitive therapy for decompression illness. Recompression reduces the volume of gas within tissues (Boyle's law), forces gas back into solution and is followed by slow decompression that allows the gas load to be excreted.

Decompression illness can be provoked by flying. Diving tables should be consulted to leave a safe gap between a final dive and a subsequent plane journey.

9

VR Tallentire,
MJ MacMahon, J Bain,
S Fadden

10

Acute medicine and critical illness

Multiple Choice Questions

10.1. A 76 year old man develops an acute kidney injury 2 days after an elective knee replacement. His past medical history includes mild chronic obstructive pulmonary disease and hypertension (controlled with an angiotensin-converting enzyme (ACE) inhibitor). He is hypotensive (80/50 mmHg), oliguric and has urea of 18 mmol/L (50.4 mg/dL), creatinine of 165 μmol/L (1.87 mg/dL), potassium of 5.1 mmol/L and a normal bicarbonate level. He has received 30 mL/kg of intravenous fluids over the past 2 hours.

Which will be the most efficacious measure to improve his renal outcome?

A. Commence renal replacement therapy
B. Further fluid challenge
C. Intravenous dopamine infusion
D. Intravenous furosemide infusion
E. Intravenous noradrenaline (norepinephrine) infusion

10.2. A 68 year old man presents with worsening exertional dyspnoea. He is known to have non-alcoholic fatty liver disease (NAFLD), with cirrhosis on a recent ultrasound scan, mild jaundice but with no ascites or encephalopathy. On examination he has normal breath sounds throughout both lung fields with no added sounds and his jugular venous pressure is not elevated. He has an oxygen saturation of 87% on air whilst standing (although this improves to 94% in the supine position). Multiple spider naevi are noted over his thorax and abdomen.

Which of the following processes are most likely to account for his hypoxaemia?

A. Low inspired oxygen concentration
B. Shunt
C. Ventilation–perfusion ($\dot{V}/\dot{Q}$) mismatch: alveolar hypoventilation
D. $\dot{V}/\dot{Q}$ mismatch: perfusion defect
E. $\dot{V}/\dot{Q}$ mismatch: central hypoventilation

10.3. A 69 year old woman is admitted to the intensive care unit (ICU) following a road traffic accident. She is known to have disseminated pancreatic cancer with metastases in the brain, liver and lung. She was intubated at the scene by the paramedics. She has sustained multiple long bone fractures, a head injury and is requiring a high inspired oxygen concentration to maintain her oxygen saturations. Which of the following statements is MOST accurate?

A. All sedatives and analgesics must be stopped to allow an accurate assessment of conscious level
B. An advance directive stating that the patient would not want to survive with severe disability should be taken into consideration
C. If a withdrawal decision has been made, it is unethical to extubate the patient as she may die from airway obstruction
D. It is unjustifiable to withdraw active treatment while there is still a chance of recovery
E. The family will need to be contacted to make a decision about ongoing treatment

10.4. A 22 year old man is admitted to the ICU with an acute exacerbation of asthma. On high-flow oxygen he has a PaO_2 of 31 kPa (233 mmHg) and a $PaCO_2$ of 16 kPa

(120 mmHg). There is respiratory effort but no audible air entry on auscultation. He is unconscious and preparations are being made to intubate and ventilate him. Other than severe asthma, he has no other past medical history.

Which of the following statements is CORRECT?

A. Large cannulae should be inserted bilaterally into the second intercostal space at the mid-clavicular line
B. Once intubated, a high respiratory rate and large tidal volumes should be used initially to clear the carbon dioxide
C. Once intubated, a respiratory rate of 12 breaths/min, a tidal volume of 6 mL/kg and a prolonged expiratory time should be used initially
D. The blood gas is likely to be erroneous as his PaO_2 is too high
E. The CO_2 will return to normal if the oxygen mask is removed

10.5. Which of the following statements best describes good practice when using sedation and analgesia in intensive care?

A. A Richmond Agitation and Sedation Score (RASS) score of 0 suggests sedation is optimal
B. Etomidate is the most cardio-stable sedative and should be used as an infusion in patients who are very unstable
C. Muscle relaxants can be used to reduce the need for sedation
D. Patients should be deeply sedated to reduce the risk of delirium
E. Sedation should not be stopped abruptly as there is an unacceptable risk of self-extubation

10.6. A 45 year old man is being ventilated for acute respiratory distress syndrome (ARDS) following a lobar pneumonia. The bedside nurse has a number of questions regarding the strategy for ventilating this man as his lung function improves.

Which of the following points is correct?

A. During weaning, patients should not be allowed to go for long periods with no mechanical ventilator support if they are showing signs of respiratory distress
B. If the patient is febrile, minute volumes will be lower and it is a good opportunity to wean the ventilatory support

C. Positive end-expiratory pressure (PEEP) should be weaned to zero before extubation is considered
D. The fraction of inspired oxygen (FiO_2) should be weaned to achieve a PaO_2 of 15 kPa (113 mmHg) and above
E. Tracheostomy should be immediately performed if the patient fails a spontaneous breathing trial

10.7. Which of the following findings suggests that ongoing intensive care treatment still has a realistic chance of a good neurological outcome following cardiac arrest?

A. A computed tomography (CT) brain showing preserved grey–white differentiation
B. Absent corneal reflexes at 72 hours after return of spontaneous circulation (ROSC)
C. Absent motor response to painful stimulus 72 hours after ROSC
D. Bilaterally absent N20 spike on somatosensory evoked potentials
E. Myoclonic jerking within the first 24 hours after ROSC

10.8. A 37 year old previously healthy man is brought into the emergency department by ambulance having stopped the car he was driving. When the paramedics arrived he was conscious but appeared confused. This progressed over the following 30 minutes to aphasia and the development of bilateral upper and lower limb weakness with bilateral cranial nerve palsies. CT head scan on arrival is reported as normal.

Which investigation is most likely to reveal the underlying pathology?

A. CT angiogram of the circle of Willis
B. CT scan of the cervical spine
C. Electrocardiogram (ECG)
D. Erythrocyte sedimentation rate (ESR)
E. Lumbar puncture

10.9. A 63 year old man is weaning from mechanical ventilation. He has been ventilated in the ICU for 3 months with Guillain–Barré syndrome and profound weakness. A percutaneous tracheostomy was placed 2 months ago. He has suddenly developed respiratory distress after a bout of coughing. He is now extremely tachypnoeic, sweating and in respiratory distress. He has no previous history of any laryngeal or tracheal problems.

10

All of the actions below would be appropriate, except for one. Which of the following actions would NOT be considered best practice in this situation?

A. Applying a facial high-flow oxygen mask
B. Applying a self-inflating bag to the tracheostomy and giving the patient several large breaths
C. Calling for help
D. Passing a suction catheter through the tracheostomy to check patency
E. Removing the inner tube of the tracheostomy

10.10. Which one of the following ventilated patients has ARDS according to the Berlin definition?

A. A man with a severe influenza pneumonia. He has bilateral infiltrates on chest X-ray and a PaO_2 of 10 kPa (75 mmHg) on an FiO_2 of 0.4
B. A man with left lower lobe pneumonia, a normal echocardiogram and a PaO_2 of 10 kPa (75 mmHg) on an FiO_2 of 0.6
C. A man with long-standing, progressive idiopathic pulmonary fibrosis. He has bilateral chest X-ray infiltrates, a normal echocardiogram and a PaO_2 of 10 kPa (75 mmHg) on an FiO_2 of 0.5
D. A woman with acute pancreatitis. She has bilateral chest infiltrates, pleural effusions, a normal echocardiogram and a PaO_2 of 14 kPa (105 mmHg) on an FiO_2 of 0.3
E. A woman with endocarditis and severe mitral regurgitation from a leaflet perforation. She has bilateral chest X-ray infiltrates and a PaO_2 of 10 kPa (75 mmHg) on an FiO_2 of 0.6

10.11. A 60 year old man becomes acutely unwell on the medical ward. He was admitted 4 days prior with non-specific symptoms (malaise, fever, coryza). On admission, his ECG showed sinus rhythm with no acute ST changes, but his serum troponin level taken 24 hours post-admission was markedly raised. A viral throat swab was positive for adenovirus.

He is tachycardic (180 beats/min), hypotensive (65/30 mmHg), pale and clammy. On examination his chest is clear but he looks very unwell and a blood gas shows a lactate of 10 mmol/L (90 mg/dL) with a haemoglobin of 120 g/L. His ECG now shows left bundle branch block and a bedside echocardiogram confirms global left ventricular dysfunction.

Which management plan is most likely to be successful?

A. Commencement of an adrenaline infusion
B. Immediate percutaneous coronary intervention (PCI)
C. Insertion of an intra-aortic balloon pump
D. Intubation and ventilation with high levels of PEEP
E. Venous–arterial extracorporeal membrane oxygenation (ECMO)

10.12. Which of the following statements is TRUE regarding gas carriage in the blood?

A. For a given $PaCO_2$, more carbon dioxide can be carried by blood with haemoglobin that is 80% saturated with oxygen in comparison to 100% saturated
B. In capillaries with a high carbon dioxide content, e.g. exercising muscle, oxygen is bound more tightly to haemoglobin, i.e. the haemoglobin–oxygen dissociation curve is shifted to the left
C. The majority of carbon dioxide is transported in the blood bound to haemoglobin
D. There is a greater oxygen than carbon dioxide content in arterial blood
E. When core temperature drops, for a given blood content of carbon dioxide, the $PaCO_2$ will increase

10.13. A 45 year old man is admitted to the ICU following coronary artery bypass surgery. He is tachycardic, hypotensive and has a high lactate. Clinical examination is unremarkable and there is no bleeding apparent. An ECG shows a sinus tachycardia with no other abnormalities. His haemodynamic data (from his pulmonary artery catheter) are as follows (reference ranges are also given):

	Patient data	Reference range
Cardiac output	10.2 L/min	4–8 L/min
Cardiac index	5.42 L/min/m²	2.5–4 L/min/m²
Pulmonary artery pressures	15/9 mmHg	15–30/5–15 mmHg
Pulmonary artery capillary wedge pressure	7 mmHg	2–10 mmHg
Central venous pressure	6 mmHg	6–12 mmHg in ventilated patients

Which of the following statements is true?

A. An infusion of an inotrope such as dobutamine is indicated

B. An intra-aortic balloon pump should be inserted immediately

C. It is likely that one of the coronary grafts has become occluded

D. The data suggest he has a cardiac tamponade

E. The data suggest that he is vasodilated

10.14. Which one of the following statements regarding daily management in intensive care is MOST accurate?

A. Blood glucose levels should be maintained in the range of 4–6 mmol/L (72–108 mg/dL)

B. Proton pump inhibitors and histamine-2 antagonists reduce the incidence of gastrointestinal bleeding

C. The haemoglobin should be kept above 10 g/L in general intensive care patients

D. Unfractionated heparin (given twice daily by subcutaneous injection) is more effective than low-molecular-weight heparin at preventing pulmonary embolus in general intensive care patients

E. When pressure is being monitored, central venous and arterial lines should be attached to a pressurised bag of 5% glucose

10.15. A 75 year old man who had been previously fit and well was admitted to hospital with shortness of breath. His chest X-ray showed a left lower lobe pneumonia and he was commenced on intravenous antibiotics. His admission ECG showed a sinus tachycardia with left ventricular hypertrophy (by voltage criteria). Approximately 12 hours after admission he acutely deteriorated with tachypnoea, tachycardia, hypotension (70/40 mmHg) and reduced oxygen saturations. On examination he is agitated, managing only incomprehensible sounds, with increased work of breathing and bilateral coarse crepitations. His ECG confirms atrial fibrillation with a ventricular rate of 120 beats/min. Which one of the following statements is most accurate?

A. Antibiotics should be switched to a carbopenem

B. DC cardioversion is likely to resolve the clinical situation

C. Intubation and ventilation is contraindicated due to advanced age

D. It is likely that this man is too unstable for anaesthetic agents to be used: if intubation

is considered appropriate it should be performed awake

E. Peripheral noradrenaline (norepinephrine) can be used in this situation while intubation and central venous access is established

10.16. A 46 year old, previously healthy man is in intensive care following an influenza pneumonia with ARDS. He was on venous–venous ECMO for 10 days and is now receiving ventilatory support via a tracheostomy. It is noted today that he has bilateral weakness of his arms and legs. This has become apparent since his sedation has been lightened. On examination he has marked proximal muscle weakness. Tone and sensation appear to be normal, deep tendon reflexes are present but reduced, and plantars are downgoing. Cranial nerves are intact and the patient is alert, orientated and obeys commands.
Which of the following diagnoses is most likely?

A. A lesion of the brainstem
B. Critical illness myopathy
C. Guillain–Barré syndrome
D. Rhabdomyolysis
E. Spinal cord lesion

10.17. A 65 year old woman is brought to intensive care after an acute deterioration on the stroke ward. She had been recovering after a left partial anterior circulation infarct when she was noted to be acutely agitated and then became drowsy. This progressed quickly to unconsciousness and she was intubated to facilitate a CT scan.
The CT head scan confirmed a large haemorrhagic transformation of the infarcted area with 10 mm of midline shift, effacement of the ventricles and downward herniation of the cerebellar tonsils. Twelve hours after arrival in intensive care she is unresponsive (Glasgow Coma Scale (GCS) score 3 despite no sedation for 4 hours), normothermic, and her pupils are fixed and dilated.
Which of the following statements is true?

A. As she is not waking up, a neurosurgeon should be asked to drain the haematoma
B. Brain-death testing should be undertaken
C. She has a good prognosis, provided she can survive the acute bleed
D. She requires an electroencephalogram (EEG) and magnetic resonance imaging brain scan to confirm brain death (under UK law)

E. She should be cooled to 28°C to reduce intracranial pressure

10.18. A 45 year old man arrives in the medical receiving unit complaining of headache, blurred vision, nausea and vomiting. His blood pressure (BP) is 256/138 mmHg. A CT head scan is normal. Which of the following is true?

A. Chest pain in this context is likely to be anxiety related
B. In this context, nausea and vomiting is unlikely to represent raised intracranial pressure
C. Shortness of breath in this context may be the result of pulmonary oedema
D. The blood pressure should be reduced rapidly, aiming for a 50% reduction in the mean arterial pressure in the first hour
E. The use of cannabis is a recognised precipitant

10.19. An 87 year old woman presents to hospital with her daughter who found her in the morning confused, incoherent and wearing yesterday's clothes. Initial examination reveals normal observations. Which of the following history and examination findings most likely suggest an alternative diagnosis other than delirium?

A. A history of progressive deterioration over several months
B. A urine dipstick positive for leucocytes and nitrites
C. Fluctuant course, with more florid confusion at night
D. Periods of severe agitation requiring pharmacological management
E. The inability to direct attention and sustain conversation

10.20. A woman is brought in the emergency department by the ambulance after being found unconscious at home. Her pupils are equal and reactive. She does not open her eyes to a painful stimulus. She is making groaning noises but no comprehensible words. She has no motor response to supra-orbital pressure but she does withdraw her arms briskly to nail-bed pressure. How would you score her GCS?

A. 5/14
B. 6/15
C. 7/15
D. 8/15
E. 11/15

10.21. A 25 year old man presents to the emergency department with a 4-day history of chest pain and mild shortness of breath. He feels that the pain is worse on lying flat, coughing and deep breathing; it is relieved by sitting forwards and has improved with ibuprofen. He has no significant past medical history but was recently unwell with a non-specific viral infection. An ECG shows widespread saddle ST elevation.

What is the most likely cause of the chest pain?

A. Aortic dissection
B. Musculoskeletal chest pain
C. Pericarditis
D. Pulmonary embolism
E. Type 1 myocardial infarction (MI)

10.22. A 39 year old man is brought in by ambulance to the emergency department. He has a 3-day history of sore throat and feeling generally unwell. He is struggling to speak and swallow saliva and has marked stridor. He is distressed and does not want to lie down. Observations show: heart rate of 115 beats/min, respiratory rate of 25 breaths/min, BP 120/74 mmHg, SpO_2 94% on 15 L oxygen, temperature 39.4°C, blood glucose of 4.7 mmol/L (84.6 mg/dL), GCS score 15. The patient is normally fit and well.

Which potential diagnosis requires most urgent recognition and management?

A. Croup
B. Epiglottitis
C. Lower respiratory tract infection
D. Nasal polyps
E. Tonsillitis

10.23. Which one of these features is associated with delirium but not dementia?

A. Anxiety
B. Cognitive impairment
C. Disorientation
D. Reversibility
E. Visual hallucinations

10.24. An 88 year old woman is referred to the acute medical admissions ward by her family physician, who was asked to review her at home by a concerned carer. The patient has a medical history of frequent falls and mild cognitive impairment, but has become increasingly confused since suffering a fall in her garden 5 weeks ago. At that time, the patient sustained a few grazes and bruises to the right side of her body, including her head. The carer reports that the patient has also become increasingly unsteady on her feet and has been complaining of having a headache and blurred vision. She has been more sleepy than usual, but only intermittently. The patient's cardiorespiratory observations are unremarkable. From the options below, what is the most likely cause of her current symptoms?

A. Chronic subdural haematoma
B. Dementia
C. Encephalopathy
D. Intracerebral haemorrhage
E. Subarachnoid haemorrhage

10.25. A 24 year old woman with a body mass index (BMI) of 38 kg/m² presents to the emergency department with a swollen and tender right calf (3.5 cm larger than the left). She has recently returned from a European holiday resort and has sunburn, but is otherwise well. She suffers from well-controlled asthma, for which uses inhalers, and is also taking the combined oral contraceptive pill. Which of the following is the most likely diagnosis?

A. Calf muscle tear
B. Cellulitis secondary to an insect bite
C. Deep vein thrombosis
D. Dependent oedema
E. First-degree burn (sunburn)

10.26. Which of the following causes a leftward shift of the haemoglobin–oxygen dissociation curve?

A. Acidosis
B. Decreased temperature
C. Increased 2,3-diphosphoglycerate (2,3-DPG)
D. Increased PCO_2
E. Increased temperature

10.27. Paramedics arrive in the emergency department resuscitation room with a 70 year old man who has multiple comorbidities, including pulmonary fibrosis and chronic obstructive pulmonary disease (COPD; on home oxygen, with oxygen saturations normally of 88–92% on air). He suddenly developed right-sided sharp chest pain and dypsnoea. The paramedics report that the patient initially had a respiratory rate of 34 breaths/min and SpO_2 of 88% on 2 L/min oxygen, which fell to

64% when he was being moved into the ambulance, and symptoms improved slightly after administration of oxygen and morphine. Clinical examination reveals respiratory rate of 28 breaths/min, SpO_2 90% on 8 L oxygen and reduced chest expansion on the right side, temperature 37.2°C, troponin and an ECG are unremarkable. A venous blood gas shows H⁺ is 51 nmol/L (pH 7.29), PCO_2 7.0 kPa (52.5 mmHg), PO_2 3.1 kPa (23.3 mmHg), HCO_3^- 25.5 mmol/L, base excess –2.0 mmol/L and pulmonary vascular markings are absent on the right on the chest X-ray. Which of the following is the most likely diagnosis?

A. Acute myocardial infarction
B. Musculoskeletal chest pain
C. Pneumonia
D. Primary spontaneous pneumothorax
E. Secondary spontaneous pneumothorax

10.28. A 20 year old man is brought to the emergency department after self-extricating from a burning block of flats. He was trapped inside the building for 15 minutes, in a flat on the floor above the source of the fire. He has sustained no obvious injuries, but has a persistent cough and feels 'dizzy'. Paramedics have applied oxygen via a face mask, and the patient's SpO_2 is 99% on 2 L oxygen. An arterial blood gas sample is taken from the patient. What additional test, not routinely requested on an arterial blood gas sample, should be done?

A. Carboxyhaemoglobin
B. Fetal haemoglobin
C. Haemoglobin A
D. Nitrous oxide
E. Superoxide

10.29. Which of the following is a 'red flag' symptom in a person presenting with a headache?

A. Associated with taking codeine tablets for a week
B. Gradual onset (over an hour or more)
C. Improved by lying down
D. Right arm weakness
E. Visual aura

10.30. A 60 year old woman with a previous head injury is admitted with collapse. Taken from the history alone, which one feature may point to a diagnosis of syncope rather than seizure?

A. Amnesia
B. Cyanosis
C. Olfactory aura
D. Rapid recovery back to baseline state
E. Tongue-biting

10.31. Which one of the following does not score points on routinely used early warning systems in the context of medical observation monitoring?

A. Capillary blood glucose
B. Glasgow Coma Scale score
C. Heart rate
D. SpO_2
E. Temperature

10.32. A 38 year old man is admitted for observation after falling over the handlebars of his pushbike. He was wearing a helmet and had no loss of consciousness, although he feels nauseated and 'faint' when standing up. You are asked to see him, as his heart rate has increased from 95 to 150 beats/min over the first hour of his admission. He is complaining of upper abdominal pain and mild shortness of breath. Non-invasive BP is 100/60 mmHg and he feels cool peripherally. His chest is clear, with no clinical evidence of pneumothorax or rib fracture. His respiratory rate is 25 breaths/min, SpO_2 99% on 4 L/min oxygen. His GCS score is 15 with normal limb movements. You have taken an arterial blood gas, full blood count, urea and electrolytes and a coagulation screen and are awaiting the results.

What is the next most useful investigation to elucidate the cause of this man's deterioration?

A. CT abdomen
B. CT head
C. ECG
D. Renal ultrasound
E. $\dot{V}/\dot{Q}$ scan

10.33. In the general medical setting, what is the earliest and most sensitive sign of clinical deterioration?

A. Blood pressure
B. Core temperature
C. Heart rate
D. Respiratory rate
E. Urine output

10.34. In the context of cardiac physiology, which of the following is stroke volume most dependent on?

A. Cardiac filling (preload) and contractility
B. Cardiac index
C. Haemoglobin and oxygen saturation
D. Heart rate and diastolic blood pressure
E. Jugular venous pressure alone

10.35. A 52 year old office worker is brought in by ambulance to the emergency department. She was found collapsed in the toilets at work, having earlier complained of a 4-day history of mild headache. She has a past medical history of well-controlled hypertension, diet-controlled type 2 diabetes mellitus and she smokes 40 cigarettes a day. Her partner reports that she drinks three glasses of wine a week and has never previously been admitted to hospital. The paramedics have been supporting her ventilation using an oropharyngeal airway and bag-valve-mask. Examination reveals heart rate of 60 beats/min, respiratory rate of 6 breaths/min (without support), BP 190/105 mmHg, SpO_2 90% on 15 L oxygen, temperature 37.1°C, blood glucose 4.8 mmol/L (86.4 mg/dL), GCS score 6 (E1, V2, M3) with no lateralising signs. There is no visible rash or external evidence of injury.

Which one of the following conditions is the most likely cause of this patient's presentation?

A. Alcohol withdrawal
B. Bacterial meningitis
C. First presentation of epilepsy
D. Hypoglycaemia
E. Subarachnoid haemorrhage

10.36. An 84 year old man is brought to hospital after a fall. He was found by his daughter and had been lying on the floor for the previous 24 hours. He has a variety of soft tissue injuries but no serious head or orthopaedic injuries. On catheterisation, his urine is dark brown. Which one of these tests is most suggestive of rhabdomyolysis?

A. 1+ blood on urine dipstick
B. Creatine kinase
C. Haemoglobin
D. Renal ultrasound
E. Urea

10.37. A 20 year old man is brought in by ambulance to the emergency department, complaining of moderate central chest pain and feeling lightheaded. These symptoms came on acutely whilst he was playing football. Observations show: heart rate of 180 beats/

min, respiratory rate of 18 breaths/min, BP 75/4 mmHg, SpO_2 94% on 15 L oxygen, temperature 36.9°C, blood glucose 4.6 mmol/L (82.8 mg/dL), GCS score 15. ECG reveals a regular narrow complex tachycardia.

Which one of these treatments would be most appropriate as initial management?

A. Adenosine 6 mg intravenous (IV) bolus
B. Amiodarone 300 mg IV bolus
C. Digoxin 500 µg orally
D. Electrolyte replacement
E. Synchronised DC cardioversion

10.38. The Third International Consensus Definitions for Sepsis and Septic Shock (Sepsis-3) gives a clear definition of sepsis as patients with suspected infection who have two or more of three particular features. Which of these features form part of that definition?

A. GCS score <15
B. Increase of one point on the Sequential Organ Failure Assessment (SOFA) score
C. Respiratory rate >20 breaths/min
D. Serum lactate >1.5 mmol/L (>13.5 mg/dL)
E. Systolic blood pressure of <110 mmHg

10.39. According to the Berlin definition of ARDS, which set of variables would denote severe ARDS?

A. PaO_2 of 9 kPa (67.5 mmHg) and FiO_2 0.8 = 11.25
B. PaO_2 of 10 kPa (75.0 mmHg) and FiO_2 0.5 = 20
C. PaO_2 of 12 kPa (90.0 mmHg) and FiO_2 0.4 = 30
D. PaO_2 of 13 kPa (97.5 mmHg) and FiO_2 0.21 = 61
E. PaO_2 of 16 kPa (120.0 mmHg) and FiO_2 0.5 = 32

10.40. A 75 year old sustains a cardiac arrest secondary to myocardial ischaemia. Return of spontaneous circulation is achieved after 15 minutes of cardiopulmonary resuscitation (CPR) and 2× DC shocks. Which one of these is a physiological target after return of circulation post-cardiac arrest?

A. A MAP of no greater than 45 mmHg
B. Core temperature of 36°C and avoidance of pyrexia
C. Glucose 11–16 mmol/L (198– 288 mg/dL)
D. $PaCO_2$ <3.5 kPa (26.3 mmHg)
E. Urine output of 0.1 mL/kg/hr

10.41. Hyperlactaemia is very rarely seen in which of the following situations?

A. Cardiogenic shock
B. Chronic renal failure
C. Major haemorrhage
D. Metformin overdose
E. Sepsis

10.42. A 49 year old woman is admitted to the acute medical ward with a severe leg cellulitis. She has type 2 diabetes with a BMI of 41 kg/m². Observations show: heart rate of 119 beats/min, respiratory rate of 20 breaths/min, BP 70/35 mmHg, SpO_2 97% on air, temperature 38.5°C, GCS score 15.

Which one of the following treatments would you initiate first?

A. Crystalloid IV bolus of up to 30 mL/kg
B. Hydrocortisone 100 mg IV
C. Peripheral IV adrenaline (epinephrine) 80–240 µg/hr
D. Peripheral IV noradrenaline (norepinephrine) 480 µg/hr
E. Vasopressin (antidiuretic hormone, ADH) 0.04 IU/min

10.43. For which of these conditions is non-invasive ventilation (bi-level positive airway pressure; BiPAP) the first-line respiratory treatment?

A. Epiglottitis
B. H1N1 influenza
C. Mild congestive cardiac failure
D. Severe pneumonia
E. Type II respiratory failure with respiratory acidosis

10.44. The following are all terms that are used in relation to complications of invasive ventilation for patients in an intensive care setting, except for one. Which is the one that is not a real term used in this context?

A. Atelectotrauma
B. Barotrauma
C. Biotrauma
D. Pulmotrauma
E. Volutrauma

10.45. A patient with a known peanut allergy presents to the emergency department with wheeze, tongue swelling and difficulty talking. He does not routinely carry an EpiPen. On examination he has an SpO_2 of 98% on 15 L/min oxygen via non-rebreathe mask, respiratory

10

rate of 25 breaths/min, heart rate of 120 beats/min, BP 130/80 mmHg. He finds talking difficult. He is otherwise fit and well. He does not yet have IV access.

Which of the following is your first treatment priority?

A. IV access and crystalloid bolus
B. 10 μg adrenaline (epinephrine) IV
C. 50 μg adrenaline intramuscularly (IM)
D. 0.5 mL 1:1000 adrenaline IM
E. 5 mL 1:10000 adrenaline sublingually

10.46. A 75 year old man presents to the hospital with a 4-day history of diarrhoea and vomiting. He has a history of moderate left ventricular failure, prostate cancer and chronic kidney disease stage 4. His regular medication includes aspirin 75 mg once daily, bisoprolol 5 mg once daily and ramipril 5 mg once daily. On admission his observations are as follows: heart rate of 60 beats/min, BP 90/45 mmHg, respiratory rate of 16 breaths/min, SpO_2 94% on air. He is lethargic and slow to respond to questions. He is oliguric after catheterisation. ECG demonstrates peaked T waves. Blood results include haemoglobin 101 g/L, white cell count 16×10^9/L, platelets 190×10^9/L, urea 20.2 mmol/L (121 mg/dL), creatinine 367 μmol/L (4.15 mg/dL), sodium 134 mmol/L, potassium 8.3 mmol/L. He receives two boluses of calcium gluconate and two infusions of insulin/dextrose to manage his potassium. After this, a venous blood gas demonstrates H^+ 84 nmol/L (pH 7.08) and potassium 8.2 mmol/L.

What would be your next step in managing this man?

A. 40 mg IV furosemide bolus
B. Critical care referral for monitoring and consideration of renal replacement therapy
C. Further bolus calcium gluconate
D. Further fluid resuscitation
E. Further insulin/dextrose infusion

10.47. A 63 year old man has been admitted to the coronary care unit after percutaneous coronary intervention for ST elevation myocardial infarction (MI). Four hours after admission he develops acute respiratory distress. Observations are as follows: heart rate of 120 beats/min, BP 100/75 mmHg, respiratory rate of 28 breaths/min, SpO_2 96% on 15 L/min oxygen. His jugular venous pressure (JVP) is elevated. He is pale and

clammy, but alert and has no chest pain. ECG demonstrates a sinus tachycardia with low-voltage QRS complexes. Which of the following is the most likely underlying diagnosis?

A. Cardiac tamponade
B. Cardiogenic pulmonary oedema
C. Extension of the original infarction
D. Neurogenic pulmonary oedema
E. Pulmonary embolism

10.48. A 67 year old woman is admitted to the ICU after cardiac arrest. She received immediate bystander CPR, and was found to be in ventricular fibrillation when the ambulance crew arrived. She received 3× DC shocks before return of spontaneous circulation, and had a total 'downtime' of 32 minutes. She was intubated and ventilated on arrival in the emergency department. Her best GCS prior to that was E1, V1, M2. Which of the following would suggest the potential for a good neurological outcome?

A. A neuron-specific enolase >33 μg/L
B. Burst suppression on EEG
C. CT head with poor grey–white matter differentiation
D. Extensor motor response
E. Immediate bystander CPR

10.49. Using checklists for interventions in the ICU is a key component of good patient care. Which of the following forms part of the 'FAST HUG' checklist?

A. Foot care
B. Gowning and gloving
C. Spinal problems
D. Teeth
E. Ulcer prophylaxis

10.50. A 56 year old man sustains a significant lower limb injury after becoming trapped between a wall and a car. He is admitted to an orthopaedic ward for observation and operative planning. You are asked to see him 12 hours later with a swollen, painful calf and suspected compartment syndrome. Which of the following is true regarding this condition?

A. A serum D-dimer is both sensitive and specific for compartment syndrome
B. Absent peripheral pulses are an early sign suggestive of developing compartment syndrome

C. His leg should be reviewed by a consultant surgeon on the morning ward round the next day
D. Pain is worse with passive stretching
E. Sensation in the leg is likely to be normal

10.51. A 62 year old man is sedated and ventilated in the ICU after a severe subarachnoid haemorrhage. He has an intracranial pressure (ICP) monitor in situ, which has been reading 15 mmHg consistently. He is being sedated and analgesed with propofol and alfentanil infusions. On a sedation break his ICP increases to 45 mmHg and his pupils increase in size bilaterally. His mean arterial pressure is 90 mmHg. Which would be your first action to manage his ICP?

A. Administer mannitol bolus
B. Administer neuromuscular blockade
C. Increase propofol and alfentanil infusion rates
D. Refer to neurosurgery for decompressive craniectomy
E. Remove the intracranial pressure monitor

10.52. A 45 year old man is admitted to the ICU after banding of oesophageal varices and significant upper gastrointestinal (GI) haemorrhage. He has alcoholic liver disease and continues to drink 1 L of vodka per day. He is haemodynamically stable with good gas exchange and is extubated 12 hours post-procedure. He is moved to a medical ward for ongoing management. Seventy-two hours later he becomes confused and agitated, with evidence of tremor and paranoid ideation. What is the best treatment for his current condition?

A. Benzodiazepines
B. IV haloperidol 2.5 mg
C. Oramorph
D. Quetiapine
E. Thiamine

10.53. Which of these statements is true regarding the use of intra-aortic balloon pump (IABP)?

A. Carbon dioxide is used to inflate the balloon
B. It is associated with improved survival in cardiogenic shock
C. It is commonly inserted via the brachial artery
D. It is designed to improve diastolic pressure proximal to the balloon
E. There is no risk of mesenteric ischaemia when inserted correctly

10.54. A 68 year old woman, who has previously been fit and well, required intubation and ventilation in the ICU with severe pneumonia. After 10 days, tracheostomy to aid ventilatory weaning proves difficult, secondary to respiratory muscle weakness, and she requires a further 19 days of ventilation before being weaned off her tracheostomy. On neurological examination she has global proximal muscle weakness with no lateralising signs. Sensory examination is normal. Reflexes are generally decreased. Nerve conduction studies demonstrate reduced amplitude of transmitted voltage action potential with preserved velocity. Muscle biopsy is normal and creatine kinase is unremarkable. What condition is most likely responsible for this woman's difficulty in weaning from ventilation?

A. Brainstem stroke
B. Critical illness myopathy
C. Critical illness polyneuropathy
D. Guillain–Barré syndrome
E. Multiple sclerosis

10.55. A 24 year old man is admitted to the ICU after sustaining a severe head injury after a fall from a height at work. CT head on admission demonstrates massive intracranial haemorrhage with midline shift, and the clinical opinion is that of brain death. His family say that he previously expressed a wish to donate his organs if this situation ever arose. Which of the following would prevent testing for brain death?

A. Administration of 10 mg morphine IV 2 hours previously
B. Administration of a bolus of atracurium 72 hours previously
C. Core temperature of 36°C
D. Normal thyroid function tests
E. Serum sodium of 133 mmol/L

10.56. Which of these is an early complication of percutaneous tracheostomy carried out in the ICU?

A. Haemorrhage
B. Laryngeal stenosis
C. Tracheal stenosis
D. Tracheomalacia
E. Wound site infection

10.57. A 67 year old man presents to the emergency department with a 3-day history of haematemesis and melaena. He has a past medical history of alcoholic liver disease and

10

mild asthma (well controlled). His observations are: heart rate of 100 beats/min, respiratory rate of 16 breaths/min, BP 85/40 mmHg (70/35 mmHg on standing), SaO_2 95% on 6 L oxygen, temperature 36.5°C, blood glucose 4.2 mmol/L (75.7 mg/dL), GCS score 15. On examination, he is pale, cool peripherally, talking in full sentences, and his chest is clear. His abdomen is soft and non-tender but fresh melaena is found on rectal examination. He is not actively vomiting currently. Initial laboratory results show haemoglobin 42 g/L, white cell count 5.7×10^9/L, platelets 41×10^9/L, sodium 132 mmol/L, potassium 5.6 mmol/L, urea 16 mmol/L (96 mg/dL), creatinine 75 μmol/L (0.85 mg/dL), lactate 4.5 mmol/L (40.5 mg/dL).

Which of the following would be your immediate next step in managing this man?

A. Arrange urgent upper GI endoscopy
B. Critical care referral for monitoring
C. Insertion of a Sengstaken–Blakemore tube
D. Large-bore IV access and red cell transfusion
E. Terlipressin 2 mg IV

Answers

10.1. Answer: E.

This man has developed multi-organ dysfunction following arthroplasty. The pathology is not well understood but may involve an inflammatory response to the cement. As the glomerular filtration rate (GFR) falls, there may also be an accumulation of antihypertensive drugs, causing a cycle of organ dysfunction. If normal physiology is not restored with 30 mL/kg of fluid in a short period of time, it is unlikely that ongoing intravenous fluid will be beneficial. Furosemide and dopamine may improve the urine output, but have no effect on the GFR in this context. Renal replacement therapy is not required at this stage and will not improve the renal outcome. A noradrenaline (norepinephrine) infusion is the best option as it will improve the mean arterial pressure (MAP) and may improve the GFR by vasoconstriction of the efferent arteriole (which is dilated by ACE inhibition).

10.2. Answer: B.

This man has orthodeoxia (arterial saturations reduce on standing). In the context of chronic liver disease and a normal chest examination, it is likely that hepato-pulmonary syndrome is the cause. The pathology involves inappropriate dilation of the pulmonary capillaries so blood flows through the lungs without becoming oxygenated. This is an example of shunt. The only treatment known to be effective is liver transplantation.

10.3. Answer: B.

This is a very difficult situation and the right course of action will depend upon the legal framework of the country and the ethical values of the patient, usually expressed through the family. This woman has severe underlying disease and a poor prognosis from the trauma, so although there is a theoretical chance of surviving the injuries, it may be ethically justifiable to withdraw active treatment (although a consensus must be reached with the family). The decision regarding withdrawal of treatment should not be made by the family in isolation – the clinical team must guide the process. An advance directive provides useful information about the values of the patient. Once a decision has been made to withdraw treatment, it is an ethical obligation to provide palliative care (sedatives and analgesia) and extubation is a reasonable course of action. If the other injuries are deemed unsurvivable, it is not strictly necessary to stop all sedation/ analgesia as this may cause a great deal of pain and suffering.

10.4. Answer: C.

This man has life-threatening asthma with type II respiratory failure. The PaO_2 is high as the patient is receiving a high inspired oxygen concentration, and the pathology is air trapping and alveolar hypoventilation. Even with very small amounts of ventilation, the PaO_2 can be maintained if there is normal gas transfer across the alveoli, but the $PaCO_2$ rises. Intubation and ventilation is indicated as he has become unconscious. Initial ventilator settings should prioritise adequate minute volume while allowing sufficient expiratory time. High tidal volumes and respiratory rates will lead to air trapping and a very high intrathoracic pressure:

this can cause cardiovascular collapse. Whilst pneumothorax is a consideration, inserting cannulae without evidence of pneumothorax is likely to be harmful.

10.5. Answer: A.
Patients should ideally be calm, able to follow commands and tolerate endotracheal intubation (a RASS score of 0). This is not always possible as the tracheal tube is very stimulating and patients may need sedation to synchronise their breathing with the ventilator. Deep sedation does not reduce the incidence of delirium or post-traumatic stress disorder following intensive care discharge: it probably increases the risk of both complications. Daily sedation breaks are used safely in many intensive care units. There are many sedative agents that are used safely; however, etomidate is not used by infusion as it causes adrenocortical suppression.

10.6. Answer: A.
Weaning should occur when the primary pathology has resolved. During a febrile episode, CO_2 production is increased and a higher minute volume is required to maintain normocapnia: not a good time to wean. During the weaning process, the PEEP is usually maintained to keep the lung bases open, while the pressure support and FiO_2 are weaned (although a PaO_2 of >10 kPa (75 mmHg) would be a more usual target). A spontaneous breathing trial with minimal or no ventilator support is frequently used to assess if a patient is ready for extubation – if it is unsuccessful, the support should be reinstituted before any lung injury is incurred and further options considered to optimise respiratory function. A tracheostomy is usually only considered when there is repeated failure to wean.

10.7. Answer: A.
The loss of grey–white differentiation on a CT scan is suggestive of a diffuse ischaemic injury to the brain. All the other signs are strongly predictive of a poor neurological outcome.

10.8. Answer: A.
The differential diagnosis here is a cerebral vascular event, a rapidly progressive encephalomyelitis or a form of seizure disorder. Given the speed of onset and the bilateral neurological deficits, it is likely that there has been a vascular event. A vertebrobasilar

infarction or bilateral cerebral infarcts are the most likely causes. A CT angiogram of the circle of Willis has the highest diagnostic yield in the acute setting. It is possible that this man has locked-in syndrome.

10.9. Answer: B.
This scenario is likely to be an obstructed or displaced tracheostomy tube. The most likely problem is that the inner tube has become blocked with secretions; this is easily remedied by removing the inner tube and exchanging it for a fresh one. A tracheostomy can become displaced whereby it passes into a false tract alongside the trachea. Initial management should focus on supplementing oxygen via the upper airway and establishing if the tracheostomy is patent (by attempting to pass a suction catheter). If it is not possible to pass a suction catheter, then the tracheostomy should be removed and the patient re-intubated via the oral route. It is dangerous to apply positive pressure to a potentially dislodged tracheostomy. It can cause a large amount of surgical emphysema, which can prevent oral intubation.

10.10. Answer: A.
ARDS is a syndrome characterised by infiltration of the lungs by an inflammatory exudate. This causes the features of hypoxaemia and reduced lung compliance. The Berlin definition of ARDS stipulates that the following must be present:

- The time of onset must be within 1 week of a known clinical insult, or new or worsening respiratory symptoms, i.e. not long-standing pulmonary disease
- Bilateral opacities present on chest X-ray, not fully explained by effusions, lobar/lung collapse or nodules, i.e. not lobar pneumonia in isolation
- Respiratory failure not fully explained by cardiac failure or fluid overload. Objective assessment (e.g. by echocardiography) must exclude hydrostatic oedema if no risk factors are present. (Therefore mitral regurgitation causing pulmonary oedema is this scenario would not classify)
- Impaired oxygenation: PaO_2/FiO_2 ratio of <40 kPa (300 mmHg)

In this question ARDS in association with influenza pneumonia is the only case that meets these criteria

10

10.11. Answer: E.
The history and investigations are all suggestive
of viral myocarditis. This can cause hyperacute
cardiogenic shock. In this case, the use of
inotropes is unlikely to modify the outcome as
the myocardium is profoundly damaged. An
intra-aortic balloon pump is unlikely to provide
adequate organ perfusion. The global
myocardial dysfunction and the presentation
more generally is not suggestive of coronary
disease, and ventilation with high PEEP will not
improve cardiac output. Venous–arterial ECMO
has been used successfully in a number of
severe myocarditis cases. Despite the severity
of the cardiogenic shock, many patients with
this condition will recover if they are adequately
supported.

10.12. Answer: A
There is a larger volume of carbon dioxide per
100 mL of arterial blood than oxygen
(approximately 50 mL vs. 20 mL). The majority
of blood carbon dioxide is carried as
bicarbonate ions, but significant quantities are
bound to haemoglobin (carbamino compounds)
and dissolved in the plasma. This is significant,
as desaturated haemoglobin has a higher
affinity for carbon dioxide than fully saturated
haemoglobin; hence the $PaCO_2$ will be lower
for a given carbon dioxide content if the oxygen
saturations are low (the Haldane effect). This
partially explains why patients with type II
respiratory failure become more acidotic when
high levels of oxygen are administered. When
temperature drops, carbon dioxide solubility
increases, so for a given content of carbon
dioxide, the partial pressure will be lower at
lower temperatures. High capillary carbon
dioxide shifts the haemoglobin–oxygen
dissociation curve to the right, improving
oxygen offloading at the tissues (Bohr
effect).

10.13. Answer: E.
The data shows a high cardiac output with low
pulmonary arterial, left atrial (wedge pressure)
and central venous pressures. This pattern
suggests vasodilatation, which is common
following cardiopulmonary bypass. Cardiac
tamponade typically causes a low cardiac
output and increased intracardiac pressures.
Graft occlusion is likely to reduce the cardiac
output, and the pulmonary artery wedge
pressure is likely to increase. Inotropes and
intra-aortic balloon pumps may increase the

cardiac output, but have little or no role in this
scenario.

10.14. Answer: B.
Controlling blood glucose levels at
6–10 mmol/L (108–180 mg/dL) is
recommended. Low-molecular-weight heparin
is more efficacious as thromboembolic
prophylaxis than unfractionated heparin.
Five-percent glucose should not be used as the
'flush' bag as it can lead to erroneous glucose
measurements and a risk of inappropriate
insulin use. Several large studies have
suggested a transfusion threshold of 70 g/L
is as safe as 100 g/L and has a lower
requirement for transfusion. Proton pump
inhibitors or histamine-2 antagonists reduce the
incidence of gastrointestinal bleeding, but may
be associated with increased nosocomial
infection.

10.15. Answer: E.
The clinical picture here may be due to
pulmonary oedema or secretion retention with
exhaustion and septic shock. It is unlikely that
DC cardioversion will correct the underlying
pathology. Critical care is not contraindicated
on the basis of age; frailty is a more important
predictor of outcome. Intubation and ventilation
can be performed with low doses of hypnotic
agents, and awake intubation would be
challenging in an agitated patient. Escalation of
antibiotics is not required unless there are
specific risk factors for resistant organisms.
Peripheral noradrenaline (norepinephrine) via a
well-sited cannula may provide enough stability
to facilitate intubation and ventilation
(Box 10.15).

> **i 10.15 Optimising safety during intubation**
>
> Intervene early in the disease process (once it has become
> clear that the disease trajectory is downward)
> Use a stable anaesthetic technique: low doses of sedative
> agents and rapidly acting paralytic agents
> Remember that intubation should be performed by the
> most experienced operator available
> Use techniques to optimise oxygenation and ventilation in
> the period around intubation, e.g. keeping non-invasive
> ventilation in situ for pre-oxygenation, leaving high-flow
> nasal cannulae on for the intubation process, and using
> a video-laryngoscope in an anticipated difficult
> intubation

10.16. Answer: B.
The most likely diagnosis accounting for these
symptoms is critical illness myopathy (CIM).
There are no features of a central nervous

system lesion. Normal sensation and present reflexes make a peripheral neuropathy unlikely. Rhabdomyolysis (and myositis) are a consideration and measuring a creatine kinase (CK) level is good practice, although this is far less common than CIM in this population. The prognosis of CIM is generally good provided the patient recovers from the primary pathology.

10.17. Answer: B.
It is likely that this patient is brain dead (given the imaging and the dilated pupils). It is appropriate to undertake formal brain-death testing, which requires a strict set of clinical criteria. If these are met, under UK law there is no requirement to undertake other investigations to demonstrate an absence of perfusion to the brain. The evidence for cooling (to 32–33°C) and neurosurgery for haemorrhagic transformation is uncertain: these treatments are not currently recommended.

10.18. Answer: C.
Hypertensive emergencies can develop in people with or without pre-existing hypertension. Precipitants may include drugs that produce a hyperadrenergic state, such as cocaine, amphetamines or monoamine oxidase inhibitors. Nausea and vomiting may be a sign of raised intracranial pressure, whilst dyspnoea may indicate pulmonary oedema. Chest discomfort may represent either myocardial ischaemia or aortic dissection. It is generally unwise to lower the blood pressure too quickly, as ischaemic damage may occur in the vascular beds that have become accustomed to a higher perfusion pressure. A rule of thumb is that, in the absence of aortic dissection or acute stroke, the mean arterial pressure should be reduced gradually by about 10 to 20% in the first hour. The mean arterial pressure at the end of the first 24 hours of treatment should be no more than 25% lower than the initial mean arterial pressure.

10.19. Answer: A.
Delirium is generally characterised by several key features: disturbance of attention and awareness that fluctuates over the course of a day, additional disturbance in cognition that is not explained by another pre-existing or evolving neurocognitive disorder, and identification of a plausible cause such as a medical condition, substance intoxication or withdrawal, or medication side-effect. Hyperactive delirium is also characterised by restlessness, agitation (which may be severe) and impairment in sleep duration and architecture. A longer disease trajectory is more suggestive of cognitive decline. A positive urine dipstick is not uncommon in older patients and is not diagnostic of a urinary tract infection but may suggest a precipitant of delirium.

i | **10.19 Risk factors for delirium**

Predisposing factors	
Old age	Sensory impairment
Dementia	Polypharmacy
Frailty	Renal impairment

Precipitating factors	
Intercurrent illness	Dehydration
Surgery	Pain
Change of environment or ward	Constipation
Sensory deprivation (e.g. darkness) or overload (e.g. noise)	Urinary catheterisation
	Acute urinary retention
	Hypoxia
Medications (e.g. opioids, psychotropics)	Fever
	Alcohol withdrawal

10

10.20. Answer: C.
The GCS is the composite score of the best eyes (out of 4), verbal score (out of 5) and motor (out of 6). This woman will score 1 point for eyes, 2 points for verbal (incomprehensible sounds) and 4 points for flexion/withdrawal, totalling 7/15.

10.21. Answer: C.
The pain associated with myocarditis or pericarditis is often also described as 'sharp' and may 'catch' during inspiration, coughing or lying flat. It typically varies in intensity with movement and the phase of respiration. Patients with myocarditis or pericarditis may describe a prodromal viral illness. The pain associated with aortic dissection is typically described as 'tearing' and may radiate to the intrascapular region. Pulmonary embolism may demonstrate different ECG features, most commonly a sinus tachycardia, and rarely the typically described '$S_1Q_3T_3$' pattern. A type 1 myocardial infarction would be unlikely in a 25 year old and musculoskeletal chest pain would not produce ECG changes.

10.22. Answer: B.
Epiglottitis is the diagnosis most likely to lead to airway obstruction and death. It requires prompt recognition and specialist airway management. Traditionally considered a

paediatric disease, the incidence is increasing in adults, whilst falling in the paediatric population after the introduction of the Haemophilus B influenza vaccine.

10.23. Answer: D.

Delirium manifests as a disturbance of arousal with global impairment of mental function causing drowsiness with disorientation, perceptual errors and muddled thinking. Unlike dementia, it is reversible when the underlying illness resolves. Cognitive impairment, visual hallucination, anxiety and disorientation may occur in both delirium and dementia – it is reversibility that is the hallmark of delirium.

10.24. Answer: A.

Chronic subdural bleeds are common in the elderly, and develop over a period of days to weeks, often after minor head trauma. The bleeding from a chronic bleed is slow, from bridging vessels in the dura. Symptoms are manifold, but include headache, increasing confusion, fluctuating consciousness and ataxia.

10.25. Answer: C.

Deep vein thrombosis (DVT) is the formation of a blood clot within a deep vein, predominantly in the legs. Signs include pain, swelling, redness, warmness, and engorged superficial veins. Risk factors for developing DVT include cancer, trauma, surgery, immobilisation, combined oral contraceptives, pregnancy and genetic factors affecting coagulation processes.

10.26. Answer: B.

The haemoglobin–oxygen dissociation curve delineates the relationship between the percentage saturation of haemoglobin with oxygen (SO_2) and the partial pressure (PO_2) of oxygen in the blood. A shift in the curve will influence the uptake and release of oxygen by the haemoglobin molecule. The curve moves to the right, increasing the offloading of oxygen in the tissues, in response to increases in temperature, 2,3-DPG, PCO_2 and acidosis. The curve moves to the left secondary to decreases in temperature, 2,3-DPG, PCO_2 and alkalosis (Fig. 10.26; upper line). Clinically, if arterial PO_2 is critically low, oxygen uptake in the lungs may be impaired by a right shift, resulting in severe tissue hypoxia and end-organ failure.

10.27. Answer: E.

A pneumothorax is an abnormal collection of air in the pleural space. A secondary pneumothorax occurs as a complication of underlying lung disease, whereas a primary spontaneous pneumothorax occurs spontaneously and in the absence of clinical lung disease. Clinical signs may be

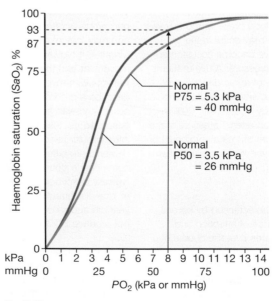

Fig. 10.26

non-specific. Chest X-ray signs include absence of pulmonary vascular markings peripherally and a rim of air between lung and chest wall may be visible.

10.28. Answer: A.
Carbon monoxide is a colourless, odourless, tasteless, poisonous gas produced by incomplete burning of carbon-based fuels. Carboxyhaemoglobin is a stable complex that forms between haemoglobin and carbon monoxide molecules. This hinders the ability of oxygen to bind to haemoglobin molecules, which will preferentially bind to carbon monoxide, resulting in tissue hypoxia even though the SpO_2 reading may be normal. The half-life of carboxyhaemoglobin can be reduced by administration of 100% oxygen or with hyperbaric chamber therapy.

10.29. Answer: D.
Focal neurological symptoms, other than those associated with migraine, may be indicative of an intracranial mass lesion. Other headache 'red flags' include: sudden onset, constitutional symptoms (such as rash), signs of raised intracranial pressure (headache worse on lying down), new onset in a person aged >60 years.

10.30. Answer: D.
Premonitory symptoms associated with syncope include nausea and lightheadedness, whereas a seizure may present initially with signs of confusion or symptoms of aura. The unconscious period of a seizure is also more obviously symptomatic, including motor seizure activity, tongue-biting or urinary incontinence (but these are not discriminatory), and is likely to entail a more prolonged recovery (post-ictal) phase.

10.31. Answer: A.
Abnormalities in respiratory rate, SpO_2, temperature, blood pressure, heart rate, neurological response and urine output form core components in common early warning systems. Each abnormality may be allocated a score from 0 to 3, with the composite score giving an indication of the severity of physiological derangement. Capillary blood glucose may be used as part of such a scoring system in specialist departments (e.g. endocrine or metabolic units) but is not included in routine early warning systems.

10.32. Answer: A.
This man most likely has concealed bleeding from an abdominal injury, given his mechanism of injury. His observations suggest hypovolaemia and a liver or splenic injury is likely. This man requires fluid resuscitation, a surgical opinion and appropriate imaging of his abdomen. A chest X-ray to rule out thoracic pathology and free air under the diaphragm would also be reasonable but would be highly unlikely to provide a definitive diagnosis.

10.33. Answer: D.
A raised respiratory rate (tachypnoea) is the earliest and most sensitive sign of clinical deterioration. Tachypnoea may be primary (i.e. a problem within the respiratory system) or secondary to pathology elsewhere in the body. All other parameters may also be affected but tend to occur later as end-organ damage occurs.

10.34. Answer: A.
Stroke volume is dependent on cardiac filling (preload) and contractility. Stroke volume is the volume of blood ejected from the left ventricle per beat. An increased preload (i.e. increased venous return) and an increase in contractility (as a result of increased sympathetic stimulation, adrenaline infusion, increased serum calcium, or glucagon infusion) will together increase stroke volume. Conversely, an increase in afterload (as a result of increased peripheral vascular resistance) will decrease stroke volume as the heart has to work harder against higher resistance. Heart rate has some effect on stroke volume as the time for ventricular filling is decreased at fast rates, decreasing the stroke volume; however, it is not the main factor. Cardiac index is a measure that relates cardiac output (stroke volume × heart rate) to body surface area; the unit of measurement is L/min/m². Haemoglobin and oxygen saturation do not directly affect stroke volume, except in very extreme situations (e.g. extreme anaemia or cellular hypoxia).

10.35. Answer: E.
The combination of hypertension, heavy smoking, sudden collapse and recent headache (possibly suggesting a herald bleed) make the diagnosis of subarachnoid haemorrhage most likely. She is not prescribed any drug for diabetes that would induce hypoglycaemia.

10

10.36. Answer: B.

A creatine kinase level of greater than 1000 U/L is highly suggestive, although it can rise to tens of thousands in severe cases. The other tests would not help in the specific diagnosis.

10.37. Answer: E.

This patient has adverse signs relating to his tachyarrhythmia (chest pain and hypotension). Therefore DC cardioversion, rather than medical management, is appropriate as per Adult Life Support guidelines.

10.38. Answer: A.

To be diagnosed with sepsis, the patient must have suspected infection and two or more of:

- Hypotension – systolic blood pressure <100 mmHg
- Altered mental status – GCS score ≤14
- Tachypnoea – respiratory rate ≥22 breaths/ min

Sepsis can also be diagnosed by suspected infection and an increase of two or more points on the SOFA score (Box 10.38).

i 10.38 Sequential Organ Failure Assessment (SOFA)
An assessment of admission characteristics (e.g. age and pre-existing organ dysfunction) and the maximum/minimum values of 12 routine physiological measurements during the first 24 hours of admission (e.g. temperature, blood pressure, GCS) that reflect the physiological impact of the illness Composite score out of 71 Higher scores are given to patients with more serious underlying diagnoses, medical history or physiological instability; higher mortality correlates with higher scores
SOFA score
A score of 1–4 is allocated to six organ systems (respiratory, cardiovascular, liver, renal, coagulation and neurological) to represent the degree of organ dysfunction, e.g. platelet count > 150 × 10^9/L scores 1 point, < 25 × 10^9/L scores 4 points Composite score out of 24 Higher scores are associated with increased mortality

10.39. Answer: A.

Severity of hypoxaemia is calculated using a Pa/FiO_2 ratio. This is a number calculated by the PaO_2 from an arterial blood gas divided by the fraction of inspired oxygen (FiO_2, expressed as a fraction). For example, a patient with a PaO_2 of 10 kPa (75 mmHg) on 50% oxygen, i.e. FiO_2 of 0.5, would have a Pa/FiO_2 ratio of 20 kPa (150 mmHg). This would be defined as moderately severe ARDS, if the other Berlin

criteria are met (Box 10.39). All measurements should be taken on a minimum of 5 cmH$_2$O of PEEP or continuous positive airway pressure (CPAP):

- Mild ARDS: 40–26.6 kPa (300–200 mmHg)
- Moderate ARDS: 26.6–13.3 kPa (200–100 mmHg)
- Severe ARDS: ≤13.3 kPa (≤100 mmHg)

i 10.39 Berlin definition of ARDS
Onset within 1 week of a known clinical insult, or new or worsening respiratory symptoms Bilateral opacities on chest X-ray, not fully explained by effusions, lobar/lung collapse or nodules Respiratory failure not fully explained by cardiac failure or fluid overload. Objective assessment (e.g. by echocardiography) must exclude hydrostatic oedema if no risk factor is present Impaired oxygenation

10.40. Answer: B.

Temperature management, i.e. maintaining a temperature of 36°C and avoidance of pyrexia, should be facilitated by the use of a cooling blanket. This should be continued for 72 hours. Muscle relaxants may be required to prevent shivering. Other physiological targets include: MAP of >70 mmHg and systolic BP >120 mmHg, blood glucose of 6–10 mmol/L (108–180 mg/dL) and oxygen saturations of 94–98% (avoiding both hypoxaemia and hyperoxia). With respect to $PaCO_2$ in the ventilated patient, the aim should be for normocapnia (4.5–6 kPa; 33–45 mmHg).

10.41. Answer: B.

All other options other than chronic renal failure are likely to result in tissue hypoperfusion or poor oxygen utilisation and thus anaerobic metabolism. This leads to a rise in lactate and is frequently used both to diagnose hypoperfusion or poor oxygen utilisation and to measure response to treatment.

10.42. Answer: A.

This woman has sepsis, the initial treatment of which includes early antibiotics and IV fluid. The other options may all be used to manage sepsis; however, they are not first line and should only be used with critical care oversight.

10.43. Answer: E.

Non-invasive ventilation is the first-line therapy in patients with type II respiratory failure usually secondary to an acute exacerbation of COPD, because it reduces the work of breathing and offloads the diaphragm, allowing it to recover strength.

10.44. Answer: D.
Volutrauma is the result of distending forces from the tidal volume; barotrauma results from excessive pressures required to inflate the lung; atelectotrauma results from alveolar collapse and re-opening throughout the respiratory cycle; the release of inflammatory cytokines in response to cyclical distension is termed biotrauma. Pulmotrauma is not used in invasive ventilation nomenclature currently.

10.45. Answer: D.
A dose of 0.5 mL 1:1000 adrenaline (epinephrine) IM forms part of the current Adult Life Support guidelines for anaphylaxis. IV adrenaline may be given by an experienced operator in anaesthesia or critical care but is not a first-line management technique.

10.46. Answer: B.
This patient has hyperkalaemia refractory to medical management and therefore the next step is renal replacement therapy. In view of his ECG changes, and potential for significant deterioration, this should take place in a critical care area.

10.47. Answer: A.
Whilst most cases of cardiogenic shock following MI are due to left ventricular dysfunction, the clinical features of a raised JVP and narrow pulse pressure, alongside low-voltage QRS complexes, suggest tamponade secondary to infarction and free wall rupture post-MI. An urgent echocardiogram should be performed, followed by pericardiocentesis.

10.48. Answer: E.
Early bystander CPR and early defibrillation are the two interventions most likely to improve survival after cardiac arrest. All other answers are markers suggestive of poor prognosis.

10.49. Answer: E.
The FAST HUG checklist for daily ward rounds includes: **f**eeding, **a**nalgesia, **s**edation, **t**hromboprophylaxis, **h**ead of bed elevation (to reduce the incidence of passive aspiration), **u**lcer prophylaxis and **g**lucose control.

10.50. Answer: D.
Compartment syndrome classically occurs following extrinsic compression of a limb due to trauma or reduced conscious level (especially when caused by drugs or alcohol). It usually presents with a tense, firm and exquisitely painful limb. The pain is characteristically exacerbated by passive muscle stretching or squeezing the compartment and altered sensation is common. Absent peripheral pulses are a late sign, and their presence does not exclude the diagnosis. Clinical suspicion of compartment syndrome should prompt CK measurement and urgent surgical review – this cannot wait until the next day. D-dimer measurement is not indicated in suspected compartment syndrome.

10.51. Answer: C.
Initial strategies to manage raised ICP include ensuring adequate sedation, sitting the patient up to ensure adequate venous drainage from the head, and ventilating to low-normal end-tidal CO_2. If this fails, further strategies include instituting neuromuscular blockade, and administering mannitol or hypertonic saline. A neurosurgical opinion may be appropriate if the above strategies are unsuccessful.

10.52. Answer: A.
Given the timescale and his past medical history, this man is most likely experiencing acute alcohol withdrawal. He is at risk of both delirium and hepatic encephalopathy (especially in view of his recent GI bleed), and these need to be considered in the differential diagnosis. Whilst benzodiazepines are still considered the most appropriate treatment for management of alcohol withdrawal, careful dosing must be used in the context of advanced liver disease.

10.53. Answer: D.
An IABP is commonly inserted via the femoral artery. Despite its effectiveness in achieving predetermined physiological goals, there is no convincing evidence for increased survival in cardiogenic shock. The balloon is inflated with helium and, even when inserted correctly under radiological screening, mesenteric ischaemia remains a risk. The balloon is inflated in diastole, augmenting the forward flow of blood to the abdominal organs and improving diastolic pressure proximal to the balloon, thus optimising coronary perfusion.

10

10.54. Answer: C.

Critical illness polyneuropathy is due to peripheral nerve axonal loss and presents as proximal muscle weakness with preserved sensation. Nerve conduction study results are as described for this patient. The clinical history is not in keeping with multiple sclerosis or brainstem stroke and, by definition, muscle biopsy must be abnormal in critical illness myopathy.

10.55. Answer: A.

Preconditions for testing for brain death include: the patient is deeply comatose, is not hypothermic, has no profound electrolyte or metabolic disturbance and that the patient is maintained on a ventilator because spontaneous respiration is inadequate or has ceased. Whilst atracurium is a muscle relaxant that would lead to cessation of respiration, it is short acting and would not cause effects 72 hours later. The administration of a large dose of IV morphine 2 hours previously raises the possibility that the coma is secondary to a narcotic drug and, therefore, brain-death testing cannot be carried out reliably.

10.56. Answer: A.

Wound site infection, tracheal stenosis and tracheomalacia are late complications of percutaneous tracheostomy. Performed correctly, laryngeal damage should not be a complication of percutaneous tracheostomy. In those patients where percutaneous tracheostomy is anticipated to be difficult, ear, nose, and throat (ENT) referral should be made for consideration of surgical tracheostomy.

10.57. Answer: D.

Whilst all of the options may be applicable to a patient with upper GI haemorrhage, the first priority must be resuscitation and maintenance of adequate haemoglobin and thus oxygen-carrying capacity.

DH Dockrell, BJ Angus

11

Infectious disease

Multiple Choice Questions

11.1. A 29 year old woman returns from a trip to Vietnam. She ignored pre-travel advice and vaccinations. She ate local foods, including several freshwater fish dishes. One month after her return she starts to note migratory nodules over her abdomen, which are itchy. Her eosinophil count is mildly elevated. What is the most likely cause of this clinical picture?

A. *Ascaris lumbricoides*
B. *Clonorchis sinensis*
C. *Fasciola hepatica*
D. *Gnathostoma spinigerum*
E. *Wuchereria bancrofti*

11.2. A 34 year old man who works as an army reservist presents with bilateral facial nerve palsy coming on over a period of a few days. Otherwise, neurological examination of cranial nerves is normal. He has been on regular army exercises in rural Wales. He does not remember any tick bites or a typical rash for Lyme disease. What is the likeliest diagnosis?

A. Botulism
B. Cerebovascular infarction
C. Complex migraine
D. Neuroborreliosis
E. Tetanus

11.3. A 42 year old businessman presents with fever and back pain. He had visited family in Pakistan 8 months previously. He has a temperature of 38.6°C. Urine dipstick is negative as is his chest X-ray. Blood tests show a mild hepatitis and mild thrombocytopenia. What test will be most likely to establish the diagnosis?

A. Blood film
B. Dengue serology
C. Hepatitis A serology
D. Hepatitis B serology
E. Leptospirosis serology

11.4. A 12 month old child presents to casualty with his father. He has been eating poorly and running a fever for the last 36 hours, after which he developed a widespread maculopapular rash on the trunk. There are no localising findings on physical examination. The father tells you that his son has had all his vaccinations, including measles, mumps and rubella (MMR). What is the potential cause of this infection?

A. Coxsackie virus
B. Enterovirus 71
C. Human herpesvirus 6
D. Parvovirus B19
E. Rubella

11.5. A 26 year old pregnant woman, in the seventh month of pregnancy, presents concerned that she was visited 5 days ago by her niece who the next day developed an itchy vesicular rash. The niece stayed in her house for 3 days. The niece saw her family physician on her return home and has been diagnosed with chickenpox. The woman is concerned because she does not remember ever having chickenpox as a child, a fact confirmed by her mother. You arrange to check a varicella zoster serology, which is negative. Which of the following should you offer to prescribe?

A. Aciclovir orally for 7 days
B. Intravenous immunoglobulin
C. Vaccination against varicella zoster virus
D. Valaciclovir orally
E. Varicella zoster immunoglobulin

11.6. A 54 year old man receives a cadaveric renal transplant. Before transplantation he is found to be cytomegalovirus (CMV) immunoglobulin G (IgG) negative and he receives a transplant from a person who is CMV IgG positive. Administration of which drug lessens his chance of developing CMV and its associated complications post-transplantation?

A. Brincidofovir
B. Cidofovir
C. Foscarnet
D. Valganciclovir
E. Zanamivir

11.7. A 28 year old man returns from a holiday to Brazil. After a short febrile illness he is diagnosed with Zika virus. What practical advice should he be given?

A. Avoid alcohol for 2 months
B. Avoid sharing towels for 1 week
C. Avoid strenuous exercise for 2 weeks
D. Condom usage for 6 months
E. Sexual abstinence for 2 weeks

11.8. A survivor from the West African Ebola virus disease outbreak presents for routine medical check-up. Which of the following is a late complication, frequently described in survivors, which it may be appropriate to assess for?

A. Anterior uveitis
B. Diabetes mellitus
C. Hypothyroidism
D. Immune thrombocytopenic purpura
E. Ulcerative colitis

11.9. A 23 year old nurse, previously fit and well, presents with fever, persistent sore throat and stridor. He is unable to eat or drink. On examination he has tonsillar enlargement and anterior and posterior cervical lymphadenopathy. A spleen tip is palpable in the abdomen. Blood tests reveal a lymphocytosis and borderline elevation of the transaminases. A blood film shows frequent atypical lymphocytes. Which of the following should be used to treat his condition?

A. Aciclovir
B. Cytotoxic T lymphocytes
C. Prednisolone
D. Rituximab
E. Valaciclovir

11.10. A 61 year old woman presents with 3 weeks' unexplained fever. She has been referred to an outpatient clinic and initial history and physical examination have revealed no obvious abnormalities. The travel history is unremarkable and she has never lived in countries with risk of tropical infections or tuberculosis. Routine bloods show normal full blood count but C-reactive protein (CRP) and erythrocyte sedimentation rate (ESR) that are elevated. Liver function tests show minor abnormalities and the urinalysis shows some protein and red blood cells. Human immunodeficiency virus (HIV) serology is negative. Routine blood cultures are negative and a chest X-ray, computed tomography (CT) abdomen and echocardiogram are all reported as normal. What would be an appropriate next step in investigation?

A. Bone marrow aspirate for culture
B. Cerebrospinal fluid examination
C. Liver biopsy
D. Mammogram
E. Positron emission tomography (PET) scan

11.11. A 29 year old man is referred to clinic because of 4 weeks' symptoms of fevers, arthralgia and sore throat. On examination he has enlarged cervical lymph nodes but the pharynx shows no erythema or purulence. There is hepatosplenomegaly and you note a pale pink macular rash over the abdomen. Initial blood tests show an increase in polymorphonuclear leucocytes and a markedly elevated ferritin. Routine cultures and autoantibodies are negative and an HIV test is pending. What would be an initial empiric treatment?

A. Antiretroviral therapy
B. Erythromycin
C. Non-steroidal anti-inflammatory drugs
D. Penicillin
E. Prednisolone

11.12. A 50 year old man is being treated for acute myelogenous leukaemia with chemotherapy. He develops neutropenic fever. Physical examination is unremarkable and the central venous catheter (CVC) tunnel site demonstrates no erythema or pus. Which of the following would be most helpful in establishing a diagnosis of a CVC line infection?

A. Differential time to positivity of CVC versus peripheral blood culture
B. Negative peripheral blood cultures

C. Positive peripheral blood cultures after <12 hours of culture

D. Urine cultures demonstrating *Pseudomonas aeruginosa*

E. Vegetations on the aortic valve on echocardiogram

11.13. A 25 year old man presents with fever, pharyngitis, oral ulceration and a severe headache. History reveals he spent the last 3 weeks working in South-east Asia and returned 3 days ago. Physical examination reveals signs of meningism. He is noted to have a solitary ulcer at his anus. Blood tests reveal lymphopenia, thrombocytopenia and abnormal liver function tests. A malaria film and rapid diagnostic test, dengue antigen and polymerase chain reaction (PCR), and monospot are all negative. Which of the following is most likely to establish a definitive diagnosis?

A. Cytomegalovirus serology

B. HIV-1 combined antigen and antibody test

C. Lumbar puncture and bacterial culture for syphilis

D. Pathergy test for Behçet's disease

E. Rectal biopsy and PCR for lymphogranuloma venereum

11.14. A 45 year old woman returns from a 2-week vacation in Mexico. She has developed diarrhoea with abdominal bloating and nausea. She has had 6–8 bowel motions a day without blood or mucus, which have persisted now for 16 days. Blood tests show normal full blood count, CRP and blood biochemistry.

Which of the following tests is most likely to establish the diagnosis?

A. Anti-transglutaminase antibodies

B. *Cyclospora cayetanensis* PCR

C. *Entamoeba histolytica* serology

D. *Shigella flexneri* cultures from the stool

E. *Yersinia entercolitica* serology

11.15. You are working as part of a medical aid organisation's team providing care in a refugee camp in sub-Saharan Africa. A 5 year old child is bought by her mother for a medical check-up. She appears small for her age and you examine a stool sample by microscopy, which shows multiple ova consistent with a diagnosis of hookworm. If a full blood count was analysed on this child, which of the following abnormalities might be apparent with a heavy burden of this parasite?

A. Atypical lymphocytes

B. Low haemoglobin with increased reticulocytes

C. Low haemoglobin with low mean corpuscular volume

D. Monocytopenia

E. Thrombocytopenia

11.16. A 13 year old Peruvian boy is evaluated by a neurologist for new-onset seizures. As part of the work-up a magnetic resonance imaging (MRI) scan of the head is performed, which shows multiple small lesions, several of which appear calcified. After establishing a diagnosis, what would appropriate therapy for this condition include?

A. Albendazole

B. Atovaquone

C. Mebendazole

D. Nifurtimox

E. Piperazine

11.17. A 6 year old child is bought into hospital by his father with fever and a petechial rash. You perform a physical examination and some initial blood tests that show evidence of leucopenia and thrombocytopenia but no evidence of malaria. A dengue PCR is positive. Which of the following signs on medical examination suggests the need for hospitalisation and intensive monitoring for complications?

A. Ankle swelling

B. Lymphadenopathy

C. Petechial rash

D. Shifting dullness on abdominal examination

E. Temperature elevation for more than 48 hours

11.18. An 18 year old student with known beta-thalassemia major that is stable with regular transfusions presents with increased fatigue and lethargy. Full blood count, blood film and a bone marrow aspirate are suggestive of aplastic crisis. He lives with his family and has five siblings, ranging in age from 3 to 16 years. During follow-up the aplasia gradually resolves without further medical intervention. Which of the following infections is the most likely cause of the aplasia?

A. Cytomegalovirus

B. Dengue

C. Human T-cell lymphotrophic virus type 1 (HTLV-1)

11

D. Mumps
E. Parvovirus B19

11.19. A 7 year old child presents with a short history of fever, tender cervical lymphadenopathy and pus on the tonsils. He is treated with penicillin and his symptoms recover. One week later his mother presents with a similar history and is also treated with penicillin. Six weeks later the child is bought back by his mother with acute pharyngitis and a throat swab confirms group A streptococcal infection. His medical history is otherwise unremarkable. In addition to prescribing penicillin what additional steps would be appropriate?

A. Aspirin prescription for 6 months
B. Blood tests for immunodeficiency
C. Clindamycin
D. Erythromycin treatment
E. Throat swabs on all the family and treatment of all carriers of group A streptococci

11.20. A 32 year old teacher presents with severe pain in her left leg, specifically excruciating pain in the calf. On examination there is an area of purplish discoloration but otherwise little to see. Temperature is 39.5°C, pulse rate 122 beats/min and blood pressure (BP) 90/60 mmHg. Which of the following is the most appropriate initial investigation to promptly establish a diagnosis?

A. CT scan leg
B. Doppler leg
C. Inspection of muscles in theatre by a surgeon
D. MRI leg
E. Ultrasound leg

11.21. A 25 year old man from Somalia presents to the hepatologist because of derangements in his liver function tests. Blood tests reveal an elevated alkaline phosphatase and bilirubin as well as a blood eosinophilia. Abdominal ultrasound shows a mass in the left lobe of the liver and some lymph node enlargement around the porta hepatis. He has been previously well and takes no regular medications and drinks no alcohol but does chew khat leaves. Serology for which parasite may be positive in this case?

A. *Enterobius vermicularis*
B. *Fasciola hepatica*
C. *Gnathostoma spinigerum*

D. *Necator americanus*
E. *Strongyloides stercoralis*

11.22. A 40 year old man from Turkey presents with a history of chronic back pain and fever. On examination an MRI scan shows sacroiliitis. He has a long history of consuming unpasteurised milk and the initial work-up includes testing with a serum agglutination test, which comes back positive at high titre. What would be an appropriate initial antimicrobial regimen?

A. Doxycycline, rifampicin and gentamicin
B. Flucloxacillin with rifampicin
C. Fluconazole with flucytosine
D. Imipenem followed by doxycycline and co-trimoxazole
E. Streptomycin with chloramphenicol

11.23. A 40 year old with HIV presents with a 3-week history of headache. He is an intravenous drug user and has not engaged with care or antiretroviral therapy. His last recorded CD4 T-cell count was 48 cells/mm^3 18 months ago. His neurological examination and a CT scan of his head are all normal. A lumbar puncture is performed. Which essential diagnostic test would help establish the diagnosis?

A. β-D-glucan assay in serum
B. Cryptococcal antibody measurement in serum
C. Cryptococcal antigen test on cerebrospinal fluid (CSF)
D. Cryptococcal PCR on CSF
E. Galactomannan enzyme-linked immunosorbent assay (ELISA) on CSF

11.24. An 84 year old nursing home resident is re-admitted with *Clostridium difficile* infection. She has been on a prolonged course of antimicrobials to treat an intra-abdominal infection that arose as a complication of a ruptured diverticular abscess but these have now stopped. Her first bout of *C. difficile* infection was severe and treated with vancomycin. She then relapsed and was treated in a clinical trial with fidaxomicin. This is her second relapse over a 3-month period. Prior to her diverticular abscess she had been well and was only on treatment for hypertension. What is a potential therapeutic option to manage her relapsing infection?

A. Ciprofloxacin
B. Glucocorticoids

C. Faecal transplantation
D. Life-long fidaxomicin
E. Life-long metronidazole

11.25. A 17 year old student presents with a short history of severe headache and photophobia. A physical examination notes neck stiffness but nothing else. A lumbar puncture is performed and shows an elevation of protein and an increase in white cells – all lymphocytes. Initial PCR for enterovirus and herpes simplex virus (HSV) are negative and blood HIV antigen and antibody are also negative. He has not lived in an area that puts him at risk of any geographically restricted or arthropod-transmitted central nervous system infections. As a child the patient moved about constantly with his parents who were musicians and does not remember having very many immunisations. He has no known risks for tuberculosis (TB), does not take any medicines or recreational drugs and has no other medical problems. Which important additional diagnostic cause of meningitis should be considered in this case?

A. Adenovirus
B. Chickenpox
C. Measles
D. Mumps
E. Rubella

11.26. A 7 year old male heart transplant recipient is referred to your clinic for advice. He receives a annual influenza ('flu') vaccine but this 'flu' season there have been a large number of 'flu' cases in individuals despite immunisation, suggesting the circulation of a strain not covered by this year's vaccine. 'Flu' cases have started to increase in your community and several children in the boy's school have started to develop 'flu'. What additional agent could be used as prophylaxis to decrease the chance of influenza infection in this boy at high risk of influenza morbidity?

A. Amantidine
B. Oseltamivir
C. Ribavirin
D. Rimantadine
E. Tenofovir

11.27. A 26 year old female botanist attends the travel clinic for advice prior to deciding whether to undertake a 6-week trip to the Amazon rainforest to study the local flora. On review,

which chronic medical condition and its treatment would most likely prevent her from having the yellow fever vaccine, and might prompt her to reconsider whether she should undertake this trip?

A. Depression, stable on a selective serotonin re-uptake inhibitor (SSRI)
B. Diabetes mellitus, on insulin
C. Epilepsy, controlled on chronic seizure medication
D. HIV on antiretroviral therapy with a high CD4 T-cell count in the normal range
E. Liver transplantation 18 months previously, receiving tacrolimus and mycophenolate immunosuppression

11.28. A 27 year old female engineer is admitted with fever, BP 80/40 mmHg and pulse rate of 120 beats/min. There is a widespread faint erythematous rash over her body and a history of a sore throat 5 days ago. Initial blood tests show a marked elevation of the neutrophil count, evidence of disseminated intravascular coagulopathy and acute kidney injury. Your region has a very low level of community-acquired meticillin-resistant *Staphylococcus aureus* (CA-MRSA). In addition to intravenous fluids, high-dose penicillin and flucloxacillin, which other antimicrobial is most often added to the initial regimen?

A. Chloramphenicol
B. Ciprofloxacin
C. Clindamycin
D. Doxycycline
E. Vancomycin

11.29. A 25 year old maize farmer from Tanzania develops high fever and lymph node enlargement in the groin. He is bought into your medical facility and noted to have tachycardia and hypotension. You perform an aspirate of the collection in the groin and then a Gram stain on this material. What are you most likely to see when you look at the slide down the microscope?

A. Bipolar staining Gram-negative coccobacilli
B. Chinese letter appearance of Gram-positive rods
C. Clusters of Gram-positive cocci
D. Drumstick appearance of Gram-positive rods
E. Filamentous pseudomycelium

11.30. A 40 year old man presents to his local clinic in India with widespread cutaneous

11

lesions and a diagnosis of leprosy (Hansen's disease) is established by slit skin smears. The presence of which of the following clinical findings suggests that he may have a high bacterial index?

A. Clearly demarcated skin lesions
B. 'Glove and stocking' sensory disturbance
C. Hypopigmented skin lesions
D. Loss of sensation over lesions
E. Loss of sweating over lesions

11.31. A 35 year old doctor returns to visit his family in rural India. Two weeks later he develops a fever, which progresses over a number of days to high-grade fever, in association with profound malaise. He develops a dry cough and subsequently diarrhoea. On examination a spleen tip is palpable. Blood cultures identify a Gram-negative rod, which is still being identified to the species level. While antimicrobial sensitivities are being determined, which one of the following antimicrobial agents should form initial empirical treatment?

A. Ceftriaxone
B. Chloramphenicol
C. Ciprofloxacin
D. Co-amoxiclav
E. Co-trimoxazole

11.32. A 43 year old Egyptian engineer attends for routine medical examination. He is noted to have haematuria and repeated urinalysis confirms this observation. He is referred for a cystoscopy and found to have squamous carcinoma of the bladder. What infection is most likely to be associated with this finding?

A. Bacille Calmette–Guérin (BCG)
B. *Escherichia coli* (enterohaemorrhagic)
C. *Salmonella* Typhi
D. *Schistosoma haematobium*
E. *Treponema pallidum*

11.33. A 50 year old former aid worker returns after working in several South Pacific islands over the last 15 years. She gave up trying to prevent mosquito bites and did not sleep under mosquito nets. She subsequently experienced several episodes a year of pain and linear streaks of erythema on her legs, and also noted the swelling of glands in her groin. She has now started to notice swelling in both legs. A full blood count reveals eosinophilia. Which of the following will be most helpful to support the diagnosis?

A. Blood film
B. Elevated IgE
C. Protrusion of a large worm from a skin nodule
D. Skin snips
E. Slit-lamp eye examination

11.34. A 33 year old Spanish female veterinarian presents with fever, headache and dry cough of 5 days' duration. She has been working long hours helping local farmers deliver lambs and calves. On examination she has crackles and decreased breath sounds in the left lower lobe. Blood tests are relatively unremarkable other than some elevation of the transaminases. Blood cultures are negative but a serological test is positive. What is the likely causative organism based on the occupational setting?

A. *Bacillus anthracis*
B. *Chlamydophila psittaci*
C. *Coxiella burnetii*
D. *Legionella pneumophila*
E. *Yersinia pestis*

11.35. A 60 year old businessman from Mumbai went on vacation to South Africa. While there he went on safari and remembers noting a tick bite. He used insect repellent and took malaria prophylaxis. On returning home he develops fever and a severe retro-orbital headache. On examination he has no signs of meningism but appears flushed. You also note several black eschars on both lower extremities but no rash. Initial blood work shows lymphopenia, but is otherwise unremarkable. Blood cultures are negative, three malaria films show no parasites and HIV tests are negative. Infection with which of the following pathogens best explains the constellation of findings and likely cause of this man's syndrome?

A. *Borrelia duttonii*
B. *Coxiella burnetii*
C. *Plasmodium knowlesi*
D. *Rickettsia africae*
E. *Salmonella* Paratyphi

11.36. A 41 year old man from a rural community in the Democratic Republic of Congo presents to his local clinic complaining of irregular bouts of fever and painless enlargement of lymph nodes, particularly in the neck. He has developed a headache and his daughter says villagers have noted a personality change. Physical examination also detects a spleen tip but no other abnormalities. The full blood count identifies a relative lymphocytosis and mild elevation of transaminases. HIV tests and malaria films are negative. What would be the best test, if available, to establish a diagnosis?

A. Blood film
B. Bone marrow aspirate
C. Liver biopsy
D. Lymph node aspirate
E. Splenic aspirate

11.37. A 26 year old woman receiving total parenteral nutrition for management of short bowel syndrome, caused as a complication of Crohn's disease, is admitted because of fever and fatigue. Blood cultures grow *Candida tropicalis* both from her peripheral blood cultures and from the lumen of her tunnelled central venous catheter, with the line cultures turning positive 4 hours before the peripheral cultures. The central venous catheter is removed, temporary venous access is established and treatment with anidulafungin is commenced. In addition, which of the following should be performed?

A. CT abdomen
B. Lumbar puncture
C. MRI head
D. Oesophagogastroduodenoscopy
E. Ophthalmological review

11.38. A 47 year old man with acute myelogenous leukaemia is admitted with neutropenic fever. There are no localising signs or symptoms. Cultures through the central venous catheter and the peripheral cultures are negative. A CT chest scan is negative, as is a galactomannan assay. Despite treatment with piperacillin–tazobactam, and subsequent addition of caspofungin and teicoplanin, he remains febrile but there are still no localising signs. His other medications include allopurinol, omeprazole and alendronic acid. Increasing lymphadenopathy is noted and there are abnormal liver function tests but no other abnormalities. Which of the following is a likely cause of this syndrome?

A. Allopurinol hypersensitivity reaction
B. Cytomegalovirus infection
C. Epstein–Barr virus infection
D. Invasive fungal infection
E. Penicillin allergy

11.39. A 25 year old man from South-east Asia presents with severe headache, photophobia and meningism. He recently returned back to his home in a rural area of Vietnam for a 3-week visit. A lumbar puncture is performed, which shows a marked increase in white cells and protein, and he commences treatment with ceftriaxone. Later that evening the laboratory contact you to say they have reviewed the white blood cells and performed some additional stains, which confirm there are significant numbers of eosinophils, in this case reported as 20% of the total white blood cells. Which of the following is a potential cause of this man's eosinophilic meningitis?

A. *Angiostrongylus cantonensis*
B. Japanese encephalitis virus
C. Non-prescription analgesics
D. *Schistosoma japonicum*
E. *Taenia solium*

11.40. A 32 year old female anthropologist was living in remote regions of the Brazilian rainforest, studying the indigenous population. While there, she lived in local dwellings. Approximately 3 months from the end of her trip she developed an illness with an indistinct rash and noted some enlarged lymph nodes. Before returning home she went to a large clinic in Brazil where she was noted to have lymphadenopathy and splenomegaly. They performed some additional tests, including xenodiagnostics with a triatomine bug, which resulted in a diagnosis. She was advised she needed treatment but she preferred to defer treatment until she was back home. Which medication is most likely to treat this condition?

A. Nelfinavir
B. Niclosamide
C. Nifurtimox
D. Nitazoxanide
E. Nystatin

11.41. A 23 year old woman attends her family physician having noticed a 'bull's eye' rash on her thigh and developing flu-like symptoms. She walks her dog regularly through local woodland in southern England. What action should be taken?

A. Ensure tetanus vaccination is up to date
B. No action required
C. Prescribe intravenous ceftriaxone for 2 weeks
D. Prescribe oral doxycycline for 2 weeks
E. Test for antinuclear antibodies

11

11.42. A 55 year old man returns from Medina in the Kingdom of Saudi Arabia. He developed a coryzal illness, which progressed rapidly to severe dyspnoea 4 days ago and he was hospitalised for 3 days in Medina before he took his own discharge and flew home. On reaching home his family were concerned he was increasingly short of breath and took him to hospital. He is known to have diabetes mellitus and chronic lymphocytic leukaemia. On examination he is febrile; his pulse rate is 106 beats/min, respiratory rate is 20 breaths/min and oxygen saturation is 90% on air. His BP is 116/78 mmHg. The examination shows bilateral crackles through both lung fields and the chest X-ray shows bilateral infiltrates. Which of the following illnesses should first be excluded in this case?

A. Acute respiratory distress syndrome (ARDS) complicating pneumonia
B. Avian influenza
C. Meningococcal sepsis
D. Middle East respiratory syndrome coronavirus (MERS-CoV)
E. Severe acute respiratory syndrome (SARS)

11.43. A 44 year old intravenous drug user is admitted with fever, tachycardia and low blood pressure. Chest X-ray shows multiple nodules in the lungs. After initial blood cultures are performed, which intravenous antimicrobial should be included in initial empirical therapy? (Local antimicrobial-resistance patterns suggest good activity can be expected.)

A. Flucloxacillin
B. Meropenem
C. Moxifloxacin
D. Piperacillin–tazobactam
E. Tigecycline

11.44. A 42 year old woman presents with fever. She returned from a holiday in India 2 months previously having spent 8 months travelling in rural areas. She has a temperature of 38.2°C. Urine dipstick is negative. Blood tests show a mild hepatitis and thrombocytopenia. A diagnosis of *vivax* malaria is made on blood film. What test will help with further treatment?

A. Antiplatelet antibodies
B. Haemoglobin electrophoresis
C. Hepatitis B serology
D. Test for glucose-6-phosphate dehydrogenase (G6PD) deficiency
E. Ultrasound of spleen

11.45. A 42 year old businessman presents with a history of seizures over the last 3 weeks. He has been previously fit and well. He lives in a large house with domestic servants. A CT scan of his head shows a number of small cystic space-occupying lesions with a characteristic appearance, some of which demonstrate an opacified area protruding into the cyst. What is the likely organism causing this presentation?

A. *Angiostrongyloides cantonensis*
B. *Taenia solium*
C. *Gnathostoma spinigerum*
D. *Toxocara* spp.
E. *Trichinella spiralis*

11.46. A 34 year old native Australian man is admitted to a hospital in Darwin, Australia, with a widespread itchy rash with crusting lesions all over his body. Some have secondary infection and he has a heart murmur. What is the likeliest diagnosis?

A. Impetigo
B. Melioidosis
C. Pustular psoriasis
D. Scabies
E. Varicella zoster

11.47. A 68 year old man is admitted to hospital complaining of abdominal pain radiating to his back, following a bout of food poisoning. Blood cultures are recurrently positive with two out of two bottles growing *Salmonella* Enteritidis. What is the investigation most likely to reveal the diagnosis?

A. CT scan abdomen
B. HIV serology
C. Serum electrophoresis
D. Transoesophageal echocardiogram
E. Transthoracic echocardiogram

11.48. A 24 year old female student returned from a trekking holiday in Nepal 25 days ago with fever and diffuse abdominal pain. She has not had diarrhoea. On examination, pulse is 56 beats/min, BP 97/54 mmHg and temperature 39.4°C. She has a tender right iliac fossa and small faint spots on her abdomen but no other skin lesions. What is the likeliest diagnosis?

A. Appendicitis
B. Cyclosporiasis
C. Dengue
D. Scrub typhus
E. Typhoid

11.49. A 21 year old man presents to an emergency department in the UK with a 3-day history of bloody diarrhoea and right iliac fossa abdominal pain. He had eaten takeaway food 2 days previously but other members of his family had also eaten the meal and were well. He has a family history of ulcerative colitis. What is the likeliest diagnosis?

A. Amoebiasis
B. *Bacillus cereus* toxin food poisoning
C. *Campylobacter* infection
D. Crohn's disease
E. Ulcerative colitis

11.50. A 21 year old student returns from a trip to Belize in Central America with a non-healing ulcer on his face. A biopsy and PCR confirm a clinical diagnosis of leishmaniasis. The organism is identified a *L. braziliensis*. What is the most appropriate treatment?

A. Cryotherapy
B. Intralesional stibogluconate
C. Liposomal amphotericin
D. No treatment indicated
E. Paromomycin

11.51. A 34 year old man is admitted to intensive care with a diagnosis of *Pneumocystis* pneumonia. He is noted to have widespread violaceous papules on his skin and hard palate. On biopsy these are Warthin–Starry silver stain positive. What is the likeliest diagnosis?

A. Bacillary angiomatosis
B. Kaposi's sarcoma
C. Malignant melanoma
D. Sporotrichosis
E. Stevens–Johnson syndrome

11.52. A 47 year old man is admitted to intensive care with a diagnosis of *Pneumocystis* pneumonia and HIV. He is noted to have widespread purple papules on his skin and hard palate. On biopsy these are human herpesvirus 8 (HHV-8) DNA positive. What is the likeliest diagnosis?

A. Bacillary angiomatosis
B. Kaposi's sarcoma
C. Malignant melanoma
D. Sporotrichosis
E. Stevens–Johnson syndrome

11.53. A 19 year old man develops a sore throat and fever; 2 days after the onset, he develops left-sided chest pain and haemoptysis with pain and tenderness on the left side of his neck. On examination he is fevered and shocked with low oxygen saturations on room air. Chest X-ray shows a blood-borne pneumonia and ultrasound shows left internal jugular vein thrombosis. What is the diagnosis?

A. Adult Still's disease
B. Haemophagocytic lymphohistiocytosis (HLH)
C. Kikuchi's disease
D. Lemierre's syndrome
E. Streptococcal toxic shock syndrome

11.54. A 44 year old truck driver was involved in a road traffic collision; this resulted in a traumatic injury to his pelvis, which was contaminated with soil from a ditch. He develops a brain abscess, which is drained, and on microscopy shows long, filamentous, branching Gram-positive rods that are weakly acid-fast. What is the likeliest organism involved?

A. *Actinomyces israelii*
B. *Clostridium perfringens*
C. *Mycobacterium chelonae*
D. *Nocardia asteroides*
E. *Sporothrix schenckii*

11.55. A 35 year old anthropology researcher returned from a trip to Sarawak studying primate behaviour 7 days previously. He had no history of monkey bites but had been working close to primates. He complains of fever, headache and diarrhoea. Examination reveals hepatosplenomegaly and his full blood count shows mild anaemia, a mildly elevated white cell count and a platelet count of 76×10^9/L. Malaria rapid diagnostic test is negative. What is the likeliest diagnosis?

A. Chesson variant *Plasmodium vivax* infection
B. Herpes B infection
C. Monkeypox
D. *Plasmodium knowlesi* infection
E. Rabies

11.56. An 18 year old female presents unwell with sudden onset of bloody diarrhoea with fever and abdominal pain. Temperature is 38.9°C, pulse 110 beats/min and BP 93/56 mmHg. She looks jaundiced and pale with diffuse abdominal pain. Blood tests show a haemoglobin of 67 g/L, white cell count 18.6×10^9/L, platelets 110×10^9/L; bilirubin 98 μmol/L (5.73 mg/dL), aspartate aminotransferase (AST) 21 U/L, creatinine

11

345 µmol/L (3.90 mg/dL). What is the likeliest diagnosis?

A. Haemolytic uraemic syndrome
B. Hantavirus infection
C. Leptospirosis
D. Toxic shock syndrome
E. Typhoid fever

11.57. A 24 year old woman is investigated for chronic bloody diarrhoea with left iliac pain by colonoscopy. Biopsy shows granulomas in the terminal ileum and CT scan shows mesenteric lymphadenopathy. A presumptive diagnosis of Crohn's disease is made; however, stool culture grows a Gram-negative organism at low temperatures. What is this likely to be identified as?

A. *Campylobacter jejuni*
B. *Mycobacterium pseudotuberculosis*
C. *Necator americanus*
D. *Salmonella* Enteritidis
E. *Yersinia enterocolitica*

11.58. A 44 year old farmer presents with fever and increasing shortness of breath after clearing out one of his barns. His symptoms progressed over the 48 hours following exposure, despite avoiding the barn. He has not had any similar symptoms previously. He is found to have widespread respiratory fine crackles and his chest X-ray reveals pulmonary oedema. Blood tests show evidence of acute kidney injury. What is the likeliest diagnosis?

A. Acute allergic bronchiolitis
B. Allergic bronchopulmonary aspergillosis
C. Goodpasture's syndrome
D. Granulomatous polyangiitis
E. Hantavirus infection

11.59. A 27 year old zoology student is on a field trip examining bats. She receives a bite. Vaccination against which of the following should be recommended?

A. Diphtheria
B. Hepatitis A
C. Mumps
D. Rabies
E. Smallpox

11.60. A 19 year old pet shop owner presents with a pustular rash on her hands and arms. She had recently received a shipment of pet Gambian pouch rats. What is the likeliest diagnosis?

A. Contact dermatitis
B. Listeriosis
C. Monkeypox
D. Palmoplantar pustulosis
E. Smallpox

11.61. A 54 year old woman presents with sudden onset of severe left-sided abdominal pain; she scores this at 10 out of 10. There is no history of wounds or trauma. The pain is constant in nature and not associated with food. On examination she has a temperature of 38.6°C and BP of 92/54 mmHg. Her left hypogastrium is extremely tender with a small bruise on the skin but she has no peritonism. Venous blood gas analysis shows an H⁺ ion concentration of 76 nmol/L (pH 7.12) and a lactate of 4.3 mmol/L (38.7 mg/dL). What is the likeliest diagnosis?

A. Gas gangrene
B. Lemierre's syndrome
C. Necrotising fasciitis
D. Perforated descending colon
E. Splenic rupture

11.62. A 23 year old intravenous drug user presents to the emergency department. He had recently been injecting heroin into his skin. He complains of double vision and has progressive difficulty in swallowing. On examination he has ptosis and divergent eye movements. What is the likeliest diagnosis?

A. Guillain–Barré syndrome
B. Myasthenia gravis
C. Staphylococcal brain abscess
D. Tetanus
E. Wound botulism

11.63. A 17 year old intravenous drug user presents with abdominal pain, vomiting and fever. On examination there is a painless black eschar on her left arm. What is the likeliest diagnosis?

A. Cutaneous anthrax
B. Gas gangrene
C. Lyme disease
D. Necrotising fasciitis
E. Staphylococcal bacteraemia

11.64. A 45 year old laboratory technician originally from India presents with a fever and unilateral swelling in his neck. He also complains of mild testicular pain. He is otherwise well and blood tests are normal. What is the likeliest diagnosis?

A. Cervical tuberculosis
B. Kikuchi's disease
C. Lymphoma
D. Mumps
E. Teratoma

11.65. A 34 year old intravenous drug user presents with painful swelling of his left arm. On examination his arm is swollen, oedematous and dusky, with apparent crepitus. A diagnosis of gas gangrene is made. What is the causative organism?

A. *Clostridium difficile*
B. *Clostridium perfringens*
C. *Clostridium septicum*
D. *Clostridium sordellii*
E. *Clostridium tetani*

11.66. A 24 year old waitress complains of flushing and tingling around her mouth after eating some left-over canned sardines for lunch and has no known occupational or recreational exposures to toxins. The symptoms resolve over an hour. What is the likeliest diagnosis?

A. Ciguatera poisoning
B. Monosodium glutamate poisoning
C. Paralytic shellfish poisoning
D. Scombroid poisoning
E. Thallium poisoning

11.67. An 84 year old man, previously fit and well, presents with a pustular painful rash in the left ophthalmic nerve distribution. He was started on intravenous aciclovir but deteriorated with headache, fever and delirium followed by sudden onset of a right hemiparesis. What is the likeliest diagnosis?

A. Acute diffuse encephalomyelitis
B. Aciclovir-induced encephalopathy
C. Cavernous sinus thrombosis
D. Granulomatous cerebral angiitis
E. Sagittal sinus thrombosis

11.68. A 54 year old Jamaican man presents with fatigue and a widespread rash. On examination he has widespread lymphadenopathy. A blood count shows a significant increase in lymphocytes and on flow cytometry these are found to be T cells. He is also found to have an elevated blood calcium. Which of the following is a potential viral cause of this syndrome?

A. Adenovirus
B. Human herpesvirus 7
C. HIV-2
D. Human T-cell lymphotropic virus type 1 (HTLV-1)
E. West Nile virus

11.69. A 44 year old Chinese businessman returns from a trip to Hong Kong with a cough, fever and myalgia. He is diagnosed as having a lower respiratory tract infection. He is worried about 'bird flu' since he visited his relatives who are farmers and keep poultry in a rural area. Which of the following viruses might be responsible for his syndrome if there is an epidemiological link to visiting the farm?

A. Bocavirus
B. H1N1 pmd2009 influenza A
C. H5N1 influenza A
D. Parainfluenza
E. SARS coronavirus

11.70. A 14 year old refugee recently arrived from South Sudan is found to have ulcerated, pustular nodules on his elbow. He also has underlying deformity of the humerus. His blood tests show him to be HIV negative but the venereal disease research laboratory (VDRL) test positive. What is the likeliest diagnosis?

A. Bejel
B. Congenital syphilis
C. Pinta
D. Podoconiosis
E. Yaws

11.71. A 34 year old woman who takes prednisolone and azathioprine for control of her Crohn's disease presents with a 10-day history of headache and double vision. On examination she has meningism and a 3rd nerve palsy. CSF shows a white cell count of 500 cells/mm^3, which are predominately lymphocytes, an elevated protein and low glucose. Special stains and antigen tests are negative. What is the likeliest infecting organism?

A. *Cryptococcus neoformans*
B. *Listeria monocytogenes*
C. *Mycobacterium tuberculosis*
D. *Neisseria meningitidis*
E. *Streptococcus pneumoniae*

11.72. A 34 year old man presents with painful ulceration on his hand after catching and skinning wild rabbits on his farm.

11

On examination he has a area of ulceration on his right hand with axillary lymphadenopathy. What is the likeliest infecting organism?

A. *Bartonella henselae*
B. *Francisella tularensis*
C. *Mycobacterium marinum*
D. *Orientia tsutsugamushi*
E. *Sporothrix schenckii*

11.73. A 73 year old man with a history of benign prostatic hypertrophy, mitral regurgitation, prior cholecystectomy and an indwelling catheter presents with a 10-day history of fever and malaise. On examination he is febrile, tachycardic and has a mitral regurgitant murmur. Blood cultures are repeatedly and rapidly positive for a Gram-positive coccus, identified as *Enterococcus faecalis*. Which of the following is most likely to establish the source of this man's enterococcal infection?

A. Catheter urine sample
B. CT abdomen
C. Echocardiogram
D. MRI cholangiogram
E. Ultrasound of biliary tree

11.74. A 44 year old truck driver was involved in a road traffic collision; this resulted in a traumatic injury to his pelvis, which was contaminated with soil from a ditch. He develops a brain abscess, which is drained, and on microscopy shows long, filamentous, branching Gram-positive rods that are weakly acid-fast. Which of the following is the most appropriate treatment?

A. Co-trimoxazole plus imipenem
B. Doxycycline plus gentamicin
C. Rifabutin and clarithromycin
D. Rifampicin, isoniazid, ethambutol and pyrazinamide
E. Vancomycin plus rifampicin

11.75. You are working in a hospital in Darwin, Northern Australia, and are asked to see a surgical emergency admission of a 13 year old refugee from New Guinea who has severe abdominal pain and on CT scan has necrotising colitis. He is obviously malnourished and very unwell. What is the likeliest causative primary organism leading to this syndrome?

A. *Ascaris lumbricoides*
B. *Clostridium difficile*
C. *Clostridium perfringens*

D. *Necator americanus*
E. *Taenia solium*

11.76. A 16 year old presents unwell with sudden onset of bloody diarrhoea with fever and abdominal pain. Her temperature is 38.4°C, pulse 112 beats/min and BP 89/54 mmHg. She appears jaundiced and pale with diffuse abdominal pain. Blood tests show a haemoglobin of 57 g/L, white cell count 19.3×10^9/L, platelets 106×10^9/L, bilirubin 95 μmol/L (5.55 mg/dL), AST 25 U/L, creatinine 467 μmol/L (5.28 mg/dL). Which of the following is the most appropriate treatment?

A. Azithromycin
B. Ciprofloxacin
C. Co-trimoxazole
D. No antimicrobial indicated
E. Vancomycin

11.77. A 24 year old student has returned from a holiday in the Canary Islands. She had noticed a black scar where she had been bitten by a tick. Since then she has felt increasingly unwell with fatigue and shortness of breath on exertion. Her blood tests show a haemolytic anaemia. What is the most likely causative organism?

A. *Babesia microti*
B. *Mycoplasma pneumoniae*
C. *Plasmodium falciparum*
D. *Plasmodium vivax*
E. *Rickettsia prowazekii*

11.78. A 47 year old man originally from Zambia presents with lymphadenopathy and lethargy. His CSF reveals trypanosomiasis. Which of the following is the most appropriate treatment?

A. Benznidazole
B. Melarsoprol
C. Miltefosine
D. Nifurtimox
E. Sodium stibogluconate

11.79. A 31 year old man presents with a 3-day history of bloody diarrhoea and cramping abdominal pain. He had eaten a takeaway meal 2 days previously but other members of his family had also eaten the meal and were well. Which of the following is the most appropriate treatment?

A. Azithromycin
B. Ciprofloxacin

C. Co-amoxiclav
D. Erythromycin
E. No antibiotics

11.80. A 21 year old woman presents having been bitten by a rhesus macaque monkey while working in a research laboratory. She is concerned about herpes B virus infection. What is the correct treatment for this infection?

A. Aciclovir
B. Foscarnet
C. Ganciclovir
D. Human normal immunoglobulin
E. No treatment available

Answers

11.1. Answer: D.
The presentation suggests exposure to a zoonotic parasite. The clinical scenario with itchy migratory nodules emerging after eating local freshwater fish dishes suggests gnathostomiasis. Ascariasis and filariasis, the latter caused by *Wuchereria bancrofti*, are not caused by zoonotic parasites while both fascioliasis and *Clonorchis sinensis* infections primarily involve the hepatobiliary system.

11.2. Answer: D.
Neurological Lyme disease can present as facial nerve palsy and not all patients remember a bite. Treatment is usually with at least 1 month of intravenous ceftriaxone. Botulism is usually a descending paralysis and tetanus causes trismus with spasm.

11.3. Answer: A.
The blood film is essential in returning travellers. *Falciparum* malaria usually present up to a month after travel, but when patients have travelled to areas where *vivax* malaria is found, they may have delayed symptoms. This patient's blood film showed typical trophozoites of *Plasmodium vivax*. The incubation period here would exclude the other infections.

11.4. Answer: C.
The history of rash after fever resolution and the age of the child make roseala infantum the likely exanthem in this case. This is caused by human herpesvirus 6 or 7. Parvovirus B19 also causes an exanthem, but typically with alternative features like a 'slapped cheek' rash. Rubella is not likely as the efficacy of live rubella vaccine is very high. Coxsackie and enterovirus infections can cause rashes, although enterovirus 71 has been primarily associated with neurological syndromes.

11.5. Answer: E.
The patient is non-immune to varicella zoster virus (VZV) and has had a significant exposure during pregnancy within the last 7 days so should receive passive immunisation with varicella zoster immunoglobulin. Immunoglobulin would not have as high levels of antibodies. Vaccination would take too long to generate immunity. Treatment with aciclovir or valaciclovir is not indicated (Box 11.5).

11.6. Answer: D.
Valganciclovir is indicated because he is high risk for CMV due to his lack of pre-existing immunity and receipt of an organ from a CMV-seropositive donor. Foscarnet and cidofovir are used to treat CMV but only when resistance arises to ganciclovir or valganciclovir; their side-effect profile makes them less suitable for use in prophylaxis. Brincidofovir is being developed as an alternative agent to cidofovir while zanamivir is used to treat influenza A virus.

11.7. Answer: D.
Zika virus may be transmitted in semen for prolonged periods after recovery. Condom use is advised for those infected for at least 6 months and for those who have returned from an endemic area for at least 2 months if they do not develop signs of infection. Alcohol and dietary interventions have not been found to alter Zika virus infection to date. Strenuous exercise is not contraindicated, although in the early recovery period of any serious virus infection it is prudent to discontinue it. Infection is not spread by body contact, so avoiding sharing towels is not necessary.

11.8. Answer: A.
Late complications of Ebola virus disease include uveitis, sensineural deafness and

11

i 11.5 Infections in pregnancy		
Infection	Consequence	Prevention and management
Rubella	Congenital malformation	Childhood vaccination and vaccination of non-immune mothers post-delivery
Cytomegalovirus	Neonatal infection, congenital malformation	Limited prevention strategies
Zika virus	Congenital malformation	Avoidance of travel, delay in pregnancy if infected
Varicella zoster virus	Neonatal infection, congenital malformation, severe infection in mother	VZ immunoglobulin
Herpes simplex virus (HSV)	Congenital or neonatal infection	Aciclovir and consideration of caesarean section for mothers who shed HSV from genital tract at time of delivery. Aciclovir for infected neonates
Hepatitis B virus	Chronic infection of neonate	Hepatitis B immunoglobulin and active vaccination of newborn
Hepatitis E virus	Fulminant hepatitis, pre-term delivery, fetal loss	Maintenance of standard food hygiene practices
HIV-1	Chronic infection of neonate	Antiretroviral drugs for mother and infant and consideration of caesarean section if HIV-1 viral load detectable. Avoidance of breastfeeding
Parvovirus B19	Congenital infection	Avoidance of individuals with acute infection if pregnant
Measles	More severe infection in mother and neonate, fetal loss	Childhood vaccination, human normal immunoglobulin in non-immune pregnant contacts and vaccination post-delivery
Dengue	Neonatal dengue if mother has infection <5 weeks prior to delivery	Vector (mosquito) control
Syphilis	Congenital malformation	Serological testing in pregnancy with prompt treatment of infected mothers
Neisseria gonorrhoeae and Chlamydia trachomatis	Neonatal conjunctivitis (ophthalmia neonatorum)	Treatment of infection in mother and neonate
Listeriosis	Neonatal meningitis or bacteraemia, bacteraemia or pyrexia of unknown origin in mother	Avoidance of unpasteurised cheeses and other dietary sources
Brucellosis	Possibly increased incidence of fetal loss	Avoidance of unpasteurised dairy products
Group B streptococcal infection	Neonatal meningitis and sepsis. Sepsis in mother after delivery	Risk- or screening-based antimicrobial prophylaxis in labour (recommendations vary between countries)
Toxoplasmosis	Congenital malformation	Diagnosis and prompt treatment of cases, avoidance of under-cooked meat while pregnant
Malaria	Fetal loss, intrauterine growth retardation, severe malaria in mother	Avoidance of insect bites. Intermittent preventative treatment during pregnancy to decrease incidence in high-risk countries

arthritis. The other conditions listed have not been reported as common late sequelae.

11.9. Answer: C.
Glucocorticoids are sometimes used to treat complications of Epstein–Barr virus (EBV) infection. Potential indications include massive tonsillar enlargement causing airway compromise, haemolytic anaemia or thrombocytopenia, and sometimes neurological complications. Antivirals such as aciclovir and valaciclovir have no role. Patients who are immunosuppressed may develop lymphoproliferative disorders with EBV infection, which may be treated with rituximab (anti-CD20

monoclonal antibody) or cytotoxic T lymphocytes, but these do not have a role in treatment for immunocompetent individuals.

11.10. Answer: E.
The patient has features of pyrexia of unknown origin and evidence of raised inflammatory markers with some abnormalities in the liver tests and urinalysis. Potential concerns, in addition to infection, include connective tissue disorders and malignancy. A PET scan may aid identification of sites of inflammation and selection of potential sites for biopsy to establish a diagnosis. Investigation for malignancy may be undertaken, but its yield is

low if there are no clues to a potential source. Bone marrow aspirate for culture, lumbar puncture and liver biopsy may be part of the work-up but the diagnostic yield is low if there are no signs localising to these sites, as in this case.

11.11. Answer: E.
The patient has presented with features of pyrexia of unknown origin (PUO). Although there is a history of sore throat there is no sign of pharyngitis and cultures are negative. The rash and markedly elevated ferritin, along with the other clinical features, make adult-onset Still's disease a consideration, which is a clinical diagnosis that requires treatment with prednisolone or alternative anti-inflammatory therapy. There is no indication that this is streptococcal pharyngitis, so antibiotics are not indicated. HIV-induced acute retroviral syndrome should always be considered with presentation with PUO and rash but should only be treated after diagnostic confirmation.

11.12. Answer: A.
Central venous catheter infections are suggested by detecting positive cultures in the sample from the CVC at least 2 hours prior to the peripheral blood sample, detecting 5- to 10-fold greater colony counts in the CVC sample versus the peripheral blood sample or detecting at least 15 colony-forming units in culture of the CVC tip. Peripheral blood cultures are frequently positive with CVC line infections and a short time to culture positivity would be suggestive of endovascular infection but not specifically CVC line infection. Although right-sided endocarditis may complicate CVC line infection, there is usually no reason for left-sided endocarditis as evidenced by vegetations on the aortic valve. A positive urine culture for *P. aeruginosa* would be more suggestive of a urinary catheter-related infection.

11.13. Answer: B.
Any traveller with an unexplained illness should have HIV infection excluded. In this case the presence of an anal lesion suggests the possibility of unprotected anal intercourse. In addition to performing a genitourinary medicine screen to establish the source of the lesion, an HIV test should be performed. In this case, since recent acquisition is a consideration, the test should combine detection of antigen with antibody since the patient may not yet have developed an antibody to HIV. Although there are several considerations in the diagnosis, the clinical features and laboratory features are compatible with acute retroviral syndrome (primary infection) from recently acquired HIV infection. All of the other diagnoses mentioned may be considered, but Behçet's is a comparatively rare cause of oral and genital ulceration, syphilis is not diagnosed by bacterial culture on cerebrospinal fluid but rather by serology, and detection of a sexually transmitted infection such as lymphogranuloma venereum would not explain all the features in this case but would indicate the need for further tests to exclude sexually acquired HIV infection.

11.14. Answer: B.
There are multiple potential causes of diarrhoea in travellers. In this case there is a relatively long history but an absence of acute inflammatory markers or evidence of dysentery. This would fit best with a parasitic cause such as cyclosporiasis, cryptosporidiosis or with giardiasis. *Shigella* spp. and *Entamoeba histolytica* cause a dysenteric illness and *Yersinia enterocolitica* often presents with abdominal pain mimicking an acute abdomen. In chronic diarrhoea – usually defined as diarrhoea lasting at least 2–4 weeks – when infective causes have been excluded, other causes such as coeliac disease, inflammatory bowel disease and malignancy should always be considered.

11.15. Answer: C.
Hookworm infection can cause iron deficiency anaemia, which would be indicated by a low mean corpuscular volume. Haemolysis, indicated by raised reticulocytes, and thrombocytopenia are associated with other parasitic infections, notably malaria. Atypical lymphocytes are typically associated with viral infections but occasionally are seen with malaria and trypanosomiasis.

11.16. Answer: A.
The scenario is suggestive of neurocysticercosis for which albendazole is most often prescribed. Praziquantel is the preferred alternative and the other anti-parasitic agents are not recommended treatment options for this infection.

11

11.17. Answer: D.
The World Health Organization has issued criteria for the identification of dengue with warning signs. These mandate intensive medical management and monitoring. The development of ascites, suggested by shifting dullness or other signs of fluid accumulation, are one of these warning signs. The other signs listed here are not regarded as warning signs.

11.18. Answer: E.
Parvovirus B19 is associated with transient aplastic crisis in patients with haemoglobinopathy or haemolytic anaemia. Dengue and CMV cause anaemia but typically not aplastic crisis, while HTLV-1 tends to cause acute T-cell leukaemia/lymphoma.

11.19. Answer: E.
Streptococcal infections are usually sensitive to penicillin, which is the treatment of choice in pharyngitis. Although clindamycin and erythromycin are alternatives and may be used in penicillin allergy, some strains show resistance. A work-up for immunodeficiency is not indicated since there have been no prior features of infection; however, since several family members appear to have developed pharyngitis, it would be appropriate to screen all family members at the same time, since streptococci can be nasopharyngeal commensals and can be passed from one family member to another. Aspirin may be used for rheumatic fever but there is no indication there are signs of rheumatic fever.

11.20. Answer: C.
The scenario is suggestive of necrotising fasciitis, which is a medical emergency. In this case there are signs suggestive of shock, and urgent surgical intervention and debridement of involved muscles is essential. Imaging modalities will only delay definitive treatment and surgical inspection will provide the most prompt diagnosis and management.

11.21. Answer: B.
Although there are several causes of deranged liver function tests with eosinophilia, including drug-related causes, the scenario in this case and the obstructive features make infection with a fluke that can infect the bile duct a consideration. Of the causes listed, only *Fasciola hepatica* is a fluke that infects the bile duct and it is associated with eating plants that may have been contaminated with the parasite, such as watercress and also the khat plant, which is commonly chewed by people who live in regions around the Horn of Africa or Arabian Peninsula.

11.22. Answer: A.
The history of living in an endemic area and of consuming unpasteurised milk makes brucellosis a potential cause; it is an agent whose diagnosis involves confirmation by a serological test such as a serum agglutination test. The regime in option A would be appropriate for this infection; the regimens in options B, C and D might be considered for bone infection due to *Staphylococcus aureus*, *Candida* spp. or in melioidosis, respectively; streptomycin is usually used in infections like plague and tularaemia where bone infection is less likely.

11.23. Answer: C.
The individual has a low CD4 T-cell count and is at risk of meningitis caused by an opportunistic infection. Cryptococcal meningitis is a leading consideration and should be excluded. The test of choice is a cryptococcal antigen test on the CSF, which is highly sensitive and specific. PCR is not routinely performed and detection of blood antibody against cryptococci is not used in the diagnosis of cryptococcal meningitis. β-D-glucan and galactomannan assays are used in the diagnosis of *Aspergillus* spp. and in the case of β-D-glucan some other fungi. Although cryptococcal infection can be detected at low levels with the β-D-glucan, this test is not routinely used to diagnose cryptococcal infection.

11.24. Answer: C.
Faecal transplantation has emerged as a potential therapy for relapsing *C. difficile* infection in those without other contraindications. Although fidaxomicin decreases the risk of relapse compared to vancomycin, it is not used long term. Metronidazole is used in short courses and vancomycin is usually used in prolonged tapering courses to prevent relapse, although, if there is no other option, it might be considered for an indefinite period. Glucocorticoids may be used in severe disease but are not used to manage relapse and ciprofloxacin has been implicated in the development rather than the prevention of *C. difficile* infection.

11.25. Answer: D.
An incomplete vaccination history or waning immunity can put young adults at risk of mumps, which can cause an aseptic or lymphocytic meningitis. Although multiple other viruses can cause aseptic meningitis, mumps is a potential consideration, especially when common causes such as enteroviruses, HSV, HIV and geographically restricted mosquito-mediated viral infections are not present and when there is no history of TB exposure, chronic medication use or medical comorbidity.

11.26. Answer: B.
When vaccination has not been performed or may have been unsuccessful due to drift in the circulating strain from the vaccine strain, prophylaxis is indicated for high-risk patients such as heart and lung transplant recipients. Prophylaxis uses the neuraminidase inhibitors oseltamivir or zanamivir rather than the M2 proton channel inhibitors amantadine and rimantidine, which were used in the past. Ribavirin and tenofovir are not used in the prophylaxis of influenza.

11.27. Answer: E.
The yellow fever vaccine is a live vaccine that can cause viscerotropic disease in those with immunosuppression. The decision to give the vaccine is based on assessing the relative balance of risks and benefits. In this case, although both HIV and organ transplantation are associated with immunosuppression, the relative risk is much greater in the scenario with liver transplantation only 18 months previously, due to its associated more significant degree of immunosuppression due to tacrolimus (a calcineurin inhibitor) and mycophenolate. In contrast, controlled HIV with a normal CD4 count is not an absolute contraindication and the vaccine may be considered if it is essential. The other conditions are not associated with significantly increased risk of side-effects from this vaccine, although they may influence other medical considerations. For example mefloquine malaria prophylaxis would not be used with a seizure history and the antimicrobial linezolid should be avoided for those on an SSRI.

11.28. Answer: C.
The scenario is suggestive of streptococcal or staphylococcal toxic shock syndrome. In addition to β-lactam antibiotics, clindamycin is usually added to decrease toxin production. There is a low likelihood of CA-MRSA, so this probably does not need to be added initially, but the decision on this would be governed by the risk of MRSA. The other antimicrobials would be added in other settings, although doxycycline is an alternative agent that may also decrease protein synthesis.

11.29. Answer: A.
The epidemiological setting and the appearance of a severe illness with a groin swelling suggestive of a bubo make plague a likely diagnosis. The causative agent *Yersinia pestis* gives the appearance of safety pins or bipolar staining with Gram stain. *Staph. aureus* appears as a cluster on Gram stain and would be in the differential of any abscess. Other characteristic appearances on Gram staining include *Corynebacterium diphtheriae*, which appear as rods at acute angles suggestive of Chinese letters. A drumstick appearance due to the presence of a terminal spore is seen with *Clostridium tetani*. *Candida albicans* can appear as a filamentous form suggestive of a mould, but this, in fact, is a pseudomycelium formed by the yeast.

11.30. Answer: B.
A high bacterial index is associated with lepromatous leprosy. The presence of widespread lesions and a 'glove and stocking' distribution sensory disturbance both suggest lepromatous leprosy. The other findings of clearly demarcated hypopigmented lesions with early loss of sensation and sweating are all more in keeping with tuberculoid leprosy, where a lower bacterial index would be expected.

11.31. Answer: A.
The likely diagnosis is typhoid fever. Antimicrobial resistance is increasing, meaning many agents formerly used are no longer active such as chloramphenicol, amoxicillin and co-trimoxazole. Ciprofloxacin resistance has also emerged as major problem, particularly in Asia, so ceftriaxone is the most reasonable initial choice.

11.32. Answer: D.
Schistosoma haematobium is associated with squamous cell bladder carcinoma, which is a less common histological type of bladder carcinoma in the developed world. BCG is

11

sometimes used in the treatment of bladder carcinoma and *Salmonella* Typhi carriage is associated with *Schistosoma mansoni* infection in particular but not bladder carcinoma. Enterohaemorrhagic *E. coli* is associated with haemolytic uraemic syndrome but not bladder carcinoma, and syphilis, caused by *Treponema pallidum*, is not associated with bladder carcinoma.

11.33. Answer: A.
The story is most suggestive of lymphatic filariasis, which would best be diagnosed by looking for microfilaria on a blood film or by serology. An elevation of IgE is often seen in lymphatic filariasis but is not of itself diagnostic. A slit-lamp examination or skin snip is used to diagnose onchocerciasis, while a protruding worm would be more suggestive of dracunculiasis.

11.34. Answer: C.
The occupation as a veterinarian and, in particular, the recent contact with animals that have been giving birth, puts this veterinarian at risk of *Coxiella burnetii* infection. Although the other microorganisms listed can all cause pneumonic illness they have distinct epidemiological settings. *Chlamydophila psittaci* is associated with exposure to sick birds such as parrots and *Legionella pneumophila* with contaminated water-cooling towers and other water systems. *Bacillus anthracis* has been associated with bioterrorism and *Yersinia pestis*, the causative agent of plague, with hunters and others exposed to endemic plaque in rural settings.

11.35. Answer: D.
Despite the precautions this patient took, tick bites can be hard to avoid. The appearance of eschars with no findings on blood film are suggestive of African tick bite fever, and the features of multiple eschars without rash are more suggestive of *Rickettsia africae* than of *Rickettsia conorii*. *Borrelia duttonii* is also transmitted by ticks but results in relapsing fever. The other infections are less likely in this scenario as they do not link to the history of tick bites, explain the eschars and would be expected to provide other laboratory findings.

11.36. Answer: D.
The patient is likely to have *Trypanosoma brucei gambiense* infection. Although blood

films may be positive, they are less likely to be positive than in *T. brucei rhodesiense* infection, except early on in the infection. Since this infection has likely been present for some time, aspiration of the lymph nodes is more likely to make a diagnosis. In addition, nothing has been noted on blood films sent for malaria testing, which should also reveal trypanosomes. Serologic responses against *T. brucei* and a lumbar puncture should also be performed. A bone marrow aspirate and splenic aspiration are tests employed in the diagnosis of leishmaniasis and a liver biopsy would not be helpful in this case to determine the cause of the liver function test abnormalities. In addition, these tests need specialist facilities, particularly splenic aspiration.

11.37. Answer: E.
Candidaemia has a propensity to lead to intraocular infection. This has resulted in the recommendation that all patients with candidaemia should be assessed by an ophthalmologist with dilated fundoscopy. Oesophagogastroduodenoscopy is used to assess *Candida* oesophagitis and the other investigations are indicated if signs or symptoms suggest infection at these sites.

11.38. Answer: A.
Drug fever is an important consideration in patients with pyrexia of unknown origin, particularly in those who are on multiple medications. Allopurinol is a potential cause of drug-related hypersensitivity and is associated with abnormal liver function tests and lymphadenopathy. Penicillins and other antimicrobials can cause fever but in this case the fever predated use of piperacillin–tazobactam. The failure to respond to broad-spectrum antimicrobial therapy and the absence of any localising features or positive microbiological tests mean that a microbiological cause remains unproven and other possibilities need to be excluded. Herpes virus aetiologies are important, particularly in solid organ transplant recipients or those who have received a haematopoietic stem cell transplant, but these are not found in this case and a patient with acute leukaemia on chemotherapy is not at particular risk of these infections. Invasive fungal infection remains a diagnostic consideration, particularly for patients with acute myelogenous leukaemia, but the fever has remained despite addition of

caspofungin, and the galactomannan and chest CT scan has been negative.

11.39. Answer: A.

Eosinophilic meningitis is seen with *Angiostrongylus* spp. infections and also with gnathostomiasis or coccidioidomycosis. The other infections listed may be found in South-east Asia but cause alternative clinical neurological syndromes.

11.40. Answer: C.

The epidemiological setting, clinical scenario and use of xenodiagnoses are consistent with a diagnosis of Chagas' disease (American trypanosomiasis), which is treated with nifurtimox. Niclosamide and nitazoxanide are used to treat other parasites.

11.41. Answer: D.

The likeliest diagnosis is acute Lyme borreliosis. This is increasing in frequency in the UK. The commonest organism responsible in Europe is *Borrelia burgdorferi*. The recommendation is for family physicians to treat with oral doxycycline or amoxicillin for uncomplicated acute disease.

11.42. Answer: D.

Any patient who has a history of recent travel to the Middle East along with fever and severe respiratory symptoms should have infection with MERS-CoV excluded before infection control measures can be relaxed. SARS is another coronavirus infection that leads to severe respiratory symptoms but circulated in 2003. There are no risk factors for avian influenza, which would require a history of contact with chickens. ARDS complicating pneumonia would be in the differential but does not have the same influence on infection control policy and therefore is not the first diagnosis to be excluded. Meningococcal sepsis has been reported after pilgrimages to the Middle East and sepsis can present with respiratory symptoms but would be expected to present with additional signs of sepsis.

11.43. Answer: A.

The empiric therapy of fever in an intravenous drug user should include coverage of *Staph. aureus*. The specific agents will be influenced by local antimicrobial resistance patterns and rates of meticillin-resistant *Staph. aureus* (MRSA). In this scenario the chest X-ray raises the possibility of haematogenous spread of septic emboli from infected thrombophlebitis or right-sided endocarditis. In an area with low rates of MRSA, flucloxacillin is a good choice for empiric coverage of a potential endovascular *Staph. aureus* infection. Meropenem and piperacillin–tazobactam might be considered in cases of sepsis but would not be first choice where *Staph. aureus* needs to be treated. Tigecycline might be used against MRSA in certain settings, such as skin and soft tissue infection, but would not be first choice when potential bloodstream infection needs to be treated. Moxifloxacin is not usually used in *Staph. aureus* infection.

11.44. Answer: D.

Radical cure of *vivax* malaria requires the use of the 8-aminoquinoline drug primaquine. This causes oxidative stress, which can result in massive haemolysis in patients who have low G6PD activity due to various inherited traits. The other tests will not impact on the treatment.

11.45. Answer: B.

Cysticercosis is caused by the pork tapeworm *Taenia solium* and results when humans ingest tapeworm ova, often from an infected household contact. The disease leads to cysts that can involve the subcutaneous tissue, muscle and brain. The lesions are visible on CT or MRI scan of the head and can have a characteristic appearance. They can result in a variety of neurological features, including new-onset seizures. Treatment is most often with albendazole.

11.46. Answer: D.

Scabies with increasing drug resistance is a huge problem in indigenous populations in Australia. This is associated with post-streptococcal rheumatic fever with rheumatic heart disease as a sequela. Ivermectin is used for large infestations. The other answers would not explain both the skin lesions and the heart murmur.

11.47. Answer: A.

Salmonellosis can invade and colonise aortic arteriosclerotic plaques and result in a mycotic aortic aneurysm in older patients. Endocarditis is uncommon with salmonellae. Persistently positive blood cultures raise the possibility of endovascular infection and while this is most

11

often associated with a central venous catheter infection or endocarditis, certain organisms are associated with other foci and require specific investigations, as in this case.

11.48. Answer: E.

This is a typical presentation of enteric fever caused by *Salmonella* Typhi. Nepal is a high-risk country for typhoid, which is contracted from contaminated water. She has signs of sepsis, which would make cyclosporiasis less likely, and the rash would not be typical for appendicitis. The incubation period is too long for dengue. Although scrub typhus causes a rash, the history with prominent abdominal symptoms and absence of an eschar and regional lymphadenopathy is less typical.

11.49. Answer: C.

Campylobacter is the commonest cause of infective colitis in the UK. Although inflammatory bowel disease should be considered, it is less common than *Campylobacter*.

11.50. Answer: C.

Mucocutaneous leishmaniasis due to *L. braziliensis* should always be treated aggressively with systemic therapy due to the risk of dissemination. The other treatments would not prevent dissemination.

11.51. Answer: A.

Bacillary angiomatosis is caused by infection with *Bartonella* species, a slow-growing Gram-negative bacillus that causes problems in immunocompromised hosts. These include endocarditis, trench fever and bacillary peliosis (widespread blood-filled cavities in major organs). Treatment is with doxycycline. Kaposi's sarcoma also can cause violaceous papules but histology should show characteristic spindle cell formations and would not be positive with Warthin–Starry silver stain, which detects the *Bartonella* species. Similarly, the histology does not show features of melanoma and this also would not have a positive Warthin–Starry stain; nor would the other conditions listed, which also would have alternative dermatological appearances.

11.52. Answer: B.

Kaposi's sarcoma is an angioproliferative tumour related to HHV-8 infection in immunocompromised hosts. The finding of

lesions on the palate usually indicates that there is deep-organ involvement, such as gut and lung, which may lead to life-threatening bleeding. Treatment is with doxorubicin and immune reconstitution.

11.53. Answer: D.

Lemierre's syndrome is due to suppurative jugular vein thrombophlebitis with bacteraemia usually secondary to a bacterial sore throat. Treatment is usually supportive with penicillin. It is often complicated by disseminated intravascular coagulopathy.

11.54. Answer: D.

Nocardia are filamentous Gram-positive branching rods that stain positive with a modified acid-fast stain. They are found in the soil and may lead to brain abscesses. *Actinomyces israelii* and *Clostridium perfringens* are also Gram-positive, but *C. perfringens* would not appear as branching rods and although *A. israelii* would have a similar microbiological appearance, *Nocardia* would be more likely to cause a brain abscess in this scenario. *Mycobacterium chelonae* would stain with an acid-fast stain and *Sporothrix* is a dimorphic fungus and would appear as a yeast form.

11.55. Answer: D.

Plasmodium knowlesi is the sixth human malaria now that *Plasmodium ovale* has been classified as two subspecies on the basis of genetic homology. *P. knowlesi* is associated with close contact with non-human primates and is usually a mild infection, which does not relapse. Its life cycle is 24 hours (as opposed to 48 hours for *falciparum*), giving rapid changes in fever. Chesson strain *vivax* is relatively resistant to primaquine and is found in Indonesia.

11.56. Answer: A.

Haemolytic uraemic syndrome is usually associated with infection with *E. coli* O157. Treatment is supportive. The other options would not give this combination of anaemia, jaundice and renal failure.

11.57. Answer: E.

Yersinia enterocolitica is commonly found in pork, causes mild to moderate gastroenteritis and can produce significant mesenteric adenitis after an incubation period of 3–7 days. It resolves slowly. The other options would not give this clinical picture.

11.58. Answer: E.

Hantavirus is a ribonucleic acid (RNA) virus associated with pulmonary and renal failure mimicking pulmonary syndrome in leptospirosis, and is associated with a history of contact with mice within a wide geographical area. Some strains of hantaviruses cause the potentially fatal diseases – hantavirus haemorrhagic fever with renal syndrome and hantavirus pulmonary syndrome – while others have not been associated with known human disease. Treatment is supportive. The other syndromes are non-infectious and while all enter the differential, the scenario means one should consider hantavirus.

11.59. Answer: D.

Bat bites have been associated with transmission of rabies and individuals who are bitten or likely to be exposed to bats should have a rabies vaccine. The other infections are not associated with bats.

11.60. Answer: C.

Monkeypox is a relatively harmless infection with a poxvirus. Although similar in appearance to smallpox, it is a mild infection. The most recent outbreak in the USA was related to importation of pet rats from The Gambia in Africa.

11.61. Answer: C.

The cardinal feature of necrotising fasciitis is pain out of keeping with clinical signs. The diagnosis is by surgical exploration with necrotic deep tissue being seen. It is usually due to a polymicrobial infection and treatment is with broad-spectrum antibiotics including a macrolide to reduce toxin production plus surgical debridement. Gas gangrene is associated with wounds, and crepitus may be detected in the skin. Splenic rupture would be associated with trauma and there is no history of this. Lemierre's syndrome presents as a pain in the neck, which results from a thrombophlebitis, typically of the internal jugular vein, complicating a sore throat. A colonic perforation would be considered with the location of the abdomen pain but would not be expected to cause the skin lesion visible over the hip, which is a key feature that raises the possibility of necrotising fasciitis.

11.62. Answer: E.

Wound botulism results from the contamination of a wound with the bacterial species *Clostridium botulinum*, which then secretes botulinum toxin into the bloodstream. It has become increasingly common in people who take drugs intradermally or subcutaneously (skin popping). Botulism is typically described as a 'triad of bulbar palsy and descending paralysis, lack of fever, and clear senses'. Staphylococcal brain abscesses and tetanus are also associated with drug injection but the patient's neurological symptoms with prominent bulbar signs and ocular involvement make these less likely. Staphylococcal brain abscess would be more associated with injection into the vein than skin popping. The other conditions may cause ocular signs but are not particularly associated with drug use.

11.63. Answer: A.

Anthrax amongst drug users is related to heroin contaminated with anthrax spores. Urgent surgical debridement (to remove dead or devitalised tissue and drain any abscess/collection) is most important. This should be performed alongside empiric antibiotic treatment to cover *Bacillus anthracis* as well as other more common causes of soft tissue infection. Antibiotic treatment may involve ciprofloxacin and clindamycin intravenously in combination with penicillin, flucloxacillin and metronidazole (i.e. a five-drug combination). Gas gangrene is not particularly associated with an eschar and is more associated with dusky skin discoloration and crepitus. Neither Lyme disease not staphylococcal bacteraemia are associated with an eschar, and necrotising fasciitis would typically be associated with more pain at the site and other skin features.

11.64. Answer: D.

Some adults may not have been immunised with MMR. The combination of neck swelling due to parotitis and orchitis is highly suggestive of mumps. The other causes listed might explain cervical swelling or the combination of cervical and testicular problems but are less consistent from the relatively healthy nature of this patient and the short history of symptoms.

11.65. Answer: B.

Gas gangrene is due to infection with *C. perfringens*. Treatment involves surgical debridement and penicillin with clindamycin.

11

12

G Maartens

HIV infection and AIDS

Multiple Choice Questions

12.1. What is human immunodeficiency virus (HIV) protease enzyme responsible for?

A. Budding of HIV from the cell
B. Cleavage of post-translational regulatory proteins
C. Fusion of HIV with the host cell surface
D. Integration of viral deoxyribonucleic acid (DNA) into the host genome
E. Reverse transcription of viral ribonucleic acid (RNA) to DNA

12.2. What is the risk of acquiring HIV during a single act of unprotected vaginal sexual intercourse when the male partner is HIV infected and not on antiretroviral therapy, and the female partner is HIV uninfected?

A. 0.001%
B. 0.01%
C. 0.1%
D. 1%
E. 10%

12.3. Which of the following is a correct statement regarding the features of primary HIV infection?

A. A maculopapular rash is a common feature
B. Atypical lymphocytosis occurs more frequently than in Epstein–Barr virus (EBV) infection
C. Primary infection is asymptomatic in most people
D. The incubation period is 5–7 days
E. Transient CD4 lymphocytosis is usual

12.4. What is the most sensitive blood test for diagnosing HIV during primary infection?

A. HIV antibodies detected by enzyme-linked immunosorbent assay
B. HIV antibodies detected by western blot
C. p24 antigen detection
D. Polymerase chain reaction (PCR) to detect HIV RNA
E. Rapid point-of-care antibody test

12.5. A 35 year old HIV-positive man presents with diarrhoea of 4 weeks' duration accompanied by tenesmus. Blood and mucus is present in the stool. He is not on antiretroviral therapy. His CD4 count is 17 cells/mm^3. Which of the following is the most likely diagnosis?

A. Cryptosporidiosis
B. Cystoisosporiasis
C. Cytomegalovirus (CMV) colitis
D. Giardiasis
E. Microsporidiosis

12.6. Which one of the following non-acquired immunodeficiency syndrome (non-AIDS) cancers has been shown to have an increased incidence in HIV-infected patients?

A. Anal cancer
B. Breast cancer
C. Melanoma
D. Ovarian cancer
E. Prostate cancer

12.7. A 45 year old man with a CD4 count of 23 cells/mm^3 presents with gradually progressive spastic paraplegia and urinary incontinence. There is impaired short-term memory. Plain X-ray of the spine is normal. What is the most likely cause of the paraplegia?

A. Cytomegalovirus polyradiculopathy
B. Human T-cell lymphotropic virus type 1 (HTLV-1) myelopathy
C. Multiple sclerosis
D. Tuberculosis of the spine
E. Vacuolar myelopathy

12.8. An HIV-infected woman with a CD4 count of 36 cells/mm³ presents with symptomatic anaemia. She is not on antiretroviral therapy. Full blood count shows: haemoglobin 26 g/L, normochromic and normocytic, with a low reticulocyte index; white cell count and platelets are normal. Bone marrow biopsy shows pure red cell aplasia. Which one of the following viral infections is likely to be responsible?

A. Cytomegalovirus
B. Epstein–Barr virus
C. Herpes simplex virus
D. JC virus (John Cunningham virus)
E. Parvovirus B19

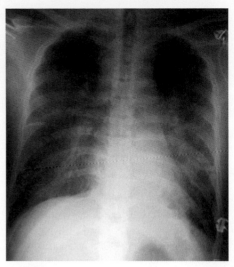

Fig. 12.11

12

12.9. Which of the following is a clinical indication for starting prophylactic co-trimoxazole in HIV-infected adults in middle- to high-income settings?

A. Enlarged parotid glands
B. Fungal nail infections
C. Generalised lymphadenopathy
D. Herpes zoster infection
E. Oral hairy leucoplakia

12.10. A 24 year old HIV-infected man presents with a 5-day history of fever, cough and right pleuritic chest pain. There are crackles and signs of consolidation in the right lung posteriorly and chest radiograph shows dense consolidation of the right lower zone. What is the most likely pathogen?

A. *Mycobacterium tuberculosis*
B. *Pneumocystis jirovecii*
C. *Pseudomonas aeruginosa*
D. *Streptococcus pneumoniae*
E. The 'atypical bacteria' (e.g. *Mycoplasma pneumoniae*, *Chlamydophila pneumoniae*, and *Legionella* species)

12.11. A 34 year old man with a CD4 count of 116 cells/mm³ presents with a 4-week history of dry cough and progressively worsening dyspnoea. On examination he has a fever of 38°C, respiratory rate of 26 breaths/min, and no focal chest signs. Chest radiograph shows a bilateral interstitial infiltrate (Fig. 12.11). Oxygen saturation is 90% on room air. White blood cell count and haemoglobin are normal. What is the most likely diagnosis?

A. Bacterial pneumonia
B. Lymphoid interstitial pneumonitis
C. *Pneumocystis jirovecii* pneumonia
D. Pulmonary Kaposi's sarcoma
E. Pulmonary tuberculosis

12.12. Which of the following statements is true about the diffuse inflammatory lymphocytosis syndrome (DILS)?

A. DILS is a recognised complication of co-infection with human herpesvirus 8
B. DILS is a risk factor for parotid gland lymphoma
C. DILS is associated with polymyositis
D. DILS is characterised by infiltration of the parotids with B lymphocytes
E. DILS is usually associated with a marked CD4 lymphocytosis

12.13. A nurse administers an intramuscular injection to an HIV-infected woman who is not yet on antiretroviral therapy. After the injection she pricks her finger on the needle. What is the approximate risk of acquiring HIV following this occupational exposure?

A. 0.003%
B. 0.03%
C. 0.3%
D. 3%
E. 30%

12.14. A 37 year old man with a CD4 count of 24 cells/mm^3 presents with painless, progressive visual loss. On fundoscopy the vitreous is clear, and haemorrhages and exudates are seen on the retina. What is the most likely diagnosis?

A. Cytomegalovirus retinitis
B. HIV retinopathy
C. Ocular syphilis
D. Ocular toxoplasmosis
E. Progressive outer retinal necrosis due to varicella zoster virus

12.15. What is the mechanism of action of the antiretroviral drugs raltegravir, dolutegravir and elvitegravir?

A. Chemokine receptor CCR5 antagonist
B. Fusion inhibitor
C. Integrase inhibitor
D. Protease inhibitor
E. Reverse transcriptase inhibitor

12.16. A 44 year old woman with a CD4 count of 73 cells/mm^3 presents with a progressive left hemiplegia and headache over a week. Her magnetic resonance imaging scan shows multiple ring-enhancing mass lesions with surrounding cerebral oedema. What is the most likely diagnosis?

A. Brain abscess
B. Cerebral toxoplasmosis
C. Cryptococcoma
D. Primary central nervous system (CNS) lymphoma
E. Tuberculoma

12.17. What is the correct statement regarding the immune reconstitution inflammatory syndrome (IRIS)?

A. Antiretroviral therapy (ART) should be stopped if IRIS is suspected
B. It is more common in patients responding poorly to ART
C. It is more common when ART is initiated with higher baseline CD4 counts (>200 cells/mm^3)
D. It usually presents within the first 3 months of initiating ART
E. The mortality is high (approximately 25%)

12.18. A 26 year old woman with newly diagnosed HIV infection and a CD4$^+$ lymphocyte count of 34 cells/mm^3 presents with dysphagia. There is no oral candidiasis. You prescribe a course of fluconazole for possible *Candida* oesophagitis. Two weeks later she returns with no improvement. What is the most likely cause of her dysphagia?

A. Cytomegalovirus oesophageal ulceration
B. Herpes simplex virus oesophageal ulceration
C. Kaposi's sarcoma of the oesophagus
D. Major aphthous ulceration of the oesophagus
E. Oesophagitis to azole-resistant *Candida* species (e.g. *C. krusei*)

12.19. A 39 year old man presents with asymmetric cervical lymphadenitis for 2 months. His CD4 count is 234 cells/mm^3. The largest node is 4×3 cm and is fluctuant. Several nodes are matted together. What is the most likely diagnosis?

A. HIV lymphadenopathy
B. Kaposi's sarcoma
C. Non-Hodgkin lymphoma
D. Pyogenic lymphadenitis
E. Tuberculosis

12.20. Which of the following statements is correct about AIDS-associated Kaposi's sarcoma?

A. It is a spindle-cell tumour of lymphoendothelial origin
B. It is associated with infection by human herpesvirus 6
C. Multiple skin lesions indicate a poor prognosis
D. The commonest site of visceral spread is the brain
E. Women are more likely than men to develop Kaposi's sarcoma

12.21. Which of the following statements on viral load in HIV infection is correct?

A. A viral load change of 15 848 to 10 000 copies/mL (difference of 0.2 log$_{10}$) is regarded as a significant reduction 4 weeks after starting antiretroviral therapy
B. The viral load should be suppressed after 6 months of effective antiretroviral therapy
C. Vaccination transiently decreases the viral load
D. Viral load measures intracellular viruses
E. Viral load reaches a relatively stable plateau 2 weeks after seroconversion

12.22. A 42 year old man presents with severe headache and vomiting of 3 weeks' duration. His CD4 count is 62 cells/mm^3. Computed tomography (CT) scan of the brain is normal. Lumbar puncture shows mild pleocytosis with positive cryptococcal antigen test and elevated opening pressure of 34 cmH₂O. You commence therapy with intravenous amphotericin B and flucytosine for the cryptococcal meningitis. What is the most appropriate management for the raised intracranial pressure?

A. Acetazolamide
B. Dexamethasone
C. Insert a ventriculo-peritoneal shunt
D. Mannitol
E. Therapeutic lumbar puncture, removing enough cerebrospinal fluid to reduce pressure to < 20 cmH₂O

12.23. Which of the following features is characteristic of HIV-associated nephropathy (HIVAN)?

A. Heavy proteinuria (> 1.5 g/24 hrs) is a usual finding
B. People of European descent are more likely to develop HIVAN
C. Severe hypertension is a characteristic feature
D. Small kidneys on ultrasound are typically seen when the creatinine clearance decreases to 30 mL/min or less
E. The course of the disease is relatively benign with few progressing to end-stage renal failure

Answers

12

12.1. Answer: B.
This is the main function of protease (Fig. 12.1). Fusion is mediated after binding to CD4 and the chemokine receptor, reverse transcriptase mediates reverse transcription, and integrase mediates integration of viral DNA.

Budding occurs after cleavage of proteins by protease.

12.2. Answer: C.
Several factors increase this risk: sexually transmitted infection (especially genital ulcers),

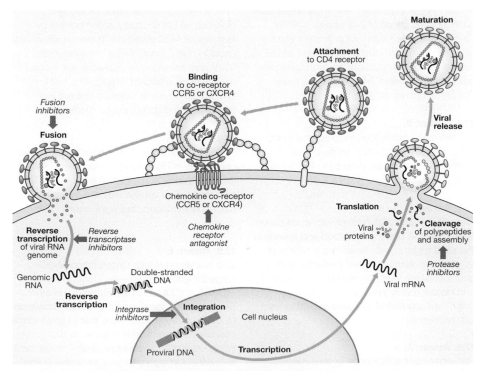

Fig. 12.1 Life cycle of HIV. Arrows indicate sites of action of antiretroviral drugs.

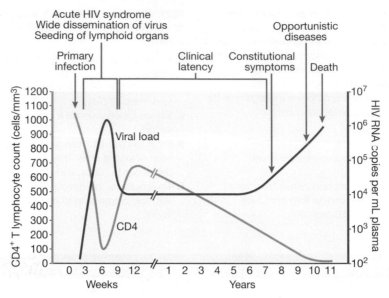

Fig. 12.3 Virological and immunological progression of untreated HIV infection.

cervical ectopy, uncircumcised male partner and menstruation.

12.3. Answer: A.
Primary HIV is a glandular fever-type illness with an incubation period of 2–4 weeks. It differs from EBV infection with less prominent atypical lymphocytosis and a rash is common (with EBV, rashes usually only occur when aminopenicillins are given). Typically CD4 lymphocytes are transiently decreased (Fig. 12.3).

12.4. Answer: D.
Nucleic acid amplification tests are the most sensitive, followed by p24 antigenaemia. Antibodies typically are detectable 2–6 weeks later.

12.5. Answer: C.
The other diseases all present with small-bowel diarrhoea. The presence of blood and mucus in the stool together with tenesmus is typical of large-bowel diarrhoea. CMV involvement of the gastrointestinal tract typically causes ulceration and occurs mainly in the oesophagus and colon, but any part of the gastrointestinal tract can be involved.

12.6. Answer: A.
HIV increases the incidence of virus-related cancers. Anal cancer is linked to human papilloma virus infection; the other cancers listed are not caused by viruses.

12.7. Answer: E.
This is a typical presentation of this HIV disorder, which is usually accompanied by features of AIDS dementia. Tuberculosis would usually cause abnormalities on spine X-rays. CMV polyradiculopathy causes lower motor neuron signs and pain. Myelopathy from HTLV-1 and multiple sclerosis are not HIV associated and do not cause memory loss.

12.8. Answer: E.
This is the commonest infectious cause of red cell aplasia in HIV infection. The antiretroviral drug lamivudine is another rare cause. CMV and some other viruses may occasionally cause pancytopenia, but not pure red cell aplasia.

12.9. Answer: E.
This is a World Health Organization (WHO) stage 3/Centers for Disease Control and Prevention (CDC) B manifestation. The others are all WHO stage 2, which is not an indication to start co-trimoxazole. Note that in low-income countries co-trimoxazole is given to all, irrespective of CD4 count or clinical stage, as it is of benefit in high infectious diseases burden settings (including areas with malaria risk).

12.10. Answer: D.
Pneumococcal pneumonia incidence is markedly increased in HIV. Atypical bacteria can present in this way, but are less common causes. *Pseudomonas* pneumonia is rare. Tuberculosis can present acutely, but is usually a more subacute illness and the chest radiograph is seldom that of dense lobar consolidation with no other features.

12.11. Answer: C.
The duration of symptoms is too long for bacterial pneumonia. The prominent dyspnoea and chest radiograph appearance is typical of *Pneumocystis jirovecii* pneumonia. Lymphoid interstitial pneumonitis can have a similar radiographic appearance but is a more chronic illness and fever is uncommon. Pulmonary tuberculosis with adult respiratory distress syndrome is possible, but this is a rare complication in tuberculosis.

12.12. Answer: C.
DILS is a benign polyclonal CD8 infiltration of tissues, especially the parotids, and is associated with human leucocyte antigen (HLA)-DRB1. A number of autoimmune disorders are seen in DILS, including polymyositis.

12.13. Answer: C.
Several factors increase this risk: high viral load in source patient, hollow-bore needle that was in source patient's vessel, visible blood on the needle.

12.14. Answer: A.
CMV retinitis is the commonest cause of visual loss in AIDS. Toxoplasmosis often causes a concomitant vitritis and HIV retinopathy does not cause visual loss.

12.15. Answer: C.
The standard combination antiretroviral regimens are two nucleoside reverse transcriptase inhibitors (NRTIs) together with a non-nucleoside reverse transcriptase inhibitor (NNRTI), protease inhibitor (PI) or integrase inhibitor (Box 12.15). Dual NRTI combinations are usually emtricitabine or lamivudine (they have the same mechanism of action and so are never combined) together with one of abacavir, tenofovir or zidovudine. See Fig. 12.1, above, for mechanisms of action of the different antiretroviral drugs.

i 12.15 Commonly used antiretroviral drugs	
Classes	Drugs
Nucleoside reverse transcriptase inhibitors (NRTIs)	Abacavir, emtricitabine, lamivudine, tenofovir, zidovudine*
Non-nucleoside reverse transcriptase inhibitors (NNRTIs)	Efavirenz*, rilpivirine (only if viral load <100 000)
Protease inhibitors (PIs)	Atazanavir, darunavir, lopinavir*
Integrase inhibitors	Raltegravir, dolutegravir, elvitegravir
Chemokine receptor inhibitor	Maraviroc

These drugs are no longer recommended as first-line options in high-income countries due to their toxicity.

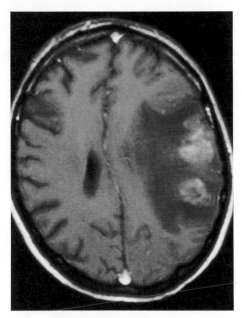

Fig. 12.16 Cerebral toxoplasmosis. Multiple ring-enhancing lesions with surrounding oedema are characteristic.

12.16. Answer: B.
This is the commonest cause of space-occupying lesions in patients with HIV infection – CD4 counts are usually < 100 cells/mm^3 and multiple lesions are typical (Fig. 12.16).

12.17. Answer: D.
IRIS is an exaggerated inflammatory response seen in the first 3 months after starting ART. It is most common in patients starting ART with low CD4 counts. It is usual to continue ART and provide symptomatic relief for IRIS manifestations; steroids may be useful with life-threatening manifestations.

12

12.18. Answer: D.

Candida oesophagitis is the commonest cause, but failure to respond in this case virtually rules this out (azole-resistant *Candida* species are usually only seen in patients with prolonged azole use). The next commonest cause is major aphthous ulceration, which responds well to steroids and ART.

12.19. Answer: E.

Tuberculosis nodes are often matted and may fluctuate. Malignant nodes rarely fluctuate, unless there is central necrosis. Persistent generalised lymphadenopathy of HIV is typically symmetrical and does not fluctuate.

12.20. Answer: A.

Kaposi's sarcoma (KS) is a spindle-cell tumour of lymphoendothelial origin. All forms of KS are due to sexually transmitted human herpesvirus 8, also known as KS-associated herpesvirus.

In Africa, the male:female ratio of AIDS-associated KS is much lower than is seen with endemic KS, but men are still more affected than women, despite the fact that the seroprevalence of human herpesvirus 8 is the same in both sexes.

AIDS-associated KS is always a multicentric disease. Early mucocutaneous lesions are macular and may be difficult to diagnose. As the disease progresses, the skin lesions become more numerous and larger. Lymphoedema is common, as lymphatic vessels are infiltrated. KS also commonly spreads to lymph nodes and viscerally, especially to the lungs and gastrointestinal tract.

12.21. Answer: B.

The level of viraemia is measured by quantitative PCR of HIV RNA, known as the viral load. Determining the viral load is crucial for monitoring responses to antiretroviral therapy. People with high viral loads (e.g. >100 000 copies/mL) experience more rapid declines in CD4 count, while those with low viral loads (<1000 copies/mL) usually have slow or even no decline in CD4 counts. Viraemia peaks during primary infection and then drops as the immune response develops, to reach a plateau about 3 months later (see Fig. 12.3, above).

Transient increases in viral load occur with intercurrent infections and immunisations, so the test should be done at least 2 weeks afterwards. Viral loads are variable; only changes in viral load of more than $0.5 \log_{10}$ copies/mL are considered clinically significant.

12.22. Answer: E.

The raised intracranial pressure is best managed by therapeutic lumbar puncture as this is a communicating hydrocephalus. Steroids and acetazolamide have been shown to be harmful. Shunting is seldom necessary. Mannitol is irrational, as the primary problem is not cerebral oedema.

12.23. Answer: A.

HIVAN typically presents with nephrotic syndrome and/or chronic kidney disease (CKD). Progression to CKD is rapid with preserved kidney size. People of African descent are more likely to develop HIVAN.

13

Sexually transmitted infections

Multiple Choice Questions

13.1. Most women with genital *Chlamydia trachomatis* are symptomless. In women who do develop symptoms, which of the following is the most common?

A. Deep dyspareunia
B. Dysuria
C. Increased vaginal discharge
D. Lower abdominal pain
E. Unexpected vaginal bleeding

13.2. A patient with confirmed infection with herpes simplex virus type 2 (HSV-2) has had symptomatic recurrences approximately every month for the last year. What is the standard first-line antiviral regime to be prescribed in this case?

A. Aciclovir 200 mg four times daily
B. Aciclovir 400 mg twice daily
C. Famciclovir 250 mg once daily
D. Famciclovir 750 mg once daily
E. Valaciclovir 500 mg once daily

13.3. A 34 year old human immunodeficiency virus (HIV)-positive man who has sex with men (MSM) complains of severe rectal pain, blood-stained discharge and tenesmus. He is taking antiretroviral therapy, has a CD4 count of 636 and an undetectable HIV viral load. Proctoscopy reveals rectal inflammation and visible mucopus. Which is the most likely cause of this presentation?

A. *Campylobacter* infection
B. Cytomegalovirus colitis

C. Gonorrhoea
D. Lymphogranuloma venereum
E. Secondary syphilis

13.4. Most of the following are complications of disseminated gonococcal infection (DGI). Which would you be UNLIKELY to see as a recognised complication of DGI?

A. Arthritis
B. Endocarditis
C. Pustular rash
D. Tenosynovitis
E. Uveitis

13.5. What is the most likely diagnosis in this 17 year old young man who has become aware of these painless "lumps"?

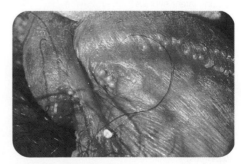

A. Coronal papillae
B. Genital warts
C. Lichen planus
D. Molluscum contagiosum
E. Sebaceous glands

13.6. Which of the following antimicrobial drugs is unlikely to be effective against genital *Chlamydia trachomatis* infection?

A. Amoxicillin
B. Ciprofloxacin
C. Erythromycin
D. Ofloxacin
E. Oxytetracycline

13.7. Which of the following statements is true of infection with human papilloma virus (HPV) types 6/11?

A. More cases of perianal warts are seen in homosexual men than in heterosexual men
B. This is associated with penile cancer
C. This is cleared by treatment with topical liquid nitrogen
D. This is prevented by vaccination with Cervarix
E. This will result in visible genital warts in less than 50% of cases

13.8. A symptomless 43 year old MSM undergoes a routine STI screen for the first time in 3 years. All tests for STIs were previously negative. His serological tests for syphilis are now as follows:

Test	Result
Antitreponemal immunoglobulin G (IgG) enzyme immunoassay (EIA)	Positive – optical density 20.3
Rapid plasma reagin (RPR)	Positive – titre 4
Treponema pallidum particle agglutination assay (TPPA)	Positive – titre >5120
Antitreponemal immunoglobulin M (IgM) EIA	Negative

Which of the following is most compatible with these results?

A. Early latent syphilis
B. Partially treated late syphilis
C. Primary syphilis
D. Secondary syphilis
E. Untreated late syphilis

13.9. A 19 year old woman complains of moderate lower abdominal pain that has been present for 2 weeks, and is particularly noticeable during sex. Which of the following actively supports a diagnosis of chlamydial salpingitis?

A. A dipstick urine test showing haematuria +++
B. A positive pregnancy test
C. A temperature of 36.3°C
D. Diarrhoea
E. Right upper quadrant tenderness

13.10. A 22 year old MSM presents for an STI screen. His only complaint is of pain on defecation. Examination reveals an anal fissure. Serological tests for syphilis are as follows:

Test	Result
Antitreponemal IgG EIA	Negative
RPR	Negative
TPPA	Positive – titre 160
Antitreponemal IgM EIA	Positive – optical density 3.4

Which of the following is the most likely explanation of the serology?

A. Early latent syphilis
B. False-positive syphilis serology
C. Primary syphilis
D. Secondary syphilis
E. Treated syphilis

13.11. A 38 year old married man tells you that he had unprotected sex exactly 1 week ago with a woman who he thinks may be an intravenous drug user (IDU). Which of the following statements is true?

A. He can safely have sex with his wife if all tests for STIs taken today are negative
B. He can safely have sex with his wife if given treatment with a single dose of azithromycin 1 g
C. He is at significant risk of acquiring hepatitis C (HCV)
D. He should be offered post-exposure prophylaxis (PEP) against HIV
E. He should be offered vaccination against hepatitis B (HBV)

13.12. A symptomless 29 year old MSM presents for an STI screen. Serological tests for syphilis are as follows:

Test	Result
Antitreponemal IgG EIA	Positive – optical density 33
RPR	Negative
TPPA	Positive – titre >5120
Antitreponemal IgM EIA	Positive – optical density 11.4

Which of the following is the most likely explanation of the serology?

A. Early latent syphilis
B. False-positive syphilis serology
C. Fully treated late latent syphilis
D. Partially treated late latent syphilis
E. Untreated late latent syphilis

13.13. The following infections are not thought of as being STIs, but which is the only one that cannot be sexually transmitted?

A. Cytomegalovirus (CMV)
B. Hepatitis A (HAV)
C. *Plasmodium vivax*
D. *Shigella sonnei*
E. Zika virus

13.14. A 27 year old woman is 24 weeks pregnant. She mentions to you that her current male partner has a previous history of genital herpes caused by herpes simplex virus type 1 (HSV-1). Although he has had few recurrences in the past, he has had no symptoms at all in the last year. Which of the following statements is most appropriate?

A. As her partner has been symptom-free for a year, she can be reassured that there is no risk of transmission to her
B. Primary genital herpes is more likely to lead to disseminated infection if it is caused by HSV-2
C. She should avoid unprotected sex for the duration of the pregnancy
D. She should be commenced on valaciclovir 500 mg once daily to prevent transmission
E. Her baby should be delivered by caesarean section

Answers

13.1. Answer: E.
Chlamydia can cause a cervicitis, and the resulting friability may present as unexpected bleeding, especially after sexual intercourse. Urethritis resulting in dysuria is less common, but may be mistaken for eubacterial cystitis. Deep dyspareunia and lower abdominal pain are symptoms of ascending infection (salpingitis/pelvic inflammatory disease), which occurs less frequently than was believed previously. Increased vaginal discharge is possible, but in most cases is probably due to an unrelated condition like bacterial vaginosis or candidiasis.

13.2. Answer: B.
Early studies using aciclovir to suppress recurrences found that 200 mg four times daily was more effective than 400 mg twice daily, but the difference is small enough to recommend the less frequent dosing regime, which is going to make adherence easier. Valaciclovir and famciclovir are more expensive and so reserved for cases where aciclovir is ineffective. The recommended dose of valaciclovir is 500 mg once daily as per option E, but the correct starting dose of famciclovir is 250 mg twice daily.

13.3. Answer: D.
Lymphogranuloma venereum is the likeliest cause of severe proctitis and is most often diagnosed in HIV-positive MSM in the UK. Gonococcal proctitis is usually less severe than in this case, as are the rare cases of syphilitic proctitis. *Campylobacter* infection is seen in MSM but diarrhoea would be a more prominent symptom. Cytomegalovirus (CMV) colitis is only seen in end-stage HIV infection, which is clearly not the case here.

13.4. Answer: E.
Typical manifestations of DGI include monoarthropathy, vasculitic rash and tenosynovitis. Endocarditis is seen rarely. The sexually transmitted infection (STI) associated with uveitis is secondary syphilis.

13.5. Answer: A.
Coronal papillae are a normal anatomical feature, which become more prominent in adolescence, and young men can mistake these normal skin appendages for an infection, especially genital warts. Warts would not be limited to the corona, and are usually either more papular or keratotic. Molluscum lesions are umbilicated. Lichen planus typically presents as violaceous flat-topped papules. Sebaceous glands, also known as Fordyce spots, are seen on the shaft and base of the penis.

13.6. Answer: B.
Erythromycin and oxytetracycline were used before the advent of azithromycin and doxycycline, respectively. Ofloxacin is a quinolone with antichlamydial efficacy, but this is not the case for ciprofloxacin. Somewhat surprisingly, amoxicillin was found to be effective in the treatment of *Chlamydia* in pregnancy, although azithromycin is much preferred now.

13

13.7. Answer: E.

The percentage of infected patients who develop visible warts is unknown, but is definitely a small minority. Although homosexual men (MSM) are relatively more likely to get perianal warts, the majority of cases present in heterosexual men. The mode of inoculation is unclear. Liquid nitrogen destroys infected tissue but does not clear HPV infection. HPV types 6/11 are not associated with genital cancer – HPV types 16/18 are the most common oncogenic types. Cervarix vaccine only protects against HPV types 16/18; Gardasil also protects against types 6/11.

13.8. Answer: B.

A diagnosis of primary or secondary syphilis is based on typical clinical findings so cannot be applied to a symptomless individual. The negative IgM makes early latent syphilis unlikely, and the RPR titre in untreated early or late latent syphilis would be expected to be much higher – at the very least 32. The titre here of 4 is more likely to represent accidental treatment – in this case, antibiotics for a dental infection. It would still be prudent to offer definitive treatment, e.g. with a course of three injections of benzathine penicillin at weekly intervals.

13.9. Answer: E.

Right upper quadrant tenderness is a feature of perihepatitis, a rare complication of ascending chlamydial infection. Diarrhoea is not a symptom suggestive of salpingitis. Haematuria would be more suggestive of a urinary tract infection. A normal temperature neither supports nor refutes the diagnosis. A positive pregnancy test would raise concerns about a possible ectopic pregnancy.

13.10. Answer: C.

The positive IgM is suggestive of early infection. False-positive IgM tests are possible, but a second positive test, in this case the TPPA, makes that unlikely. The low TPPA titre is compatible with very early infection. Although the chancre of primary syphilis is usually painless, this is not necessarily so for an anal chancre, so primary infection is most likely. The RPR would be strongly positive in secondary or early latent syphilis. In treated infection, the IgG EIA would remain positive, but the IgM would become negative.

13.11. Answer: E.

A rapid course of vaccination against hepatitis B – with inoculations today, and in 1 and 3 weeks' time – would give good protection against this infection that is more common in IDUs. PEP for HIV is only effective if given up to 72 hours following risk. Female to male sexual transmission of HCV is extremely rare. One week after exposure is too soon to rely upon negative tests for any STI. Negative tests for *Chlamydia* and gonorrhoea become reliable at 2 weeks, negative fourth-generation HIV tests become reliable at 4 weeks, and negative tests for HBV and HCV are reliable at 3 months. Azithromycin is only reliably curative for chlamydial infection, less so for syphilis and gonorrhoea, and would have no effect upon viruses such as HIV or HBV.

13.12. Answer: A.

Three of the four tests are positive, so this is not a false-positive scenario. The negative RPR is almost certainly false and represents a prozone phenomenon where the very high antibody titre prevents formation of the antibody–antigen lattice necessary to observe flocculation in the test. Diluting the serum will allow this to be observed. The strongly positive IgM test makes late infection extremely unlikely.

13.13. Answer: C.

Male to female transmission of Zika virus is described. Outbreaks of shigellosis and HAV are seen in MSM. CMV is shed in genital secretions. *Plasmodium vivax* (malaria) is not known to be sexually transmitted.

13.14. Answer: C.

Both HSV-1 and HSV-2 have a greater risk of causing disseminated disease in pregnancy, so it is important that she is counselled effectively to prevent acquisition. Symptomless shedding of virus can continue in the absence of clinical episodes, so there is a risk of transmission in this scenario. Valaciclovir has been shown to reduce HSV transmission in sero-discordant couples, is probably safe to take in pregnancy, but would be a suboptimal strategy. Caesarean section would only be considered if she developed primary infection around the time of delivery. Avoidance of sex or consistent condom use represents the safest strategy in this case.

A Mather, D Burnett,
DR Sullivan

14

Clinical biochemistry and metabolic medicine

Multiple Choice Questions

14.1. What is a particular advantage of obtaining a test analysis and result using a point-of-care test (POCT) system rather than using a traditional central laboratory?

A. POCT analysers often have a wider menu of available tests than central laboratories
B. POCTs avoid the need to use the laboratory or the medical records
C. POCTs provide test results at the time of seeing the patient
D. POCTs are generally cheaper than traditional testing
E. POCTs use newer technology and are generally more accurate and precise

14.2. Which of the following is an autosomal recessive Inherited disorder, often diagnosed through newborn screening programmes and treated with dietary modification, which can present with wide-ranging clinical manifestations, including vascular disorders, skin hypopigmentation, ectopia lentis, and disorders of the central nervous or skeletal systems?

A. Cystathionuria
B. Cystinosis
C. Cystinuria
D. Homocystinosis
E. Homocystinuria

14.3. There have been many different lysosomal storage diseases (LSDs) discovered, and some of these have been included in successful population-wide community genetic screening

programmes. What is the most common form of inheritance of these LSDs?

A. Autosomal dominant
B. Autosomal recessive
C. Multifactorial
D. X-linked dominant
E. X-linked recessive

14.4. In the investigation of glycogen storage diseases (glycogenoses), which of the following is a commonly used non-invasive test or finding that may be useful in diagnosing this condition?

A. Cataract in the lens of the eye
B. 'Cherry-red spot' in the fundus of the eye
C. Dislocated lens (ectopia lentis) in the eye
D. Exercise-induced fatigue or pain in muscles
E. Hypopigmentation of the skin

14.5. A 59 year old man presents for cardiovascular risk assessment, but he has not fasted for the blood collection that was to be performed during his appointment. Which of the following plasma lipid or lipoprotein levels is most likely to be affected by his recent consumption of food?

A. Calculated low-density lipoprotein (LDL) cholesterol
B. High-density lipoprotein (HDL) cholesterol
C. Lipoprotein (a)
D. Non-HDL cholesterol
E. Total cholesterol

14.6. The same 59 year old man returns with a set of fasting results that include: total cholesterol 6.7 mmol/L (259 mg/dL), fasting triglyceride 3.3 mmol/L (292 mg/dL), HDL cholesterol 0.9 mmol/L (35 mg/dL), calculated LDL cholesterol 4.3 mmol/L (166 mg/dL), non-HDL cholesterol 5.8 mmol/L (224 mg/dL) and fasting serum glucose 6.9 mmol/L (124 mg/dL). What is the best indicator of the metabolic component of his cardiovascular risk?

A. Calculated LDL cholesterol
B. Fasting plasma glucose
C. HDL cholesterol
D. Non-HDL cholesterol
E. Total cholesterol

14.7. The same 59 year old man fails to improve his lipid profile following diet and exercise advice, and pharmacological treatment is deemed necessary. Which of the following medications may have a detrimental effect on the triglyceride component of his lipid profile?

A. An anti-PCSK9 monoclonal antibody
B. Cholestyramine
C. Ezetimibe
D. Niacin
E. Rosuvastatin

14.8. The same 59 year old man commences atorvastatin 20 mg every evening. His follow-up lipid profile and glucose reveals: total cholesterol 3.7 mmol/L (143 mg/dL), fasting triglyceride 1.1 mmol/L (97 mg/dL), HDL cholesterol 1.1 mmol/L (42 mg/dL), calculated LDL cholesterol 2.1 mmol/L (81 mg/dL), non-HDL cholesterol 2.6 mmol/L (100 mg/dL) and fasting serum glucose 8.9 mmol/L (160 mg/dL). A subsequent glucose tolerance test is diagnostic of new-onset type 2 diabetes. What best describes the relationship between the onset of diabetes and the use of statins?

A. Diabetes development is more likely in those with pre-existing impaired fasting glucose
B. The development of diabetes is inconsistent with the fact that fasting triglyceride has improved
C. The development of diabetes is unrelated to the dose or potency of the statin
D. The development of diabetes means that statins are now contraindicated in that individual
E. The onset of diabetes and the use of statins are completely unrelated

14.9. A 57 year old man is having a blood test and the resident doctor finds it difficult to take

blood. When she receives the results she is worried that the test is inaccurate due to haemolysis of the cells whilst performing venepuncture. What is the dominant intracellular cation that may be inaccurately reported in this situation?

A. Bicarbonate
B. Calcium
C. Magnesium
D. Potassium
E. Sodium

14.10. One litre of normal saline is given to a patient in the emergency department. How is this fluid likely to be distributed between the fluid compartments?

A. Intracellular fluid 0 mL, extracellular fluid 1000 mL, plasma volume 1000 mL
B. Intracellular fluid 0 mL, extracellular fluid 1000 mL, plasma volume 200 mL
C. Intracellular fluid 1000 mL, extracellular fluid 0 mL, plasma volume 0 mL
D. Intracellular fluid 500 mL, extracellular fluid 500 mL, plasma volume 500 mL
E. Intracellular fluid 666 mL, extracellular fluid 334 mL, plasma volume 68 mL

14.11. In comparison to the ultrafiltrate found in Bowman's capsule, which of these terms best describes the filtrate that leaves the proximal tubule?

A. Hyperosmolar
B. Hypertonic
C. Hypo-osmolar
D. Hypotonic
E. Isotonic

14.12. Amino acids are almost entirely reabsorbed from the glomerular filtrate via active transport in which section of the nephron?

A. Collecting duct
B. Early distal tubule
C. Late distal tubule
D. Loop of Henle
E. Proximal tubule

14.13. A 35 year old man has been hiking in hot weather. He collapses and is brought into the emergency department. He is found to have a blood pressure of 95/62 mmHg with a postural drop of 15 mmHg. His pulse rate is 112 beats/min, his jugular venous pressure is not visible and he has a dry tongue. Which statement describes an element of his physiological response to this clinical scenario?

A. Increased atrial natiuretic peptide release
B. Increased catecholamine release
C. Increased glomerular filtration rate
D. Reduced renin release
E. Vasoconstriction of renal efferent arterioles

14.14. Which statement best explains why loop diuretics are the most effective at promoting salt and water excretion?

A. Vasopressin (antidiuretic hormone, ADH) acts on the ascending limb of the loop of Henle to increase water permeability
B. Loop diuretics block the triple co-transporter that prevent the reabsorption of potassium
C. The ascending limb of the loop of Henle is permeable to both water and sodium
D. The ascending limb of the loop of Henle is the last segment to reabsorb sodium
E. The sodium reabsorptive capacity of the segments distal to the ascending limb of the loop of Henle is limited

14.15. An 83 year old woman presents to the emergency department delirious and disorientated. She has a history of hypertension, treated with a thiazide diuretic. Her blood tests reveal the following: serum sodium 116 mmol/L; serum osmolality 239 mmol/kg; urinary osmolality 385 mmol/kg.

Which of the following abnormalities is responsible for her inability to maximally dilute her urine?

A. Abnormal function of the early distal tubule
B. Inadequate vasopressin in the circulation
C. Inadequate response of the collecting duct to vasopressin
D. Inadequate solute delivery to the early distal tubule
E. Inadequate solute delivery to the loop of Henle

14.16. A 67 year old man with hypertension and diabetes has chronic kidney disease with a stable serum creatinine of 267 μmol/L (3.02 mg/dL). Amongst other symptoms, he complains of nocturia. Which of the following abnormalities is responsible for his inability to maximally concentrate his urine?

A. Abnormal function of the early distal tubule
B. Excess vasopressin release into the circulation

C. Excess aldosterone release into the circulation
D. Inadequate solute delivery to the early distal tubule
E. Inadequate solute delivery to the loop of Henle

14.17. A 17 year old male presents to the emergency department with poorly controlled type 1 diabetes. He is found to be hyponatraemic with the following results: sodium 123 mmol/L and plasma glucose 35 mmol/L (630 mg/dL). Which one of the following is the most likely cause of the abnormal sodium reading?

A. Autoimmune hypothyroid disease
B. Hyperosmotic hyponatraemia secondary to hyperglycaemia
C. Hypoglycaemic agent-induced hyponatraemia
D. Loss of water in excess of sodium
E. Osmotic diuresis-induced hypovolaemic hyponatraemia

14.18. A 32 year old man who has been diagnosed with chronic schizophrenia lives with his mother and has been managing well in the community on stable medications for some time. An ambulance was called to the house when he started having seizures and his bloods on presentation to the emergency department are as follows: sodium 116 mmol/L; potassium 4.0 mmol/L; chloride 88 mmol/L; bicarbonate 20 mmol/L; urea 9 mmol/L (54 mg/dL); creatinine 66 μmol/L (0.75 mg/dL). His mother cannot recall any changes to his medications or in his behaviour but does comment that he has been drinking up to 8 L of water per day.

Which of the following results are most likely to be found on further investigation?

A. Serum osmolality 235 mmol/kg; urine osmolality 74 mmol/kg; urine sodium 24 mmol/L
B. Serum osmolality 262 mmol/kg; urine osmolality 112 mmol/kg; urine sodium 5 mmol/L
C. Serum osmolality 270 mmol/kg; urine osmolality 135 mmol/kg; urine sodium 42 mmol/L
D. Serum osmolality 290 mmol/kg; urine osmolality 84 mmol/kg; urine sodium 34 mmol/L
E. Serum osmolality 280 mmol/kg; urine osmolality 64 mmol/kg; urine sodium 44 mmol/L

14

14.19. In which one of the following clinical scenarios is urine sodium excretion likely to be less than 20 mmol/24 hrs?

A. Acute diarrhoea
B. Adrenal insufficiency
C. Hypothyroidism
D. Renal disease
E. Syndrome of inappropriate antidiuretic hormone (vasopressin) secretion (SIADH)

14.20. A 57 year old man with hypertension is found to have a tumour arising in the zona glomerulosa of the adrenal gland that leads to uncontrolled secretion of a hormone that is responsible for his hypertension.

Which of the following would you expect to decrease in this scenario?

A. Extracellular fluid volume
B. Plasma concentration of bicarbonate
C. Plasma concentration of potassium
D. Thyroid-stimulating hormone
E. Tubular reabsorption of sodium

14.21. A 12 year old boy is being investigated for fatigue. A physical examination, including blood pressure, is normal. Blood results show: sodium 135 mmol/L, potassium 3.1 mmol/L, bicarbonate 35 mmol/L; 24-hour urine results: potassium 245 mmol/24 hrs, calcium 12 mmol/24 hrs (N < 7.5).

What is the most likely diagnosis?

A. Bartter's syndrome
B. Gitelman's syndrome
C. Laxative abuse
D. Primary hyperaldosteronism
E. Type 1 renal tubular acidosis (RTA)

14.22. Metabolic acidosis is seen in conjunction with which cause of hypokalaemia?

A. Diarrhoea
B. Gitelman's syndrome
C. Loop diuretics
D. Primary hyperaldosteronism
E. Vomiting

14.23. Hypokalaemia may be seen in association with normal blood pressure in which of the following conditions?

A. Bartter's syndrome
B. Cushing's syndrome
C. Gordon's syndrome
D. Liddle's syndrome
E. Primary hyperaldosteronism

14.24. The amount of potassium excreted by the kidneys will decrease in which of the following situations?

A. When dietary intake of potassium increases
B. When distal tubule sodium delivery increases
C. When plasma aldosterone concentration increases
D. When the patient has acute metabolic acidosis
E. When the patient has respiratory alkalosis

14.25. A 42 year old patient has the following bloods. Arterial blood gases: H^+ 57.5 nmol/L (pH 7.24); PaO_2 11.1 kPa (83 mmHg); $PaCO_2$ 4.3 kPa (32 mmHg); bicarbonate 15 mmol/L. Serum biochemistry: sodium 134 mmol/L; potassium 2.4 mmol/L; chloride 109 mmol/L. Urine pH 5.2; following administration of intravenous sodium bicarbonate, urine pH is 5.8.

What is the likely underlying cause of these abnormalities?

A. Loop diuretic abuse
B. Thiazide diuretic abuse
C. Type 1 (distal) renal tubular acidosis
D. Type 2 (proximal) renal tubular acidosis
E. Type 4 renal tubular acidosis

14.26. A 38 year old man presents with a 1-week history of arthralgia, rash, haematuria and mild peripheral oedema. Blood tests taken in the emergency department show that his serum creatinine is 620 μmol/L (7.01 mg/dL).

What pattern of acid–base disorder is most likely to occur in this clinical scenario?

A. Metabolic acidosis with no respiratory compensation
B. Metabolic acidosis with respiratory compensation
C. Metabolic alkalosis with respiratory compensation
D. Respiratory acidosis with metabolic compensation
E. Respiratory alkalosis with metabolic compensation

14.27. A 42-year-old homeless man is brought into the emergency department. He is known to have a history of alcohol abuse and presents on this occasion with delirium, shortness of breath and blurred vision. Initial investigations show the following. Arterial blood gases (ABG): H^+ 58.9 nmol/L (pH 7.23); $PaCO_2$ 3.6 kPa (27 mmHg); bicarbonate 12 mmol/L. Blood results: sodium 130 mmol/L; potassium

4.3 mmol/L; urea 7.2 mmol/L (43 mg/dL); creatinine 113 μmol/L (1.28 mg/dL); chloride 97 mmol/L; glucose 4.2 mmol/L (76 mg/dL).
What is the most likely diagnosis?

A. Acute kidney injury
B. Diabetic ketoacidosis
C. Ethylene glycol ingestion
D. Methanol ingestion
E. Severe ethanol intoxication

14.28. Which of the following is the most important buffer in the blood?

A. Ammonia
B. Bicarbonate
C. Haemoglobin
D. Hydrogen phosphate
E. Proteins

14.29. A high school student is nervous about an upcoming exam and breathes rapidly with anxiety before fainting. If you were to take an ABG at this point, what would you most likely find?

A. High pH; high HCO_3^-, high PCO_2
B. High pH; normal HCO_3^-, low PCO_2
C. High pH; low HCO_3^-, low PCO_2
D. Low pH; high HCO_3^-, high PCO_2
E. Low pH; low HCO_3^-, high PCO_2

Answers

14.1. Answer: C.
The key advantage of POCT testing over central laboratory testing is that rapid availability of the result enables immediate medical decisions and actions. POCTs are generally more expensive than the equivalent test performed in a central laboratory. While POCT instruments often use new technology, the requirement for portability or miniaturisation may involve design or engineering compromises that result in less accuracy or precision than the equivalent standard laboratory test. Most POCT instruments are designed for a specific environment or group of tests, and so their menu is usually more restrictive than standard laboratory analysers. All laboratory and pathology results, including POCT, should always be recorded in the medical records.

14.2. Answer: E.
Homocystinuria is inherited in an autosomal recessive manner. It is most commonly caused by loss of function of the cystathionine β-synthase (*CBS*) gene. This affects the metabolism of the amino acid methionine and causes accumulation of the related amino acids homocysteine and methionine. It is often diagnosed through newborn screening programs. Dietary treatment is available, designed to correct the imbalance in the amino acids caused by the missing enzyme function.
    There is no condition called homocystinosis. This should not be confused with homocystinuria (see option E). Cystinuria is an aminoaciduria, inherited in an autosomal

recessive pattern. It is characterised by high concentrations of cysteine in the urine, leading to cysteine stone formation in the urinary tract. Cystinosis is a lysosomal storage disease and is also inherited in an autosomal recessive manner. There is accumulation of cystine within tissues. It is one of the causes of Fanconi's syndrome, in which there is abnormal renal tubular function. Cystathionuria (also called cystathionase deficiency) is also an autosomal recessive disorder, in which there is abnormal accumulation of plasma cystathionine, leading to increased urinary excretion. It is often considered to be a benign biochemical anomaly.

14.3. Answer: B.
Most lysosomal storage diseases exhibit an autosomal recessive pattern of inheritance, although a few can be X-linked recessive (e.g. Fabry's disease).

14.4. Answer: D.
Exercise-induced fatigue or pain in muscles is associated with several of the glycogenoses. An ischaemic lactate forearm test can be used as a clinical diagnostic test for some forms of glycogen storage disease. The cherry-red spot in the fundus is typically associated with Tay–Sachs disease, one of the inherited GM2 gangliosidoses. Hypopigmentation, ectopia lentis and cataracts can be associated with many conditions, some of which are inherited, but the glycogenoses are not typically part of this group.

14

14.5. Answer: A.
Calculated LDL cholesterol is correct because the calculation includes the triglyceride level, which increases following food consumption. The effect of food consumption on the other measurements is small by comparison, especially in relative terms.

14.6. Answer: D.
Non-HDL cholesterol is correct because it allows for the presence of small dense LDL and other atherogenic lipoproteins. This is particularly relevant in hypertriglyceridaemia, with or without accompanying elevation of fasting plasma glucose. It is more strongly associated with cardiovascular disease (CVD) in studies where comparison has been made with the other alternatives.

14.7. Answer: B.
Cholestyramine reduces recirculation of bile acids, down-regulates the farnesoid X receptor (FXR) and stimulates the replacement of the bile acids by conversion of cholesterol via 7 alpha-hydroxylase. The response to the down-regulation of FXR includes increased synthesis and secretion of triglyceride and very low-density lipoproteins (VLDLs). The other agents have neutral or favourable effects on triglyceride levels.

14.8. Answer: A.
Type 2 diabetes following statin therapy is likely in those with pre-existing impaired fasting glucose. It is proportional to the dose and potency of the statin, but the CVD benefit of the response clearly outweighs the CVD risk of the diabetes. Statins modestly improve triglyceride, even in the presence of diabetes.

14.9. Answer: D.
The dominant intracellular cation is potassium. If cells haemolyse during venepuncture, increased potassium will be released from the cells and a patient may be erroneously diagnosed with hyperkalaemia.

14.10. Answer: B.
Total body water is about one-third extracellular fluid (ECF) and two-thirds intracellular fluid. ECF is about one-fifth plasma and four-fifths interstitial fluid. Fluids that contain neither sodium nor protein (such as 5% dextrose) will distribute in all the body fluid compartments in proportion to the normal distribution of total body water, as in option E. Fluids that are rich in proteins (such as concentrated albumin) will remain in the plasma volume, as in option A. Normal saline distributes within only the extracellular compartment as in option B.

14.11. Answer: E.
In the proximal tubule, water reabsorption closely matches sodium reabsorption, meaning that the fluid that enters the loop of Henle is isotonic with the fluid that leaves the Bowman's capsule.

14.12. Answer: E.
The proximal tubule reabsorbs filtered sodium by coupling re-entry of sodium into the proximal tubular cell with amino acids as well as glucose, phosphate and other organic molecules.

14.13. Answer: B.
This man has hypovolaemia and sodium depletion as evidenced by his symptoms and signs on presentation. The kidneys respond to this scenario by activating mechanisms that will increase sodium reabsorption, thereby restoring sodium and fluid balance. Mechanisms that will increase sodium reabsorption include increased catecholamine release and increased renin release. In order to restrict fluid loses the kidneys will reduce glomerular filtration rate in part by vasoconstriction of renal afferent arterioles.

14.14. Answer: E.
Loop diuretics inhibit the Na,K,2Cl triple co-transporter in the ascending limb of the loop of Henle and are the most effective diuretics as this transporter reabsorbs about 25% of the sodium load. More distal reabsorption by the sodium–chloride transporter in the distal tubule only accounts for about 5% of sodium reabsorption and increased delivery to this segment when using a loop diuretic overwhelms the reabsorptive capacity of that transporter. Option C is incorrect as the ascending limb is permeable only to sodium; the triple co-transporter does transport potassium as in option B, but this is not relevant to the diuretic effect; in option D, the ascending limb of the loop of Henle is not the last segment to reabsorb sodium, as outlined above; and in option A, vasopressin acts on the collecting ducts to increase water permeability.

14.15. Answer: A.

In order to maximally dilute urine, there needs to be normal function of both the loop of Henle and the early distal tubule. Thiazide diuretics inhibit the normal function of the early distal tubule by blocking the sodium–chloride co-transporter. An inability to maximally dilute urine can also result from options D and E but this is not the mechanism of thiazide diuretics. Absence of vasopressin is required for maximal dilution of the urine.

14.16. Answer: E.

Chronic kidney disease results in poor solute delivery to the loop of Henle causing a failure to generate the medullary concentration gradient. Adequate solute delivery to and function of the early distal tubule is required for maximal dilution of urine but not concentration. Failure of vasopressin effect, either through inadequate release or blunted action at the level of the collecting duct (rather than excess vasopressin), contributes to poor urinary concentration.

14.17. Answer: B.

Hyperglycaemia causes osmotic shifts of water from the intracellular to the extracellular space, causing a relative dilutional hyponatraemia. The serum sodium corrects to 131 mmol/L when using the correction factor of 1.6 mmol/L for every 5.5 mmol/L increase in serum glucose. The other causes of hyponatraemia are possible but would result in a genuine reduction in sodium concentration and option D would cause hypernatraemia.

14.18. Answer: A.

These results are consistent with primary polydipsia which is the likely diagnosis here. The serum osmolality is low, confirming hypotonic hyponatraemia and the urinary osmolality is also low suggesting relative excess water intake. Option B, which demonstrates low urinary sodium, is seen in patients with low effective arterial volume due to either extrarenal losses or hypervolaemic states. The high urinary sodium and osmolality seen in option C is consistent with SIADH or renal sodium loss. Option D is consistent with hyperosmotic hyponatraemia, as seen in hyperglycaemia, and option E suggests isosmotic hyponatraemia such as with hyperlipidaemia.

14.19. Answer: A.

Acute diarrhoea would result in extrarenal sodium and water loss and the normal renal response of sodium conservation. In the other scenarios urine sodium would be high or normal due to effects of limited sodium reabsorption in the nephron secondary to vasopressin, or lack of cortisol/thyroxine response.

14.20. Answer: C.

Aldosterone is produced in the zona glomerulosa of the adrenal gland and acts on the mineralocorticoid receptors in the distal tubules and collecting ducts of the nephron. It acts to reabsorb sodium and excrete potassium. In excessive quantities, such as in Conn's syndrome as described here, it causes hypertension and hypokalaemia.

14.21. Answer: A.

Metabolic alkalosis associated with hypokalaemia and urinary potassium wasting is typical of diuretic use, or in this case Bartter's syndrome, which mimics loop diuretic use. Gitelman's or thiazide diuretics would also present like this, but are associated with low, not high, urinary calcium. Laxative abuse would be associated with renal conservation of potassium and therefore low urinary potassium level. Primary hyperaldosteronism is associated with hypertension and RTA with acidosis.

14.22. Answer: A.

Loop and thiazide diuretics, Bartter's syndrome and Gitelman's syndrome, and primary hyperaldosteronism are all associated with metabolic alkalosis. As outlined in Fig. 14.22, vomiting is also associated with metabolic alkalosis while diarrhoea causes loss of bicarbonate thereby resulting in a normal anion gap acidosis.

14.23. Answer: A.

Answers B–E are associated with hypertension while Bartter's syndrome is associated with low or normal blood pressure readings.

14.24. Answer: D.

A number of factors alter potassium secretion in the distal nephron segments. Increased distal sodium delivery and increased plasma aldosterone concentration will result in greater luminal sodium entry through epithelial sodium channels, thereby increasing potassium

14

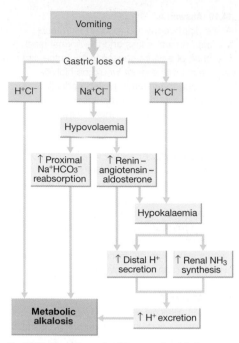

Fig. 14.22 Generation and maintenance of metabolic alkalosis during prolonged vomiting. Loss of HCl⁻ generates metabolic alkalosis, which is maintained by renal changes.

secretion. Acid–base disturbances have complex effects on renal potassium excretion. Alkalosis is generally associated with increased potassium secretion while acute metabolic acidosis is associated with reduced renal potassium excretion. However, over time, acidosis will cause an increase in distal sodium delivery and an increase in aldosterone production that will result in an increase in potassium secretion.

14.25. Answer: D.
The patient has a metabolic acidosis with a low pH, low bicarbonate and compensatory low $PaCO_2$. Acidosis with a low potassium, makes type 1 or 2 renal tubular acidosis (RTA) the only possible answers. Type 4 renal tubular acidosis would be associated with hyperkalaemia and diuretic abuse is associated with metabolic alkalosis. The urine pH is initially normal, but becomes alkalotic when bicarbonate is administered. This is consistent with poor

bicarbonate reabsorption, which makes type 2 (proximal) RTA the most likely diagnosis.

14.26. Answer: B.
Acute kidney injury as seen in this patient with nephritic syndrome is associated with metabolic acidosis with respiratory compensation.

14.27. Answer: D.
Looking first at the ABG, there is a low pH suggesting an acidosis. Bicarbonate and carbon dioxide are both low, consistent with a metabolic acidosis with respiratory compensation. The anion gap = $(Na^+ + K^+) - (Cl^- - HCO_3^-)$ is 23, which is high. This indicates the presence of unmeasured anions. A high anion gap acidosis is commonly caused by an endogenous acid load as seen in diabetic ketoacidosis or kidney injury, but in this patient the absence of hyperglycaemia or significant renal impairment make these diagnoses unlikely. Other causes of an increased anion gap acidosis are related to exogenous acid loads from poisoning. Methanol poisoning typically presents with visual impairment and in severe cases results in permanent blindness.

14.28. Answer: B.
As outlined in the above questions, the most important buffer system in blood and tissues involves the reaction of hydrogen ions (H⁺) with bicarbonate (HCO_3^-) to form carbonic acid (H_2CO_3) and ultimately CO_2 and H_2O. Hydrogen phosphate (HPO_4) and ammonia are important urinary buffers that associate with H⁺ ions secreted into the luminal space, thereby reducing luminal H⁺ concentration and allowing for continued acid secretion.

14.29. Answer: C.
The student would have a respiratory alkalosis, best represented by option C. Given the acute nature of the respiratory alkalosis, a small change in bicarbonate concentration occurs, but if respiratory alkalosis persists over days to weeks, the kidneys would have time to make adjustments to acid secretion and produce further compensation and reduction in HCO_3^- concentration.

B Conway, P Phelan,
GD Stewart

15

Nephrology and urology

Multiple Choice Questions

15.1. A 45 year old man presents with a 6-week history of bilateral ankle swelling. On examination his pulse was 72 beats/min, blood pressure (BP) 126/68 mmHg, jugular venous pressure (JVP) was not elevated and auscultation of heart and lungs was unremarkable. He had no stigmata of chronic liver disease. Which of the following is the most appropriate initial investigation?

A. Abdominal ultrasound scan
B. D-dimer
C. Echocardiogram
D. Urinalysis
E. Urinary sodium

15.2. A 72 year old man is found to have acute kidney injury (AKI). Urine microscopy reveals the presence of red cell casts. What is the most likely aetiology of his renal failure?

A. Acute tubular necrosis
B. Haemolytic uraemic syndrome
C. Microscopic polyangiitis
D. Sclerodermic renal crisis
E. Tubulointerstitial nephritis

15.3. Which of the following is maintained in the circulation when transiting through the kidney and not freely filtered across the normal glomerular filtration barrier?

A. Free light chains
B. Glucose
C. Glutamine
D. Immunoglobulin A (IgA)
E. Lithium

15.4. The following subjects all have a Modification of Diet in Renal Disease (MDRD)

formula-derived estimated glomerular filtration rate (eGFR) of 40 mL/min/1.73 m^2. Which person below is likely to have the lowest measured (true) glomerular filtration rate (i.e. the eGFR is falsely reassuring)?

A. A 25 year old male body builder
B. A 40 year old African American man with hypertension
C. A 45 year old woman currently taking trimethoprim for a urinary tract infection
D. A 56 year old man with type 2 diabetes and an above-knee amputation
E. An 85 year old woman with hypertension and type 2 diabetes

15.5. A 46 year old man with a 10-year history of type 2 diabetes presents with a 6-week history of bilateral leg swelling. He reports that he had been taking non-steroidal anti-inflammatory drugs (NSAIDs) for osteoarthritis regularly for the past 3 months. Investigations reveal: eGFR >60 mL/min/ 1.73 m^2; urinalysis: protein 4+, blood negative; protein : creatinine ratio 1680 mg/mmol; and a serum albumin of 14 g/L. Serum albumin and urinary albumin : creatinine ratios 4 months previously were 36 g/L and 25 mg/mmol, respectively. What is the most likely diagnosis?

A. Amyloidosis
B. Diabetic nephropathy
C. IgA nephropathy
D. Minimal change disease
E. Tubulointerstitial nephritis

15.6. A 25 year old man presents with visible haematuria. He reports that he had a very sore throat 2 weeks previously, but is otherwise well.

His blood pressure and renal function are both normal. Protein:creatinine ratio was elevated (100 mg/mmol). What is the most likely diagnosis?

A. Bladder cancer
B. IgA nephropathy
C. Polycystic kidney disease (PKD)
D. Post-infectious glomerulonephritis
E. Renal calculus

15.7. A 69 year old man is diagnosed with streptococcal endocarditis and commenced on benzylpenicillin and gentamicin. His renal function is normal on admission, but 1 week later it has deteriorated (eGFR 28 mL/min/1.73 m^2). Investigations reveal: urinalysis: blood 3+, protein 3+; ultrasound scan: normal-sized kidneys with no hydronephrosis; serum complement level (C3 and C4) is low. What is the most likely diagnosis?

A. Acute interstitial nephritis
B. Acute tubular necrosis
C. Infection-related glomerulonephritis
D. Microscopic polyangiitis
E. Pre-renal failure

15.8. A 76 year old woman attends her family physician complaining of bilateral leg swelling and vague aches and pains. Initial investigations reveal: urinalysis: protein 4+, trace blood; haemoglobin 79 g/L; white cell count 1.9×10^9/L; platelet count 46×10^9/L; sodium 131 mmol/L; potassium 4.6 mmol/L; urea 15 mmol/L (90.1 mg/dL, BUN 42.0 mg/dL); creatinine 176 µmol/L (1.99 mg/dL); albumin 23 g/L. What is the most likely finding on renal biopsy?

A. Amyloidosis
B. Cast nephropathy
C. Interstitial nephritis
D. Minimal change disease
E. Thrombotic thrombocytopenic purpura (TTP)

15.9. A 49 year old male presents with deafness, shortness of breath, haemoptysis, reduced urinary output and ankle swelling. On examination: BP is 170/100 mmHg; JVP is 4 cm above the sternal angle, there are bibasal crepitations in the lungs and he has bilateral leg swelling to the mid-calves. Initial investigations reveal: haemoglobin 92 g/L, white cell count 9×10^9/L; platelet count 460×10^9/L; sodium 142 mmol/L; potassium 6.8 mmol/L; urea 45 mmol/L (270 mg/dL); creatinine 1260 µmol/L (14.25 mg/dL); albumin 32 g/L. Chest X-ray: bi-basal air space shadowing; ultrasound: normal-sized kidneys, no evidence of hydronephrosis. No urine is available for urinalysis. What is the most appropriate initial investigation from the list below?

A. Anti-glomerular basement membrane (GBM)/antineutrophil cytoplasmic antibody (ANCA)/antinuclear antibody (ANA) serology
B. Computed tomography (CT) pulmonary angiography
C. Genetic testing for Alport's disease
D. Plasma protein electrophoresis
E. Renal biopsy

15.10. A 32 year old man is referred to the nephrology clinic for investigation of persistent non-visible haematuria initially detected at an insurance medical examination. He is otherwise well, with no personal or family history of renal disease. His BP is 126/68 mmHg. Preliminary investigations reveal: urinalysis: blood 3+, protein negative; creatinine 100 µmol/L (1.13 mg/dL); eGFR >60 mL/min/1.73 m^2. What is the most likely diagnosis?

A. Alport's disease
B. Bladder tumour
C. IgA nephropathy
D. Membranous nephropathy
E. Vesico-ureteric reflux

15.11. A 75 year old woman has peripheral vascular disease and stage 3 CKD with proteinuria due to IgA nephropathy. Her BP is 136/80 mmHg on lisinopril 40 mg, amlodipine 10 mg and bendroflumethiazide 2.5 mg (all once daily). Her renal function has been relatively stable over the past 2 years with current eGFR 39 mL/min/1.73 m^2. Ultrasound scan revealed that her left kidney length at 9 cm was smaller than the right kidney at 11.5 cm. Magnetic resonance angiography confirmed a 90% stenosis at the ostium of the left renal artery. What is the most appropriate management from the list below?

A. Check plasma renin activity
B. Commence a statin
C. Discontinue lisinopril
D. Perform angiography and stenting to her left renal artery
E. Start warfarin

15.12. A 62 year old man presents with a large myocardial infarction and undergoes primary coronary angiography and stenting. Two days later he develops a low-grade fever and dusky discolouration of the toes on both feet, although peripheral pulses are palpable. eGFR was 52 mL/min/1.73 m^2 pre-procedure and falls to 25 mL/min/1.73 m² 2 days later. Other investigations reveal: urinalysis: blood 1+, protein 1+; haemoglobin 12 g/L; white cell count 10.6×10⁹/L with eosinophilia; platelet count 70×10⁹/L. Creatine kinase is elevated at 640 U/L. What is the most likely cause of his acute kidney injury?

A. Cholesterol embolisation
B. Contrast nephropathy
C. Haemolytic uraemic syndrome
D. Renal artery thrombosis
E. Rhabdomyolysis

15.13. A 17 year old male returns from an Outward Bound centre holiday and falls ill with vomiting and bloody diarrhoea. His acute illness subsides, but 3 days later he notices that his urinary output has declined and his ankles begin to swell. He attends his family physician where his temperature is 38.2°C, BP is 164/92 mmHg and he has bilateral ankle oedema, but no other clinical signs. The following investigation results are obtained: urea 36 mmol/L (216 mg/dL); creatinine 640 μmol/L (7.24 mg/dL); sodium 129 mmol/L; potassium 6.4 mmol/L; haemoglobin 64 g/L; white cell count 9.6×10⁹/L; platelet count 36×10⁹/L; blood film shows schistocytes; urinalysis: blood 1+, protein negative; stool cultures negative for *Escherichia coli* O157. What is the most likely diagnosis?

A. Haemolytic uraemic syndrome
B. Lupus nephritis
C. Malignant hypertension
D. Pre-renal failure
E. Thrombotic thrombocytopenic purpura

15.14. A 60 year old man with long-standing stage 4 chronic kidney disease presents with vague bony pain. Blood tests reveal eGFR 17 mL/min/1.73 m²; calcium 2.92 mmol/L (11.70 mg/dL); phosphate 1.82 mmol/L (5.64 mg/dL), parathyroid hormone (PTH) is elevated at 156 pmol/L (1471 pg/mL), alkaline phosphatase 470 U/L. What is this picture consistent with?

A. Excess vitamin D consumption
B. Milk alkali syndrome
C. Primary hyperparathyroidism
D. Secondary hyperparathyroidism
E. Tertiary hyperparathyroidism

15.15. A 62 year old man with stage 3 CKD (eGFR 39 mL/min/1.73 m²) is noted to have haemoglobin of 79 g/L, white cell count 8.9×10⁹/L; platelet count 146×10⁹/L; mean corpuscular volume (MCV) 76 fL. What is the most appropriate investigation?

A. Bone marrow biopsy
B. Serum erythropoeitin level
C. Serum folate studies
D. Serum iron studies
E. Ultrasound scan of abdomen

15.16. The Reciprocal creatinine plot shown of a 48 year old man would be consistent with the natural history of progression of which of the following causes of kidney failure?

15

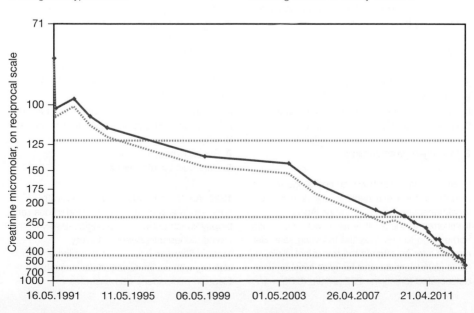

A. Adult polycystic kidney disease
B. Microscopic polyangiitis
C. Multiple myeloma
D. Post-infectious glomerulonephritis
E. Renovascular disease

15.17. A 42 year old woman with IgA nephropathy and stage 3 CKD (eGFR 45 mL/min/1.73 m^2) is developing proteinuria (protein:creatinine ratio is 120 mg/mmol). BP is 158/86 mmHg and she is commenced on an ACE inhibitor (lisinopril 10 mg daily). Two weeks later her eGFR has fallen to 37 mL/min/1.73 m^2 and her potassium has risen from 5.2 to 5.9 mmol/L, although BP and protein:creatinine ratio have fallen to 146/82 mmHg and 30 mg/mmol, respectively. She is already on a low-potassium diet. What is the most appropriate management?

A. Add a thiazide diuretic
B. Add a β-adrenoceptor antagonist (β-blocker)
C. Commence calcium resonium
D. Increase the lisinopril dose
E. Stop the lisinopril

15.18. Which of the following is true regarding peritoneal dialysis?

A. Fluid removal is achieved by increasing the concentration of sodium in the dialysate
B. Hyperkalaemia is less common than for haemodialysis
C. It is associated with improved patient survival compared with haemodialysis
D. It is unsuitable for elderly patients
E. Peritonitis is usually caused by gut bacteria traversing the bowel wall

15.19. Which of the following is typical of the development of pre-eclampsia?

A. Low serum urate level
B. Maternal history of cigarette smoking
C. Occurrence in the mother's first pregnancy
D. Onset of hypertension in the second trimester
E. Prolonged prothrombin time

15.20. A 14 year old boy with end-stage renal disease due to reflux nephropathy received a renal transplant from his mother. Aged 17 he transferred to the adult renal service and he left home to go to university the following year. Six months later he attends the transplant clinic. He is asymptomatic, but his graft function has deteriorated (creatinine 297 μmol/L (3.36 mg/dL), increased from 126 μmol/L (1.43 mg/dL) 3 months previously). Urinalysis: blood 1+, protein 2+, no leucocytes; ultrasound scan of graft revealed no hydronephrosis. What is the most likely explanation for the deterioration in renal function?

A. Acute pyelonephritis
B. Acute rejection due to non-adherence with immunosuppression
C. Anti-glomerular basement membrane disease
D. Chronic allograft injury
E. Thrombosis in the artery to the graft

15.21. A previously fit 17 year old male presents with a 2- to 3-week history of arthralgia and more recently has developed a skin rash on the lower legs. Just prior to admission to hospital he developed abdominal discomfort with blood-stained stool. On examination, he has a widespread non-blanching rash over his limbs. Initial investigations reveal: urinalysis: blood 3+; protein 3+; eGFR 46 mL/min/1,73 m^2; protein:creatinine ratio 220 mg/mmol; haemoglobin 120 g/L, white cell count 12.9×10^9/L; platelet count 259×10^9/L; C-reactive protein 62 mg/L. What is the most likely diagnosis?

A. Anti-glomerular basement membrane disease
B. Haemolytic uraemic syndrome
C. Henoch–Schönlein purpura
D. Post-streptococcal glomerulonephritis
E. Systemic lupus erythematosus

15.22. A 62 year old man presents with sudden anuria on a background history of several weeks of 'not passing much urine'. He denies dysuria or haematuria but admits to having a poor stream for many years. He is normotensive and otherwise looks well and has no systemic symptoms. What is the best initial diagnostic investigation?

A. Blood test for electrolytes and renal function
B. CT of kidneys and urinary tract with contrast
C. Renal biopsy
D. Renal ultrasound scan
E. Urinalysis for red cell casts

15.23. An 18 year old male presents with haematuria and proteinuria. He undergoes renal biopsy which shows a mesangiocapillary glomerulonephritis pattern of injury. Immunofluorescence shows complement C3 staining with no immunoglobulin deposition. Electron microscopy demonstrates electron-dense deposits in a ribbon-like pattern in the glomerular basement membrane (so called 'dense deposits'). What is the most likely underlying cause of his mesangiocapillary glomerulonephritis?

A. Autoimmune disease
B. Genetic defect of alternative complement pathway
C. Hepatitis B infection
D. Hepatitis C infection
E. Monoclonal gammopathy

15.24. A 49 year old woman presents with acute kidney injury after an acute illness manifested by myalgia, diarrhoea and vomiting. Her BP is 84/50 mmHg and she has dry mucous membranes. She was taking ibuprofen, paracetamol and domperidone during the illness. Her renal function improves rapidly with intravenous (IV) fluids. Which one of the following findings are likely to be present?

A. Dense granular ('muddy brown') casts on urinalysis
B. Hypercalcaemia
C. Hyponatraemia
D. Low (<1%) fractional excretion of sodium
E. Low urine specific gravity

15.25. A 68 year woman develops malaise and a low-grade fever. She has no rash and appears euvolaemic. She takes atorvastatin, omeprazole, amlodipine and digoxin regularly and takes ibuprofen intermittently. Urinalysis shows some leucocytes but no casts, haematuria or proteinuria. She has a creatinine of 320 μmol/L (3.62 mg/dL), which has been 68 μmol/L (0.77 mg/dL) 1 year previously. What is the likely cause of renal injury?

A. Acute interstitial nephritis
B. ATN due to rhabdomyolysis
C. Glomerulonephritis
D. Pre-renal injury due to NSAIDs
E. Urinary obstruction

15.26. A 55 year old man with significant cardiovascular disease and diabetes has acute kidney injury in the context of a viral illness. He was at a social gathering where he consumed alcohol and woke the next morning unwell. He had fever, aches and pains, headache and felt thirsty. He takes atorvastatin, lansoprazole, amlodipine, bisoprolol, warfarin, digoxin regularly. He passed a small amount of dark urine. His creatinine is 190 μmol/L (2.15 mg/

dL), potassium 6.8 mmol/L, corrected calcium 1.97 mmol/L (7.90 mg/dL), international normalised ratio (INR) 2.0. Urine dipstick shows haematuria but no proteinuria. Direct urinalysis revealed no cells or casts. What is the likely cause of his kidney injury?

A. Acute interstitial nephritis
B. ATN due to viral infection
C. Haemorrhage into the kidneys
D. Pre-renal injury due to dehydration from alcohol
E. Rhabdomyolysis

15.27. A patient with acute kidney injury has been anuric for 12 hours despite fluid challenges. Potassium is 5.2 mmol/L, urea is very high and a pericardial rub is audible. The patient appears euvolaemic. A decision is made to commence haemodialysis due to concerns regarding uraemia and specifically uraemic pericarditis. What will the first dialysis session involve?

A. A large surface area dialyser
B. A short 2-hour session initially
C. Heparin anticoagulation
D. High blood flow rate of 400 mL/min
E. Ultrafiltration of 2 L (fluid removal)

15.28. In a patient presenting with renal impairment, which of the following is most helpful in discriminating between AKI and a late presentation of CKD?

A. Anaemia
B. Hyperphosphataemia
C. Hyponatraemia
D. Renal biopsy showing interstitial fibrosis and tubular atrophy
E. Small echogenic kidneys on ultrasound

15.29. A 32 year old man with IgA nephropathy since the age of 18 received a well human leucocyte antigen (HLA)-matched kidney transplant from his older brother. He had no pre-formed anti-HLA antibodies and the kidney functioned immediately. One week later his urine output is noted to be lower than the previous days and his creatinine is increased, having previously dropped to normal in the first few days post-transplant. His BP is 180/90 mmHg, he has dipstick-positive blood on urinalysis and he looks euvolaemic. What is the likely diagnosis?

A. Acute cellular rejection
B. BK polyomavirus nephropathy

15

C. Hyperacute rejection

D. Recurrent IgA nephropathy

E. Renal artery stenosis

15.30. A 56 year old woman with polycystic kidney disease received her second kidney transplant. She had pre-formed anti-HLA antibodies (from the first transplant) but the cross-match was negative so she proceeded to transplant using induction therapy (anti-thymocyte globulin; ATG). She had immediate function of the transplant but suffered an acute rejection after 2 months, which was successfully treated with IV glucocorticoids. She developed a urinary tract infection (UTI) in the week after the steroids were administered, which cleared with oral antibiotics. Her renal function has deteriorated again at 4 months and her serum shows BK polyomavirus on polymerase chain reaction testing. A biopsy reveals BK polyomavirus nephropathy. Risk factors for BK polyomavirus include which of the following?

A. Augmented immunosuppression (ATG and high-dose steroids)

B. Polycystic kidney disease

C. Presence of anti-HLA antibodies

D. Previous UTI

E. Second transplant

15.31. What is the pathogenesis of 'myeloma kidney' (cast nephropathy)?

A. Glomerular light chain deposition due to light chains, and rarely heavy chains, often giving a nodular pattern of injury

B. Light chain misfolding, creating glomerular deposits that are Congo red positive

C. Light chains precipitating with Tamm–Horsfall protein in the tubular lumen

D. Proximal tubular injury and dysfunction due to light chain deposition in tubular epithelial cells

E. Tubular damage due to hypercalcaemia

15.32. A patient with known sarcoidosis has developed renal impairment over the past 2 months. Corrected serum calcium is slightly high (2.7 mmol/L; 10.82 mg/dL). A renal biopsy is performed and glucocorticoids are commenced. Renal function gradually normalised over a period of several weeks. What would the likely initial renal biopsy findings show?

A. A granulomatous interstitial nephritis

B. Calcium deposition in the tubules

C. Focal segmental glomerulosclerosis (FSGS)

D. Necrotising cresentic glomerulonephritis

E. Widespread interstitial fibrosis and tubular atrophy

15.33. Patients with advanced liver disease are at risk of developing AKI, termed hepatorenal syndrome. Which of the following is true of this syndrome?

A. Aggressive dialysis may prevent hepatic encephalopathy

B. IgA deposition is a common cause

C. Kidney biopsy should be performed for an accurate diagnosis

D. Outcomes are good with haemodialysis

E. The aetiology is haemodynamically mediated, so urine sodium will be reduced

15.34. Which of the following is true in diabetic nephropathy?

A. ACE inhibitors generally cause resolution of proteinuria and stabilisation of renal function

B. Biopsy is generally needed to confirm the diagnosis

C. It is an uncommon cause of end-stage renal disease (ESRD) outside of North America

D. Sodium–glucose co-transporter-2 (SGLT2) inhibitors, such as empagliflozin, may be associated with improved cardiovascular and renal outcomes and work by improving insulin sensitivity

E. The natural history is of slow development of microalbuminuria over years, with overt proteinuria and renal impairment at a late stage

15.35. A 23 year woman presents with a facial rash and arthralgia soon after getting married. She is found to have an eGFR of 106 mL/min/1.73 m^2, red cell casts in her urine and 5.5 g/24 hrs of proteinuria. Renal biopsy confirms lupus nephritis. Which of the following is true in this patient?

A. Best treatment for this patient is with cyclophosphamide and glucocorticoids

B. Mycophenolate mofetil would be the induction agent of choice, along with glucocorticoids

C. She probably has mild lupus nephritis that can be managed with an ACE inhibitor alone

D. She should be referred immediately to the transplant team

E. She would be at high risk for recurrence after a renal transplant causing allograft loss

15.36. A 42 year old woman from China presents with slowly progressive renal failure in the context of taking herbal remedies for years containing aristolochic acid. Which of the following clinical characteristics is likely in this patient?

A. Biopsy demonstrating focal segmental glomerulosclerosis

B. Bland urine sediment with interstitial fibrosis on biopsy

C. Heavy proteinuria in the nephrotic range

D. High anion gap metabolic acidosis

E. Large kidneys on ultrasound scanning

15.37. A 22 year old man develops diabetes and is found to have renal impairment with small kidneys on scanning, in addition to noted pancreatic atrophy. He has a history of gout for 2 years and his father developed ESRD aged 38. His father also had 'renal failure' due to cystic disease and has diabetes. A mutation in which gene is likely?

A. COL4A5

B. HNF1-beta

C. PKD1

D. PKD2

E. UMOD

15.38. In patients with Alport's syndrome (hereditary nephritis), which of the following statements is true?

A. After kidney transplant, patients may develop anti-GBM disease

B. All patients harbouring pathogenic COL4A mutations develop progressive chronic kidney disease

C. Deafness may occur due to otosclerosis

D. Female carriers of X-linked disease (COL4A5 mutations) do not manifest disease

E. It is always an X-linked condition

15.39. A 20 year old woman has a history of autosomal dominant polycystic kidney disease (APKD) on her father's side. Her paternal grandmother and her father's brother both died suddenly in their 50s. What was the likely cause of death?

A. Mitral valve prolapse

B. Myocardial infarction

C. Pulmonary embolism

D. Ruptured berry aneurysm

E. Ruptured hepatic cyst

15.40. A 65 year man presents with flank discomfort and haematuria. He is found to have bilateral polycystic kidneys and some liver cysts on ultrasound scan. His renal function is normal, with an eGFR of 90 mL/min/1.73 m^2. He gives a family history on his mother's side of 'cysts in the kidney' but no family member ever needed dialysis or a transplant. Which of the following is true about his disease?

A. Any offspring have a 50% chance of developing the condition

B. He is a good candidate for tolvaptan to slow cyst growth

C. He is at high risk of liver failure due to a polycystic liver

D. He probably has a mutation in PKD1

E. He will probably develop end-stage renal disease within 5 years

15.41. A 75 year old man with hypertension, heart failure, peptic ulcer disease and osteoarthritis presents with acute kidney injury after being prescribed ibuprofen. His usual medicines are lisinopril, furosemide, omeprazole and atorvastatin. He has 1+ proteinuria and no haematuria on dipstick. What is the mechanism underlying his renal failure?

A. Afferent arteriolar vasoconstriction with ibuprofen (in context of efferent vasodilatation with lisinopril)

B. Afferent arteriolar vasoconstriction with lisinopril (in context of efferent vasodilatation with ibuprofen)

C. Afferent arteriolar vasodilatation with ibuprofen (in context of efferent vasoconstriction with lisinopril)

D. Afferent arteriolar vasodilatation with lisinopril (in context of efferent vasoconstriction with ibuprofen)

E. Rhabdomyolysis from the statin

15.42. A 64 year old man has osteoarthritis in his knees and is prescribed ibuprofen regularly for 3 months. He notices some swelling in his ankles and his family physician finds his urine dipstick reveals 4+ protein with no blood or white cells. His creatinine is normal and his serum albumin is 190 g/L. A renal biopsy is performed. What is the light microscopy likely to reveal?

A. Fibrin microthrombi in glomerular capillary loops

15

B. Intense interstitial inflammation, with infiltration of the tubules by neutrophils, lymphocytes and some eosinophils
C. Necrotising cresentic glomerulonephritis
D. Normal glomeruli
E. Tubular dilatation, breaks in the tubular basement membrane, interstitial oedema and sloughing of necrotic tubular cells into the tubular lumen

15.43. Regarding micturition, which of these statements is correct?

A. A low-compliance bladder is required for voiding to be initiated
B. Contraction of the pelvic floor commences micturition
C. Micturition is initiated when the compliance limit of the bladder is reached
D. Voiding is controlled by the cerebellum
E. Voiding is coordinated by the pontine micturition centre

15.44. What is the optimal imaging to rule out bone metastases in a man with prostate cancer?

A. Contrast-enhanced CT urogram
B. Dimercaptosuccinic acid (DMSA) static radionuclide scan
C. Non-contrast CT of kidneys, ureters and bladder (CTKUB)
D. Pelvic magnetic resonance imaging (MRI) scan
E. Technetium-labelled methylene diphosphonate (^{99m}Tc-MDP) radionuclide scan

15.45. A 25 year old woman from Uganda who has recently delivered a baby presents with new continuous incontinence. What is she likely to be suffering with?

A. Duplex kidney with insertion of upper pole moiety into the vagina
B. Overflow incontinence
C. Stress urinary incontinence
D. Urge incontinence
E. Vesicovaginal fistula

15.46. What is the most likely cause of painless, visible haematuria in a 60 year old man?

A. Ureteric stone
B. Bladder cancer
C. IgA nephropathy
D. Systemic lupus erythematosus
E. Upper urinary tract urothelial cancer

15.47. A 27 year old woman presents as an emergency with rigors, flank pain and fever. Non-contrast CTKUB reveals an 8-mm stone in the left mid-ureter. Which is the optimal management option?

A. Extracorporeal shockwave lithotripsy (ESWL)
B. Percutaneous nephrolithotomy (PCNL)
C. Ureteric stent insertion
D. Ureterolysis
E. Ureteroscopy and laser fragmentation of stone

15.48. In which of the following situations would you consider treating an asymptomatic patient identified to have $>10^5$ E. coli/mL urine?

A. Healthy 14 year old girl
B. 24 year old woman, normal ultrasound and flexible cystoscopy in the past
C. 32 year old pregnant woman
D. 67 year old man with a urethral catheter in situ
E. 78 year old woman with a ureteric stent in place for retroperitoneal fibrosis

15.49. Following a trial of treatment with α-adrenoceptor antagonist (α-blocker) medication, a 65 year old man is referred by his family physician to urology with poor flow, terminal dribbling and hesitancy. Which of the following is the most relevant investigation?

A. Cystoscopy
B. MRI pelvis
C. Prostate biopsy
D. Ultrasound prostate
E. Urinary flow test

15.50. A 49 year old woman presents with visible haematuria. A cystoscopy is normal, but a contract-enhanced CT scan of chest, abdomen, pelvis reveals a 17-cm left renal mass, consistent with a renal cell cancer. What is the best treatment option for this woman?

A. Cryotherapy
B. External beam radiotherapy
C. Open radical nephrectomy
D. Robotic partial nephrectomy
E. Tyrosine kinase inhibitor (TKI)

15.51. A 72 year old fit ex-smoking man is identified on flexible cystoscopy to have a 4-cm bladder tumour. Cystoscopy and transurethral resection of bladder tumour provides tissue that on pathological examination shows a G3pT2 urothelial cell cancer. What is the optimal management for this muscle-invasive cancer?

A. Brachytherapy
B. Chemotherapy (gemcitabine and cisplatin)
C. Observation with regular flexible cystoscopy
D. Partial cystectomy
E. Radical cystectomy

15.52. A healthy 81 year old man presents with back pain to his family physician. A PSA is undertaken, which measures 2350 ng/mL. The patient is referred to a urologist who identifies a craggy, hard prostate gland and undertakes a bone scan, which shows multiple bone metastases. What is the best treatment option for this man?

A. Active surveillance
B. External beam radiotherapy to pelvis
C. Gonadotrophin-releasing hormone (GnRH) agonist therapy
D. High-frequency focused ultrasound
E. Radical prostatectomy

15.53. What is the most appropriate set of investigations for a 71 year old male smoker who presents with dysuria and the family physician identifies persistent non-visible haematuria?

A. DMSA static scan, mid-stream urine (MSU) for microbiology culture, renal tract ultrasound
B. MRI pelvis and MSU
C. MSU, flexible cystoscopy, renal tract ultrasound
D. Nil, only investigate when visible haematuria
E. Non-contrast CTKUB, transrectal ultrasound scan and biopsy

15.54. An 18 year old male presents with long-standing mild left testicular pain, with a hard 1-cm lump in the testicle. What is the most appropriate course of action?

A. Analgesia and observation
B. CT scan
C. Intravenous antibiotics and observation
D. Nuclear medicine scan
E. Scrotal ultrasound

15.55. In a 67 year old man with benign prostatic hypertrophy (BPH) who has a large prostate (70 cc) and is already treated with an α-blocker but with ongoing bothersome symptoms of hesitancy and poor flow, which of the following options is most appropriate?

A. 5α-reductase inhibitor such as finasteride
B. High-intensity focused ultrasound therapy
C. Open prostatectomy
D. Robot-assisted laparoscopic radical prostatectomy
E. Transurethral resection of the prostate

15.56. A 81 year old man attends as an emergency having passed nothing more than 50 mL of urine for 2 days. He has nocturnal enuresis, a palpable bladder and a creatinine of 378 μmol/L (4.28 mg/dL). What is the most appropriate initial management?

A. Bilateral ureteric stent insertion
B. Haemodialysis
C. Start an α-blocker, i.e. tamsulosin
D. Transurethral resection of the prostate
E. Urethral catheterisation

15.57. A 54 year old female has stress incontinence proven by urodynamics. What is the most appropriate initial management?

A. Anticholinergic medication
B. Botulinum neurotoxin type A
C. Pelvic floor exercises
D. Sacral nerve stimulation
E. Tension-free vaginal tape

15.58. Which of the following statements is true regarding erectile dysfunction (ED)?

A. Intracavernosal alprostadil should be considered as a first-line treatment option
B. Perineal trauma is the most common cause
C. PSA should be checked in all men
D. Pudendal artery angiography is useful in early assessment
E. Risk factors for cardiac disease should be assessed

15

Answers

15.1. Answer: D.
He has no clinical evidence of heart failure (JVP not elevated, no basal crepitations, no third heart sound) or chronic liver disease and there is no history of obstructive urinary symptoms; therefore there is no indication to perform

echocardiogram/abdominal ultrasound at this point. Bilateral leg swelling is unlikely to be due to a deep vein thrombosis (DVT), unless it affects the inferior vena cava. This raises the possibility of either renal failure or nephrotic syndrome and urinalysis may be helpful in either circumstance.

15.2. Answer: C.
Red cell casts indicate the presence of a glomerulonephritis and are not observed in tubulo-interstitial disease or haemolytic uraemic syndrome/sclerodermic renal crisis.

15.3. Answer: D.
Small molecules such as glucose, amino acids (glutamine) and lithium are freely filtered. Most free light chains are also filtered and may be taken up by tubules, causing tubular damage. Immunoglobulins are too big to cross the normal glomerular barrier, but may do so in nephrotic syndrome, leading to increased risk of infection.

15.4. Answer: D.
The MDRD equation estimates GFR based on the serum creatinine level, and hence it will be inaccurate in patients whose muscle bulk is atypical for someone of that sex and age. The body builder and African American male will have greater muscle bulk and hence higher creatinine for a given level of renal function compared to what would be expected for a sedentary Caucasian male; hence the MDRD eGFR will underestimate the true GFR (for this reason a correction factor of 1.21 should be applied to the eGFR in those of African American descent). Trimethoprim competes with creatinine for excretion in the distal tubule and hence will increase serum creatinine; thus the MDRD eGFR will underestimate true GFR. Loss of muscle bulk following amputation will lead to a lower creatinine and hence the MDRD equation will overestimate the true GFR. The MDRD eGFR should approximate to true eGFR in the elderly woman with chronic kidney disease (CKD).

15.5. Answer: D.
Minimal change disease classically presents with sudden onset of nephrotic syndrome and is associated with consumption of NSAIDs. Although NSAIDs may also cause tubulo-interstitial nephritis, the heavy proteinuria implies a glomerular rather than a tubulo-interstitial disease process and the absence of haematuria renders a glomerulonephritis such as IgA nephropathy unlikely. The rapid rise in proteinuria is too sudden to be accounted for by diabetic nephropathy alone. Amyloid is less likely, as it is associated with rheumatoid arthritis and not osteoarthritis, and the rapid onset of nephrosis in a relatively young man would be atypical for amyloid.

15.6. Answer: B.
The proteinuria renders bladder cancer, polycystic kidney disease and renal calculi less likely. Furthermore, bladder cancer would be rare in this age group. Post-infectious glomerulonephritis typically presents with non-visible haematuria after the infection is resolved. In addition, hypertension and renal failure are common. Visible haematuria is a common presentation of IgA nephropathy, typically during an upper respiratory tract infection. The haematuria settles spontaneously and the renal prognosis is typically good.

15.7. Answer: C.
Acute tubular necrosis due to gentamicin and interstitial nephritis due to amoxicillin and pre-renal failure related to sepsis are all common in this scenario; however, the 3+ blood and 3+ protein on urinalysis would point towards a glomerulonephritis. Microscopic polyangiitis is a possibility, but this is not associated with low complement levels, which are observed in infection-related glomerulonephritis.

15.8. Answer: A.
This is a presentation of nephrotic syndrome, which is consistent with amyloid or minimal change disease. The pancytopenia could not be explained by minimal change disease, but raises suspicion of a bone marrow disorder such as myeloma. While myeloma could cause cast nephropathy, this would present with AKI rather than nephrotic syndrome. While haemolytic uraemic syndrome (HUS)/TTP may cause low platelets, they do not cause pancytopenia and do not present with nephrotic syndrome.

15.9. Answer: A.
The presence of haemoptysis and kidney injury indicates a pulmonary renal syndrome, most

commonly due to granulomatosis with polyangiitis (previously known as Wegener's granulomatosis), anti-glomerular basement membrane disease or lupus. Pulmonary embolus may cause haemoptysis, but it would not explain the renal failure in the context of hypertension. While Alport's disease can cause deafness, it does not account for the haemoptysis, nor the acute nature of the process. Renal biopsy is likely to be required, but the risk of bleeding is very high at this point due to hypertension and uraemia. Serological testing should be performed urgently given the high risk of one of the above causes of pulmonary renal syndrome (most likely granulomatosis with polyangiitis given the deafness).

15.10. Answer: C.
Asymptomatic non-visible haematuria is a common presentation of IgA nephropathy. Alport's disease is a possibility, although the absence of deafness and a family history of renal disease renders this less likely. Membranous nephropathy presents with nephrotic syndrome and vesico-ureteric reflux would rarely cause isolated haematuria with no evidence of proteinuria or CKD. Ultrasound scan and cystoscopy to exclude uroepithelial tumour would need to be considered if he were over 40 years old.

15.11. Answer: B.
The Study of Heart and Renal Protection (SHARP) provides evidence for reduced cardiovascular events with statins in patients with CKD with or without renal artery disease. The patient's renal function is stable and blood pressure is well controlled and she has proteinuria, and therefore her lisinopril should be continued; however, she should be informed to discontinue lisinopril transiently should she develop vomiting, diarrhoea or fever. The Angioplasty and Stenting for Renal Artery Lesions (ASTRAL) and Cardiovascular Outcomes in Renal Atherosclerotic Lesions (CORAL) trials have not found any benefit from renal artery revascularisation in this context and similarly there is no evidence for the use of warfarin. Plasma renin activity does not help discriminate those who might benefit from angioplasty and will be difficult to interpret in the context of angiotensin-converting enzyme (ACE) inhibition.

15.12. Answer: A.
The dusky toes (sometimes called trash foot) raise clinical suspicion of cholesterol emboli in the microvasculature (especially if peripheral pulses are intact) and this diagnosis is supported by the low-grade fever and eosinophilia. Contrast nephropathy is the other main differential diagnosis; however, it would not account for the trash foot or eosinophilia, nor would renal artery thrombosis. Although the creatine kinase is elevated, either due to myocardial ischaemia or mild leg muscle damage, at this level there is likely to be insufficient myoglobinuria to cause AKI. While low platelets and AKI are consistent with haemolytic uraemic syndrome, the haemoglobin is only mildly reduced and this does not fit the clinical picture.

15.13. Answer: A.
The combination of low haemoglobin, low platelets and schistocytes on blood film suggest microangiopathic haemolytic anaemia, which may be due to a number of conditions, including haemolytic uraemic syndrome or thrombotic thrombocytopenic purpura. The antecedent bloody diarrhoea and predominant renal versus neurological complications are consistent with HUS rather than TTP. The negative *E. coli* O157 stool cultures do not rule out HUS as they have been taken after the diarrhoeal phase of the illness. Malignant hypertension may also cause microangiopathic haemolytic anaemia; however, the blood pressure is typically much higher than observed here. Scleroderma renal crisis, but not lupus, may cause microangiopathic haemolytic anaemia and AKI. While vomiting and diarrhoea predispose to pre-renal failure, his high blood pressure and leg swelling would indicate that he is hypervolaemic, not hypovolaemic.

15.14. Answer: E.
High serum calcium due to excess calcium or vitamin D consumption should suppress the PTH level. The PTH level here is inappropriately elevated, indicating hyperparathyroidism. Serum phosphate should be low in primary hyperparathyroidism. In patients with CKD, calcium is initially maintained in the normal range by elevated PTH (secondary hyperparathyroidism); however, as here, eventually the gland may become autonomous and the PTH level will be very high, resulting in

an elevated serum calcium concentration (tertiary hyperparathyroidism).

15.15. Answer: D.
While erythropoietin (EPO) deficiency is common in patients with chronic kidney disease, the haemoglobin level here is disproportionately low for this level of renal failure. Haemoglobin <10 g/L is not usually observed until stage 4 CKD. Serum EPO levels may be difficult to interpret in this context, although if they are low or indeed normal, this is inappropriate in the context of anaemia and makes renal EPO insufficiency more likely. The MCV is low, indicating potential iron rather than folate deficiency, and white cell and platelet counts are normal, rendering a bone marrow problem or hypersplenism less likely.

15.16. Answer: A.
The slow and very consistent rate of decline in renal function illustrated here is consistent with polycystic kidney disease. Post-infectious glomerulonephritis is rapidly progressive, and microscopic polyangiitis is also typically more rapidly progressive than here and may be associated with remissions and relapses. Progression of renovascular disease typically occurs in a step-wise manner. Myeloma typically affects an older age group and does not explain slow progression over 20 years.

15.17. Answer: A.
There is good evidence that ACE inhibitors are the drug of choice to treat hypertension and reduce proteinuria in patients with CKD and protein:creatinine ratio >100 mg/mmol, and initiation of lisinopril has been partially effective in this patient. The fall in eGFR of <20% is acceptable and all alternative measures should be taken to reduce potassium before stopping the ACE inhibitor. Calcium resonium is only suitable for short-term management of hyperkalaemia due to risk of bowel perforation. While BP is suboptimal, increasing the lisinopril or adding a β-blocker are not recommended at this level of potassium. A thiazide would be more appropriate as this will have the combined benefit of reducing BP and lowering potassium.

15.18. Answer: B.
Hyperkalaemia is less common than for haemodialysis where potassium oscillates from high values pre-dialysis to low values post-dialysis. Fluid removal is achieved by altering the glucose concentration in the dialysate. Peritoneal dialysis may be the most appropriate modality for renal replacement therapy for elderly patients who may not tolerate the fluid and electrolyte shifts associated with haemodialysis. There is no evidence of a survival benefit when haemodialysis and peritoneal dialysis have been compared, although transplantation does confer improved survival. Peritonitis is typically caused by skin contaminants translocating through the lumen or along the tract of the peritoneal catheter.

15.19. Answer: C.
Pre-eclampsia is more common in first pregnancies or first pregnancy with a new partner. Serum urate level may be elevated, which may be helpful in diagnosis. Pre-eclampsia typically presents in the third trimester, and onset of hypertension prior to this raises the possibility of pre-existing renal disease. Maternal history of smoking may actually reduce the risk of pre-eclampsia. Prolonged prothrombin time suggests the development of disseminated intravascular coagulation.

15.20. Answer: B.
Unfortunately, the age group with the lowest graft survival includes adolescence. The transition from paediatric to adult care and to more independent living away from the parental home is a high-risk period for non-adherence. The rate of decline in renal function here is too rapid to be explained by chronic allograft nephropathy. The absence of symptoms or leucocytes in the urine makes acute pyelonephritis in the graft unlikely. Graft thrombosis is rare outside of the early transplant phase or during very severe dehydration. Anti-GBM disease may occur in patients with Alport's disease who receive a kidney with a normal collagen IV isoform.

15.21. Answer: C.
A purpuric rash with renal impairment, abdominal and joint pain is typical of Henoch–Schönlein purpura. Haemoglobin and platelets are normal; therefore haemolytic uraemic syndrome is unlikely. Anti-glomerular basement membrane disease, post-streptococcal glomerulonephritis and systemic lupus

erythematosus could account for the renal failure and urinary findings, but not the purpura.

15.22. Answer: D.
Anuria in this setting is probably caused by bladder outflow obstruction: hence an ultrasound is the correct answer. A CT scan would likely diagnose this too, but ultrasound is the best, quickest and cheapest test. A catastrophic vascular event is a less common cause in which a contrast CT may be helpful. Red cell casts could indicate a rapidly progressive glomerulonephritis, although this is much less common. Bloods for urea and electrolytes will not be helpful in diagnosis, although they should obviously be performed, and a biopsy should not be needed if the cause is obstruction.

15.23. Answer: B.
A mesangiocapillary glomerulonephritis pattern of injury has two broad causes based on the immunofluorescence findings: complement deposition, which is caused by inherited alternative pathway complement gene mutations with unregulated complement activation; and immunoglobulin deposition, which may be caused by chronic infections (frequently viral hepatitis), autoimmune diseases and monoclonal gammopathy. 'Dense deposit disease', with a mesangiocapillary pattern of injury, is due to inherited complement mutations.

15.24. Answer: D.
This is pre-renal injury, without evidence of acute tubular necrosis (ATN), as renal function improved fully with fluids. Therefore she would likely manifest low urine sodium, low urine fractional excretion of sodium and concentrated urine (high specific gravity). Dense granular casts would probably be present in ATN. There is no particular reason she should be hyponatraemic or hypercalcaemic.

15.25. Answer: A.
This patient likely has allergic acute interstitial nephritis due to her proton pump inhibitor (omeprazole) as she has a mild fever and her urine has some white cells but nothing else to suggest glomerulonephritis. Pre-renal injury/ATN is a possibility but, given euvolaemia and lack of an apparent insult, it is unlikely.

15.26. Answer: E.
Rhabdomyolysis is the most likely diagnosis given the dark urine and risk factors, including a statin, viral illness and alcohol use. Many cases will have several risk factors and rhabdomyolysis may occur after being on a statin for some time. The dipstick 'haematuria' without red cells being visible is due to urine myoglobin. Intracellular ions (potassium, phosphate) tend to be particularly high with rhabdomyolysis and calcium may be low (precipitates with phosphate).

15.27. Answer: B.
The first dialysis is designed to be a short, incomplete treatment due to the risks of dialysis disequilibrium syndrome if the uraemia is corrected too quickly. Therefore a short session is performed, using a small surface area dialyser with low blood and dialysate flows. Anticoagulation is generally not used for the first session, as a dialysis catheter will recently have been placed, and in this case also due to concerns regarding uraemic pericarditis, which may be haemorrhagic precipitating tamponade.

15.28. Answer: E.
Hyperphosphataemia and anaemia are frequently considered signs of likely CKD but they may occur early in the course of AKI (and are common in certain causes of AKI such as haemolytic uraemic syndrome) so are not very helpful discriminators. Hyponatraemia has no value in this setting. Small kidneys are a non-invasive, helpful indication of chronic renal injury. It is rarely necessary to perform a renal biopsy for the presence of interstitial fibrosis and tubular atrophy, which will be a universal finding in small atrophic kidneys.

15.29. Answer: A.
Acute cellular rejection is commonest from day 6–7 to week 12 post-transplant. Hyperacute rejection is rare with modern cross-matching techniques and occurs immediately post-transplant and this patient had no preformed anti-HLA antibodies. Renal artery stenosis manifests after several months with hypertension and slowly deteriorating transplant function. BK polyomavirus nephropathy may occur as early as 1–2 months post-transplant but not this early. Recurrent IgA nephropathy happens often but is often not clinically significant and would perhaps be a late cause of transplant dysfunction. Causes not listed that

15

would need to be ruled out include a urine leak causing obstruction and a vascular thrombosis (transplant artery or vein).

15.30. Answer: A.
BK polyomavirus causes an interstitial nephritis in renal transplant patients. It appears to be much less common in non-renal solid organ recipients. It appeared as an entity in the era of modern immunosuppression with tacrolimus and mycophenolate. Risk factors are augmented immunosuppression such as ATG or high-dose glucocorticoids given for acute rejection.

15.31. Answer: C.
Cast nephropathy is a tubular injury as described in option C and presenting with renal impairment. Option A refers to monoclonal immunoglobulin deposition disease (usually light chain deposition disease). Option B refers to amyloidosis, which may occur with multiple myeloma and presents with proteinuria or nephritic syndrome. Option D refers to Fanconi's syndrome, a proximal tubulopathy.

15.32. Answer: A.
Sarcoidosis typically causes a granulomatous interstitial nephritis. It is not associated with the FSGS lesion. Option D refers to a rapidly progressive glomerulonephritis such as ANCA vasculitis or anti-GBM disease. A chronic interstitial nephritis may manifest as widespread 'scarring' (interstitial fibrosis and tubular atrophy) but the process described above is relatively acute and resolved with treatment. While sarcoidosis frequently causes hypercalcaemia, calcium does not deposit in tubules, but larger-scale nephrocalcinosis may be seen on an ultrasound scan.

15.33. Answer: E.
Hepatorenal syndrome should be considered a pure form of pre-renal injury, mediated by reduced renal perfusion, due to splanchnic vasodilatation and up-regulation of the renin–angiotensin system among others. Therefore urine sodium is classically low. It is a diagnosis of exclusion and renal biopsy is generally not performed, and may be dangerous in a coagulopathic liver patient. Hepatorenal syndrome portends a dismal prognosis and dialysis is only performed if the liver disorder is remediable or a liver transplant is likely. If dialysis is performed, slow

continuous treatments are better tolerated with a reduced risk of precipitating encephalopathy. IgA nephropathy is associated with chronic liver disease but is not the cause of hepatorenal syndrome.

15.34. Answer: E.
SGLT2 inhibitors work by inducing glycosuria via impaired glucose reabsorption at the proximal tubule. Diabetic nephropathy is the commonest cause of ESRD in the developed world and likely worldwide. Biopsy is generally not performed when the diagnosis is clear from the patient history and the patient has overt proteinuria, but may be performed if atypical features present (e.g. short history of well-controlled diabetes, haematuria). ACE inhibitors generally decrease proteinuria and slow, but do not halt, progression of the disease.

15.35. Answer: B.
The presence of red cell casts and heavy proteinuria indicates severe glomerular injury and a likely proliferative lupus nephritis that needs immunosuppression. Mycophenolate mofetil and glucocorticoids have been shown to be as effective as the traditional treatment of cyclophosphamide and steroids for both induction and maintenance treatment. As this woman likely wants to preserve her fertility, mycophenolate mofetil is a better choice for her. Most patients who develop ESRD go into remission. If transplanted, recurrence may occur post-transplant, but usually does not cause significant nephritis, possibly due to post-transplant immunosuppression.

15.36. Answer: B.
This patient has chronic interstitial nephritis, which manifests as progressive renal failure, small kidneys and urine showing no blood and minimal to no proteinuria. Biopsy will often have no glomerular changes but will demonstrate interstitial fibrosis and tubular atrophy. Patients with chronic interstitial nephritis may have a renal tubular acidosis, which is a hyperchloraemic (i.e. non-anion gap) acidosis.

15.37. Answer: B.
HNF1-beta mutations may cause several renal phenotypes, which may differ within the same family (including interstitial nephritis, cystic kidneys, vesico-ureteric reflux), maturity-onset diabetes of the young, pancreatic atrophy,

gout, hypomagnesaemia and abnormal liver function tests. *COL4A5* mutations cause X-linked Alport's syndrome, which would not fit here (male-to-male transmission, cystic disease, other features). He likely has an autosomal dominant condition but he does not have polycystic kidney disease as no cysts are evident on scanning. *UMOD* mutations may cause a chronic interstitial nephritis and gout, but would not explain the other features (diabetes, pancreatic atrophy).

15.38. Answer: A.
Anti-GBM antibodies may develop due to normal type IV collagen subunits expressed on the donor kidney. Female carriers of X-linked disease may be symptomatic, although milder than males, due to random inactivation of the X chromosome. Deafness may occur due to the presence of abnormal cochlear type IV collagen. Some patients with type IV collagen mutations develop subtle abnormalities manifested clinically by haematuria only (thin basement membrane disease). Alport's syndrome is usually X-linked (*COL4A5* mutations) but autosomal recessive and dominant disease may occur (*COL4A3* and *COL4A4* mutations).

15.39. Answer: D.
Patients with APKD are at risk of liver cysts, cerebral berry aneurysms and mitral valve prolapse. A ruptured liver cyst would not cause sudden death but a berry aneurysm certainly would. Mitral valve prolapse is usually asymptomatic but may lead to mitral regurgitation; however, it would be a rare cause of sudden death.

15.40. Answer: A.
The patient has APKD. It is an autosomal dominant condition, so offspring have a 50% chance of inheriting it. Given his preserved renal function and good prognosis in affected family members, the mutation is likely located in the *PKD2* gene. While liver cysts are common, liver failure is very rare in APKD, particularly in men. Tolvaptan is indicated for patients deemed to be high risk for progression, which this man is not, given his preserved renal function well into his 60s and good prognosis in affected family members.

15.41. Answer: A.
NSAIDs cause prostaglandin-induced afferent arteriolar vasoconstriction, which drops glomerular perfusion. ACE inhibitors cause efferent arteriolar vasodilatation, further dropping intra-glomerular pressure and hence GFR. The diuretic may cause volume depletion, adding to the insult. Rhabdomyolysis is not the cause, as the atorvastatin is not a recent medicine, and urine myoglobin causes a false-positive dipstick for blood.

15.42. Answer: D.
This patient has developed the nephrotic syndrome after taking NSAIDs so the possibilities are minimal change disease, characterised by normal light microscopy, or membranous nephropathy. Option D refers to minimal change disease and none of the answers describe membranous nephropathy. Option A refers to thrombotic microangiopathy, which NSAIDs do not cause. Options B and E refer to acute interstitial nephritis and acute tubular necrosis. Both may be caused by NSAIDs, but do not cause the nephrotic syndrome. Option C refers to rapidly progressive glomerulonephritis such as ANCA vasculitis.

15.43. Answer: E.
The micturition cycle has a storage (filling) phase and a voiding (micturition) phase. During the filling phase, the high compliance of the detrusor muscle allows the bladder to fill steadily without a rise in intravesical pressure. As bladder volume increases, stretch receptors in its wall cause reflex bladder relaxation and increased sphincter tone. At approximately 75% bladder capacity, there is a desire to void. Voluntary control is now exerted over the desire to void, which disappears temporarily. Compliance of the detrusor allows further increase in capacity until the next desire to void. Just how often this desire needs to be inhibited depends on many factors, not the least of which is finding a suitable place in which to void.

The act of micturition is initiated first by voluntary and then by reflex relaxation of the pelvic floor and distal sphincter mechanism, followed by reflex detrusor contraction. These actions are coordinated by the pontine micturition centre.

15.44. Answer: E.
Although MRI and CT scanning may identify some large bone metastases in the area scanned, they will not identify smaller deposits

15

(which may be multiple). The injection of Tc-labelled methylene diphosphonate (^{99m}Tc-MDP) to undertake a whole-body bone scan is needed to definitively identify bone metastases.

15.45. Answer: E.

This description is pathognomonic of a vesicovaginal fistula secondary to a prolonged obstructed labour. Similar symptoms may occur in an infant with congenital ectopic ureter inserting into the vagina but this would not present for the first time in a woman in her 20s.

15.46. Answer: B.

The commonest causes of visible haematuria are: urinary tract infection, bladder cancer and urinary tract stones. Ureteric stones are usually painful rather than painless; nephrological causes of visible haematuria are less common than urological causes. Upper urinary tract urothelial cell cancer is rare relative to bladder cancer. Of these choices, bladder cancer is the most likely pathology.

15.47. Answer: C.

This patient has an infected, obstructed left kidney secondary to an obstructing ureteric stone. The critical step here is to unobstruct the kidney and allow recovery of the sepsis with antibiotics and resuscitation. The key urological interventions to unobstruct the kidney are a ureteric stent or percutaneous nephrostomy tube insertion. Definitive treatment options (ESWL, PCNL or ureteroscopy) are not appropriate at this time and should be deferred to a later date when the patient has recovered from sepsis.

15.48. Answer: C.

Asymptomatic bacteriuria is defined as $> 10^5$ organisms/mL urine in healthy, asymptomatic patients. It is commonly identified in patients with indwelling catheters and stents. This condition should be treated with antibiotics in infants, pregnant women and those with urinary tract abnormalities.

15.49. Answer: E.

This man has lower urinary tract symptoms, most likely secondary to bladder outlet obstruction. His family physician has correctly trialled him on treatment with an α-blocker. On attending the urology department he should initially be assessed by digital rectal examination (DRE), International Prostate Symptom Score (IPSS) questionnaire and flow test with residual volume of urine assessment by ultrasound. Prostate biopsy would be undertaken if prostate cancer was suspected by DRE and/or raised prostate-specific antigen (PSA). MRI pelvis is mainly used to assess the prostate for presence of cancer, not assessment of lower urinary tract symptoms (LUTS). Cystoscopy is not an initial investigation for voiding LUTS. Prostate ultrasound is useful to assess the exact size, presence of calcification or abscess of the prostate, but is not routinely used to assess LUTS.

15.50. Answer: C.

This woman may be cured by a total nephrectomy. In a tumour of this size, an open approach is likely to be undertaken by most surgeons. The lesion is too large for a partial nephrectomy or ablative approach such as cryotherapy. Radiotherapy is not a treatment option for renal cancer. TKIs are used in metastatic disease.

15.51. Answer: E.

This fit patient is best managed with radical cystectomy to try and cure the high-grade (G3) muscle-invasive (T2) bladder cancer. The other options are not appropriate in this setting.

15.52. Answer: C.

This man's grossly elevated PSA, DRE findings and bone scan result indicate he has metastatic prostate cancer. This is incurable but controllable with GnRH agonist injections (androgen flare covered by initial androgen receptor blocker treatment for 3–4 weeks). The other therapies are not appropriate for metastatic disease, nor is observation in a man with symptoms of metastatic disease.

15.53. Answer: C.

Persistent non-visible haematuria is 2 of 3 urine dipstick tests positive for at least 1+ blood. Investigations should be undertaken in patients who have associated symptoms (such as dysuria) that would indicate a possible intravesical lesion. Additionally, this man is a smoker, putting him at higher risk for bladder cancer. The most appropriate initial investigations are MSU to rule out infection, cystoscopy and upper tract imaging to visualise the urinary tract.

15.54. Answer: E.

This man has a testicular cancer until proven otherwise. He should be seen urgently and, following examination, undergo an urgent ultrasound, which is the gold standard investigation to rule out a testicular cancer. Testicular cancer is almost always treated with an initial inguinal orchidectomy.

15.55. Answer: A.

This man should initially be escalated to combination medical therapy for BPH with a 5α-reductase inhibitor. Further suitable treatments for symptoms that are refractory to medical therapy include: transurethral resection of the prostate, laser prostatectomy or open prostatectomy (Millen's procedure). High-intensity focused ultrasound therapy or robot-assisted laparoscopic radical prostatectomy are treatments used for prostate cancer.

15.56. Answer: E.

These symptoms indicate high-pressure chronic urinary retention for which the initial management is insertion of a urinary catheter; this will result in improvement in renal function. Bilateral ureteric stent insertion will not relieve the more distal prostatic obstruction of the urinary tract. The patient may be managed thereafter with bladder outlet surgery such as a transurethral resection of the prostate, long-term urethral catheterisation or intermittent self-catheterisation. Haemodialysis is not a curative treatment option in the setting of high-pressure urinary retention. Medical management, such as an α-blocker, is contraindicated.

15.57. Answer: C.

The first-line treatment of stress incontinence is pelvic floor exercises taught by a urophysiotherapist. If unsuccessful, further management options include tension-free vaginal tape. Anticholinergic medication, botulinum toxin injection and sacral nerve stimulation are all treatment options for urge incontinence.

15.58. Answer: E.

In men presenting with new-onset erectile dysfunction it is vital to ensure that they do not have previously undiagnosed coronary artery disease that has manifest as ED. Risk factors for vascular disease such as hypertension and hyperlipidaemia should be evaluated. Perineal trauma is a rare cause of ED. Pudendal artery angiography is rarely performed. Phosphodiesterase type 5 inhibitors are the first-line treatment options for ED, not intracavernosal alprostadil. Depending on the characteristics of the patient, the consultation for a man with ED may be a good opportunity to discuss lower urinary tract symptoms and a PSA test; however, this is not essential to the assessment of the ED component.

15

Cardiology

Multiple Choice Questions

16.1. A 55 year old man with a history of poorly controlled hypertension presents with a history of sudden-onset central chest pain. There are no diagnostic electrocardiogram (ECG) abnormalities, and an interval troponin concentration is not diagnostic of myocardial infarction. What diagnosis should be confirmed or excluded next?

A. Anxiety
B. Aortic dissection
C. Myocarditis
D. Pericarditis
E. Pneumothorax

16.2. The term 'orthopnoea' refers to breathlessness (dyspnoea) in a particular situation. Which answer below describes that situation?

A. After several hours of sleep
B. Due to asthma
C. Immediately on lying flat
D. On exertion
E. On sitting upright

16.3. A 75 year old woman presents to her family physician with a 24-hour history of rapid, irregular palpitations accompanied by fatigue. In an elderly patient, what is the most likely cause of palpitations?

A. Atrial ectopic (premature) beats
B. Atrial fibrillation
C. Supraventricular tachycardia
D. Ventricular ectopic (premature) beats
E. Ventricular tachycardia

16.4. A 74 year old woman presents with breathlessness. She is found to have an elevated jugular venous pressure (JVP). Which of the following conditions is most likely to explain this physical finding?

A. Aortic stenosis
B. Dehydration
C. Exacerbation of asthma
D. Increased left atrial pressure
E. Recurrent pulmonary embolism

16.5. A 56 year old man presents with a history of headache. He is noted to have a loud second heart sound on auscultation. Which of the following pathologies could explain this finding?

A. Aortic incompetence
B. Essential hypertension
C. Mechanical mitral valve replacement
D. Mitral incompetence
E. Postural hypotension

16.6. Which of the following pathologies can be associated with an early diastolic murmur?

A. Long QT syndrome type 1
B. Marfan's syndrome
C. Mitral valve prolapse
D. Myotonic dystrophy
E. Wolff–Parkinson–White syndrome

16.7. An 80 year old woman with a history of palpitation presents with a painful left leg. On examination, pulse rate is 80 beats/min and irregular, blood pressure (BP) 170/96 mmHg. The left leg is pale, cold, and sensation is reduced. The popliteal, dorsalis pedis and posterior tibial pulses cannot be felt. Her only regular medications are aspirin and digoxin. What is the most likely diagnosis?

A. Acute arterial plaque rupture with lower limb ischaemia
B. Deep venous thrombosis with secondary reduction of arterial blood flow
C. Dissection of the femoral artery due to uncontrolled hypertension
D. Peripheral embolism with lower limb ischaemia
E. Reduced lower limb perfusion due to cardiac failure

16.8. A 50 year old man is assessed because of 3 weeks of fever and influenza-like symptoms. Examination findings are tachycardia (heart rate 105 beats/min), and a large pulse pressure, BP 140/45 mmHg. Initially it was thought a murmur was present but repeat examination reveals no murmur. Investigations reveal no evidence of chest or urinary infection. What are these findings most compatible with?

A. Acute myocarditis
B. Acute viral pericarditis
C. Infective endocarditis affecting the aortic valve
D. Infective endocarditis affecting the tricuspid valve
E. Influenza

16.9. You assess a 62 year old woman 2 days after treatment for anterior myocardial infarction. On examination she is tachycardic and tachypnoeic, and has a harsh systolic murmur radiating to the right side of the chest. There are fine inspiratory crepitations audible at the lung bases. What is the most likely explanation for these findings?

A. Acute aortic incompetence
B. Left ventricular free wall rupture
C. Papillary muscle rupture and mitral incompetence
D. Post-infarction pericarditis with pericardial rub
E. Rupture of the interventricular septum

16.10. Which of the following physical signs is associated with left ventricular failure?

A. A gallop rhythm with a fourth heart sound
B. A gallop rhythm with a third heart sound
C. A loud second heart sound
D. A quiet first heart sound
E. Fixed splitting of the second heart sound

16.11. A 55 year old man with type 2 diabetes presents with a 1-hour history of severe central chest pain. Which of the following statements is true?

A. A normal baseline troponin and elevated 6-hour troponin level is suspicious of myocardial infarction
B. A normal ECG excludes myocardial infarction
C. A normal initial troponin level excludes myocardial infarction
D. Failure of chest pain to resolve with nitrates confirms myocardial infarction
E. T-wave inversion on the ECG confirms myocardial infarction

16.12. A 72 year old hypertensive woman presents with a history of sudden-onset, rapid, irregular palpitation. She has had several episodes over the previous 3 months, which have resolved within 1 hour. She feels tired and slightly lightheaded during episodes. From this history, which of the following most likely explains her symptoms?

A. Atrial fibrillation
B. Sinus arrhythmia
C. Supraventricular tachycardia
D. Ventricular ectopic beats (extrasystoles)
E. Ventricular tachycardia

16.13. In the management of cardiac arrest, which of the following most accurately describes basic life support (BLS)?

A. Administration of intravenous drugs and external defibrillation (the two 'D's)
B. External cardiac massage only
C. Support of airway, breathing and circulation (ABC)
D. Support of airway, breathing and circulation, and assessment of disability and exposure (ABCDE)
E. Support of airway, breathing and circulation, and assessment of disability and exposure, treatment of fibrillation (ABCDEF)

16.14. Which of the following statements is true of a pulseless electrical activity (PEA) cardiac arrest?

A. Cardiopulmonary resuscitation (CPR) should be carried out for 1 minute before the rhythm is reassessed
B. Intravenous amiodarone will restore cardiac output
C. It is initially managed with immediate defibrillation
D. Reversible causes include hyperthyroidism and hypercalcaemia
E. Reversible causes include hypothermia and hypoxia

16

16.15. A 65 year old female presents with chest pain, and the 12-lead ECG shows evidence of acute inferior myocardial infarction complicated by hypotension. An echocardiogram is performed and shows markedly reduced movement of the right ventricular walls, indicating that right ventricular infarction has occurred. Left ventricular function is only mildly impaired. Which of the following physical signs would be expected in this situation?

A. Tachycardia, a late systolic murmur and ascites
B. Tachycardia, and absent jugular venous pulse because of inability to develop right heart pressure
C. Tachycardia, acute development of peripheral oedema and acute ascites
D. Tachycardia, basal crepitations and a third heart sound
E. Tachycardia, elevated jugular venous pulse due to failure of right ventricular pump function, and hepatomegaly

16.16. What relationship does Starling's Law of the heart describe?

A. Between blood pressure and cardiac output
B. Between cardiac filling and blood pressure
C. Between cardiac filling and cardiac output
D. Between heart rate and blood pressure
E. Between heart rate and cardiac output

16.17. What underlying pathophysiological changes is chronic cardiac failure associated with?

A. Activation of the renin–angiotensin–aldosterone system (RAAS)
B. Inhibition of the RAAS
C. Inhibition of the sympathetic nervous system
D. Reduced production of brain natriuretic peptide (BNP)
E. Systemic vasodilatation

16.18. Loop diuretics such as furosemide and bumetanide have which of the following effects?

A. Diuresis due to inhibition of potassium and water reabsorption
B. Diuresis due to inhibition of sodium and water reabsorption
C. Diuresis due to inhibition of water reabsorption only
D. Increased serum potassium levels due to enhanced distal tubule function
E. Osmotic diuresis

16.19. β-Adrenoceptor antagonists (β-blockers) are used in which of the following situations?

A. Acute left ventricular failure
B. Cardiac failure associated with bradycardia
C. Cardiogenic shock
D. Chronic left ventricular systolic dysfunction
E. High-output cardiac failure

16.20. A 71 year old woman with a history of hypertension presents with fatigue and rapid, irregular palpitations. She normally takes enalapril for blood pressure control. Clinical examination reveals an irregularly irregular pulse, rate 125 beats/min, and BP 128/86 mmHg. Cardiovascular examination is otherwise normal. A 12-lead ECG is performed, which shows atrial fibrillation with poor ventricular rate control, but no other abnormality. Which of the following drugs is the most suitable agent to control heart rate in this patient?

A. Adenosine
B. Amiodarone
C. β-blocker
D. Flecainide
E. Lidocaine

16.21. An 85 year old man presents with a 6-month history of sudden episodes of lightheadedness, which last up to 15 seconds. He is admitted to hospital with an episode of syncope resulting in facial injury. Examine the rhythm strip below. Which conduction abnormality does this show?

A. Complete (third-degree) AV block
B. Left bundle branch block
C. Mobitz type II second-degree AV block
D. Sinus bradycardia
E. Wenckebach (Mobitz type I) second-degree AV block

16.22. Which of the following rhythms is NOT commonly associated with sick sinus syndrome (sinoatrial disease)?

A. Atrial fibrillation
B. Atrial tachycardia
C. Sinus bradycardia
D. Sinus pauses
E. Ventricular tachycardia

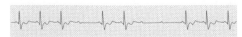

Fig. 16.21

16.23. A 75 year old woman has a history of hypertension and diabetes. She presents with atrial fibrillation. What is her CHA$_2$DS$_2$-VASc score?

A. 2
B. 3
C. 4
D. 5
E. 6

16.24. Which of the following drugs is known to be effective in preventing stroke in patients with atrial fibrillation?

A. Amiodarone
B. Apixaban
C. Aspirin
D. β-blocker
E. Clopidogrel

16.25. The ECG below shows a regular, narrow complex tachycardia in a patient presenting with sudden-onset, rapid palpitation. Which of the following should be used first in attempting to terminate this rhythm?

A. Direct current cardioversion
B. Intravenous adenosine
C. Intravenous β-blocker
D. Oral β-blocker
E. Vagal manoeuvres, e.g. Valsalva manoeuvre

16.26. For which of the following scenarios would a permanent pacemaker be an appropriate treatment?

A. Paroxysmal atrial fibrillation
B. Prevention of sudden death due to ventricular fibrillation
C. Sick sinus syndrome associated with syncope
D. Sinus bradycardia in an athlete
E. Supraventricular tachycardia

16.27. Which of the following patients is a suitable candidate for an implantable cardiac defibrillator?

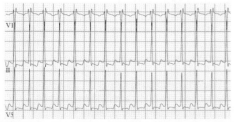

Fig. 16.25

A. A 26 year old man with polymorphic ventricular tachycardia (torsades de pointes) occurring after cocaine use
B. A 48 year old man who presents with acute inferior myocardial infarction complicated within the first 6 hours by ventricular fibrillation
C. A 55 year old woman with syncope; ECG monitoring shows sinus rhythm with third-degree atrioventricular block
D. A 75 year old man with syncope; ambulatory ECG shows sinus bradycardia and daytime sinus pauses of up to 5 seconds
E. An 80 year old man with a history of anterior myocardial infarction 6 months previously; he is fit, has never experienced arrhythmia, and a cardiac magnetic resonance scan shows poor left ventricular function (left ventricular ejection fraction 28%)

16.28. A 17 year old male presents to the emergency department with an episode of collapse. Witnesses report he became extremely blue at the time of collapse, which occurred on walking. The patient tells you he has a history of congenital heart disease. On examination you note he is centrally cyanosed. Which of the following congenital conditions is the most likely explanation for this presentation?

A. Coarctation of the aorta
B. Congenital heart block
C. Patent foramen ovale
D. Tetralogy of Fallot
E. Wolff–Parkinson–White syndrome

16.29. Which of the following is true of Eisenmenger's syndrome?

A. Breathlessness and fatigue are uncommon symptoms
B. It occurs in patients with patent foramen ovale
C. Left to right shunting occurs because of pulmonary hypertension
D. Life expectancy is markedly reduced
E. Patients are peripherally but not centrally cyanosed

16.30. A 48 year old woman registers with a new family physician. She tells the doctor she had a small hole in her heart from birth but that it did not require any treatment. On examination, pulse is 70 beats/min and regular; BP 122/76 mmHg. You detect a loud, high-pitched systolic murmur at the left sternal border, accompanied by a thrill. Which of the

16

following conditions would explain the history and physical findings?

A. Anterior mitral leaflet prolapse
B. Atrial septal defect
C. Patent foramen ovale
D. Persistent ductus arteriosus
E. Ventricular septal defect

16.31. A 21 year old man presents with a recent history of an influenza-like illness initially characterised by fever, myalgia and headache. He develops pleuritic-type chest discomfort and breathlessness. On examination, pulse is 105 beats/min and regular; BP 105/60 mmHg. The JVP is not elevated. Heart sounds 1 and 2 are present with a loud to-and-fro harsh sound present in systole and diastole. Which of the following conditions explains this clinical presentation?

A. Acute viral pericarditis
B. Aortic valve endocarditis
C. Mitral valve endocarditis
D. Persistent ductus arteriosus
E. Pulmonary embolism

16.32. What is the appropriate initial treatment for the symptoms of acute pericarditis?

A. Intravenous glucocorticoids
B. Intravenous morphine
C. Oral amiodarone
D. Oral aspirin
E. Rectal diclofenac

16.33. Which of the following best describes dilated cardiomyopathy?

A. A disease of the myocardium characterised by chamber enlargement and thinning of the left and right ventricular walls
B. A disease of the myocardium characterised by disproportionate thickening of the interventricular septum
C. A disease of the myocardium characterised by infiltration of myocardial tissue resulting in restricted contraction and relaxation
D. Isolated dilatation of the atria, causing atrial fibrillation
E. Isolated dilatation of the right ventricle, causing ventricular tachycardia

16.34. Which of the following is a cause of dilated cardiomyopathy?

A. A high-cholesterol diet
B. Heavy alcohol consumption
C. Mutation in cardiac sodium channel gene

D. Obesity
E. Recreational cannabis use

16.35. By which of the following features is hypertrophic cardiomyopathy usually characterised?

A. Asymmetric left ventricular hypertrophy with marked thickening of the interventricular septum
B. Asymmetric left ventricular hypertrophy with marked thickening of the anterior left ventricular wall
C. Hypertrophy of both atria and both ventricles
D. Hypertrophy of the left ventricle and atrophy of the right ventricle
E. Symmetrical left ventricular hypertrophy

16.36. Cardiac transplantation is considered in which group of patients with cardiomyopathy?

A. Asymptomatic patients
B. Frail elderly patients with end-stage heart failure
C. Patients who do not wish to take life-long medication
D. Patients who have poor quality of life despite optimal drug therapy
E. Patients who have symptoms but good quality of life on optimal drug therapy

16.37. A 48 year old woman with no significant previous medical history collapses while running a marathon. Despite attempts at resuscitation, she does not survive. Postmortem examination reveals asymmetric left ventricular hypertrophy with disproportionate thickening of the interventricular septum. A postmortem diagnosis of hypertrophic cardiomyopathy is made. What is the most likely cause of this patient's sudden collapse?

A. Atrial fibrillation
B. Left ventricular failure
C. Pulmonary embolism
D. Right ventricular failure
E. Ventricular arrhythmia

16.38. A 30 year old woman has recently been diagnosed with dilated cardiomyopathy. Her diagnosis was made with echocardiography, which showed moderate left ventricular dilatation and impairment. She has noticed herself becoming increasingly fatigued on moderate exertion. Her younger sister died suddenly the previous year and she is very worried about the risk of sudden death. Which of the following treatments is known to reduce her risk of sudden death?

A. Aspirin
B. β-blocker (e.g. metoprolol)
C. Calcium channel blocker (e.g. verapamil)
D. Loop diuretic (e.g. furosemide)
E. Percutaneous coronary intervention (PCI)

16.39. A 55 year old woman presents with a history of acute, severe, constricting central chest pain associated with anterior ST segment elevation on the 12-lead ECG. She immediately undergoes coronary angiography, which shows no evidence of coronary artery disease and no coronary occlusion. An echocardiogram shows left ventricular apical dilatation, with normal left ventricular basal contraction. Which of the following factors is most likely to have precipitated this illness?

A. Acute emotional stress
B. Cigarette smoking
C. Excessive alcohol consumption
D. Genetic factors
E. Viral infection

16.40. Which of the following is associated with excessive alcohol consumption?

A. Atrial fibrillation
B. Diverticulitis
C. Hypertrophic cardiomyopathy
D. Hypotension
E. Supraventricular tachycardia

16.41. Atrial myxoma is the most common primary cardiac tumour. Which of the following is true of atrial myxoma?

A. Atrial myxomas are usually malignant
B. It occurs more commonly in the right atrium than in the left atrium
C. Surgery is not indicated because atrial myxomas are benign
D. Surgery is usually indicated to prevent embolic complications such as stroke
E. The tumour commonly obstructs the aortic valve

16.42. Which of the following conditions may result in chronic pericardial constriction?

A. Acute myocardial infarction
B. Dilated cardiomyopathy
C. Excessive alcohol consumption
D. Osteoarthritis
E. Tuberculosis

16.43. A 75 year old male smoker presents with a 6-week history of progressive exertional breathlessness and fatigue. Latterly he has noticed his ankles swelling in the afternoon. On examination, pulse is 100 beats/min and regular; BP 92/60 mmHg. The JVP is elevated and rises on inspiration. Heart sounds are quiet and there are no added sounds. There is bilateral pitting oedema to the knees. A chest X-ray is requested, which shows apparent cardiomegaly with a globular cardiac silhouette. You suspect a possible pericardial effusion. Which of the following statements is true?

A. A large effusion can be a sign of malignancy
B. A pericardial rub is always heard if the effusion is large
C. An ECG is the best investigation to confirm the diagnosis
D. High-dose diuretic therapy will resolve the pericardial effusion
E. In symptomatic patients, cardiac surgery is required to remove the pericardial fluid

16.44. An 18 year old man presents with sudden onset of sharp chest pain. The pain is made worse by deep inspiration or lying down flat. It is relieved by sitting forward and taking shallow breaths. He presents to the emergency department and an ECG is recorded because the attending doctor suspects acute pericarditis. What is the most specific ECG change in pericarditis?

A. PR interval prolongation
B. PR segment depression
C. ST depression
D. ST elevation
E. T-wave inversion

16.45. A 46 year old man has recently fractured his leg, which is in a plaster cast. He suddenly becomes very breathless, unwell and collapses. The attending doctor suspects a pulmonary embolus from a deep vein thrombosis. The doctor performs an ECG. What is the most common ECG change in patients with pulmonary embolism?

A. Anterior T-wave inversion
B. Atrial fibrillation
C. 'S1Q3T3'
D. Sinus tachycardia
E. ST elevation

16

16.46. In patients with a pericardial effusion, what is the most important clinical sign to determine whether there is cardiac tamponade?

A. Cyanosis
B. Haematuria
C. Peripheral oedema
D. Pulsus paradoxus
E. Raised JVP

16.47. The following medical treatments are all associated with improved symptoms in patients with heart failure due to left ventricular systolic dysfunction. However, which of the treatments has NOT been shown to also improve survival?

A. Bisoprolol
B. Enalapril
C. Furosemide
D. Sacubitril–valsartan
E. Spironolactone

16.48. Which of the following antiplatelet drugs is a phosphodiesterase inhibitor?

A. Cangrelor
B. Clopidogrel
C. Dipyridamole
D. Prasugrel
E. Ticagrelor

16.49. A 54 year old security guard who is obese and enjoys drinking alcohol and cigarette smoking with his friends has a diet high in saturated fats. He has an acute myocardial infarction. Which lifestyle risk factor has the strongest association with myocardial infarction?

A. Excess alcohol
B. High-saturated fat diet
C. Obesity
D. Sedentary activity
E. Smoking

16.50. A 36 year old smoker has sudden onset of chest pain whilst out walking in a remote island of Scotland. He attends the local hospital and is found to have ST segment elevation myocardial infarction. Which treatment has the strongest time-dependent benefit (i.e. the quicker received, the better the outcome) for ST segment elevation myocardial infarction?

A. Aspirin
B. β-blocker
C. Heparin
D. Percutaneous coronary intervention
E. Tissue plasminogen activator

16.51. An 80 year old woman presents with shortness of breath and swollen ankles. Her ECG showed some poor R-wave progression. She was referred for an echocardiogram and was found to have a high ejection fraction. Which of these conditions is the most likely cause of her presentation?

A. Acute myocarditis
B. Aortic stenosis
C. Dilated cardiomyopathy
D. Ischaemic cardiomyopathy with extensive infarction
E. Restrictive cardiomyopathy

16.52. Neuroendocrine system activation is a feature of heart failure. Abnormalities of which hormone can cause heart failure rather than result from heart failure?

A. Aldosterone
B. Angiotensin II
C. Catecholamines
D. Thyroxine
E. Vasopressin (antidiuretic hormone, ADH)

16.53. Which of the following biomarkers is a structural protein rather than a cardiac enzyme?

A. Aspartate aminotransferase
B. Creatine kinase
C. Creatine kinase MB
D. Lactate dehydrogenase
E. Troponin I

16.54. A patient has a stent placed in his right coronary artery. On return to the ward, he gets severe chest pain and becomes very unwell. The nurse undertakes an ECG and calls the interventional cardiologist to review the patient because she is concerned that he has a thrombosed stent. What ECG features would suggest the stent has become occluded?

A. Anterior T-wave inversion
B. Atrial fibrillation
C. Atrioventricular block
D. ST elevation in I, aVL and V_6
E. ST elevation in V_2–V_5

16.55. A 72 year old woman has had 'indigestion' for 4 days with vomiting and sweating. She presents to the emergency department where a delayed presentation inferior ST segment elevation myocardial infarction is diagnosed. She has already developed Q waves in leads II, III and aVF. One day after admission to hospital, she suddenly deteriorates with severe breathlessness, low blood pressure and sudden onset of pulmonary oedema. What is the most likely cause?

A. Acute papillary muscle rupture
B. Acute pericarditis
C. Atrial septal defect
D. Free wall rupture
E. Mural thrombus

16.56. A patient admitted to the emergency department with severe chest pain and ST segment deviation suddenly collapses and is found not to be breathing or have a pulse. A cardiac arrest call is made. What is the most likely cause of his collapse?

A. Asystole
B. Complete heart block
C. Free wall rupture
D. Pulseless electrical activity
E. Ventricular fibrillation

16.57. A 75 year old man is incidentally found to have a pulsatile swelling in his abdomen on a routine health check. He is sent for an abdominal ultrasound scan, which confirms the presence of an abdominal aortic aneurysm. Which risk factor is protective against the formation and expansion of an abdominal aortic aneurysm?

A. Diabetes mellitus
B. Family history of aneurysm disease
C. Hypercholesterolaemia
D. Hypertension
E. Smoking

16.58. A 39 year old heavy smoker presents with calf pain on walking and is referred to a vascular surgeon for assessment. Which clinical feature would be most reassuring?

A. Capillary refill <2 seconds
B. Cold temperature
C. Hair loss
D. Pallor
E. Pulselessness

16.59. A 65 year old smoker with hypertension is found to have an abdominal aortic aneurysm on population screening with ultrasound. Which intervention will most reduce his future risk of aortic aneurysm rupture?

A. Angiotensin-converting enzyme (ACE) inhibitor
B. β-blocker

C. Smoking cessation
D. Statin
E. Warfarin

16.60. Limb ischaemia can take many forms and has varied causes. This may result in sudden acute vessel occlusion from arterial spasm or thrombosis, or more chronic processes. What is the most likely underlying cause of severe limb ischaemia in an otherwise well, thin 30 year old heavy smoker?

A. Atherosclerosis
B. Atrial fibrillation
C. Buerger's disease
D. Diabetes mellitus
E. Raynaud's disease

16.61. A 65 year old man with known hypertension presents with severe central chest pain that radiates between his shoulder blades. He is sweaty with a BP of 200/100 mmHg in his right arm, a pale left arm and an ECG showing sinus tachycardia. His chest X-ray shows mediastinal widening and a computed tomography scan shows a type A aortic dissection. Which of the following is known to reduce mortality?

A. Anticoagulation
B. Control of the blood pressure
C. Emergency repair of the ascending aorta
D. Intravenous β-blockade
E. Prevention of limb or renal ischaemia

16.62. A short young woman presents with severe chest pain, vomiting and a sinus tachycardia. She is in the last trimester of pregnancy and has had normal blood pressure and observations at antenatal care. She is admitted for observation but is later found collapsed and in cardiac arrest. Despite attempts at resuscitation, mother and child die. Postmortem reveals an aortic dissection. What is the most likely underlying cause for the dissection?

A. Coarctation of the aorta
B. Intramural haematoma
C. Marfan's syndrome
D. Pregnancy
E. Undiagnosed hypertension

16.63. A 50 year old woman with diabetes, who smokes, presents with jaw pain, severe nausea, autonomic arousal and vomiting. An ECG is performed in the emergency department and

16

shows anterior ST segment elevation. What is the best immediate reperfusion therapy?

A. Coronary artery bypass graft surgery
B. Morphine
C. Primary percutaneous coronary intervention
D. Streptokinase
E. Tissue plasminogen activator

16.64. An 81 year old non-smoker presents with chest pain and an ECG with ST segment depression. His troponin concentration is 456 ng/L (reference range <34 ng/L). He is treated with an angioplasty and stent 2 days later. At the same time, a 60 year old smoker with diabetes has a large anterior ST segment elevation myocardial infarction, has ventricular fibrillation in the ambulance and has immediate defibrillation. He undergoes immediate percutaneous coronary intervention on arrival at hospital and has a troponin concentration of >50 000 ng/L. A medical student asks who has the better prognosis. What is the biggest predictor of mortality following acute myocardial infarction?

A. Age
B. Cardiac arrest
C. ECG changes
D. Smoking
E. Troponin concentration

16.65. A 35 year old executive has a reproducible BP of 180/100 mmHg. She is referred for assessment in the clinic. You perform a range of tests to determine whether there is an underlying cause for her hypertension. What is the commonest cause of secondary hypertension?

A. Congenital adrenal hyperplasia
B. Conn's syndrome
C. Phaeochromocytoma
D. Renal disease
E. Thyrotoxicosis

16.66. A 60 year old man is referred by his family physician because despite four drugs he continues to have uncontrolled blood pressure. The doctor feels that the patient needs further investigation for a potential secondary cause of hypertension. What is the commonest cause of poorly controlled hypertension?

A. Conn's syndrome
B. Glucocorticoid-suppressible hyperaldosteronism
C. Hyper-reninaemia

D. Poor adherence with medication
E. Renal failure

16.67. An 18 year old woman presents with a sore throat and suspected acute rheumatic fever. Which of the following is a minor manifestation of acute rheumatic fever?

A. Carditis
B. Chorea
C. Erythema marginatum
D. Raised C-reactive protein
E. Subcutaneous nodules

16.68. An 18 year old woman has a raised C-reactive protein, a rash consistent with erythema marginatum and pyrexia. However, the clinician remains uncertain about the diagnosis of acute rheumatic fever. Rapid response to which treatment will help to confirm the diagnosis?

A. Aspirin
B. Bed rest
C. Diuretics
D. Glucocorticoids
E. High-dose antibiotics

16.69. A 34 year old woman presents with symptoms of breathlessness on exertion, a malar flush and has a past history of rheumatic fever. She is in sinus rhythm and has an echocardiogram that confirms mitral stenosis. Which physical sign is she likely to have?

A. Ejection systolic murmur
B. Mid-systolic click
C. Pre-systolic accentuation
D. Quiet second heart sound
E. Thrusting apex beat

16.70. An 80 year old man presents with an incidental ejection systolic murmur. His family physician notices a parasternal thrill. What is the likely underlying reason for the thrill?

A. Aortic stenosis
B. Large atrial septal defect
C. Mitral stenosis
D. Pulmonary hypertension
E. Right ventricular hypertrophy

16.71. A 43 year old man undergoes a routine health check with his employers. He is found to have a murmur, isolated systolic hypertension (180/60 mmHg) and left ventricular hypertrophy on his ECG. A significant regurgitant blood flow is noticed across the aortic valve on echocardiogram. Which of the following clinical signs is likely to be observed?

A. Crescendo–decrescendo murmur
B. Palpable thrill in the aortic area
C. Prominent pulsation in the neck (de Musset's sign)
D. Quiet second heart sound
E. Slow rising pulse

16.72. A 65 year old man presents with a 4-week history of general malaise and lethargy. He has had two courses of antibiotics that have temporarily improved his symptoms but he continues to feel worse over time. His family physician notices he has become anaemic. He attends the emergency department and he is admitted to hospital with a fever. He has some blood cultures taken and he undergoes an echocardiogram, which shows a mass on his mitral valve. What is the most likely organism that will be grown from his blood cultures?

A. *Staphylococcus aureus*
B. *Staphylococcus epidermidis*
C. *Streptococcus faecalis*
D. *Streptococcus gallolyticus*
E. Viridans streptococci

16.73. Considering the patient in Question 16.72, before the blood culture results are known, the junior doctor reviews the 65 year old man and examines him for evidence of endocarditis. What is the commonest sign that the doctor is likely to find?

A. Haematuria
B. Osler's nodes
C. Roth's spots
D. Splinter haemorrhages
E. Subconjunctival haemorrhages

16.74. Considering the patient in Questions 16.72 and 16.73, blood cultures demonstrate viridans streptococci. What is the most appropriate antibiotic regime to commence the patient on?

A. Intravenous ampicillin and gentamicin
B. Intravenous benzylpenicillin and gentamicin
C. Intravenous flucloxacillin
D. Intravenous vancomycin and gentamicin
E. Oral benzylpenicillin

16.75. An army recruit is referred for assessment because there is a family history of sudden cardiac death and an uncle was diagnosed with hypertrophic cardiomyopathy.

In what manner is hypertrophic cardiomyopathy commonly inherited?

A. Autosomal dominant
B. Autosomal recessive
C. Never inherited
D. X-linked dominant
E. X-linked recessive

16.76. A 23 year old woman is referred for evaluation because she is very tall, has problems with her vision and has a heart murmur. Her family physician is concerned that she may have Marfan's syndrome. What structural gene is associated with an abnormality in Marfan's syndrome?

A. Fibrillin
B. Myosin heavy chain
C. Myosin-binding protein
D. Titan
E. Troponin

16.77. A patient presents with an incidental finding of a mass in the left atrium whilst undergoing an echocardiogram for hypertension. What is the most likely cardiac tumour in this situation?

A. Angiosarcoma
B. Atrial myxoma
C. Fibroelastoma
D. Fibroma
E. Lipoma

16

16.78. A 43 year old man has an extensive anterior myocardial infarction and has received antiplatelet, anticoagulant and statin therapy. He is referred for an echocardiogram. What will transthoracic echocardiography most usefully assess in this setting?

A. Cardiac arrhythmia
B. Future prognosis
C. Left ventricular function and the presence of mural thrombus
D. Myocardial scar formation
E. Thrombus in the left atrium

16.79. The man with an extensive anterior myocardial infarction in Question 16.78 undergoes coronary angiography and is found to have coronary artery disease. Which features on angiography predict the best outcome/improvements with coronary artery bypass graft surgery?

A. Diabetes mellitus and diffuse three-vessel coronary heart disease

B. Left main stem stenosis and significant left ventricular systolic dysfunction
C. Severe proximal disease of the left anterior descending coronary artery
D. Three-vessel coronary heart disease with good left ventricular function
E. Two-vessel coronary heart disease

16.80. The man with an extensive anterior myocardial infarction in Questions 16.78 and 16.79 has left main stem and triple-vessel disease and is referred for coronary artery bypass graft surgery. However, the surgeon is concerned that the anterior wall is completely infarcted and is no longer viable. The surgeon wants to know if the anterior wall has significant amounts of scar tissue. Which imaging modality is best to identify the scar of acute myocardial infarction?

A. Computed tomography
B. Coronary angiography
C. Echocardiography
D. MRI
E. Stress echocardiography

16.81. An 83 year old woman presents with acute pulmonary oedema, BP of 180/100 mmHg and a SaO_2 of 85%. Which treatment is UNLIKELY to be helpful in this setting?

A. Furosemide
B. Intravenous dobutamine
C. Intravenous nitrates
D. Non-invasive ventilation
E. Supplementary oxygen therapy

16.82. A 43 year old woman with a past history of breast cancer is referred with a gradual onset of breathlessness. An echocardiogram demonstrates a dilated poorly contracting left ventricle. You wish to investigate potential causes of her dilated cardiomyopathy. Which of the following would be an irreversible cause of her dilated cardiomyopathy?

A. Alcohol excess
B. Anthracycline chemotherapy
C. Haemochromatosis
D. Hypothyroidism
E. Thyrotoxicosis

16.83. A 56 year old man presents with sudden onset of chest pain radiating down his left arm, ST segment depression of the ECG and a plasma troponin concentration of 4365 ng/L

(reference range <34 ng/L). Which of the following treatments is likely to worsen his prognosis?

A. Aspirin
B. Fondaparinux
C. Intravenous tissue plasminogen activator (tPA)
D. Metoprolol
E. Ticagrelor

16.84. An anaesthetist is seeking advice regarding a patient with coronary heart disease, diabetes mellitus and a murmur. Which of the following is NOT a significant risk factor for perioperative myocardial infarction during non-cardiac surgery?

A. Aortic stenosis with a peak gradient of 25 mmHg
B. Diabetes mellitus treated with insulin and associated with renal failure
C. Recent (within 4 weeks) stenting of a severe proximal stenosis in the left anterior descending coronary artery
D. Recent acute coronary syndrome
E. Severe left ventricular dysfunction

16.85. A 67 year old woman presents with predictable exertional angina pectoris when climbing steep inclines. She has been commenced on aspirin, statin and a β-blocker. She attends your clinic for assessment. Which of the following suggests the patient is at low risk of future events?

A. Poor exercise tolerance
B. Poor left ventricular function
C. Post-infarct angina
D. Recent onset of symptoms
E. ST segment depression during stage 3 of the Bruce Protocol

16.86. You review a 50 year old smoker 2 months after successful treatment for a myocardial infarction. Which intervention has the greatest benefit to prevent a recurrence of myocardial infarction?

A. ACE inhibitor therapy
B. Aspirin
C. Regular and frequent aerobic exercise
D. Smoking cessation
E. Statin therapy

Answers

16.1. Answer: B.
In a patient with poorly controlled hypertension, aortic dissection should be considered as a potential cause of acute chest pain. While *interscapular* pain is a common feature of acute aortic dissection, the presentation is highly variable and central chest pain commonly occurs. If antiplatelet or antithrombotic drugs are given before excluding this diagnosis, fatal bleeding may occur.

16.2. Answer: C.
Orthopnoea refers to breathlessness occurring immediately on lying flat, whereas the term 'paroxysmal nocturnal dyspnoea' refers to sudden episodes of breathlessness occurring at night-time. It can occur with respiratory pathologies such as chronic obstructive pulmonary disease but is most often associated with heart failure. It is caused by gravity-dependent changes in pulmonary capillary hydraulic pressure leading to alveolar oedema.

16.3. Answer: B.
The most common cause of a rapid, irregular rhythm in the elderly is atrial fibrillation. In patients with very frequent atrial or ventricular ectopic beats, the pulse is also very irregular but a regular pattern can usually be perceived within it.

16.4. Answer: E.
The internal jugular vein is in direct continuity with the right atrium, and there is no venous valve between the two. The JVP therefore is a reflection of right atrial pressure, which becomes elevated in conditions where either there is increased resistance to right ventricular ejection (e.g. pulmonary hypertension due to chronic lung disease, or recurrent pulmonary embolism) or mechanical dysfunction of the right heart (e.g. right ventricular infarction, right-sided valve disease).

16.5. Answer: B.
The second heart sound, which occurs at the beginning of ventricular diastole, occurs when the aortic and pulmonary valves close. When either aortic or pulmonary artery diastolic pressure is high (e.g. in essential or pulmonary hypertension), the second heart sound may be loud. Postural hypotension will have little effect on the intensity of heart sounds at rest. Aortic incompetence is often associated with a quiet second heart sound, and mitral incompetence with a quiet or absent first heart sound. A mechanical mitral valve replacement will produce a loud mechanical first heart sound.

16.6. Answer: B.
Marfan's syndrome is a connective tissue disorder that is associated with abnormal production of elastic tissues. This can affect the aorta, aortic root and aortic valve. Aortic root dilatation can lead to aortic regurgitation and is also associated with increased risk of aortic dissection. Aortic regurgitation occurs with onset at the beginning of diastole, as soon as the aortic valve closes, and produces an early diastolic murmur. Myotonic dystrophy is associated with dilated cardiomyopathy and conducting system problems, which can lead to atrioventricular block and ventricular arrhythmias. Long QT syndrome is an inherited arrhythmia syndrome that is not usually associated with any structural cardiac abnormality. Mitral valve prolapse produces a late systolic murmur. Wolff–Parkinson–White syndrome is rarely associated with structural cardiac abnormalities (which are Ebstein's anomaly and rarely hypertrophic cardiomyopathy) and is not associated with aortic incompetence.

16.7. Answer: D.
Clinical features of acute limb ischaemia include pallor, pain, pulselessness, paraesthesia and 'perishing-with-cold' – the five 'P's. Deep venous thrombosis would cause limb swelling, venous engorgement, and a dusky blue discoloration, and this does not affect arterial flow. In cardiac failure, peripheral blood flow is not sufficiently reduced to cause limb ischaemia except in cardiogenic shock. In a patient with a history of atrial fibrillation, embolisation from the left atrial appendage is the most likely cause of limb ischaemia. Aspirin does not provide effective prophylaxis against this and current guidelines recommend the use of warfarin or a direct oral anticoagulant such as apixaban.

16

16.8. Answer: C.

Infective endocarditis is often diagnosed relatively late in its clinical course. It may initially present with non-specific symptoms that lead to a diagnosis of influenza or viral infection. Any patient with unexplained fever and a cardiac murmur, especially if changing, should be assessed for possible endocarditis, with urinalysis, an ECG, echocardiogram, blood cultures, and blood testing for white cell count and C-reactive protein concentration. In this case the wide pulse pressure is suggestive of aortic incompetence which, if severe, may occur without a murmur.

16.9. Answer: E.

After myocardial infarction, haemodynamic compromise associated with a new murmur may be caused by either papillary muscle rupture, or rupture of the interventricular septum (acquired ventricular septal defect; VSD). With acquired VSD the murmur often radiates to the right sternal border because of left-to-right shunting across the interventricular septum, whereas the murmur of acute mitral incompetence would be more likely to radiate to the axilla or the back. Acute left ventricular free wall rupture is almost always fatal and would not cause a murmur. While pericarditis may cause a sound that could be confused for a murmur, serious haemodynamic compromise is rare, as the associated pericardial effusion is usually small. Aortic incompetence is not a complication of myocardial infarction.

16.10. Answer: B.

Clinical signs of left ventricular failure are tachycardia, a gallop rhythm with a third heart sound (which is the sound of abrupt left ventricular filling due to high left atrial pressure), and bi-basal inspiratory fine crepitations at the lung bases. A fourth heart sound occurs during atrial systole because of increased left ventricular stiffness in patients with left ventricular hypertrophy. A loud second heart sound is usually caused by systemic or pulmonary hypertension. A quiet first heart sound may accompany mitral regurgitation.

16.11. Answer: A.

Troponin testing is an important component in the assessment of patients with chest pain. In patients with acute myocardial infarction, plasma troponin concentration takes time to become detectable. The admission troponin level may be normal if the patients attends soon after the onset of symptoms. If the 6-hour troponin level is normal then acute coronary syndrome is not likely to explain the patient's chest pain and other causes should then be considered. An elevated troponin level is suspicious of myocardial infarction but should be interpreted in the context of the clinical presentation. Some non-cardiac pathologies (e.g. sepsis, pulmonary embolism) are also commonly associated with minimal myocardial injury and therefore troponin release.

16.12. Answer: A.

Atrial fibrillation is the most common tachyarrhythmia encountered in older patients and is seen in approximately 2% of patients aged over 70 years, and in some studies up to 10% of those aged over 80 years. Ventricular ectopic beats would not produce episodic symptoms of this type and sinus arrhythmia is a normal variant and would not cause any symptoms. Supraventricular tachycardia normally causes *regular* palpitation.

16.13. Answer: D.

Basic life support describes the interventions that can be carried out with minimal equipment in the event of a cardiac arrest. It does not include defibrillation or administration of intravenous drugs. It does include chest compression and mouth-to-mouth resuscitation, but the ABCDE mnemonic is a helpful *aide mémoire* for these and the other components of basic life support.

16.14. Answer: E.

Pulseless electrical activity means that there is an organised cardiac rhythm seen on the ECG, but no discernible cardiac output. Defibrillation is not appropriate, as this is a treatment for ventricular fibrillation. Amiodarone can cause hypotension and is not an appropriate treatment. In current resuscitation protocols, CPR should be carried out for *2 minutes* before the rhythm is reassessed. Reversible causes of PEA include hypothermia, hypoxia, hypovolaemia, hypo-/hyperkalaemia (the four 'H's), and thrombosis (coronary or pulmonary), tension pneumothorax, tamponade and toxins (the four 'T's).

16.15. Answer: E.
While peripheral oedema and ascites are signs of right-sided cardiac failure, they typically take days or weeks to develop. Acute right ventricular failure is characterised by hypotension, a compensatory sinus tachycardia, elevation of the jugular venous pulse because of ineffective right ventricular ejection, and hepatomegaly can develop quite quickly because of hepatic venous congestion.

16.16. Answer: C.
Starling's Law describes the relationship between cardiac filling (preload) and cardiac output. Low preload causes inadequate ventricular filling and low output. Moderate preload causes optimal cardiac filling and cardiac output. Very high preload causes ventricular stretch and reduces the efficiency of contraction, resulting in reduced cardiac output. Patients with decompensated cardiac failure have high preload pressure, and diuretics and vasodilator medication can reduce this and improve cardiac function.

16.17. Answer: A.
Cardiac failure is associated with activation of the sympathetic nervous system and RAAS. The resulting production of noradrenaline (norepinephrine) and angiotensin II cause peripheral vasoconstriction. BNP production *increases* in cardiac failure in response to ventricular stretch.

16.18. Answer: B.
Loop diuretics interfere with the countercurrent sodium exchanger in the loop of the nephron. This prevents water reabsorption and results in loss of sodium and water (natriuresis).

16.19. Answer: D.
β-Blockers have several beneficial effects in chronic cardiac failure – improvement of diastolic filling, reduction of myocardial ischaemia, and prevention of ventricular arrhythmias and atrial fibrillation. β-Blockers reduce heart rate so should not be used if the patient is already bradycardic. In acute cardiac failure (e.g. acute left ventricular failure or cardiogenic shock), in which left ventricular systolic function is acutely compromised, β-blockers should not be used as they may further impair systolic function.

16.20. Answer: C.
First-line therapy for rate control in atrial fibrillation consists of β-blockade (or, if contraindicated, a rate-limiting calcium channel blocker such as verapamil can be used). In this case, the β-blocker could be prescribed in place of enalapril, as it may provide quite effective blood pressure control, as well as limiting the heart rate. None of the other agents are appropriate for rate control in atrial fibrillation. Lidocaine is used to treat ventricular arrhythmias. Flecainide and amiodarone are used for rhythm control (i.e. maintenance of sinus rhythm) and not rate control, in atrial fibrillation. Adenosine is an ultra-short-acting atrioventricular (AV) node blocker and is not used to treat atrial fibrillation.

16.21. Answer: C.
In Mobitz type II second-degree AV block, most P waves conduct normally to the ventricles and are associated with a QRS complex. Some P waves do not conduct and there is no preceding increase in the P–R interval before the blocked P wave. This reflects block in the His–Purkinje system where conduction is 'all-or-nothing'. In contrast, Mobitz type I second-degree AV block is characterised by progressive lengthening of the P–R interval block. This reflects block in the AV node itself, where conduction is 'decremental', i.e. the AV node exhibits signs of 'fatigue' with each successive beat.

16.22. Answer: E.
Sinoatrial disease is characterised by abnormalities of sinus rate, and atrial arrhythmias such as atrial flutter, atrial tachycardia and atrial fibrillation. Ventricular arrhythmias are not commonly associated with this condition.

16.23. Answer: D.
The CHA$_2$DS$_2$-VASc score is used to assess stroke risk in patients with atrial fibrillation (and atrial flutter). The mnemonic takes account of clinical risk factors for stroke (C, congestive heart failure = 1 point; H, hypertension = 1 point; A$_2$, age ≥75 years = 2 points; D, diabetes mellitus = 1 point; S$_2$, previous stroke or transient ischaemic attack = 2 points; V, vascular disease = 1 point; A, age 65–74 years = 1 point; Sc, sex category female = 1 point). In this case, the score is 5 points (2 points for age ≥75 years, 1 point each for

16

female gender, diabetes and hypertension). This is associated with quite a high risk of stroke (approximately 5% annual risk if untreated) and this patient should be considered for oral anticoagulation.

16.24. Answer: B.

Antiplatelet drugs are no longer recommended for stroke prevention in atrial fibrillation, although they are effective at preventing stroke due to carotid vascular disease. Amiodarone and β-blockers can help prevent atrial fibrillation episodes but are not known to reduce stroke risk. Apixaban is an oral factor Xa inhibitor, which has been shown in large-scale clinical trials to be effective at preventing stroke in patients with atrial fibrillation and moderate-to-high stroke risk.

16.25. Answer: E.

This ECG shows a narrow, complex tachycardia with no obvious P waves. The P waves may be concealed in the QRS complex or ST segment. The term 'supraventricular tachycardia' is used to describe this rhythm. The two most likely mechanisms are atrioventricular nodal re-entrant tachycardia (AVNRT) or atrioventricular re-entrant tachycardia (AVRT). The key to terminating these tachycardias is to cause transient block in the AV node and the quickest and least invasive way of doing this is by using vagal manoeuvres such as carotid sinus pressure or the Valsalva manoeuvre.

16.26. Answer: C.

Pacemakers are used to treat or prevent bradycardia and the main indications are symptomatic sinoatrial disease and AV nodal disease. Pacemakers are not effective at preventing atrial fibrillation or supraventricular tachycardia. Sinus bradycardia in an athlete is a normal, physiological finding that requires no treatment. An implantable cardiac defibrillator (ICD), not a permanent pacemaker, is used to prevent sudden death due to ventricular arrhythmias in vulnerable patients.

16.27. Answer: E.

ICDs are indicated for primary prevention in patients with previous myocardial infarction who have chronically impaired left ventricular function. It is thought that the scar burden in these patients predisposes them to ventricular arrhythmias, which, when they occur, are poorly tolerated. As long as there are no

comorbidities, age is not a barrier to implantation. ICDs are not indicated for patients who have experienced ventricular arrhythmias due to reversible factors (e.g. drug misuse) or in the acute phase of myocardial infarction, as subsequent risk of similar arrhythmias is generally low. Patients with sinoatrial disease or AV nodal block without ventricular arrhythmia are treated with a permanent pacemaker, not an ICD.

16.28. Answer: D.

The only one of these conditions associated with a significant intracardiac shunt is tetralogy of Fallot. Central cyanosis occurs because of shunting of blood through a ventricular septal defect, and this is exacerbated by the over-riding aorta (i.e. the aorta over-rides the defect, causing blood from the right ventricle to be ejected directly into the aorta) and by muscular right ventricular outflow obstruction. Cyanotic episodes may be precipitated by fever or by dehydration. In most cases the condition is recognised and corrected in infancy.

16.29. Answer: D.

Eisenmenger's syndrome occurs in patients with untreated intracardiac shunts such as atrial or ventricular septal defects. Initially shunting is from the left to the right side of the heart, and central cyanosis does not occur. The response to increased pulmonary blood flow is pulmonary vasoconstriction, which leads to permanent sclerotic changes in the pulmonary microvasculature. This causes right heart pressure to increase to the point it exceeds left heart pressure. Shunt reversal and central (and peripheral) cyanosis then occur. Breathlessness and fatigue are common symptoms. Patients with Eisenmenger's syndrome have markedly reduced life expectancy because of cardiac failure and cardiac arrhythmias. Patent foramen ovale is not a cause of Eisenmenger's syndrome and it does not cause significant intracardiac shunting.

16.30. Answer: E.

Ventricular septal defect (VSD) causes a harsh systolic murmur that may radiate to the right side of the sternum. Small VSDs do not cause significant shunting but can produce a loud murmur. Atrial septal defect might cause a quiet systolic flow murmur. Persistent ductus arteriosus causes a continuous murmur throughout systole and diastole. Patent foramen ovale produces no abnormal auscultatory findings. Mitral valve prolapsed causes a late systolic murmur and is not referred to as a 'hole' in the heart.

16.31. Answer: A.
Pericarditis is associated with friction between the epicardial surface of the heart and the pericardial sac. This causes a scratchy to-and-fro sound in time with the cardiac cycle, which is distinct from a murmur. It is associated with pleuritic chest pain, which may be affected by sitting forward or backward. Heart sounds are either normal or, if there is a large pericardial effusion, diminished. It may occur in the context of flu-like illness and a viral aetiology is common. Endocarditis is not associated with pleuritic chest pain. Persistent ductus arteriosus is a congenital (rather than acute) condition, which is associated with a continuous murmur.

16.32. Answer: D.
Aspirin, through its anti-inflammatory effects, is a very effective symptomatic treatment for pericarditis. Non-steroidal anti-inflammatory drugs such as diclofenac can also be used orally. Steroids are rarely required. Amiodarone is an anti-arrhythmic drug and has no role in the management of acute pericarditis.

16.33. Answer: A.
Dilated cardiomyopathy is characterised by dilatation of the atria and ventricles, and thinning of ventricular walls. Hypertrophic cardiomyopathy causes disproportionate thickening of myocardium, particularly the interventricular septum. Myocardial infiltration (e.g. with amyloid protein) can cause restrictive cardiomyopathy, which does not cause cardiac dilatation but does restrict myocardial contraction and relaxation.

16.34. Answer: B.
Cigarette smoking is a leading cause of cardiovascular disease but its main influence is on the genesis of atherosclerosis and coronary artery disease. Likewise, obesity is associated with risk of hypertension and type 2 diabetes mellitus, but is not a risk factor for cardiomyopathy. Hypercholesterolaemia may have dietary and genetic components and is a risk factor for coronary artery disease, not cardiomyopathy. Dilated cardiomyopathy can be caused by genetic defects of sarcomeric

proteins such as troponins, tropomyosin, myosin heavy chain, actin and actin-binding proteins, among many, but cardiac sodium channel gene mutations predispose to cardiac arrhythmias by causing long QT syndrome or Brugada syndrome.

16.35. Answer: A.
Hypertrophic cardiomyopathy is characterised by left ventricular hypertrophy. This is often asymmetric with the interventricular septum classically affected. There are other variants, such as apical hypertrophic cardiomyopathy.

16.36. Answer: D.
Cardiac transplantation is limited by the availability of donor organs, the need for life-long immunosuppressive therapy to prevent rejection, and the risks of surgery and the drugs used afterwards. Therefore it is only offered to patients with cardiac failure who remain symptomatic despite adherence with optimal pharmacological therapy and, where appropriate, cardiac resynchronisation therapy.

16.37. Answer: E.
Hypertrophic cardiomyopathy is associated with disorganisation and fibrosis of left ventricular myocardial tissue. This can predispose patients to sudden ventricular arrhythmias, and these may occur without warning during intense exercise. The risk is highest in patients with gross hypertrophy or left ventricular outflow tract obstruction. Some genetic variants are also associated with high risk, such as troponin T mutations. Right ventricular failure and pulmonary embolism are not common in patients with hypertrophic cardiomyopathy. Atrial fibrillation occurs and may cause symptoms but is rarely life-threatening.

16.38. Answer: B.
Loop diuretics have no effect on mortality in patients with cardiac failure. Rate-limiting calcium channel blockers such as diltiazem and verapamil are usually avoided, as they have a negative inotropic effect, which may aggravate cardiac failure. Aspirin and percutaneous coronary intervention are treatments for coronary artery disease, not cardiomyopathy.

16.39. Answer: A.
Takotsubo (stress) cardiomyopathy occurs most often in females and is associated with emotional stress. It can occur due to

16

bereavement, acute non-cardiac illness, natural disasters and other major life events. It is characterised by chest pain and ECG changes that mimic myocardial infarction. Troponin elevation is common but coronary angiography does not show occlusive coronary artery disease or intracoronary thrombus. Echocardiography shows a characteristic left ventricular appearance of apical dilatation, giving the appearance of an octopus trap or takotsubo!

16.40. Answer: A.
Alcohol has many negative effects on health. These include liver disease, pancreatitis, hypertension and cognitive dysfunction. It also causes many behavioural and social problems, particularly if alcohol dependency occurs. Cardiac effects include atrial fibrillation and dilated cardiomyopathy, both of which may be reversible if the patient abstains early enough.

16.41. Answer: D.
Atrial myxoma is the most common cardiac tumour and 75% or more occur in the left atrium. Large tumours may partially obstruct the mitral valve, affecting cardiac output and causing a tumour 'plop' on auscultation. Tumours are benign but can be associated with cerebral and peripheral embolism (which is how they often first present), so surgery is usually indicated to prevent this.

16.42. Answer: E.
Chronic pericardial constriction is a late complication of tuberculous and viral pericarditis and is caused by pericardial fibrosis, contraction and adhesion to the epicardium. It can also complicate chronic inflammatory disorders such as rheumatoid disease. Acute myocardial infarction can lead to acute post-infarct pericarditis, but this almost never leads to pericardial constriction.

16.43. Answer: A.
Large pericardial effusions are normally not associated with a pericardial rub as the pericardium and epicardium are well separated by pericardial fluid and friction does not occur. The ECG may show small complexes but is not a sensitive test, and an *echocardiogram* is required to make the diagnosis. The chest X-ray may show a spherical or globular cardiac silhouette. In symptomatic patients, percutaneous pericardial drainage is used to

relieve symptoms and to obtain fluid for laboratory analysis. Patients with pericardial effusion are very dependent on high preload pressure to maintain cardiac output, so diuretics may cause significant hypotension. Large effusions may occur because of malignancy, usually metastatic disease from lung or breast cancer.

16.44. Answer: B.
'Saddle' ST segment elevation is a common feature of acute pericarditis, but it can be confused with an ST segment elevation myocardial infarction, Brugada syndrome, and a normal variant in some ethnic groups such as those of African or Caribbean descent. In contrast, PR interval depression is very specific to pericarditis and, when seen, is usually diagnostic.

16.45. Answer: D.
Sinus tachycardia is the most common ECG abnormality in pulmonary embolism, although atrial fibrillation may also occur. The next commonest ECG change is anterior T-wave inversion due to right ventricular wall stress. The S1Q3T3 (large S wave in lead I, Q-wave and T-wave inversion in lead III) pattern is commonly absent but, when present, is more specific to massive pulmonary embolism.

16.46. Answer: D.
Although elevation of the JVP and peripheral oedema often occur with chronic pericardial effusion, they are not specific signs of cardiac tamponade. Here, pulsus paradoxus and Kussmaul's sign (the JVP falling on inspiration) are specific signs. Pulsus paradoxus is an exaggeration of physiological variation in blood pressure caused by compression of the heart in the pericardial sac, and is characterised by a large fall in blood pressure during inspiration.

16.47. Answer: C.
All of the agents listed except furosemide have been shown to improve survival in patients with heart failure due to left ventricular systolic dysfunction. Loop diuretics such as furosemide are important for symptom control, but so far, no large-scale randomised trial has shown survival benefit.

16.48. Answer: C.
P2Y12 receptor antagonists inhibit adenosine diphosphate (ADP)-dependent platelet

activation and all of the agents listed except dipyridamole act via this receptor. Dipyridamole is a phosphodiesterase inhibitor, which blocks the response to ADP by inhibiting breakdown of cyclic adenosine monophosphate (cAMP) and inhibits the re-uptake of adenosine into platelets.

16.49. Answer: E.
Smoking is by far the strongest modifiable risk factor for coronary artery disease. Obesity is associated with hypertension, type 2 diabetes and unfavourable lipid profile, and is thus associated with risk of myocardial infarction. High levels of dietary saturated fat (e.g. from red meat and processed meat products) are also known to be associated with increased cardiovascular risk.

16.50. Answer: E.
Both percutaneous coronary intervention and fibrinolytic drug therapy are treatment modalities for acute ST elevation myocardial infarction. Both treatments aim to re-open the culprit coronary vessel to restore perfusion to the infarct territory. In randomised studies, administration of tPA or other fibronolytic drugs had a strongly time-dependent beneficial effect. If administered more than 8–10 hours after the onset of symptoms, risk of treatment begins to outweigh benefit. As fibrinolytic drugs take time to work, and may not completely restore flow in the culprit vessel, they are best administered early. Percutaneous coronary intervention and the other therapies described do not have such a time-dependent effect on outcome. When primary percutaneous coronary intervention cannot be provided within 2 hours, fibrinolytic therapy should be administered immediately.

16.51. Answer: E.
Dilated cardiomyopathy, myocarditis and myocardial infarction all reduce left ventricular systolic function and are associated with low left ventricular ejection fraction (LVEF), a measure of the percentage of left ventricular blood ejected in systole. Aortic stenosis is associated with either normal LVEF, or if severe, sometimes low LVEF. Restrictive cardiomyopathy is associated with myocardial infiltration and sometimes reduction in left ventricular cavity size, but normal systolic function. LVEF is high but stroke volume low due to small cavity size. Heart failure is caused

by diastolic dysfunction – the inability of the left ventricle to fill properly in diastole.

16.52. Answer: D.
Both the sympathetic nervous system and the RAAS systems are activated in heart failure. Vasopressin may also be released from the posterior pituitary in response to reduced cardiac output. Thyroid hormone levels are generally unaffected in cardiac failure but profound hypo- or hyperthyroidism can cause heart failure.

16.53. Answer: E.
Troponin I is a structural myocardial protein subunit, and not an enzyme. Along with the other markers listed, it is released into the blood stream after acute myocardial infarction from injured myocardial tissue.

16.54. Answer: C.
If the patient has occluded his stent, then the ECG will show an acute inferior ST segment elevation myocardial infarction. Electrocardiographic features of acute inferior myocardial infarction include ST segment elevation in the inferior leads (II, III and aVF) and sometimes atrioventricular block.

16.55. Answer: A.
Sudden, severe pulmonary oedema after myocardial infarction may be a sign of a mechanical complication. Acute papillary muscle rupture causes sudden and very severe mitral regurgitation, which, in turn, is complicated by pulmonary oedema. Acute pericarditis causes sharp chest pain but does not cause pulmonary oedema. Free wall rupture usually causes pulseless electrical activity (PEA) cardiac arrest and is almost always fatal. Atrial septal defect is not a complication of myocardial infarction. Left ventricular mural thrombus is usually asymptomatic, and is detected on echocardiography. It can lead to stroke and peripheral embolism.

16.56. Answer: E.
Ventricular fibrillation is an early complication of acute myocardial infarction and is the leading preventable cause of death. Early recognition of myocardial infarction is therefore important. Sudden death rates may be reduced by education of the public about symptoms of myocardial infarction and the need to seek immediate medical help, and by the

16

now-ubiquitous placement of external defibrillators in emergency ambulances. Community first responder programmes and public access defibrillation are other strategies that allow a more rapid response to myocardial infarction and cardiac arrest in rural areas.

16.57. Answer: A.
Diabetes mellitus has been shown in large cohort studies to be protective against the risk of development of abdominal aortic aneurysm, and where aneurysm is present, the rate of enlargement is slower than in non-diabetics. The reason for this negative association is unclear.

16.58. Answer: A.
Acute limb ischaemia leads to pallor, pain, pulselessness, paraesthesia and 'perishing-with-cold' – the five 'P's. Chronic limb ischaemia is associated with hair loss in the affected limb. Capillary refill time is a measure of peripheral perfusion and is tested by squeezing the skin over the fingers or toes until it blanches, then assessing the time taken for colour to fully return. A capillary refill time of <2 seconds is a sign of good peripheral perfusion and if >3 seconds is a sign of reduced peripheral perfusion.

16.59. Answer: C.
β-Blockers and ACE inhibitors help reduce arterial wall stress and, through their role in controlling hypertension, may help reduce risk of aortic aneurysm expansion and rupture. Statins reduce the rate of progression of atherosclerosis and may help reduce risk of rupture through cholesterol-dependent and cholesterol-independent effects. However, of all interventions, smoking cessation has the greatest effect in reducing the risk of aneurysm rupture.

16.60. Answer: C.
Atherosclerotic peripheral vascular disease is the most common cause of limb ischaemia. Buerger's disease is a form of obliterative arteritis affecting small and medium-sized vessels, strongly associated with cigarette smoking. It causes limb ischaemia and gangrene, and presents at a relatively young age. Raynaud's disease is a vasospastic condition associated with some connective tissue disorders. It can cause digital ischaemia and in some cases infarction. Atrial fibrillation

can cause limb ischaemia because of its association with stroke and peripheral embolism. Diabetes mellitus is associated with atherosclerotic and microvascular disease and is strongly linked with limb ischaemia; however, it would be unusual in a normal-weight individual of this age without symptoms.

16.61. Answer: C.
While control of blood pressure is important in type A aortic dissection, through use of β-blockers or other antihypertensive agents, it is early surgery that has the greatest effect on mortality. Type A aortic dissection involves the ascending aorta and patients may die because of cardiac tamponade, aortic rupture, or dissection into downstream arteries resulting in ischaemia of limbs or organs. The most effective way of preventing this is to repair the entry point of the dissection in the ascending aorta. Anticoagulation is contraindicated in acute aortic dissection as it may cause fatal bleeding.

16.62. Answer: D.
Hypertension, because of its population prevalence, is the leading cause of aortic dissection; however, this would have been picked up on antenatal checks in this case. Marfan's syndrome (usually associated with tall stature) and coarctation of the aorta are relatively uncommon conditions, but both have a strong association with aortic dissection. Intramural haematoma refers to spontaneous bleeding into the aortic wall and may be the precursor to aortic dissection. Pregnancy-associated dissection is rare, but when it occurs it is usually in the third trimester or postpartum period, and is more likely to occur in patients with predisposing conditions such as Marfan's syndrome.

16.63. Answer: C.
Primary percutaneous coronary intervention (PPCI) is more effective at reperfusing the infarct-related territory than fibrinolysis with streptokinase or tPA. Fibrinolytic drugs may not reach the site of vessel occlusion if there is no flow, and will do nothing to treat the culprit occlusive atherosclerotic lesion. PPCI usually completely restores blood flow by fragmenting the clot and by opening up the site of stenosis. It is associated with lower mortality and lower rates of subsequent angina and re-infarction.

Coronary artery bypass surgery is not used to treat acute myocardial infarction but is an effective treatment for some patients with chronic coronary artery disease.

16.64. Answer: A.

There is a strong association between age and risk of death after myocardial infarction. In-hospital mortality is three times greater in individuals aged over 80 years than it is in those aged 60–65 years. While risk of myocardial infarction is much higher in smokers than in non-smokers to start with, the risk of death in smokers after myocardial infarction is lower than in non-smokers, probably because their main risk factor is modifiable. ECG changes and troponin concentration are not good predictors of mortality risk. Cardiac arrest within 24 hours of myocardial infarction is an effect of acute ischaemia and does not predict risk of sudden death after discharge from hospital.

16.65. Answer: D.

There are many uncommon endocrine causes of hypertension, including those listed, but renal disease is the most common cause.

16.66. Answer: D.

All other options given apart from D describe recognised causes of secondary hypertension. Antihypertensive drug therapy, along with lifestyle changes, effectively controls blood pressure in most patients with hypertension. The most common cause of poor blood pressure control is therefore poor adherence with antihypertensive therapy. This may be because of side-effects, and also because of the asymptomatic nature of the condition.

16.67. Answer: D.

The revised Jones criteria are used to diagnose rheumatic fever. The condition is diagnosed if two major criteria are met, or one major and two minor criteria are met. Carditis, subcutaneous nodules, erythema marginatum and chorea are all major criteria, whereas elevation of C-reactive protein (or erythrocyte sedimentation rate) is a minor criterion.

16.68. Answer: A.

Aspirin is the drug of choice in rheumatic fever and is used in high doses compared with those used in common analgesia. Glucocorticoids are not used in this condition.

16.69. Answer: C.

Mitral stenosis is characterised by the presence of a tapping apex beat, reflecting a palpable opening snap, accompanied by a low-pitched mid-diastolic murmur. If the patient is in sinus rhythm, pre-systolic accentuation of the murmur may occur because of atrial contraction. A loud second heart sound may be heard due to secondary pulmonary hypertension, which often accompanies mitral stenosis.

16.70. Answer: A.

A thrill is indicative of aortic stenosis or hypertrophic obstructive cardiomyopathy, both of which are *not* associated with a parasternal heave. A parasternal heave occurs because of right ventricular hypertrophy and does not cause a thrill. Conditions which lead to pulmonary hypertension (e.g. mitral stenosis, chronic lung disease and atrial septal defect) may therefore cause right ventricular hypertrophy and a parasternal heave.

16.71. Answer: C.

Aortic regurgitation is associated with a large-volume, collapsing pulse and an early diastolic murmur associated with a systolic 'flow' murmur. In severe aortic regurgitation, the pulse pressure may be so large as to cause prominent neck pulsation. A slow rising pulse, crescendo–decrescendo murmur, quiet second heart sound and palpable thrill in the aortic area are signs of aortic *stenosis*.

16.72. Answer: E.

Viridans streptococci are the most common cause of endocarditis on a native heart valve. *Staphylococcus aureus* is the most common organism to infect prosthetic valves.

16.73. Answer: A.

Cutaneous signs of endocarditis (options B, D and E) are not seen in most patients with the condition, but when present, are highly diagnostic of it. Roth's spots (seen on fundoscopy) are also relatively uncommon. Haematuria (often microscopic) is a common manifestation of endocarditis.

16.74. Answer: B.

Viridans streptococci are usually very sensitive to benzylpenicillin, and this agent works synergistically with gentamicin. Bactericidal blood concentrations can only be achieved with

16

frequent intravenous dosing. Ampicillin is not as effective, and flucloxacillin and vancomycin are principally used to treat staphylococcal infections.

16.75. Answer: A.
Hypertrophic cardiomyopathy is often familial, and the most common mode of inheritance is autosomal dominant.

16.76. Answer: A.
Mutations in myosin heavy chain, troponin and myosin-binding protein most often lead to hypertrophic cardiomyopathy. Titan mutations (and some myosin-binding protein mutations) may cause dilated cardiomyopathy. It is mutations in fibrillin, a glycoprotein critical to production of elastic tissue, that most often leads to Marfan's syndrome.

16.77. Answer: B.
Atrial myxoma is the most common cardiac tumour. It is a benign tumour that usually occurs in the left atrium and is associated with increased risk of stroke and peripheral embolism.

16.78. Answer: C.
Transthoracic echocardiography is a form of ultrasound imaging that has limitations. It is good for assessing heart valve and myocardial function but has limited value in characterising tissues (e.g. for fibrosis). The left atrial appendage is the most common site for thrombus formation in atrial fibrillation and this structure is not visible during transthoracic echocardiography. The *electrocardiogram*, not echocardiogram, is used to assess cardiac arrhythmias. Whilst poor left ventricular function is associated with a poor future prognosis, in isolation, echocardiography gives limited information about prognosis.

16.79. Answer: B.
The decision between percutaneous coronary intervention (PCI) and coronary artery bypass graft surgery is an important one in patients with angina or after myocardial infarction. The patients who have the most to gain from surgery are those with left main stem disease and left ventricular impairment.

16.80. Answer: D.
Gadolinium-enhanced MRI is currently the most sensitive imaging modality for the identification

of myocardial fibrosis. In addition to assessing scar burden and distribution after myocardial infarction, it is also helpful in the diagnosis of and risk stratification in cardiomyopathies, because of the association between myocardial fibrosis, these conditions, and risk of ventricular arrhythmias. It is also useful to help guide the likelihood of success from coronary artery bypass graft surgery.

16.81. Answer: B.
The main components in the management of acute pulmonary oedema are bed rest, oxygen therapy, intravenous nitrates and intravenous diuretics. Non-invasive continuous positive airway pressure (CPAP) ventilation is helpful in resistant cases. Dobutamine is an inotrope that increases cardiac work; it is sometimes used in the management of cardiogenic shock, but is not appropriate in a patient with high blood pressure and cardiac failure.

16.82. Answer: B.
Endocrine causes of dilated cardiomyopathy, and alcohol-related cardiomyopathy, are often reversible as long as the underlying problem is treated early enough. Anthracycline chemotherapy can cause acute or late-onset dilated cardiomyopathy that responds only in a limited manner to β-blockers and ACE inhibitors and which may cause permanent cardiac dysfunction.

16.83. Answer: C.
Non-ST segment myocardial infarction is normally initially managed with dual antiplatelet therapy (e.g. aspirin and ticagrelor), and an antithrombotic agent (e.g. fondaparinux or enoxaparin). β-Blockade is often used as prophylaxis against angina and arrhythmias. Intravenous tPA is a treatment for *acute ST elevation myocardial infarction* and has not been shown to improve outcome in patients with non-ST segment elevation myocardial infarction. Indeed, patients with ST segment depression have a worse outcome with thrombolytic therapy.

16.84. Answer: A.
Surgery is associated with activation of platelets and coagulation pathways, so patients who have had recent myocardial infarction or recent percutaneous coronary intervention are at increased risk of thrombosis in the affected vessel, resulting in myocardial infarction.

Patients with left ventricular impairment are at increased risk of acute cardiac failure and haemodynamic problems in the perioperative phase. Insulin-treated diabetic patients and those with renal failure may have occult coronary artery disease and are at increased risk of perioperative myocardial infarction. Aortic stenosis with a relatively small peak pressure gradient is not likely to cause haemodynamic problems during or after surgery.

16.85. Answer: E.

Exercise tolerance testing can be used to identify patients with coronary artery disease who have a low threshold for myocardial ischaemia. Patients who can exercise into stage 3 of the Bruce Protocol before ECG abnormalities develop are likely to have a high ischaemic threshold and are not at high risk of major cardiovascular events. Conversely, patients with new-onset, rapidly progressive, or limiting symptoms may have critical coronary artery disease. Patients with poor left ventricular function have poor cardiac reserve and carry higher than average risk because they tolerate myocardial ischaemia poorly.

16.86. Answer: D.

Smoking is the strongest risk factor for the development of coronary artery disease. More than any other lifestyle modification, or any other preventative therapy, smoking cessation makes the largest difference to cardiovascular risk.

16

17

Respiratory medicine

Multiple Choice Questions

17.1. A 46 year old woman has a recent diagnosis of adenocarcinoma of the lung made at bronchoscopy 1 week ago. She presents to the emergency department acutely short of breath with a non-productive cough. She has an ache in the centre of her chest that is made worse by breathing in. She is apyrexial. Oxygen saturations are 91% on 40% oxygen. Respiratory rate is 30 breaths/min. Blood pressure (BP) is 100/65 mmHg and pulse is 110 beats/min.

Examination reveals decreased expansion of the right side with dullness to percussion throughout the right side. Her trachea is deviated to the right and the apex beat is not palpable. Breath sounds are reduced on the right. What is the most likely diagnosis?

A. Collapse of the right lung
B. Pericardial effusion
C. Right-sided pleural effusion
D. Right-sided pneumonia
E. Right-sided pneumothorax

17.2. An 83 year old woman was passenger in a car that collided with a lamppost in the city centre. She was initially complaining of pain in her right hip and ribs but has become increasingly drowsy since the paramedics administered 2 mg of morphine. She is brought to the emergency department by ambulance. Urgent X-rays reveal a pelvic fracture, and a single right-sided rib fracture.

Having, initially been drowsy but responsive she is now unresponsive. Oxygen saturations are 87% on 2 L/min oxygen via nasal cannulae. She is apyrexial. BP is 110/66 mmHg, pulse is 65 beats/min. There are no new findings on examination. An urgent CT brain reveals only

small vessel disease. Arterial blood gas: H$^+$ 60 nmol/L (pH 7.22), PaO_2 8.7 kPa (65 mmHg), $PaCO_2$ 10 kPa (75 mmHg), HCO_3^- 26 mmol/L. What is the most likely cause of her deteriorating conscious level?

A. Cholesterol embolism – ventilation/perfusion ($\dot{V}/\dot{Q}$) mismatch
B. Chronic obstructive pulmonary disease (COPD) with oxygen toxicity – loss of hypoxic drive
C. Flail segment due to rib fracture – loss of elastic recoil
D. Opiate toxicity – suppression of the respiratory centre
E. Undetected fracture of C3 – diaphragmatic failure

17.3. A 55 year old man has smoked 30 cigarettes per day since he was 15 years old. He is a taxi driver. He finds he is increasingly breathless on exertion. Oxygen saturations are 98% on room air. Examination reveals tracheal tug, reduced cricosternal distance and a barrel chest. He has reduced cardiac dullness and symmetrically reduced air entry. CXR reveals hyperinflation and spirometry reveals moderate airways obstruction. The patient walks 300 m on an incremental walk test before becoming breathless; oxygen saturations are maintained.

What pathological change best explains why he is breathless on exertion?

A. Activation of central chemoreceptors
B. Exercise-induced bronchospasm
C. Loss of elastic recoil
D. Paradoxical diaphragm movement
E. Pulmonary hypertension

17.4. A 52 year old man presents with 4 days of haemoptysis. Over the last 2 months he has lost weight without experiencing night sweats. He has smoked 30 cigarettes per day for 40 years and worked in construction. He thinks it is likely that he encountered asbestos at work but cannot recall any specific exposure. He returned home from holiday in Guyana 1 week ago. What is most likely to cause the CXR findings shown below.

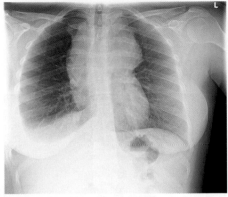

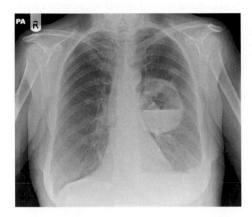

A. Bronchial carcinoma
B. Granulomatous polyangiitis
C. Lung abscess
D. Pulmonary and pleural tuberculosis (TB)
E. Pulmonary infarct

17.5. A 26 year old woman presents with 24 hours of central chest pain and progressive shortness of breath over a month. Examination reveals pulse 105 beats/min, BP 105/65 mmHg, oxygen saturations 96% on room air, apyrexial, respiratory rate 16 breaths/min. Chest clear; heart sounds dual, no murmurs. Electrocardiogram (ECG): sinus tachycardia; no other abnormalities.

Blood tests: haemoglobin 110 g/L, white cell count (WCC) 9×10^9/L, platelets 340×10^9/L, urea and electrolytes normal range, C-reactive protein (CRP) 67 mg/L.

Given the CXR below, what should the next test be?

A. Bronchoscopy
B. CT chest, abdomen, pelvis
C. D-dimer
D. Echocardiogram
E. Positron emission tomography (PET) scan

17.6. A 52 year old man presents with a 1-week history of fever, left-sided pleuritic chest pain and increasing shortness of breath. He has a past medical history of alcohol dependency, alcoholic liver disease and chronic pancreatitis. He has smoked 10 cigarettes per day for 30 years and still drinks 28 units a week. He worked as a casual labourer on building sites where asbestos was removed when he was in his 20s.

What is most likely to be causing the CXR shown below?

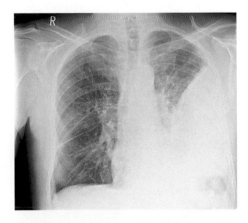

A. Bronchial carcinoma
B. Empyema
C. Hepatic hydrothorax
D. Mesothelioma
E. Pleural effusion secondary to pancreatitis

17

17.7. A 63 year old woman had a CT pulmonary angiogram (CTPA) when she presented with left-sided pleuritic chest pain to the medical assessment unit. There was no pulmonary thromboembolism but the appearance below was noted on CT scan.

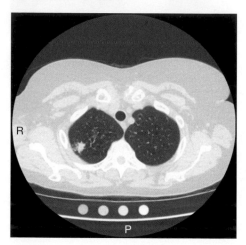

The patient recovered spontaneously over 24 hours and had no other symptoms or past medical history. She has smoked 10 cigarettes per day for 40 years. What is the best next step?

A. Bronchoscopy
B. Commence antibiotics
C. CT-guided biopsy
D. Interferon-gamma release assay
E. PET scan

17.8. A 63 year old woman had a pulmonary nodule identified incidentally during a CTPA examination. She has a 20 pack-year smoking history but no past medical history and is asymptomatic with performance status 0. She has had pulmonary function testing, including lung volumes and gas transfer, with no abnormalities identified. She went on to have the test below and the only abnormality identified is shown.

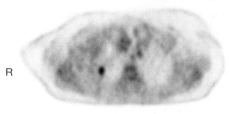

What should be the next step?

A. Antituberculous chemotherapy
B. Further follow-up scan in 3 months
C. Palliative chemotherapy
D. Palliative radiotherapy
E. Right upper lobectomy

17.9. A 51 year old woman presents to the emergency department with sudden-onset breathlessness and right-sided pleuritic chest pain. She is a non-smoker with no significant occupational exposures and no significant past medical history. She requires 40% oxygen to maintain her saturations at 92%, apyrexial, BP 101/62 mmHg, pulse 112 beats/min, respiration rate 30 breaths/min.
What is shown on the CXR?

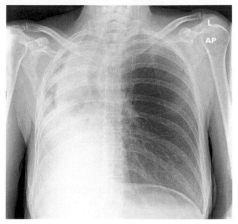

A. Dextrocardia
B. Left-sided tension pneumothorax
C. Right-sided lung collapse
D. Right-sided pleural effusion
E. Right-sided pneumothorax

17.10. A 53 year old woman has had asthma for 30 years. It had been well controlled until the last year. Despite escalation of her inhaled therapies and intermittent oral corticosteroids she has an ongoing cough productive of copious volumes of green sputum, breathlessness and wheeze. After review in the respiratory clinic she is sent for a CT scan. What is shown on the image here?

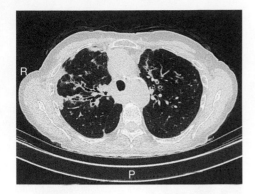

A. Bronchiectasis
B. Chronic bronchitis and emphysema
C. Cystic fibrosis
D. Honeycombing and interstitial fibrosis
E. Typical changes of asthma

17.11. A 71 year old man presents with increasing shortness of breath with no cough or systemic symptoms. He has atrial fibrillation for which he takes apixaban. A recent echocardiogram suggests preserved left ventricular systolic function and no valvular abnormalities. He has no significant respiratory exposures and has always worked in an office. He has only ever holidayed in North America.
    What does his CXR show?

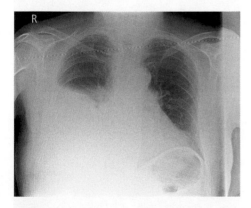

A. Right middle and lower lobe collapse
B. Right-sided bronchial carcinoma
C. Right-sided consolidation
D. Right-sided mesothelioma
E. Right-sided pleural effusion

17.12. For the patient described in Question 17.11, what would be the best next step in his management?
A. Bedside thoracic ultrasound and pleural aspiration
B. Diuretic therapy
C. Repeat echocardiogram
D. Stop apixaban
E. Thoracic ultrasound scan-guided intercostal chest drain

17.13. A 35 year old man has been unwell for a week. He has experienced fever, productive cough, rhinitis and aching muscles. He now presents with left-sided pleuritic chest pain to the emergency department. Observations include temperature 39°C, oxygen saturations 94% on room air, BP 134/76 mmHg, pulse 101 beats/min, respiratory rate 24 breaths/min. His CXR is below.

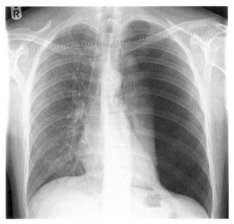

What is shown on the CXR?
A. Bilateral hilar lymphadenopathy
B. Collapse/consolidation of the lingula
C. Diffuse right-sided infiltrates
D. Left hilar consolidation
E. Left-sided pneumothorax

17

17.14. A 29 year old man presents with progressive shortness of breath over a week and a new central chest discomfort. He has a productive cough. He works in telemarketing and smokes cannabis recreationally. He has no other past medical history of note. Observations include temperature 38.5°C, oxygen saturations 93% on room air, BP 112/87 mmHg, pulse 106 beats/min, respiratory rate 24 breaths/min. His CXR is shown.

What would be the next step in his management?

A. Admit for observation
B. CT scan
C. Human immunodeficiency virus (HIV) test
D. Intercostal chest drain
E. Therapeutic aspiration

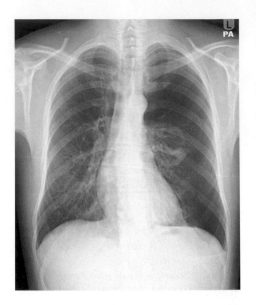

17.15. A 54 year old woman attends the rapid-access lung cancer clinic with haemoptysis and an abnormal CXR. CT scanning confirms a large cavitating right upper lobe mass and bronchoscopic biopsy confirms a squamous lung cancer. The PET scan below was arranged.

What does the CT-PET scan show?

A. Uptake confined to the right upper lobe lesion
B. Uptake in the right upper lobe lesion and a spinal metastasis
C. Uptake in the right upper lobe lesion and physiological uptake in large vessels
D. Uptake in the right upper lobe lesion and right hilar lymph node
E. Uptake in the right upper lobe lesion, a spinal metastasis and a sternal metastasis

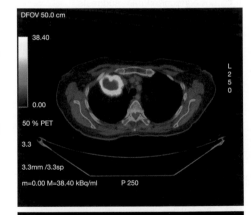

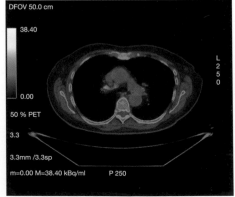

17.16. A 73 year old woman has struggled with increasing shortness of breath on exertion over the last year. In addition, she has a dry cough. She worked in an office until she retired. She has a pet dog. She has osteoarthritis, osteoporosis and hypothyroidism. She takes regular paracetamol, a bisphosphonate and calcium/vitamin D supplementation. Her sister was treated for TB when they were children and she had X-ray screening that she thinks was clear. Examination reveals finger clubbing and bi-basal crackles. Her CT scan is shown below.

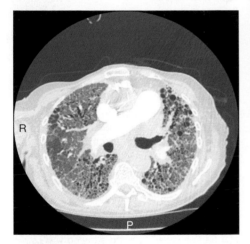

What is the likely cause of the CT appearance?

A. Bronchiectasis
B. Emphysema
C. Idiopathic pulmonary fibrosis
D. Lymphangitis carcinomatosa
E. Scarring related to pulmonary tuberculosis

17.17. A 45 year old man has returned home from a holiday in Spain with a dry cough, left-sided pleuritic chest pain and fever. He had started some amoxicillin he bought whilst in Spain. He has been sent to the medical assessment unit after a family physician visit at home where he was found to be quite muddled. He has a fever of 39.5°C and oxygen saturations of 85% on air. Respiratory rate is 26 breaths/min, BP 103/63 mmHg, pulse 112 beats/min. Examination reveals left-sided bronchial breathing with increased vocal resonance.

Blood tests reveal: haemoglobin 143 g/L, WCC 12 × 10⁹/L (neutrophilia), platelets 435 × 10⁹/L, urea 9 mmol/L (54 mg/dL), creatinine 102 μmol/L (1.15 mg/dL), sodium 128 mmol/L, bilirubin 12 μmol/L (0.70 mg/dL), alanine transaminase (ALT) 243 U/L, γ-glutamyl transferase (GGT) 354 U/L, alkaline phosphatase 250 U/L, CRP 334 mg/L. His CXR is below.

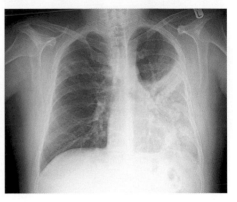

What abnormality is seen on his CXR?

A. Extensive left-sided consolidation
B. Large left-sided pleural effusion
C. Left-sided bronchial carcinoma
D. Left-sided empyema
E. Left-sided pulmonary infarct

17.18. For the same patient described in Question 17.17, what is his CURB-65 score?

A. 0
B. 1
C. 2
D. 3
E. 4

17.19. For the same patient described in Question 17.17, which of the following is the causative organism likely to be?

A. *Chlamydia pneumoniae*
B. *Haemophilus influenzae*
C. *Legionella pneumophila*
D. *Mycoplasma pneumoniae*
E. *Streptococcus pneumoniae*

17

17.20. A 38 year old man presents with cough productive of blood-streaked sputum, fever and left-sided pleuritic chest pain. In addition he has developed troublesome cold sores. His past medical history includes appendicectomy. He works in a bank. His CXR is below.

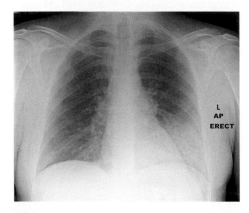

What does his CXR show?

A. Left-sided apical pneumothorax
B. Left-sided basal consolidation
C. Left-sided collapse
D. Left-sided pleural effusion
E. Left-sided reticulonodular opacification

17.21. An 82 year old man presents with increasing shortness of breath on exertion over the last 2 years. He has finger clubbing and bi-basal inspiratory crackles within the chest. His CT chest reveals bilateral, diffuse fibrotic change and basal honeycombing. The radiologist feels the appearance is in keeping with usual interstitial pneumonia. The patient is keen that everything be done to ensure the diagnosis is accurate. Which one of the following statements is true?

A. A typical CT appearance is sufficient for diagnosis
B. Blind transbronchial needle aspiration would likely give the diagnosis because of diffuse nodal involvement
C. Bronchoscopy with cytopathological analysis of washings would help characterise the nature of his pulmonary fibrosis
D. Endobronchial ultrasound of his subcarinal node would exclude more diffuse disease
E. Transbronchial lung biopsy would give a tissue diagnosis because idiopathic pulmonary fibrosis is diffuse

17.22. A 75 year old man with no past medical history presents with increasing shortness of breath over 6 months. He previously worked at a shipyard where he had significant exposure to asbestos. He has a large right-sided pleural effusion. Pleural aspiration is performed and reveals an exudate but cytopathological examination identifies no malignant cells. CT scanning reveals circumferential pleural thickening but no other abnormalities.
   Which test is most likely to give a diagnosis?

A. Abrams needle biopsy
B. Bronchoscopy
C. Echocardiogram
D. Repeat pleural aspiration
E. Thoracoscopy

17.23. A 59 year old smoker presents with a new cough. CXR is abnormal and subsequent CT scanning identifies a 4-cm tumour peripherally in the left lower lobe and an enlarged hilar lymph node on the ipsilateral side. The tumour is surrounded by emphysematous change and the radiologist feels CT-guided biopsy would have a high risk of pneumothorax. PET scanning reveals high FDG avidity in the presumed tumour and indeterminate uptake in the hilar lymph node but no other significant uptake. The patient has a forced expiratory volume in 1 second (FEV_1) of 1.5 L (predicted 3.2) and a forced vital capacity (FVC) of 3.0 L (predicted 3.4).
   What should be the next investigation?

A. CT-guided biopsy
B. Endobronchial ultrasound-guided fineneedle aspiration (EBUS-FNA)
C. Flexible bronchoscopy
D. Repeat CT scanning
E. Thoracoscopy

17.24. A 37 year old asthmatic woman presents with difficult asthma control despite maximal inhaled therapy and montelukast. Her asthma control consistently deteriorates in April and May. During this time the patient experiences streaming eyes and nasal secretions. The patient is an enthusiastic runner but finds it difficult to complete a run during these months. The patient has no exposure to animals or birds and works in an office. Serum allergy testing reveals the following results:
   Total IgE 1241 kU/L
   Specific IgE to dog 24 kU/L
   Specific IgE to cat 3.4 kU/L

Specific IgE to tree pollen 0.2 kU/L
Specific IgE to oilseed rape 34 kU/L
Specific IgE to grass pollen 25 kU/L

What is the likely explanation for the patient's presentation?

A. The patient has exercise-induced asthma (IgE testing irrelevant)
B. The patient has lied about exposure to animals (specific IgE to cats and dogs elevated)
C. The patient is non-adherent with medication (total IgE remains high)
D. The patient is sensitised to montelukast (IgE results represent cross-reactivity)
E. The patient's asthma is triggered by seasonal pollens (specific IgE to oilseed rape and grass positive)

17.25. A 49 year old patient returns from a holiday in Portugal with fever, a dry cough, increasing shortness of breath. His wife has brought him to hospital because he had an episode where he became very muddled and seemed not to recognise his family members. In Spain he stayed in a hotel and on his return he was exposed to a nephew who has since been diagnosed with influenza and has been admitted to the local paediatric hospital with breathing difficulties.

Observations on arrival include: temperature 39.3°C, BP 110/55 mmHg, pulse 102 beats/min, oxygen saturations 89% on room air. Blood tests reveal an inflammatory response and a CXR shows bilateral infiltrates. What is the most useful diagnostic test likely to be?

A. Differential cell count in bronchial lavage
B. High-resolution CT chest (HRCT)
C. Nucleic acid amplification testing for respiratory pathogens
D. Paired serology for mycoplasma and legionella
E. Sputum cytology

17.26. A 45 year old smoker is sent for pulmonary function testing because of breathlessness, wheeze and productive cough. There are no other significant respiratory exposures. The family physician has trialled a salbutamol inhaler, which has been somewhat helpful. Spirometry reveals:

FEV$_1$ 2.6 L
FVC 4.4 L
FEV$_1$/FVC 0.59

Following nebulisation of 2.5 mg salbutamol:

FEV$_1$ 3.2 L
FVC 4.4 L
FEV$_1$/FVC 0.73

What does the respiratory function testing reveal?

A. A mixture of obstruction and restriction
B. A restrictive defect
C. A reversible obstructive defect
D. An irreversible obstructive defect
E. Inhaled salbutamol has confounded testing

17.27. A 62 year old woman attends the family practice surgery with increasing shortness of breath on exertion and is sent for full pulmonary function testing. She is an ex-smoker of 25 pack years and works caring for horses at a riding stable. Respiratory function testing reveals:

FEV$_1$ 3.2 L
FVC 3.8 L
FEV$_1$/FVC 0.84
Total lung capacity (TLC) 4.1 L
Residual volume (RV) 0.6 L
Transfer factor for carbon monoxide (TL$_{CO}$) 1.5 (44%)
Transfer coefficient (K$_{CO}$) 1 (56%)

How should the respiratory function testing be interpreted?

A. Gas transfer reduction indicates emphysema
B. Gas transfer reduction indicates hypersensitivity pneumonitis
C. No evidence of airways obstruction
D. There is a restrictive picture
E. There is an obstructive picture

17.28. A 53 year old man presents with a 3-month history of non-productive cough. He has no other symptoms but is finding the cough tiresome and frustrating. He is a non-smoker and works in an office. He is on omeprazole 20 mg once a day, which has controlled his acid reflux for the last 2 years. He has trialled a nasal spray and cough linctus without improvement. Spirometry is normal.

Which of the following statements is true?

A. A CXR should be performed
B. A trial of an inhaled corticosteroid (ICS) is warranted
C. He should see an ear, nose and throat (ENT) surgeon
D. His cough has become a habit and he must get used to it
E. His reflux medication should be increased

17

17.29. A 75 year old woman has been referred with a daily, chronic non-productive cough that has been present for at least 10 years. She has no nocturnal and no nasal symptoms. Her only other symptom is of back pain following a further vertebral fracture in the last month.

Her past medical history includes: osteoporosis (multiple vertebral fractures and kyphosis), previous duodenal ulcer, TB meningitis as a child. She is a life-long non-smoker. Her medication includes: omeprazole 20 mg once daily, alendronic acid once a week, calcium and vitamin D, and cod liver oil capsules. CXR reveals a large hiatus hernia and significant kyphosis.

What is the most likely cause of her cough?

A. Asthma
B. Gastro-oesophageal reflux
C. Hypercalcaemia
D. Lung cancer
E. Tuberculosis

17.30. A 42 year old woman presents with a 4-month history of breathlessness that occurs at rest and on exertion, exclusively in the daytime. She has no other symptoms and is a non-smoker. The breathlessness started following an episode of upper respiratory tract infection where she had significant nasal blockage. She has no nasal symptoms now but often has the feeling that she cannot get a satisfying breath, like she cannot extract enough oxygen from the air. Sometimes this becomes very frightening and on one occasion she was admitted to the emergency department after nearly passing out. Her D-dimer was positive but a CTPA was normal and she was discharged home with a salbutamol inhaler, which she sometimes finds helpful. Her father was a smoker and died of lung cancer in his 60s.

Examination is unremarkable, spirometry is normal, oxygen saturations are 98% on room air. What should be the next investigation?

A. Arterial blood gas
B. Bronchoscopy
C. Dysfunctional breathing studies and a Nijmegen questionnaire
D. Echocardiogram
E. Lung volume and gas transfer studies

17.31. A 67 year old woman has been progressively breathless over the last year.

She has never been an active person but now struggles with breathlessness on exertion, especially walking uphill or when carrying shopping bags. She stopped smoking 15 years ago when her husband had a heart attack. She had smoked 20 cigarettes per day before that.

Her spirometry is within normal limits but her CXR suggests a hilar abnormality. A subsequent CT scan demonstrates that this was a projectional anomaly and excludes a sinister cause. The image below is from the CT scan performed 2 months previously.

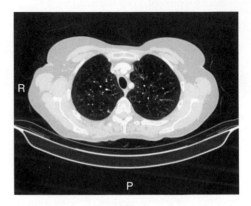

What is the most likely cause of this woman's breathlessness?

A. Asthma
B. Cardiac failure
C. COPD
D. Interstitial lung disease
E. Pulmonary thromboembolism

17.32. A 64 year old woman with COPD presents with right-sided pleuritic chest pain that came on suddenly and left her feeling very breathless. She had felt very well until that point, having been away on holiday for 3 weeks in North America. She was well on the flight, which lasted 5 hours. Her last exacerbation of COPD was 4 months ago, when she was admitted to hospital and received oxygen, nebulised bronchodilators and prednisolone.

Observations: oxygen saturations 84% on room air, BP 151/81 mmHg, pulse 110 beats/min; apyrexial. Examination reveals globally decreased air entry and mild bipedal oedema.

Investigations: CXR hyperinflation, nil focal. CRP 15 mg/L, D-dimer 865 ng/mL, WCC

11×10^9/L; ECG: sinus tachycardia with a rightward axis.

What is the most likely cause of her chest pain?

A. Bronchospasm
B. Malignant pleural disease
C. Pneumonia
D. Pneumothorax
E. Pulmonary thromboembolism

17.33. An 84 year old man has had a nagging ache in his left chest that has slowly built up over 3 months. The pain is worst in his axilla but radiates posteriorly towards the spine. The patient smoked a pipe for 50 years and worked initially in the merchant navy before taking up a job in a brewery.

Examination reveals: dullness to percussion from the left lung base to the mid-zone and *erythema ab igne* of the posterior chest wall. Which of the following is the most likely cause of this chest pain?

A. Chronic thromboembolic disease
B. Herpes zoster
C. Mesothelioma
D. Pneumonia
E. Tictze's syndrome

17.34. A 45 year old man attends his family physician with a sprained wrist following a mistimed punch at his karate class. The doctor notices that he has clubbed fingers. The patient has no past medical history of note, is a non-smoker and, apart from his painful wrist, is asymptomatic. He says people have always commented on his fingers and that his father's fingers are similar in appearance. On checking the patient's record the doctor notes finger clubbing was first recorded in his teenage years.

What is the next step the family physician should take?

A. Check bloods (including LFTs, thyroid function tests and erythrocyte sedimentation rate)
B. CXR to exclude cancer
C. Reassurance
D. Referral to respiratory clinic
E. Sweat test to exclude cystic fibrosis

17.35. A patient presents acutely having coughed up 50 mL of fresh red blood suddenly that morning. He is well known to the respiratory department because of recurrent exacerbations of bronchiectasis. The cause of the bronchiectasis was tuberculosis treated 20 years ago. The patient has had a large apical cavity on the right side of the CXR for at least 10 years.

CXR today appears to show that this cavity has partially filled in. What is the likely cause of his haemoptysis?

A. Carcinoma
B. Mycetoma
C. Pulmonary infarction
D. Suppurative pneumonia
E. Tuberculosis

17.36. A 32 year old cystic fibrosis patient presents with massive haemoptysis in the form of 250 mL of fresh red blood. The patient is actively coughing more blood but is haemodynamically stable (BP 145/72 mmHg, pulse 98 beats/min). The most useful investigation is likely to be:

A. Bronchial artery angiography
B. Bronchoscopy
C. Coagulation studies
D. CTPA
E. Sputum culture

17.37. A 67 year old man has a CT colonogram as a screening test for iron-deficiency anaemia. No colonic abnormality is identified but a 6-mm nodule is identified in the right lower lobe of the lung. The radiologist suggests referral to the respiratory team for ongoing follow-up.

With regard to pulmonary nodules, the risk of malignancy increases with which of the following?

A. A smooth margin
B. Central deposition of calcification
C. Lack of smoking history
D. Size < 4 mm
E. Upper lobe distribution

17.38. A 65 year old woman with rheumatoid arthritis has a CT scan to determine whether she has an associated interstitial lung disease. She has mild basal interlobular septal thickening in keeping with early interstitial lung disease (ILD). The radiologist also identifies a speculated, 1.5 cm-diameter right upper lobe nodule that he suggests may require further investigation.

17

Which of the following statements is true with regard to PET scanning for pulmonary nodules?

A. It always detects bronchoalveolar carcinoma
B. Inflammatory nodules are reliably excluded
C. It has replaced tissue biopsy
D. It is not useful in nodules < 1 cm in diameter
E. It offers no more information than a standard CT

17.39. Which of the following is a cause of a transudative pleural effusion?

A. Drug-induced pleural effusion
B. Hypothyroidism
C. Pulmonary infarction
D. Rheumatoid arthritis
E. Tuberculosis

17.40. Which one of the following statements is true? Light's criteria includes:

A. Pleural fluid:serum protein ratio > 0.6
B. Pleural fluid lactate dehydrogenase (LDH) > two-thirds of the upper limit of normal serum LDH
C. Pleural fluid LDH < two-thirds of the upper limit of normal serum LDH
D. Pleural fluid LDH:serum LDH ratio > 0.5
E. Pleural fluid:serum protein ratio < 0.5

17.41. A 64 year old man presents with fever, sweats, right-sided pleuritic chest pain and breathlessness. He is an ex-smoker and drinks 2 L of cider a day. The CXR (A) and thoracic ultrasound (B) are shown below.

Pleural fluid aspiration is performed under ultrasound guidance. Which one of the following values might be expected?

A. Pleural fluid glucose 5.6 mmol/L (101 mg/dL)
B. Pleural fluid LDH 150 U/L
C. Pleural fluid pH 6.9 (H+126 nmol/L)
D. Pleural fluid protein 27 g/L
E. Pleural fluid triglycerides 5.4 mmol/L (478 mg/dL)

17.42. In which of the following conditions might acute type I respiratory failure be expected?

A. Flail chest injury
B. Lobar collapse
C. Lymphangitis carcinomatosa
D. Obstructive sleep apnoea (OSA)
E. Opioid toxicity

17.43. A 27 year old woman with severe atopic asthma is 26 weeks pregnant. She has been awake at night coughing and short of breath for 48 hours. She has been trying to avoid using her salbutamol inhaler but nonetheless has had to take it 6 to 8 times in the last 24 hours. She has no nasal symptoms and no reflux.

Observations: oxygen saturations 94% on room air, respiratory rate 22 breaths/min, BP 110/65 mmHg, pulse 96 beats/min, apyrexial; peak expiratory flow rate (PEFR) 240 L/min (best 450 L/min).

Examination of the chest reveals bilateral wheeze, mild bilateral pedal oedema, heart sounds dual, no murmur.

The patient's current medications include: regular high-dose ICS/long-acting β_2-agonist (LABA) and oral montelukast; inhaled short-acting β_2-agonist (SABA) as required. She insists she has been adherent with medication,

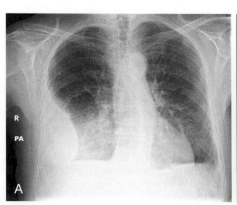

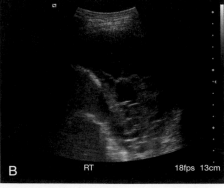

although she is very worried about taking any medications whilst pregnant.

What should be the next step in her management?

A. Low-molecular-weight heparin (LMWH)
B. Oral amoxicillin
C. Oral prednisolone
D. Reduce high-dose ICS/LABA
E. Stop montelukast

17.44. A 48 year old asthmatic is referred to clinic because of increased frequency of asthma exacerbations. He has been waking at night with cough and breathlessness that require extra doses of inhaled salbutamol.

Spirometry reveals an obstructive defect and blood tests reveal an eosinophilia of 0.67×10^9/L. CXR is clear. The patient's current therapy includes Flixotide 500 µg/salmeterol 25 µg 1 puff twice a day; salbutamol 2 puffs, as required. The patient has started prednisolone 40 mg for 5 days as prescribed by his family physician today.

In line with British Thoracic Society guidelines, what should be suggested in order to step-up therapy?

A. Add amoxicillin
B. Add montelukast
C. Double prednisolone dose
D. Provide home nebuliser
E. Start omalizumab

17.45. A 65 year old man with known COPD and mild airways obstruction on spirometry presents with increasing shortness of breath on exertion. He mainly struggles walking on inclines or climbing stairs. He does not experience exacerbations of COPD and he has had no courses of oral prednisolone or antibiotics in the last 2 years.

His current inhaled therapy includes a long-acting muscarinic antagonist (LAMA) and an SABA. Examination reveals decreased air entry bilaterally, with loss of cardiac dullness on percussion. The patient does not desaturate on an incremental walk test.

What would be a reasonable addition for this patient to escalate therapy?

A. Ambulatory oxygen
B. Inhaled corticosteroid (ICS)/LABA combination inhaler
C. LAMA/LABA combination inhaler
D. Oral prednisolone
E. Salbutamol nebuliser

17.46. A 57 year old woman has been coughing for 3 years. She always carries tissues with her to collect the phlegm she coughs up throughout the day. Sometimes her phlegm can be green and she feels run-down and unwell. Antibiotics seem to help but she only feels better for 2–3 weeks.

The patient is a non-smoker who works in an office. She finds her cough embarrassing and work colleagues have been giving her a hard time. What would be the best investigation for this patient?

A. α_1-Antitrypsin levels
B. Bronchoscopy
C. CXR
D. High-resolution CT chest
E. Immunoglobulin levels

17.47. A patient who attends the asthma clinic has been experiencing significant deterioration in control. The main problem is a cough productive of green sputum that is difficult to expectorate and a right-sided pleuritic chest pain that has developed in the last 48 hours. Since then breathing has been more difficult.

Blood tests reveal: haemoglobin 136 g/L, WCC 14×10^9/L (neutrophils 7×10^9/L, lymphocytes 1.46×10^9/L, monocytes 0.8×10^9/L, eosinophils 4.7×10^9/L), platelets 340×10^9/L, CRP 120 mg/L. CXR is shown below.

17

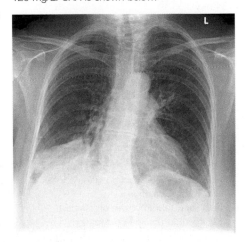

What is the likely cause of the deterioration in control?

A. Bacterial infection
B. Fungal infection
C. Mycobacterial infection
D. Parasitic infection
E. Viral infection

17.48. A 24 year old man with cystic fibrosis has recently moved into the area. He keeps relatively well and missed some appointments at his previous service. He has had two exacerbations of bronchiectasis in the last year and is disappointed with his most recent lung function measures. He has heard about a new medicine called ivacaftor that is only beneficial to some patients with cystic fibrosis and wonders if he qualifies.

Ivacaftor is a small-molecule drug that corrects the function of which of the following cystic fibrosis transmembrane regulator (*CFTR*) gene defects?

A. ΔF508
B. G542X
C. G551D
D. R117H
E. W1282X

17.49. A 24 year old cystic fibrosis patient has failed to recover from a recent exacerbation of her bronchiectasis. Previously *Haemophilus influenzae* and *Staphylococcus aureus* have been isolated from her sputum. A 2-week course of co-amoxiclav followed by 2 weeks of doxycycline have failed to improve spirometry or reduce sputum load. CXR is unchanged and blood tests are unrevealing, apart from CRP of 134 mg/L.

The microbiology team have isolated *Pseudomonas aeruginosa* in the most recent sample provided. Which one of the following statements is true of *P. aeruginosa* in cystic fibrosis?

A. Intravenous antibiotic therapy is rarely required
B. It is a benign coloniser of the bronchiectatic airways
C. It is one of the earliest bacteria isolated in sputum from CF patients
D. Nebulised azithromycin 3 times a week suppresses infection
E. Nebulised tobramycin is an effective treatment in chronic colonisation

17.50. Acute coryza is most commonly caused by which of the following?

A. *Bordetella pertussis*
B. *Haemophilus influenzae*
C. *Mycoplasma pneumoniae*
D. Rhinovirus
E. *Streptococcus pneumoniae*

17.51. A 32 year old man presents with a 5-day history of left-sided pleuritic chest pain, fever and cough productive of rusty sputum. Observations include: BP 100/60 mmHg, pulse 105 beats/min, temperature 38.2°C, respiratory rate 21 breaths/min, oxygen saturations 87% on room air. Examination reveals dullness to percussion and bronchial breathing on the left. Nasolabial cold sores are noted.

Which organism is likely to be responsible for this presentation?

A. *Aspergillus fumigatus*
B. Herpes simplex virus (HSV)
C. *Mycobacterium tuberculosis*
D. *Pneumocystis jirovecii*
E. *Streptococcus pneumoniae*

17.52. A 53 year old businessman presents with fever, chills, cough and shortness of breath. He has recently returned from a trip to the Middle East where he visited a number of countries and spent time in the city as well as visiting more rural areas.

Examination reveals temperature of 40°C, pulse 115 beats/min, BP 100/50 mmHg, oxygen saturations 80% on room air. CXR shows diffuse infiltrates.

Which of the following statements is most accurate?

A. *Burkholderia pseudomallei* needs to be covered
B. He should be isolated and tested for carbapenemase-producing Enterobacteriaceae (CPE)
C. He should be isolated and tested for Middle East respiratory syndrome (MERS)
D. He should be isolated and tested for severe acute respiratory syndrome (SARS)
E. Local antibiotic protocol for community-acquired pneumonia (CAP) should be followed

17.53. A 73 year old man has been in hospital for 3 days having undergone elective hip surgery. He is acutely confused in the middle of the night with a temperature of 38.3°C. Urinalysis is negative but blood testing reveals raised inflammatory markers. A CXR clearly shows a new right-sided infiltrate.

Which of the following approaches is appropriate?

A. A CTPA should be ordered
B. Blood cultures should be taken and a watch-and-wait policy favoured

C. Local antibiotic guidelines for CAP should be followed

D. Local antibiotic policy for hospital-acquired pneumonia (HAP) should be followed

E. Local antibiotic policy for ventilator-associated pneumonia (VAP) should be followed

17.54. A 72 year old man initially improves following treatment for an exacerbation of COPD. He has been in hospital for 10 days when he spikes a temperature of 39°C, his oxygen saturations drop and he starts to expectorate green sputum with blood-streaking. A CXR reveals dense left-sided consolidation.

Late-onset HAP is often attributable to which of the following microorganisms?

A. *Acinetobacter*
B. *Chlamydia*
C. *Haemophilus*
D. *Legionella*
E. *Streptococcus*

17.55. The mortality from HAP is approximately which of the following?

A. 10%
B. 20%
C. 30%
D. 40%
E. 50%

17.56. A 34 year old woman has been unwell with high fever, pleuritic chest pain and cough productive of foul sputum. She is an intravenous drug-user and has noted that her usual injection site in the groin has developed a fluctuant swelling.

CXR shows multiple nodules and a CT shows a predominantly basal distribution and notes that some of the nodules are cavitating. What is the likely explanation for these findings?

A. Aspiration pneumonia
B. Infective endocarditis
C. Metastatic cancer
D. Pulmonary thromboembolism
E. Tuberculosis

17.57. A 28 year old student of Chinese origin has begun treatment for pulmonary tuberculosis that presented with a typical clinical picture and CXR. Sputum was positive for acid- and alcohol-fast bacilli, and polymerase chain reaction (PCR) for *Mycobacterium tuberculosis* has detected no resistance to isoniazid or

rifampicin. He is receiving the standard treatment regimen. Two weeks into therapy, he phones the specialist nursing team as he has painful eyes and is worried that the therapy is not working.

What is the likely cause of this presentation?

A. Drug resistance to ethambutol and pyrazinamide
B. Ethambutol
C. Immune reconstitution
D. Intercurrent viral infection
E. Non-tuberculous *Mycobacterium*

17.58. A 54 year old man is due to start a monoclonal antibody-based therapy for active Crohn's disease but the radiologist has noted a minor abnormality on the patient's recent CXR. The patient had a bacille Calmette–Guérin (BCG) vaccine in childhood and has no known TB contacts. He has no respiratory symptoms. Local guidance suggests checking an interferon-gamma release assay (IGRA) on a peripheral blood sample.

Which one of the following statements is true with regard to the IGRA?

A. A positive result should prompt the clinician to start antituberculous chemotherapy
B. It is more specific than tuberculin skin testing
C. It is now the first-line test for diagnosis of active TB
D. It is only positive where there is systemic mycobacterial infection
E. It measures the release of interferon-alpha from sensitised T cells

17.59. A 64 year old woman presents with back pain, weight loss and a palpable mass in her loin that extends into the buttock. She is reviewed by the orthopaedic team and imaging suggests the mass is of fluid consistency. They aspirate pus easily and send it to the laboratory for culture and cytopathological examination. They ask for advice about further testing.

Which of the following would be an important additional test?

A. Bronchoscopy
B. Echocardiogram to exclude septic embolus
C. Flow cytometry
D. Fluid biochemistry
E. Mycobacterial testing

17.60. A 34 year old haematology patient has been receiving cytotoxic chemotherapy for acute myeloid leukaemia. He is isolated with neutropenic sepsis thought to be secondary to pneumonia. He has fever, pleuritic chest pain and haemoptysis. CT scanning has revealed multiple nodules with what is described as surrounding inflammatory change. The radiological differential includes infection, inflammation and malignancy. The patient has made no response to standard antibiotics for neutropenic sepsis.

What should be the next step in management?

A. Antituberculous chemotherapy
B. Bronchoscopy
C. CTPA
D. Respiratory virus throat swab
E. Voriconazole

17.61. A 63 year old female non-smoker presents to her family physician with a new cough. Her CXR is abnormal with a 5-cm lesion in the right mid-zone. She has since undergone bronchoscopy at which an endobronchial tumour was biopsied. Which is the most common histological type of lung cancer?

A. Adenocarcinoma
B. Large cell carcinoma
C. Mesothelioma
D. Small cell carcinoma
E. Squamous carcinoma

17.62. A 73 year old woman with metastatic non-small cell lung cancer is considering palliative chemotherapy. Although she has lost weight and been more tired she has not experienced any other symptoms. Her cancer was discovered when she had a CT scan because of a combination of weight loss, smoking habit and finger clubbing.

She has developed increasingly painful wrists. What is the most likely cause for this problem?

A. Bone metastases
B. Finger clubbing
C. Horner's syndrome
D. Hypercalcaemia
E. Hypertrophic pulmonary osteoarthropathy (HPOA)

17.63. A 56 year old smoker presents with increasing shortness of breath. A CXR shows a left-sided pleural effusion and CT scanning has demonstrated a 3-cm tumour in the left lung but no evidence of lymphadenopathy. Pleural

fluid aspiration reveals an adenocarcinoma. What is the correct staging of this lung cancer?

A. I
B. II
C. III
D. IV
E. Staging not yet complete

17.64. A 36 year old non-smoker presents with isolated haemoptysis. She has no systemic symptoms but has been expectorating small amounts of fresh blood most mornings in the last 2 weeks. She denies epistaxis and is quite clear she has been coughing blood rather than vomiting.

A CT scan identifies an area of collapse in the left upper lobe (LUL) and a possible small tumour in the main bronchus. Bronchoscopy reveals a vascular-looking tumour emerging from the LUL orifice.

What is the most likely tumour type for this lesion?

A. Adenocarcinoma
B. Breast
C. Carcinoid
D. Small cell
E. Squamous

17.65. A 56 year old, non-smoking man presents with a 3-month history of an irritating non-productive cough. CXR is abnormal and subsequent CT scanning reveals metastatic disease in the bones and a 4-cm left-sided peripheral mass. Bronchoscopy achieves biopsy and cytopathological examination identifies adenocarcinoma, which proves to be EGFR (epidermal growth factor receptor) positive on molecular analysis.

What would be the treatment of choice for this man?

A. Adjuvant chemotherapy and lobectomy
B. Best supportive care
C. Cisplatin and pemetrexed
D. Erlotinib
E. Radiotherapy

17.66. A 64 year old woman with breast cancer metastatic to liver, lungs and bone has been receiving second-line chemotherapy but has become increasingly breathless over 3 months. She received antibiotics for a presumed pneumonia after CXR identified bilateral infiltrates but made no improvement.

Subsequent CT scanning has identified diffuse interstitial thickening radiating from the hilar regions.

What is the likely diagnosis?

A. Drug-induced pneumonitis
B. Lymphangitis carcinomatosa
C. *Pneumocystis* pneumonia
D. Pulmonary oedema
E. Venous thromboembolism

17.67. A 28 year old woman presents to the acute receiving unit with a vague chest discomfort that seems to move through into her back. CXR appears to show mediastinal widening. A CT angiogram is requested to rule out aortic dissection but it identifies a large mass in the anterior mediastinum and some cervical, supraclavicular and axillary lymphadenopathy.

What is the most likely diagnosis?

A. Bronchogenic cyst
B. Lymphoma
C. Neurogenic tumour
D. Oesophageal tumour
E. Retrosternal goitre

17.68. A 79 year old woman has been increasingly short of breath over 6 months. She has no significant past medical history and is on no medication. She has no significant respiratory exposures. Examination reveals bilateral, fine basal crackles and finger clubbing. An HRCT demonstrates bilateral basal, peripheral reticulation with honeycomb cysts.

What is the most likely diagnosis?

A. Acute interstitial pneumonia
B. Idiopathic pulmonary fibrosis
C. Lymphocytic interstitial pneumonia
D. Non-specific interstitial pneumonia
E. Sarcoidosis

17.69. Respiratory bronchiolitis–interstitial lung disease (RBILD) is more common in which of the following groups?

A. Non-smokers
B. Patients > 65 years of age
C. Patients with connective tissue diseases
D. Smokers
E. Women

17.70. A 28 year old woman develops a painful rash on her lower limbs, arthralgia and fever. She feels run-down and unwell. Her family

physician arranges a CXR, below, and refers to the respiratory clinic.

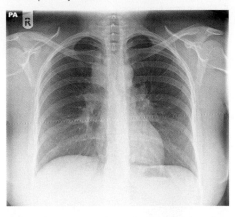

At review 4 weeks later she feels back to her usual self apart from a persistent mild lethargy. What is the most likely cause for this presentation?

A. HIV
B. Lymphoma
C. Pneumonia
D. Sarcoidosis
E. Tuberculosis

17.71. A 55 year old man presents with increasing breathlessness over 2 years. He has a dry cough. Examination of the chest is unremarkable. Pulmonary function testing reveals a restrictive defect. HRCT identifies mild bilateral hilar lymph node enlargement, nodules in a bronchovascular distribution and extensive fibrotic change.

What is the most likely diagnosis?

A. Sarcoidosis stage 0
B. Sarcoidosis stage I
C. Sarcoidosis stage II
D. Sarcoidosis stage III
E. Sarcoidosis stage IV

17.72. A 72 year old woman has had rheumatoid arthritis for 20 years. She recently had a chest infection but fully recovered. A CXR was ordered to exclude pneumonia but revealed multiple smooth nodules. CT scanning also identifies four smooth nodules of varying size. A CXR recovered from storage shows that these nodules have been present for at least 5 years.

What is the likely cause of these nodules?

A. Bronchiectasis
B. Metastatic cancer

17

C. Pulmonary embolism
D. Pulmonary fibrosis
E. Rheumatoid nodules

17.73. A 64 year old man presents with high fever, left-sided pleuritic chest pain and shortness of breath. His CXR is below.

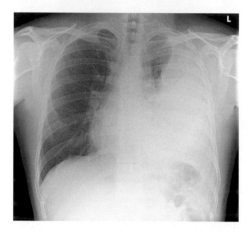

A chest drain is sited and excellent resolution is achieved. The pleural fluid characteristics are as follows: pH 6.9 (H+126 nmol/L); protein 38 g/L; LDH 800 U/L; glucose 0.3 mmol/L (5.4 mg/dL). Two weeks later he re-presents with CXR changes on the other side, with right-sided pleuritic chest pain and fever. He is still taking antibiotics. In addition he has bilateral, symmetrical arthritis with joint swelling.
What is the likely diagnosis?

A. Empyema
B. Lung cancer
C. Lymphoma
D. Mesothelioma
E. Rheumatoid arthritis

17.74. A 61 year old woman is receiving intravenous daptomycin for staphylococcal discitis. She has required intravenous fluids for a mild acute kidney injury (AKI) secondary to sepsis and dehydration. Her clinical condition and inflammatory markers had been improving with this therapy. After 2 weeks of antibiotics she spikes a fever to 39°C, her WCC rises and she develops an oxygen requirement (oxygen saturations 94% on 35% oxygen).
Blood tests: haemoglobin 102 g/L, WCC 16 × 10⁹/L (neutrophils 9 × 10⁹/L, eosinophils 5 × 10⁹/L, lymphocytes 1 × 10⁹/L, monocytes 0.8 × 10⁹/L), CRP 150 mg/L, urea 8 mmol/L (48 mg/dL), creatinine 89 µmol/L (1.01 mg/dL).

CXR bilateral peripheral, especially upper-zone consolidation.
What should the treatment be for this patient?

A. Antibiotics to cover hospital-acquired pneumonia
B. Antituberculosis chemotherapy
C. Continue current therapy
D. Intravenous furosemide
E. Stop daptomycin and give prednisolone

17.75. A 45 year old non-smoking man presents with fever, weight loss and breathlessness. On the night of his admission he has developed stridor. CXR reveals multiple, bilateral pulmonary nodules. His past medical history includes sinusitis and conductive deafness.
Blood tests reveal: urea 7 mmol/L (42 mg/dL), creatinine 165 µmol/L (1.87 mg/dL), haemoglobin 102 g/L, WCC 15 × 10⁹/L (neutrophils 12 × 10⁹/L), CRP 145 mg/L.
What is the most likely diagnosis?

A. Acute eosinophilic pneumonia
B. Bronchial carcinoma
C. Chronic eosinophilic pneumonia
D. Eosinophilic granulomatosis with polyangiitis
E. Granulomatous polyangiitis

17.76. A 70 year old woman has been coughing, short of breath, intermittently feverish and run-down over 6 weeks. Her past medical history includes transient ischaemic attack and recurrent urinary tract infections. Her medications include aspirin, simvastatin, amlodipine and nitrofurantoin. She is a non-smoker and has a pet cat.
Examination reveals oxygen saturations of 91% on room air, BP 121/76 mmHg, pulse 89 beats/min, apyrexial, respiratory rate 18 breaths/min. Her CXR shows bi-basal infiltrates.
What is the most likely diagnosis?

A. Atypical pneumonia
B. Cryptogenic organising pneumonia
C. Idiopathic pulmonary fibrosis
D. Nitrofurantoin lung disease
E. Non-specific interstitial pneumonia (NSIP)

17.77. A 26 year old non-smoking woman presents for the second time with pneumothorax. She has no other past medical history. Good resolution is achieved with chest drainage but a CT scan identifies multiple cysts throughout the lung parenchyma. The CT chest catches an abnormality on the upper pole of the right kidney, which is incompletely imaged and the radiologist suggests an MRI for better characterisation of the lesion.

What diagnosis should be considered and further investigated?

A. Alveolar microlithiasis
B. Alveolar proteinosis
C. Lymphangioleiomyomatosis
D. Lymphocytic interstitial pneumonia
E. Pulmonary Langerhans cell histiocytosis (histiocytosis X)

17.78. A 43 year old woman presents with cough, shortness of breath and wheeze. She is a smoker, has no past medical history and no exposure to birds or animals. She had been off work for 2 weeks but made an improvement after starting inhaled beclometasone and a short-acting bronchodilator as required. On return to work, things seemed to be fine but deteriorated after about 3 weeks. She works behind the counter in a local bakery.

The patient would like to know if she has occupational asthma. Which test would be most helpful in making the diagnosis?

A. Histamine challenge test
B. Peak expiratory flow rate diary
C. Specifc IgE to flour
D. Spirometry with reversibility
E. Sputum eosinophils

17.79. A 55 year old geologist has been coughing, breathless and experiencing arthralgia since renovation started at her home. The work was started because of damp and has involved some structural work. Her home always seems to be dusty currently. Her husband is a stonemason and has been working on a new piece at home in their garage. At work she has been preparing beryllium samples for a PhD project, which has been quite stressful as deadlines for submission approach.

CXR shows bilateral hilar lymphadenopathy with some soft nodularity in the mid-zones.

What is the most likely diagnosis?

A. Berylliosis
B. Dysfunctional breathing
C. Hypersensitivity pneumonitis
D. Sarcoidosis
E. Silicosis

17.80. Which of the following statements is true with regard to progressive massive fibrosis (PMF)?

A. Characterised by small radiographic nodules
B. Chyloptysis is associated
C. Finger clubbing and basal crackles are characteristic
D. It has no impact on lung function
E. It may progress even after exposure ceases

17.81. A 41 year old stonemason admits to shortness of breath on exertion. A screening CXR and pulmonary function testing are both abnormal so he has been referred to the respiratory clinic. Silicosis results from the inhalation of which of the following?

A. Coal
B. Cotton
C. Quartz
D. Silicone
E. Tin

17.82. A 72 year old man presents with progressive breathlessness over 6 months; more recently he has had a vague ache in the right side of his chest that has kept him awake at night.

His past medical history is significant for two separate episodes of 'benign asbestos pleurisy' in his 50s. He has pleural plaques and received compensation. He had worked in the construction industry and had frequent, heavy exposure to asbestos. He stopped smoking 20 years ago during a bout of pleurisy, having started age 12 years and smoked an average of 20 cigarettes per day.

CXR reveals a right-sided pleural effusion and pleural plaques. It is not possible to see the right-sided costophrenic angle.

CT scanning reveals pleural plaques, right-sided pleural effusion and mild thickening of the pleura that extends onto the mediastinum anteriorly.

What is the most likely reason for his presentation?

A. Asbestos pleural plaques
B. Asbestosis
C. Benign asbestos pleurisy
D. Diffuse pleural thickening
E. Mesothelioma

17.83. A 69 year old woman has progressive breathlessness on exertion. Because she described a vague feeling of her chest

17

tightening during one of these episodes, her family physician started aspirin and glyceryl trinitrate spray and referred to cardiology. She underwent CT coronary angiogram. This identified no coronary artery disease but diffuse ground glass and some centrilobular nodules were picked up incidentally in the lungs.

The patient has no past medical history, worked as a secretary and was a non-smoker. She has kept a pet parrot at home for the last year.

What is the likely diagnosis?

A. Aspirin sensitivity
B. Breathing artefact
C. Hypersensitivity pneumonitis
D. Idiopathic pulmonary fibrosis
E. Sarcoidosis

17.84. A 72 year old man presents with cough and weight loss. He smoked 20 cigarettes per day until 5 years ago. In addition, he worked lagging pipes with 'monkey dung' during his apprenticeship.

Examination reveals a supraclavicular lymph node but no significant chest findings. His CT scan notes the supraclavicular lymph node but also suggests there is a peripheral 5 cm peripheral mass in the left lung and an enlarged left-sided hilar lymph node. There is an indeterminate lesion in the liver and MRI is suggested for clarification.

What should the next diagnostic test be?

A. CT-guided biopsy
B. Endobronchial ultrasound
C. Flexible bronchoscopy
D. Liver biopsy
E. Supraclavicular lymph node biopsy

17.85. Which of the following associations in relation to lung disease is correct?

A. Anthrax and inadequately pasteurised milk
B. *Chlamydia psittaci* and hide factory workers
C. *Coxiella burnetii* and sewage workers
D. *Francisella tularensis* and muskrat contact
E. Leptospiral pneumonia and welding

17.86. A 45 year old man presents to the acute receiving unit with sudden-onset right-sided pleuritic chest pain, shortness of breath and a swollen, painful right calf. He recently had right-sided anterior cruciate ligament reconstruction abroad (following a skiing accident) and flew home from Canada in the last week. He has a past medical history of spontaneous VTE (treated with 6 months of warfarin) and a family history of VTE (mother and uncle).

Observations: oxygen saturations 88% on room air, respiratory rate 22 breaths/min, pulse 110 beats/min, BP 110/65 mmHg. Chest is clear. Right calf is greater in circumference than left by 3 cm. Heart sounds dual, no murmurs.

Investigations: CXR reveals marginally elevated right hemidiaphragm; ECG: sinus tachycardia; CRP 35 mg/L, D-dimer 200 ng/mL.

What should the next test be for this patient?

A. CT pulmonary angiogram
B. Echocardiogram
C. Fluoroscopy of the diaphragm
D. Respiratory virus throat swab
E. Sputum microscopy culture and sensitivity

17.87. A 28 year old woman has an anterior cruciate ligament repair and is recovering at home in an above-knee cast when she starts to feel like she will pass out every time she stands up. She attends the emergency department.

Examination reveals BP 80/45 mmHg, pulse 110 beats/min, oxygen saturations 92% on air, respiratory rate 22 breaths/min, apyrexial. Chest is clear.

Investigations: CXR is clear. Bloods are as follows: haemoglobin 100 g/L, WCC 11×10^9/L, platelets 200×10^9/L, D-dimer 1200 ng/mL, urea 10 mmol/L (60 mg/dL), creatinine 92 μmol/L (1.04 mg/dL). ECG reveals sinus tachycardia. As the investigations are being reviewed the patient has a cardiac arrest.

What should the immediate management include?

A. Apixaban
B. Intravenous heparin infusion
C. LMWH
D. Thrombolysis
E. Warfarin

17.88. A 26 year old woman has been increasingly short of breath over 2 years. She attends the emergency department and is noted to be hypoxaemic with swollen ankles. Her ECG shows right bundle branch block. An echocardiogram is arranged.

Pulmonary hypertension is defined as a mean pulmonary artery pressure measured at right heart catheterisation of at least which of the following?

A. 15 mmHg
B. 25 mmHg
C. 35 mmHg
D. 45 mmHg
E. 55 mmHg

17.89. A 24 year old woman presents with breathlessness and palpitations that has become worse over the preceding year. She has had significant social stress because of the end of a relationship and the death of her mother. Examination reveals an elevated jugular venous pressure but no other abnormalities. An ECG has a rate of 76 beats/min and a rightward axis. CXR reveals a paucity of peripheral vasculature.

What would be the most appropriate next investigation?

A. D-dimer
B. Dysfunctional breathing studies and Nijmegen questionnaire
C. HRCT
D. Spirometry
E. Transthoracic echocardiography

17.90. A 23 year old woman has been diagnosed with primary pulmonary hypertension following right heart catheterisation and extensive investigation to exclude alternative causes of her presentation at a specialist unit.

Which of the following therapies may be indicated in primary pulmonary hypertension?

A. Bosentan
B. Cyclizine
C. Etanercept
D. Infliximab
E. Isosorbide mononitrate

17.91. A 45 year old woman presents with cough that appears in May and is gone by autumn. In addition, she experiences nasal discharge and watering eyes. Examination is unremarkable and spirometry is normal.

What is the likely diagnosis?

A. Allergic asthma
B. Allergic rhinitis
C. *Bordetella pertussis*
D. Perennial rhinitis
E. Viral upper respiratory tract infection

17.92. Which of the following statements is true with regard to breathing during sleep?

A. Abnormal ventilatory drive is present in obstructive sleep apnoea
B. During sleep muscle tone increases
C. Forty per cent of middle-aged women snore
D. Hypoventilation accompanies normal sleep
E. Palatoglossus and genioglossus contract actively during expiration

17.93. A 55 year old man has been increasingly sleepy during the daytime. He is having trouble at work as he has been found asleep at his desk and has taken to napping during his breaks. He had a near-miss in his car. His Epworth sleepiness score is 18. His BMI is 36.

What is the result of his sleep study likely to be?

A. 5 apnoea/hypopneas per hour of sleep
B. 10 apnoea/hypopneas per hour of sleep
C. 20 apnoea/hypopneas per hour of sleep
D. Central sleep apnoea
E. Narcolepsy

17.94. A 55 year old woman has an apical lung cancer on the left side with lymph node involvement. She receives radiotherapy following a mediastinoscopy. She has a hoarse voice and is worried this is because of her lung tumour. Bronchoscopy reveals no vocal cord paralysis.

What is the likely cause?

A. Chronic laryngitis
B. Endotracheal intubation during mediastinoscopy
C. Laryngeal tuberculosis
D. Left recurrent laryngeal nerve involvement by the tumour
E. Psychogenic aphonia

17.95. A 34 year old man presents with acute-onset shortness of breath and left-sided pleuritic chest pain. Examination reveals oxygen saturations of 94% breathing room air, decreased air entry on the left side of the chest with hyper-resonant percussion note. CXR reveals large left-sided pneumothorax. A therapeutic aspiration is performed and 2.5 L of air is aspirated with no change in the X-ray appearance.

What should be the next step?

A. Admit for observation and oxygen
B. Bronchoscopy
C. Cardiothoracic surgery

17

D. Continue therapeutic aspiration
E. Intercostal chest drain

17.96. A 72 year old man is increasingly breathless and has woken in the night breathless. He can no longer go for his regular weekly swim. His past medical history includes ischaemic heart disease, hypertension and polio in childhood.

His CXR is under-inspired despite three attempts. A sleep study reveals significant hypoventilation and a morning arterial blood gas identifies decompensated type II respiratory failure. What is the likely diagnosis?

A. Bronchial carcinoma
B. Eventration of the diaphragm

C. Hernia through foramen of Bochdalek
D. Idiopathic diaphragmatic paralysis
E. Post-polio syndrome

17.97. Which of these associations between pathophysiological features and conditions is correct?

A. Diaphragmatic rupture and ankylosing spondylitis
B. Eventration of diaphragm and foramen of Bochdalek
C. Pectus carinatum and poliomyelitis
D. Pectus excavatum and asthma
E. Thoracic kyphoscoliosis and tuberculosis

Answers

17.1. Answer: A.
The examination findings point towards collapse of the right lung because the trachea is pulled to that side (the opposite would be the case with pleural effusion). The collapse must be significant because the apex beat is not palpable, suggesting the heart is pulled towards the right side by mediastinal shift. The patient's diagnosis was made at bronchoscopy, suggesting a central tumour. Pneumothorax is less likely than if the patient had a peripheral tumour that had been biopsied using computed tomography (CT) guidance. Pericardial effusion would not explain the respiratory examination findings. The presentation is too acute for pneumonia and the patient is apyrexial. An urgent chest X-ray (CXR) would be an important test and the patient may require urgent radiotherapy or interventional bronchoscopy to re-inflate the lung.

17.2. Answer: E.
The patient has type II respiratory failure following a road traffic accident that caused multiple fractures. It seems very likely that she would have sustained a whiplash-type injury to the neck. C3, 4 and 5 innervate the diaphragm via the phrenic nerve and a fracture at this level can cause respiratory failure. The patient has type II respiratory failure with a normal alveolar–arterial gradient. Opiate toxicity is unlikely given the dose involved. A flail segment requires multiple rib fractures. A normal alveolar–arterial gradient is against $\dot{V}/\dot{Q}$

mismatch and would be more likely to cause type I respiratory failure. There are no examination findings in keeping with COPD and the oxygen involved (although delivered in an uncontrolled fashion) is low flow.

17.3. Answer: C.
In COPD, loss of elastin fibres results in small airway collapse and air trapping during expiration. This dynamic hyperinflation is initially noticed on exertion because expiration time is shortened during exercise. Exercise-induced bronchospasm would be more likely in asthma. There are no examination findings that suggest sufficient pulmonary hypertension to cause breathlessness. There is no reason for the diaphragm to move paradoxically in this case. Central chemoreceptors are stimulated by a rise in CO_2, which might be expected in more advanced disease.

17.4. Answer: A.
The CXR shows a large central cavitating mass with a smaller nodule immediately superior to the mass and a further nodule at the lower pole of the right hilum. There is a small left-sided pleural effusion. The possible answers given represent a reasonable differential diagnosis for this appearance. The history strongly favours a bronchial carcinoma.

17.5. Answer: B.
The CXR shows significant widening of the mediastinum and a small right-sided pleural

effusion. Given the age of the patient, the imaging and the subacute presentation, the likely diagnosis is lymphoma and CT scanning is required to identify the extent of disease and identify a possible site for obtaining a tissue diagnosis. Echocardiogram might be helpful if aortic dissection or pericardial effusion were suspected. PET scan might be useful in staging or to assess treatment response. D-dimer is less relevant with the obvious CXR abnormality. Bronchoscopy is unlikely to be a useful test, although endoscopic ultrasound/endobronchial ultrasound would allow nodal sampling.

17.6. Answer: B.
The CXR shows the classic D-shaped appearance of an empyema. Thoracic ultrasound and diagnostic aspiration should be undertaken as an emergency. Insertion of an intercostal chest drain is a priority and CT scanning to plan an insertion site may be required if the ultrasound scan appearance is very complicated. Mesothelioma and bronchial carcinoma are less likely because of the acute presentation. There is no abdominal element to the presentation on this occasion, although pancreatitis can cause large (usually left-sided) pleural effusion. Hepatic hydrothorax usually causes a simple, right-sided effusion, so the D-shape configuration would be very unusual.

17.7. Answer: E.
We do not have measurements for the small pulmonary nodule at the apex of the right lung but repeat CT scanning is not an option, so we must presume it is > 8 mm in maximum diameter, and we note the patient is an asymptomatic smoker, so a PET scan to assess nodule activity is the best answer. The patient is asymptomatic (the initial pain was on the left and the lesion is on the right), so commencing antibiotics and interferon-gamma release assay (IGRA) is irrelevant. Further risk assessment prior to an invasive test is required as CT-guided biopsy is difficult in this area and the nodule is likely to be too small to allow this. Standard flexible bronchoscopy would not allow access to the nodule.

17.8. Answer: E.
The PET scan image reveals a fludeoxyglucose (FDG) avid right upper lobe pulmonary nodule that must be presumed to be an early-stage bronchial carcinoma. Given the patient's performance status and normal pulmonary

function testing, she should be referred to the cardiothoracic surgery team.

17.9. Answer: C.
The CXR shows total collapse of the right lung with the heart and mediastinum shifted to the right and tracheal deviation. This appearance is likely to have been caused by a proximal obstructing lesion such as a tumour.

17.10. Answer: A.
The CT scan shows evidence of bilateral, proximal bronchiectasis and an area of varicose bronchiectasis in the right upper lobe and non-specific inflammatory change. The clinical picture and radiology point towards allergic bronchopulmonary aspergillosis, although further investigation (e.g. peripheral blood eosinophilia, total immunoglobulin E (IgE), *Aspergillus* precipitins – IgE specific to *Aspergillus*) would be required to confirm this.

17.11. Answer: E.
The CXR shows right-sided pleural effusion with a meniscus appreciable. The trachea is relatively central as the right lung is compressed by the pleural effusion. The meniscus and homogenous opacification make consolidation unlikely. This is not collapse because the trachea is not pulled towards the opacification and there is a meniscus. Right-sided bronchial carcinoma might cause pleural effusion but the CXR does not give us this diagnosis. Right-sided mesothelioma cannot be diagnosed based on CXR but is a cause of pleural effusion.

17.12. Answer: D.
The CXR shows an isolated right-sided pleural effusion. It seems unlikely that this relates to cardiac failure given the normal echocardiogram. It will be important to further investigate this with a diagnostic aspiration but this cannot be performed safely given the apixaban therapy.

17.13. Answer: E.
The CXR shows a left-sided pneumothorax. It seems likely the patient has a concurrent respiratory tract infection that may be viral but requires further investigation.

17.14. Answer: E.
The patient has a large left-sided pneumothorax (> 2 cm depth measured at hilum) and is

17

symptomatic. He probably has a concurrent respiratory infection that may require investigation. The first step in management of a primary spontaneous pneumothorax would be therapeutic aspiration.

17.15. Answer: D.

The CT-PET shows significant uptake in the right upper lobe cancer and in an ipsilateral right hilar node, suggesting T4N2M0 disease. There is apparent uptake in the marrow of the spine and sternum but this is physiological and not typical of metastatic deposit. The CT-PET has upstaged the patient as the hilar lymph node was not obviously pathologically enlarged on standard CT scanning.

17.16. Answer: C.

The patient has finger clubbing and bi-basal crackles and presents with shortness of breath and dry cough late in life. The CT scan shows bilateral peripheral lung cysts in a honeycomb pattern with some traction bronchiectasis. This clinical presentation and CT pattern is typical of idiopathic pulmonary fibrosis but should be confirmed by the assessment of an interstitial lung disease multidisciplinary team.

17.17. Answer: A.

The CXR shows extensive left-sided consolidation. The left costophrenic angle is clear so pleural effusion is unlikely. Loculated pleural fluid could give this appearance but the likeliest cause is a pneumonia given the examination findings.

17.18. Answer: C.

The CURB-65 score was originally developed to predict mortality in community-acquired pneumonia and is now widely used for the assessment of disease severity. The components are C = confusion, U = urea > 7 mmol/L (42 mg/dL), R = respiratory rate ≥ 30 breaths/min, B = blood pressure systolic < 90 mmHg or diastolic ≤ 60 mmHg, 65 = age ≥ 65 years. His CURB-65 score is 2. He scores points for confusion and urea.

17.19. Answer: C.

The patient has pneumonia with delirium, hyponatraemia, deranged liver function tests (LFTs) and high fever. He requires investigation for legionella and antibiotics to cover this organism. It may be that his LFT derangement relates to amoxicillin therapy but this antibiotic

might have been expected to improve his symptoms if pneumonia was related to a more common pneumonia-causing organism (e.g. *S. pneumoniae*).

17.20. Answer: B.

The patient presents with classic symptoms of pneumonia and might be expected to isolate *S. pneumoniae* on sputum examination given the rusty sputum, pleuritic chest pain and cold sores. The CXR shows left-sided basal consolidation.

17.21. Answer: A.

A typical clinical presentation and CT appearance should allow an interstitial lung disease multidisciplinary meeting to reach a diagnosis of idiopathic pulmonary fibrosis (IPF) without a tissue sample. Bronchoscopy has no specific diagnostic features but may be useful in the setting of intercurrent infection or atypical CT scans/presentations. Transbronchial lung biopsy would be risky and likely to be non-diagnostic. There are no diagnostic lymph node features in IPF.

17.22. Answer: E.

Direct visualisation and targeted biopsy of any pleural lesion provides the best chance of a tissue diagnosis. Mesothelioma cannot be diagnosed on cytopathological examination of pleural fluid. Bronchoscopy would not help with pleural disease but may be helpful if there were an endobronchial lesion with pleural metastases. Echocardiogram is not considered helpful because there is pleural thickening as well as a right-sided pleural effusion, so heart failure is an unlikely cause.

17.23. Answer: B.

The patient requires a diagnostic test to confirm lung cancer, determine histological type and complete staging. It seems likely he has T2a, N1, M0 disease. EBUS-FNA will meet all these requirements. Flexible bronchoscopy might give histological type but would not confirm disease in the hilar lymph node. CT-guided biopsy is perhaps more likely than flexible bronchoscopy to confirm histological type but would have an attendant risk of pneumothorax. Thoracoscopy has no role as there is no evidence of pleural disease. Repeat CT scanning would delay diagnosis in a scenario where curative treatment may be possible.

17.24. Answer: E.
Seasonal deterioration in asthma control is a common presentation and it seems likely that the patient encounters these allergens when she is out running. It will be important in future to monitor the pollen counts and to avoid areas of high antigen density (e.g. near oilseed rape fields). The patient may be allergic to cats and dogs but it would not explain this presentation. It is possible to have positive specific IgEs but no clinical phenotype on antigen exposure. The history is as important as the serological testing. Total IgE cannot be used to monitor medication adherence. Exercise-induced asthma would not have such strong seasonality.

17.25. Answer: C.
Nucleic acid amplification testing of sputum or throat swab would differentiate between legionella and influenza in this case. The test result would be available quickly. Sputum cytology has a limited role in respiratory diagnostics. HRCT would be unlikely to offer more information than the CXR. Paired serology would determine whether the patient had been infected by legionella but would not be available in a timely fashion. Differential cell count would not give a specific answer about the causative pathogen.

17.26. Answer: C.
The patient has an obstructive defect that entirely resolves following nebulised bronchodilator; this is in keeping with asthma despite the patient's smoking history. Inhaled therapy taken on the morning of reversibility testing can confound the test but in this instance there is a clear result with strong evidence of reversibility.

17.27. Answer: C.
The gas transfer is reduced and partially corrects for lung volume. There is no evidence of airways obstruction. The respiratory function tests are non-diagnostic and further clinical details and, potentially, imaging studies are likely to be required. FEV_1, FVC and FEV_1/FVC are within normal limits.

17.28. Answer: A.
Chronic cough has many causes but it is important not to miss parenchymal lung disease or bronchial carcinoma and a CXR ought to be performed. Physicians should be very careful about attributing chronic cough to 'habit'. Reflux may be at the root of this cough but at this stage it is important to rule out parenchymal disease/bronchial carcinoma. A trial of steroid medication would usually be given if there was a suspicion of asthma or eosinophilic bronchitis, but further testing would be useful prior to this. ENT surgeons may be consulted when there is chronic rhinitis/sinusitis as part of a cough presentation, which does not respond to standard therapies.

17.29. Answer: B.
Given the CXR findings and history, reflux is the most likely cause even though the patient is asymptomatic (proton pump inhibitor started following a duodenal ulcer, so no ongoing heartburn). TB is unlikely as the cough is non-productive and there are no systemic symptoms. Asthma is less likely because there is no nocturnal element. Hypercalcaemia does not cause cough, although if it were present alongside cough it should raise the suspicion of malignancy. Lung cancer is unlikely because of the duration of the cough.

17.30. Answer: C.
This is a very typical presentation of dysfunctional breathing. The patient had an initial illness, which may have altered the breathing pattern by preventing nasal breathing, and has a reasonable fear of lung cancer because a close relative died of it. A CTPA has ruled out an acute venous thromboembolism and parenchymal lung disease (including lung cancer) as a cause. Echocardiogram might be useful if there was a murmur, background of congenital heart disease or if there were signs of right heart dysfunction (CTPA would not necessarily exclude chronic venous thromboembolism (VTE) or pulmonary hypertension). Normal CT scan makes ILD or emphysema unlikely. Arterial blood gas would not necessarily be abnormal in dysfunctional breathing (although almost certainly would have shown respiratory alkalosis during the emergency department presentation).

17.31. Answer: C.
Although this woman has stopped smoking, she accumulated a significant total number of pack years. Her history is of chronic breathlessness, typical of COPD, and her CT scan shows emphysema. It is often difficult for patients to accept that although they have

17

stopped smoking, their lung function continues to decline. Spirometry is within normal limits because she has emphysema-dominant disease with no evidence of airways obstruction on testing. She would have an abnormal gas transfer.

17.32. Answer: E.
The most likely cause of this pain is pulmonary thromboembolism because she has recently been on a long-haul flight, is hypoxaemic, tachycardic and has a positive D-dimer. Malignant pleural disease would be unlikely to have such a sudden onset. Pneumothorax and pneumonia are not supported by the X-ray findings. Bronchospasm can give a central chest tightness but not a peripheral pleuritic chest pain. Central chest tightness is a common finding in exacerbations of COPD because of coughing and strain on costal cartilages and intercostal muscles.

17.33. Answer: C.
The most likely cause is mesothelioma because of the patient's employment history (asbestos was often found in the boiler rooms of older ships), the insidious nature of the pain and its nagging quality. It seems likely the patient has a pleural effusion or perhaps pleural thickening. Chronic thromboembolic disease might present with recurrent pleuritic chest pain but more commonly is associated with progressive breathlessness. Pneumonia might be expected to present with more systemic symptoms over a shorter time period. Tietze's syndrome presents more acutely and is usually self-terminating with supportive measures.

17.34. Answer: C.
It seems very likely that this man has familial clubbing. There is documented evidence of the presence of finger clubbing for approximately 30 years and the patient is asymptomatic. Interestingly, his father probably has finger clubbing too. There is no need for further investigation or onwards referral.

17.35. Answer: B.
The likely cause of haemoptysis here is a mycetoma developing in an old cavity caused by tuberculosis. Carcinoma is less likely than mycetoma in this scenario but scar carcinomas can develop in areas of the lungs previously damaged by infection. Tuberculosis is likely to have been adequately treated and a patient regularly attending with exacerbations of bronchiectasis is likely to have had sputum screened for mycobacteria intermittently. There are no systemic symptoms to suggest a pneumonia and the haemoptysis is solely fresh blood (not mixed in with purulent sputum) and of sudden onset. Pulmonary infarction is less likely because of the lack of other symptoms (pleuritic chest pain and shortness of breath) and the CXR changes.

17.36. Answer: A.
Bronchial artery angiography will demonstrate abnormally dilated areas of bronchial vasculature and with active bleeding can isolate the leaking point. This can be difficult to interpret in chronic suppurative lung disease as the bronchial vasculature is often diffusely abnormal. Sputum culture is unlikely to be helpful in isolated massive haemoptysis although infection may be a precipitant in chronic lung disease (such as cystic fibrosis (CF) bronchiectasis). Bronchoscopy may be helpful in the presence of a central lung tumour and can sometimes determine whether the bleeding point is in the right or left lung (CXR or CT can be helpful here too), but bronchial artery angiography is increasingly favoured because of the potential to perform embolisation of the aberrant artery. A CTPA may determine the source of bleeding (e.g. tumour or pulmonary arteriovenous malformation) in some cases but is unlikely to be helpful here. Coagulation studies should be performed as CF patients may be deficient in vitamin K and can have liver disease, but the more likely cause is abnormal bronchial vasculature.

17.37. Answer: E.
Nodules greater than 4 mm require careful follow-up unless they have benign characteristics such as central deposition of calcification (which may suggest hamartoma). Spiculated margins are more typical of malignant lesions. Malignant nodules are more common in upper lobes; benign nodules distribute evenly. Smoking is a very strong risk factor for lung cancer.

17.38. Answer: D.
PET scanning is useful for nodules > 1 cm in diameter. It detects metabolic activity, which is usually higher in malignant disease. However, metabolic activity can be high in inflammatory

nodules, which can lead to false positives. Tissue diagnosis must still be pursued even with a positive PET scan to identify the best treatment option. False-negative PET scans can occur in very slow-growing cancers or in neuroendocrine cancers. Metabolic activity is assessed by PET scan, which is not detected by a single CT scan, although could be inferred by nodule growth on serial CT scans.

17.39. Answer: B.
Transudative effusions include organ failure: cardiac, renal, liver and thyroid. Hypothyroidism is therefore the correct answer, although it is relatively rare.

17.40. Answer: B.
Light's criteria suggest an exudate where two of the three criteria are met. It is nonetheless important to take a holistic overview of the case as the criteria misclassify transudates as exudates 25% of the time.

17.41. Answer: C.
The presentation and imaging are highly suggestive of empyema. As such, we would expect a high pleural fluid protein and LDH and a low pleural fluid glucose and pH. Elevated pleural fluid triglycerides would be expected in chylothorax.

17.42. Answer: B.
Acute type I respiratory failure might be expected in lobar collapse where the collapsed lobe is underventilated but perfused and CO_2 is cleared in the neighbouring functional lung units but haemoglobin saturation does not allow augmentation of oxygen uptake. If lobar collapse was associated with more widespread mucus plugging and bronchospasm (e.g. in asthma or allergic bronchopulmonary aspergillosis), type II respiratory failure might occur because of generalised $\dot{V}/\dot{Q}$ mismatch. OSA usually causes chronic type II respiratory failure. Flail chest injury might cause acute type II respiratory failure, as might opioid toxicity. Lymphangitis carcinomatosa would cause chronic type I respiratory failure.

17.43. Answer: C.
This patient is on maximal therapy for atopic asthma but has features of poor control suggesting a significant exacerbation. She needs to have oral corticosteroid therapy,

nebulised bronchodilator and be admitted for observation. Her therapy should not be reduced because the greater risk to patient and fetus is uncontrolled asthma. Antibiotics would only be considered where there was strong objective evidence of infection (fever, sputum culture positive, CXR infiltrate). The presentation is not suggestive of pulmonary thromboembolism.

17.44. Answer: B.
The scenario does not provide enough information to advocate initiation of omalizumab (we do not know patient's body mass index (BMI), total IgE, sensitisation to allergens). Montelukast and oral theophylline preparations are recommended as additional therapy at this stage. Doubling the prednisolone would increase side-effects without increasing efficacy. There is no indication for an antibiotic here. Home nebulisers are not recommended in asthma because of the risk of late presentation with significant exacerbation.

17.45. Answer: C.
The patient's main complaint is of increased shortness of breath on exertion. ICS would be indicated if there was an increase in exacerbation frequency. Oral prednisolone would be useful in the context of a current exacerbation of COPD. Ambulatory oxygen is not indicated without desaturation on exertion. Whilst a nebuliser might well improve the patient's symptoms, an escalation of inhaled therapy would be a better approach. LABA/LAMA combination inhalers offer enhanced bronchodilatation and improvements in exercise tolerance.

17.46. Answer: D.
A chronic productive cough should raise a suspicion of bronchiectasis. HRCT would show the thickened, dilated airways characteristic of the disease. CXR might show bronchiectatic changes but would not be as sensitive. Bronchoscopy may be useful if sputum samples are not definitive (e.g. intermittent non-tuberculous *Mycobacterium* isolation). α_1-Antitrypsin deficiency is a rare cause of bronchiectasis but this test would follow CT diagnosis. Immunoglobulin levels can be low where an immunodeficiency is a cause of bronchiectasis (IgA, IgM, IgE and IgG with subclasses should be measured).

17

17.47. Answer: B.
The diagnosis is likely to be allergic bronchopulmonary aspergillosis. This is an allergic reaction to *Aspergillus*, which can drive excess sputum production, bronchiectasis and lobar collapse (this would explain the pleuritic chest pain and CXR findings). The key tests would be *Aspergillus* serology, sputum mycology and HRCT. The management would include oral corticosteroids, an antifungal agent, nebulised bronchodilators and chest physiotherapy. Bronchoscopy to remove thick secretions may be required to promote lung re-inflation.

17.48. Answer: C.
Ivacaftor corrects the G551D-mutant *CFTR*. G551D is present in 4% of the CF population, whereas ΔF508 is present in 70%.

17.49. Answer: E.
Pseudomonas aeruginosa is a significant pathogen in CF bronchiectasis. It tends to emerge as patients move towards adulthood. Intravenous antibiotics are often administered in exacerbations caused by *P. aeruginosa*, frequently by implanted subcutaneous venous access ports. Oral azithromycin therapy 3 times a week is an effective therapy but is not nebulised.

17.50. Answer: D.
The common cold is most frequently caused by the rhinovirus. *Bordetella pertussis* causes whooping cough, which can be very prolonged in adults.

17.51. Answer: E.
The above presentation is typical of a lobar pneumonia caused by *Streptococcus pneumoniae*. HSV is likely to be the cause of the cold sores that frequently accompany this presentation but would be a rare cause of a lobar pneumonia. *Pneumocystis jirovecii* is an important cause of pneumonia in immunocompromised individuals. *Mycobacterium tuberculosis* rarely presents so acutely but should be considered in upper zone pneumonias, in the immunocompromised and in patients with relevant travel or exposure histories. *Aspergillus* can cause a lobar pneumonia but usually in the context of underlying lung disease.

17.52. Answer: C.
The patient has recently returned from the Middle East and has a serious respiratory infection. Isolation and exclusion (or diagnosis) of MERS are priorities. *Burkholderia pseudomallei* is endemic to South-east Asia and Northern Australia. Local antibiotic protocol is irrelevant here because of the patient's travel history. CPE testing is important when patients have been hospitalised in countries with a high prevalence of this organism.

17.53. Answer: D.
The patient has been in hospital for > 2 days and has a clinical and radiological presentation consistent with pneumonia. The priority is to start treatment for HAP.

17.54. Answer: A.
Late-onset HAP is most often attributable to Gram-negative bacteria (e.g. *Escherichia*, *Pseudomonas*, *Klebsiella* spp. and *Acinetobacter baumannii*), *Staphylococcus aureus* (including meticillin-resistant *Staph. aureus*, MRSA) and anaerobes.

17.55. Answer: C.
The mortality from HAP is high, at approximately 30%.

17.56. Answer: B.
The patient has developed haematogenous lung abscesses from an infected injection site. It is likely that the right side of the heart (pulmonary and tricuspid valves) is affected and the patient has infective endocarditis.

17.57. Answer: B.
This presentation is most likely to be to be optic neuritis secondary to ethambutol (although isoniazid can also cause this). Patients starting this drug should be warned to report all eye-related symptoms to their clinical team and to stop ethambutol until advised otherwise.

17.58. Answer: B.
IGRA is less likely to give a false-positive response in patients who have had the BCG or have opportunistic mycobacterial infection. It may be positive in active TB but also in latent TB and should not be used as a first-line diagnostic test or as a guide to therapy. The

test relies on the release of interferon-gamma from sensitised T cells.

17.59. Answer: E.
This presentation is consistent with psoas abscess and, whilst there may be a bacteriological cause, this would be a typical extrapulmonary presentation of TB. Malignancy is a major differential diagnosis. The type of imaging utilised above is not identified, but a CT/magnetic resonance imaging (MRI) would be invaluable to assess for spinal disease and potentially cord involvement.

17.60. Answer: E.
The clinical presentation and radiology findings are suggestive of invasive pulmonary aspergillosis and treatment with an antifungal agent should not be delayed for further testing (although mycological culture would be indicated – induced sputum/bronchoscopy). An intercurrent VTE is thought less likely given the scenario, but pleuritic chest pain and haemoptysis should bring this to mind in other contexts. Voriconazole is currently first-line therapy.

17.61. Answer: A.
Adenocarcinoma has recently become the commonest cause of lung cancer.

17.62. Answer: E.
The most likely cause is HPOA, a painful periostitis of the distal radius and ulna. Finger clubbing is not painful. Bone metastases are possible but less likely. Hypercalcaemia can certainly cause bone pain and measuring calcium levels is always indicated when there is bone pain. Horner's syndrome can cause pain in the inner aspect of the arm and small muscle wasting in the hand.

17.63. Answer: D.
The presence of a cytology-positive pleural effusion automatically makes this lung cancer stage IV. If the pleural effusion had an alternative cause such as intercurrent infection and was cytology-negative, the tumour could be stage Ib.

17.64. Answer: C.
A young non-smoker with isolated haemoptysis and a localised, vascular tumour is likely to have a bronchial carcinoid. These tumours are rare but have an excellent outcome. They are

not associated with the usual features of the carcinoid syndrome.

17.65. Answer: D.
Significant survival benefits are conferred by treatment with tyrosine kinase inhibitor drugs in patients with *EGFR* mutation, even in the presence of metastatic disease. The presence of these mutations is more common in non-smoking patients with adenocarcinoma.

17.66. Answer: B.
The possible answers reflect a sensible differential diagnosis for this presentation. The most likely cause, however, is lymphangitis given the insidious onset, the presence of metastatic disease in the lungs and the CT findings.

17.67. Answer: B.
The most likely diagnosis is lymphoma because of the tumour location and the lymphadenopathy.

17.68. Answer: B.
Insidious breathlessness in a woman in her eighth decade with typical examination and CT findings mean that this woman is likely to receive a diagnosis of idiopathic pulmonary fibrosis without further invasive investigation after discussion at an interstitial lung disease multidisciplinary meeting. Lung biopsy adds little information and may be associated with significant morbidity and even mortality.

17.69. Answer: D.
RBILD is a smoking-associated idiopathic interstitial pneumonia that is more common in men and presents between the ages of 40 and 60 years.

17.70. Answer: D.
The symptom complex, combined with a typical CXR appearance (bilateral hilar lymph node and paratracheal lymph node enlargement) is sufficient for a diagnosis of sarcoidosis and this presentation usually has an excellent prognosis.

17.71. Answer: E.
The presence of extensive fibrosis even in the presence of enlarged lymph nodes is suggestive of sarcoidosis stage IV. The patient's breathlessness and abnormal lung

17

function suggest the patient has respiratory failure from a silent progression of pulmonary sarcoidosis. The absence of inspiratory crackles on examination suggests the fibrotic change is due to sarcoidosis.

17.72. Answer: E.
Rheumatoid arthritis has many respiratory complications including nodules, pleural effusion, bronchiectasis and interstitial lung disease. In addition, medications given for rheumatoid arthritis also have respiratory complications and leave patients prone to a range of respiratory infections.

17.73. Answer: E.
The patient's CXR appearance and pleural fluid characteristics are typical of empyema. However, the recurrence on the opposite side in the presence of antibiotic therapy and development of arthritis make rheumatoid arthritis more likely. Lung cancer can produce pleural effusions but the joint findings are not typical of HPOA. Mesothelioma does not tend to present so acutely and is usually unilateral at presentation. Lymphoma often presents with pleural effusions but the pH and glucose levels would not be typical.

17.74. Answer: E.
The high peripheral blood eosinophil count, peripheral X-ray shadowing and potential causative agent (daptomycin) make drug-induced chronic eosinophilic pneumonia the likely diagnosis. As the patient has become systemically unwell with an oxygen requirement it is reasonable to start prednisolone as well as stopping the causative agent. The high eosinophil count makes HAP unlikely. TB should be considered (it can also cause a discitis) but does not cause a peripheral blood eosinophilia. Fluid overload is considered less likely because of the presence of fever and atypical radiology.

17.75. Answer: E.
The presentation here is of multisystem granulomatous polyangiitis. The patient has multiple nodules on CXR and the presentation with stridor suggests subglottic stenosis. It seems likely the patient also has renal involvement. Sinusitis and conductive deafness are also suggestive of granulomatous polyangiitis.

17.76. Answer: D.
The answers above are a reasonable differential diagnosis for the presentation. A progressive pneumonitis is a side-effect of nitrofurantoin taken long term for prevention of urinary tract infections. The subacute onset with systemic symptoms mitigates against IPF or NSIP, whilst atypical pneumonia would be expected to be more acute. A cryptogenic organising pneumonia should not be assumed whilst a potential cause is evident.

17.77. Answer: C.
The recurrence of pneumothorax in the presence of a multicystic lung disease and the possibility of a renal tumour in a young woman suggests lyphangioleiomyomatosis may be the underlying diagnosis. Pulmonary Langerhans cell histiocytosis is strongly associated with smoking. Lymphocytic interstitial pneumonia is usually associated with connective tissue disease or HIV. The other conditions do not cause lung cysts and are not associated with pneumothorax.

17.78. Answer: B.
All of these tests might be useful in investigating this patient's case. However, a detailed PEFR diary that measures a minimum of 4 times per day for at least 3 weeks and during a period away from work would be most informative about whether the patient is experiencing occupational asthma.

17.79. Answer: A.
A patient who works with beryllium and presents with a sarcoid-like clinical picture and imaging should have berylliosis excluded as a priority. Her husband's work should not influence her respiratory status unless she is spending significant amounts of time assisting him. It is possible that where there is damp, mould is also present, but hilar adenopathy would be uncommon in hypersensitivity pneumonitis. Although she has some work stress, dysfunctional breathing would not explain her arthralgia, cough or X-ray appearances.

17.80. Answer: E.
Finger clubbing and basal crackles are characteristic of idiopathic pulmonary fibrosis. Melanoptysis (black sputum) is associated. Simple coal worker's pneumoconiosis has no impact on lung function but PMF may lead to

respiratory failure. PMF is characterised by large conglomerate masses.

17.81. Answer: C.
Silicosis results from the inhalation of crystalline silica usually in the form of quartz.

17.82. Answer: E.
The diagnosis of exclusion here is mesothelioma. The patient has a pleural effusion, extension of pleural thickening onto the mediastinum, chest wall pain that keeps him awake at night and significant asbestos exposure. Although he has had benign asbestos pleurisy in the past, the presentation here is more sinister. Asbestosis is a fibrosing lung condition that would be picked up on CT. Although the patient has pleural plaques, these should not affect his respiratory function or clinical condition.

17.83. Answer: C.
The patient has exposure to a parrot and a CT in keeping with hypersensitivity pneumonitis. It is very likely she has bird fancier's lung. Although the CT was focused on the coronary arteries, the image quality is not likely to have created these findings by artefact. Aspirin sensitivity presents differently and her shortness of breath was present prior to starting aspirin. Sarcoidosis is possible (it is nearly always in the differential for abnormal CT chest) but the history of a parrot at home needs to be explored first. Idiopathic pulmonary fibrosis has a different CT appearance. It would be important to ensure a CT scan focused on the lungs was arranged to ensure optimal imaging available at baseline. Removal of the parrot and deep cleaning of the room it resided in are likely to lead to complete resolution of the clinical and radiological findings.

17.84. Answer: E.
The patient is at significantly increased risk of lung cancer because of his smoking and his occupation ('monkey dung' is a form of asbestos). The least invasive test that will give a histological diagnosis is peripheral lymph node biopsy. Endobronchial ultrasound would be a reasonable test but is more invasive. Liver biopsy may not give an answer as the lesion may not be related to the primary cancer. Flexible bronchoscopy is less likely to give an answer in a peripheral tumour.

17.85. Answer: D.
Chlamydia psittaci infects birds (e.g. parrots and budgerigars).
Coxiella burnetii is the causative agent of Q fever, and farm workers, abattoir workers and hide factory workers may be exposed. Anthrax may occur in workers exposed to infected hides, hair, bristle, bone meal and animal carcasses.

17.86. Answer: A.
This is a clear case of pulmonary thromboembolism (PTE) in a high-risk patient. D-dimer has been inappropriately checked as the patient is high risk and this test only safely excludes VTE in low-to-moderate risk patients. Echocardiogram may show right heart strain but cannot diagnose PTE. Sputum microscopy, culture and sensitivity, and respiratory virus throat swab would be appropriate if the history and CXR were in keeping with respiratory infection. The elevated diaphragm here is likely to reflect pleuritic pain or potentially atelectasis in keeping with PTE. Diaphragmatic studies are not indicated here.

17.87. Answer: D.
The patient's presentation is typical of a large, central pulmonary thromboembolism and she has suffered a cardiac arrest. The immediate management should include resuscitation and thrombolysis. Thrombolysis is indicated in hypotension unresponsive to fluid resuscitation and in cardiac arrest.

17.88. Answer: B.
Pulmonary hypertension is defined as mean pulmonary artery pressure of at least 25 mmHg at rest, as measured at right heart catheterisation.

17.89. Answer: E.
This presentation could be compatible with primary pulmonary hypertension, although this would require further investigation. A transthoracic echocardiogram is a good initial test. Dysfunctional breathing should not be assumed because of social stress, especially in the presence of physical examination findings and abnormal investigations. HRCT might identify enlarged pulmonary arteries but would not be the ideal study. D-dimer would not be appropriate as it would not rule out chronic thromboembolic disease as the cause of pulmonary hypertension. Spirometry would not

17

necessarily show an abnormality, although gas transfer is often reduced.

17.90. Answer: A.
Endothelin inhibitors such as ambrisentan and bosentan are therapies used in primary pulmonary hypertension. Cyclizine and nitrates are contraindicated. There is no role for anti-tumour necrosis factor agents.

17.91. Answer: B.
The seasonal presentation with prominent nasal symptoms and watering eyes suggests allergic rhinitis.

17.92. Answer: D.
Palatoglossus and genioglossus contract actively during inspiration. Abnormal ventilatory drive is present in central sleep apnoea. Forty per cent of middle-aged men snore. During sleep muscle tone decreases.

17.93. Answer: C.
The patient's presentation is typical of obstructive sleep apnoea and 15 or more apnoea/hypopnoeas per hour of sleep is diagnostic.

17.94. Answer: B.
There is no vocal cord paralysis, so local trauma during intubation is the likely cause of the acute-onset hoarseness.

17.95. Answer: E.
This is a primary spontaneous pneumothorax (PSP). Therapeutic aspiration was the appropriate first step but has failed. An intercostal chest drain would be the next step as most PSPs will resolve without the need for referral to cardiothoracic surgery. An intervention is required to treat the pneumothorax, although observation and oxygen would be useful whilst awaiting a skilled intercostal chest drain practitioner. Bronchoscopy has no role here but may be useful in lung/lobar collapse, which should not be confused with pneumothorax.

17.96. Answer: E.
This man has a past history of polio and he seems to have bilateral diaphragmatic weakness that is significantly impairing his respiratory function. A diaphragmatic defect or eventration would be unlikely to cause respiratory failure. Bronchial carcinoma would be more likely to cause unilateral diaphragmatic paralysis. A history of polio means that this is unlikely to be idiopathic.

17.97. Answer: E.
Thoracic kyphoscoliosis is caused by vertebral disease, trauma, neuromuscular disease or can be a congenital abnormality. Asthma is associated with pectus carinatum.

AJ Anderson

18

Endocrinology

Multiple Choice Questions

18.1. A 22 year old woman presents with a few weeks' history of malaise and weight loss. On clinical examination she has palmar hyperpigmentation. With which investigation should she be followed up?

A. Dexamethasone suppression test
B. Magnetic resonance imaging (MRI) abdomen
C. MRI pituitary
D. Synacthen test
E. Thyroid function tests

18.2. A 52 year old South Asian man is found to have thickened pigmented skin at the back of his neck and in the axillae. His body mass index (BMI) is elevated at 38 kg/m². Acanthosis nigricans in this setting is due to which of the following pathology?

A. Axillary perspiration and friction
B. Hyperinsulinaemia
C. Increased fibroblast growth factor activation

D. Increased growth hormone (GH)
E. Increased transforming growth factor-alpha (TGF-α)

18.3. A 28 year old woman presents with secondary amenorrhoea and galactorrhoea. An MRI scan of her brain is likely to show a lesion in which area?

A. Anterior pituitary
B. Hypothalamus
C. Lactiferous ducts
D. Pars intermedia
E. Posterior pituitary

18.4. A 38 year old man is referred with a history of polydipsia and polyuria passing over 3 L of urine in 24 hours. He undergoes a water deprivation test, which shows the following results:

Time/result	Plasma sodium (mmol/L)	Plasma osmolality (mOsm/kg)	Glucose (mmol/L)	(mg/dL)	Urine osmolality (mOsm/kg)	Urine volume (L)
0 hours	144	303	5.1	92	223	0.04
2 hours	144	301	5.2	94	346	0.08
Desmopressin (DDAVP) 2 µg intramuscular						
1 hour post-DDAVP	138	292	4.8	86	528	0.02

What is the underlying cause?

A. Cranial diabetes insipidus
B. Diabetes mellitus
C. Nephrogenic diabetes insipidus
D. Normal response to water deprivation
E. Psychogenic polydipsia

18.5. Where does arginine vasopressin (AVP) exert its maximum effect in the kidney?

A. Collecting ducts
B. Distal convoluted tubule
C. Glomerulus
D. Loop of Henle
E. Proximal tubule

18.6. A 21 year old student is found to have hyperthyroidism. She is counselled on treatment options including radioactive iodine and antithyroid medications. Carbimazole acts on which part of the thyroid hormone synthesis pathway?

A. Cleavage of thyroglobulin by proteolysis
B. Coupling of monoiodotyrosine (MIT) and diiodotyrosine (DIT) forming triiodothyronine (T_3) and thyroxine (T_4)
C. Dehalogenation of iodinated tyrosine to recycle iodide
D. Organification of iodide by thyroid peroxidase incorporating tyrosine forming MIT and DIT
E. Thyroglobulin synthesis

18.7. A 56 year old woman is reviewed in clinic. She was diagnosed with hypothyroidism 15 years previously and has been on levothyroxine 100 µg once daily ever since. Recent thyroid function tests have shown thyrotrophin (thyroid-stimulating hormone; TSH) 8.2 mIU/L and free thyroxine (free T_4) of 15.6 pmol/L (1.21 ng/dL). TSH secretion by the hypothalamus is increased by which of the following?

A. A decrease in thyroxine-binding globulin levels
B. A large increase in free T_4 beyond the normal reference range
C. During early hours of the morning
D. A fall in free T_4 of 5 pmol/L (0.39 ng/dL)
E. An increase in circulating free T_3

18.8. A 23 year old asymptomatic woman attends her family physician for thyroid function testing as her mother has recently been commenced on levothyroxine. Thyroid function tests (TFTs) show TSH 6 mIU/L, and free T_4 of 12.4 pmol/L (0.96 ng/dL). Her serum thyroid peroxidase antibodies are strongly positive. What is the most appropriate management plan?

A. Arrange a scintigraphy scan
B. Check thyroglobulin antibodies
C. Reassure and discharge
D. Repeat TFTs in 4–6 months
E. Start levothyroxine and recheck TFTs in 6 weeks

18.9. A 26 year old woman presents 12 weeks post-partum with symptoms of weight loss, palpitations and troublesome tremor. Her thyroid function is checked, revealing free T_4 24.2 pmol/L (1.88 ng/dL), free T_3 7.1 pmol/L

(0.46 ng/dL) and TSH <0.01 mIU/L. TSH receptor antibody (TRAb) levels are not elevated. What is the most appropriate management?

A. Commence propranolol
B. Consent for radioactive iodine
C. Perform ultrasound scan
D. Screen the infant for hyperthyroidism
E. Treat with selenium

18.10. A 40 year old male smoker presents with weight loss and blood tests suggesting biochemical primary hyperthyroidism. Which of the following features would suggest that the hyperthyroidism is due to Graves' disease?

A. Eyelid retraction
B. Gynaecomastia
C. Lack of orbitopathy
D. Male gender
E. Palpable smooth goitre with bruit

18.11. A 74 year old woman is admitted to hospital with a 3-month history of lethargy, weight gain and increasing shortness of breath. Hypothyroidism can result in which of the following cardiovascular effects?

A. Diastolic hypertension
B. High cardiac output
C. Low cholesterol
D. Reduced peripheral vascular resistance
E. Systolic hypertension

18.12. A 34 year old woman presents to her family physician with weight loss, palpitations and amenorrhoea. Thyroid function tests confirm thyrotoxicosis with free T_4 30.2 pmol/L (2.35 ng/dL) and TSH <0.01 mIU/L. TRAb levels are not elevated. A thyroid scintigraphy scan is performed revealing the following pattern of uptake.

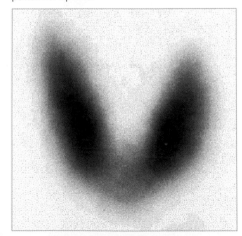

What is the most likely diagnosis?

A. Exogenous thyroxine intake
B. Graves' disease
C. Iodine deficiency
D. Toxic multinodular goitre
E. Transient thyroiditis

18.13. A 28 year old man presents to his family physician with a 6-month history of neck swelling. On examination he has a 2×3 cm palpable lump on the left side of his neck, which moves with swallowing. He has no associated clinical symptoms. He undergoes a scintigraphy scan that reveals the following image.

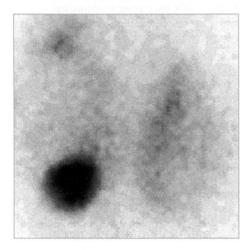

What is the most likely underlying diagnosis?

A. Hashimoto's thyroiditis
B. Thyroglossal duct cyst
C. Thyroid carcinoma
D. Toxic adenoma
E. Toxic multinodular goitre

18.14. A 28 year old man is referred to the endocrinology clinic with a relapse of Graves' disease. Thyroid function tests reveal free T$_4$ 28.4 pmol/L (2.21 ng/dL), TSH <0.01 mIU/L and TRAb 7.6iU/L. He is considering radioactive iodine (^{131}I) treatment. Which of the following statements is TRUE about this treatment?

A. ^{131}I is given as an intravenous infusion
B. He has a 10% risk of developing hypothyroidism in the first 12 months
C. He is likely to lose weight following ^{131}I
D. He is safe to father a child within 6 months of treatment
E. It may cause deterioration of active Graves' ophthalmopathy

18.15. A 23 year old white woman presents with a 6-month history of increasing neck swelling and discomfort on swallowing. On examination she has a smooth diffuse symmetrical goitre. Thyroid function tests are normal and thyroid antibody levels are undetectable. Ultrasound shows a diffuse and symmetrical echogenic pattern, with no significant nodularity. Which of the follow statements is correct in this scenario?

A. Associated lymphadenopathy is normal
B. Radioactive iodine treatment should be used to shrink the gland
C. She is likely to experience symptoms of lethargy and weight gain
D. The goitre may enlarge during pregnancy
E. There is a high risk of malignancy

18.16. A 53 year old woman whose thyroid function tests have been stable and within the normal range on 200 µg of levothyroxine for the last 6 months is found to have a TSH <0.01 mIU/L. You ask her about her current medications including those bought over the counter. Which of the following is associated with increased bioavailability of levothyroxine?

A. Calcium
B. Colestyramine
C. Iron
D. Phenytoin
E. Vitamin C

18.17. A 25 year old woman was commenced on levothyroxine 3 weeks ago for primary hypothyroidism. She is concerned about ongoing symptoms of dry skin and dry hair. She has been otherwise well with nil else to report on systemic enquiry. What is the most appropriate management plan?

A. Add in liothyronine
B. Check her anti-tissue transglutaminase antibody levels
C. Check her TRAbs
D. Increase levothyroxine dose now
E. Reassure and organise for repeat thyroid function test in a further 3 weeks

18.18. Thyroid function tests are performed on a patient who has been on levothyroxine replacement for several years. The following results are observed. TSH 8.2mIU/L, free T$_4$ 21.6 pmol/L (1.68 ng/dL) and free T$_3$ 4.2 pmol/L (0.27 ng/dL). What is the most likely underlying diagnosis?

18

A. Non-thyroidal illness
B. Non-functioning pituitary tumour
C. Thyroiditis
D. Treatment with amiodarone
E. Variable treatment adherence

18.19. A 32 year old woman attends her family physician with symptoms of tremor and vague anterior neck discomfort. Initial blood tests reveal a free T_4 14 pmol/L (1.09 ng/dL) and TSH 0.12 mIU/L. Subsequent TFTs 4 weeks later show TSH 89.8 mIU/L and free T_4 <5 pmol/L (0.39 ng/dL). Scintigraphy scan shows the following:

What is the most likely underlying cause?

A. Graves' disease
B. Primary hypothyroidism
C. Subacute thyroiditis
D. Toxic adenoma
E. Toxic multinodular goitre

18.20. A 75 year old man with a past medical history of ischaemic heart disease is admitted to hospital following a fall at home. He becomes increasingly delirious on the ward. As part of his work-up, thyroid function is checked showing TSH 0.2 mIU/L, free T_4 26.2 pmol/L (2.04 ng/dL) and free T_3 3.3 pmol/L (0.21 ng/dL). What is the most appropriate management plan?

A. Check for TRAbs
B. Commence carbimazole treatment
C. Consent for radioactive iodine treatment
D. Discontinue cardiac medications
E. Repeat thyroid function tests when the patient has fully recovered

18.21. A 72 year old man was commenced on amiodarone for atrial fibrillation 6 months previously. He is referred with a history of weight loss, tremor and sweating. Blood tests reveal TSH <0.01 mIU/L, free T_4 26.1 pmol/L (2.03 ng/dL) and free T_3 4.1 pmol/L (0.27 ng/dL). What is a scintigraphy scan likely to show?

A. Diffuse increased uptake
B. Diffuse low uptake
C. Multinodular goitre
D. Normal uptake
E. Solidary toxic nodule

18.22. What is the correct treatment for type II thyrotoxicosis secondary to amiodarone?

A. Carbimazole
B. Discontinue amiodarone only and allow resolution of thyroid function
C. Glucocorticoids
D. Levothyroxine
E. Radioactive iodine

18.23. A 62 year old woman is referred with a 3-month history of diffuse swelling in her neck and weight loss. On palpation she has a large, firm nodular goitre and non-tender cervical lymphadenopathy. She complains of hoarseness of her voice. What is her likely diagnosis?

A. Anaplastic carcinoma
B. Follicular cell carcinoma
C. Medullary carcinoma
D. Papillary cell carcinoma
E. Toxic adenoma

18.24. A 34 year old woman is reviewed in the thyroid cancer clinic following total thyroidectomy and neck dissection with lymph node clearance for a confirmed (pT4, N1, M0) papillary thyroid cancer. Follow-up management post-surgery should include which of the following?

A. Levothyroxine replacement aiming to keep TSH within the normal range
B. Radioactive iodine treatment when TSH is fully suppressed
C. Regular computed tomography (CT) scans of the neck
D. Screening of family members for thyroid cancer
E. Thyroglobulin measurement at regular intervals

18.25. A 32 year old woman attends her family physician with a 12-month history of inability to conceive. She has been having regular periods every 28 days. Ovulation can be confirmed by which of the following tests?

A. Day 10 rise in follicle-stimulating hormone (FSH)
B. Day 13 surge in oestradiol
C. Day 14 surge in progesterone
D. Day 14 surge in luteinising hormone (LH)
E. Regular menses

18.26. You review a 21 year old woman in the reproductive endocrinology clinic. She has a history of secondary amenorrhoea and anorexia since she was 18 years old. She is keen to know why she has stopped having periods. Functional hypothalamic amenorrhoea is underpinned by which process?

A. A high LH-to-FSH ratio
B. Gonadotrophin-releasing hormone (GnRH) resistance
C. High circulating leptin
D. Hyperprolactinaemia
E. Reduced pulsatility and secretion of GnRH

18.27. A 16 year old girl presents to her family physician having never had a period. She is noted to be of short stature. Blood tests reveal FSH 26.2 IU/L (5.9 µg/L), LH 18.5 IU/L (2.0 µg/L) and oestradiol <50 pmol/L (13.6 pg/mL). What is the next most appropriate investigation?

A. CT scan ovary and adrenal glands
B. Karyotype
C. MRI pituitary
D. Synacthen test
E. Ultrasound scan ovaries

18.28. A 12 year old boy attends his family physician as it has been noticed that he is falling behind in school and is considerably shorter than his classmates. Which of the following is consistent with the diagnosis of constitutional delay?

A. Bone age consistent with chronological age
B. More common in females
C. Occurs as young as 3–6 months of age
D. Smaller adult height than predicted
E. Upper-to-lower body ratio <1

18.29. A 56 year old man is referred to the endocrinology clinic with a history of poor libido and erectile dysfunction. Blood tests reveal

total testosterone 5.6 nmol/L (162 ng/dL), SHBG 42.1 nmol/L (4.00 µg/mL), FSH 2.1 IU/L (0.5 µg/L) and LH 1.76 IU/L (0.2 µg/L). He has no other past medical history of note and has not fathered any children. On examination visual fields are normal, testes are 5 mL volume and soft on palpation. He has little in the way of pubic or axillary hair. He has not noticed any problem with his sense of smell. Which of the following is the most likely underlying diagnosis?

A. Kallmann's syndrome
B. Klinefelter's syndrome
C. Previous trauma to the testes
D. Reduced testosterone secondary to obesity
E. Reduced testosterone with age

18.30. An 18 year old woman with a BMI of 31 kg/m^2 attends her family physician with troublesome hirsutism, acne and irregular periods. Hyperandrogenism as a sequela of polycystic ovary syndrome (PCOS) may result from which of the following?

A. Genetic mutation in 3β-hydroxysteroid dehydrogenase
B. Higher FSH compared with LH synthesis by the pituitary gland
C. Increased pulsatility of GnRH
D. Reduced aromatisation of androgens by theca cells
E. Reduction in circulating SHBG

18.31. A 23 year old student with known karyotype 45X attends the clinic seeking advice as she is wanting to achieve pregnancy. Which of the following should she be counselled about?

A. Child is more likely to have low IQ
B. Increased risk of ovarian cancer
C. She will require anti-androgen therapy
D. She will require screening for aortic dissection
E. There is a high chance of her becoming pregnant spontaneously

18.32. A 17 year old boy is referred with delayed puberty. He has noticed that he is taller than his classmates. On clinical examination he is found to have sparse facial and body hair as well as small pre-pubertal-sized testes and penis. Blood tests reveal testosterone 7.5 nmol/L (216 ng/dL), FSH 12 IU/L (2.8 µg/L), LH 11 IU/L (1.2 µg/L). What is the most appropriate next test?

18

A. Chromosomal analysis
B. GH measurement
C. Karyotype
D. Prolactin level
E. Thyroid function test

18.33. What is the principal pathological abnormality in Klinefelter's syndrome?

A. Defect in transforming growth factor-β (TGF-β) signalling pathway
B. Disordered migration of GnRH-producing neurons
C. Dysgenesis of the seminiferous tubules
D. Dysregulated testosterone synthesis
E. LH resistance

18.34. A 62 year old man has noticed that his breasts have been swollen and tender to touch. He is on a long list of medications. Which of the following medications can cause gynaecomastia?

A. Bendroflumethiazide
B. Dihydrotestosterone
C. Finasteride
D. Metolazone
E. Tamoxifen

18.35. A 72 year old man with a history of chronic kidney disease stage 4 is admitted with perioral paraesthesia and cramping in his hands. Blood tests reveal calcium 1.7 mmol/L (6.81 mg/dL) and parathyroid hormone (PTH) level 8.7 pmol/L (82 pg/mL). PTH has which of the following effects?

A. Absorption of calcium from the gut
B. Absorption of phosphate from the gut
C. Conversion of 25-hydroxyvitamin D to 1,25-dihydroxyvitamin D
D. Excretion of magnesium from the distal convoluted tubule
E. Increases phosphate reabsorption from proximal tubule

18.36. A 32 year old man is admitted to hospital with gastroenteritis. Blood tests reveal total calcium 2.72 mmol/L (10.9 mg/dL), potassium 3.7 mmol/L, magnesium 1.2 mmol/L (2.92 mg/dL), urea 4.7 mmol/L (28.2 mg/dL), creatinine 76 μmol/L (0.86 mg/dL) and PTH 6.0 pmol/L (57 pg/mL). He states that his mother is currently being investigated for hypercalcaemia, which was picked up on a routine blood test. What is the most likely underlying cause of his blood results?

A. Dehydration secondary to gastroenteritis
B. Malignancy
C. Mutation in calcium-sensing receptor gene
D. Mutation in the *MENIN* gene (MEN 1)
E. *RET* oncogene mutation (MEN 2/3, also known as MEN 2a/2b)

18.37. A 36 year old woman is admitted to hospital with abdominal pain. Blood tests reveal calcium 3.01 mmol/L (12.1 mg/dL), phosphate 0.5 mmol/L (1.55 mg/dL), magnesium 0.8 mmol/L (1.94 mg/dL), urinary calcium 12.8 mmol/24 hrs (512 mg/24 hrs; 32.0 mmol/L) (elevated), PTH 12.3 pmol/L (116 pg/mL). What is the most appropriate follow-up management plan?

A. Commence loop diuretic
B. Commence thiazide diuretic
C. Monitor calcium levels
D. Refer for parathyroid surgery
E. Vitamin D replacement

18.38. A 52 year old woman is referred to the clinic with a 4-month history of lethargy, generalised weakness and pains in her hands and feet. Blood tests reveal TSH 1.3 mIU/L (normal), total free T_4 18.4 pmol/L (1.43 ng/dL), calcium 2.2 mmol/L (8.81 mg/dL), phosphate 0.6 mmol/L (1.86 mg/dL), PTH 6.4 pmol/L (60 pg/mL), alkaline phosphatase 158 IU/L, creatinine 73 μmol/L (0.83 mg/dL). What is the likely underlying diagnosis?

A. Autoimmune polyendocrine syndrome
B. Haemochromatosis
C. Magnesium deficiency
D. Parathyroid adenoma
E. Vitamin D deficiency

18.39. A 33 year old man is found to have a significant postural hypotension with a drop in systolic blood pressure from 130/75 to 100/60 mmHg. Further investigations reveal elevated renin levels but low aldosterone levels on sitting. Where in the adrenal gland is the enzyme aldosterone synthase located?

A. Chromaffin cells
B. Medulla
C. Zona fasciculata
D. Zona glomerulosa
E. Zona reticularis

18.40. A mother seeks advice for her 7 year old daughter who has started developing pubic hair and body odour, and her voice has become deeper. A diagnosis of congenital adrenal hyperplasia (CAH) is being considered. What is the commonest enzyme deficiency in CAH?

A. 11β-hydroxysteroid dehydrogenase
B. 17α-hydroxylase
C. 17β-hydroxysteroid dehydrogenase
D. 18-hydroxylase
E. 21-hydroxylase

18.41. A 63 year old man presents to his family physician with a 1-month history of weight gain and difficulty climbing stairs. On clinical examination he is found to have a blood pressure of 182/85 mmHg, abdominal striae and bruising on his arms. An overnight dexamethasone test reveals a morning serum cortisol level of 153 nmol/L (5.55 µg/dL). Which of the following would be an appropriate next investigation?

A. 24-hour urine free cortisol
B. Adrenal vein sampling
C. Bilateral inferior petrosal sinus sampling
D. CT adrenals
E. High-dose dexamethasone suppression test

18.42. A 56 year old man with recently diagnosed lung cancer has noticed weight gain, easy bruising of his skin, increased thirst and difficulty climbing stairs. Which type of lung cancer is associated with this endocrinological picture?

A. Adenocarcinoma
B. Carcinoid tumour
C. Large cell carcinoma
D. Mesothelioma
E. Squamous cell carcinoma

18.43. Hypokalaemia associated with Cushing's syndrome is due to which underlying mechanism?

A. Activation of mineralocorticoid receptors
B. Adipocyte proliferation
C. Increased glycogen synthesis
D. Increased protein breakdown
E. Insulin resistance

18.44. An incidental finding of an adrenal mass is discovered when a 72 year woman has a CT scan. Which of the following parameters is associated with an increased likelihood of malignancy?

A. Bilateral lesions
B. Hounsfield units <10HU
C. Retention of contrast
D. Size <4 cm
E. Smooth surface

18.45. A 24 year old man is admitted to the emergency department having collapsed at the gym. He describes symptoms of headache, feeling flushed with associated palpitations and sweating. He was observed by his friends to become pale before he collapsed. He is persistently hypertensive and a 24-hour urine collection shows elevated metadrenalines (metanephrines). First-line treatment for this condition should be with which of the following?

A. Bisoprolol
B. Dexamethasone
C. Fludrocortisone
D. Ketoconazole
E. Phenoxybenzamine

18.46. A 28 year old man is referred having been found, on home blood pressure monitoring, to have hypertension. His serum potassium at diagnosis was 2.9 mmol/L. He has been commenced on antihypertensive therapy and is referred in for investigation of mineralocorticoid excess. Which of the following antihypertensive therapies may interfere with these investigations by increasing plasma renin concentrations?

A. Amlodipine
B. Bendroflumethiazide
C. Bisoprolol
D. Diltiazem
E. Doxazosin

18.47. Glucose-stimulated insulin secretion by the pancreas is augmented by which of the following?

A. Dipeptidyl peptidase-4
B. Glucagon-like peptide-1
C. Insulin-like growth factor-1
D. Leptin
E. Somatostatin

18.48. An 18 year old woman with no past medical history and on no regular medications is admitted to hospital following a collapse at home. She describes prodromal symptoms of palpitations, weakness and diplopia. Plasma glucose concentration is measured at

18

2.3 mmol/L (41 mg/dL). Plasma samples are taken on admission, showing C-peptide <0.66 nmol/L (<2 ng/mL) and insulin 104 pmol/L (15 µIU/mL). What is the most likely diagnosis?

A. Alcohol
B. Critical illness
C. Exogenous insulin
D. Insulinoma
E. Sulphonylurea ingestion

18.49. A 56 year old man presents with a 5-year history of chronic right-sided lower abdominal pain and altered bowel habit. More recently he has developed symptoms of increased shortness of breath, diarrhoea and intermittent flushing. A CT scan shows a calcified mass in the mesentery with a surrounding desmoplastic response and multiple hepatic metastases. Which of the following would be the next initial investigation?

A. 5-hydroxyindoleacetic acid (5-HIAA) concentration in urine
B. Capsule endoscopy
C. Colonoscopy
D. Plasma insulin concentrations
E. Plasma somatostatin concentrations

18.50. A 72 year old man with known pituitary adenoma is admitted as an emergency with sudden-onset headache, and visual disturbance. He is found to have bilateral ptosis. MRI imaging shows expansion of the tumour size secondary to haemorrhage, with invasion of the cavernous sinus. Which of the following sets of cranial nerves (CNs) are found in the cavernous sinus?

A. CN II and III
B. CN III and IV
C. CN III, IV, V and VI
D. CN IX, X, and XI
E. CN X, XI and XII

18.51. A 17 year old who was diagnosed with craniopharyngioma at the age of 2 years is reviewed in clinic. His parents are concerned about a recent dramatic increase in his weight as well as polydypsia and polyuria. He is sent for an MRI pituitary to assess any interval change in tumour size. Craniopharyngiomas arise from remnants of Rathke's pouch. In embryological development of the pituitary gland, which structure does Rathke's pouch develop into?

A. Adenohypophysis
B. Diaphragma sellae
C. Infundibulum
D. Neurohypophysis
E. Sella turcica

18.52. A 62 year old man attends the diabetes clinic and is noted to have large hands and prognathism. He complains of headaches of increasing frequency and severity over the preceding 6 months since his last visit to the clinic. Which endocrine investigation should be performed to investigate the cause of his symptoms?

A. 24-hour urinary steroid profile
B. Dexamethasone suppression test
C. Insulin tolerance test
D. Oral glucose tolerance test
E. Saline suppression test

18.53. A 42 year old woman is referred with galactorrhoea. Her periods have become irregular. She has two children who are 16 and 21 years old and has been more stressed at work than previously. She is not on any regular medication. Blood tests reveal a prolactin level of 12 124 mIU/L (570 ng/mL) with no evidence of macroprolactin. What is the most appropriate treatment?

A. Monitor prolactin levels every year
B. Reassure and discharge
C. Refer for pituitary surgery
D. Start on cabergoline 0.25 mg twice weekly
E. Start on carbimazole 40 mg once daily

18.54. A 53 year old man who is currently under investigation for bitemporal quandrantanopia presents to the emergency department with sudden acute severe headache. What is the most likely cause of his headache?

A. Cerebrospinal fluid leak
B. Meningitis
C. Migraine
D. Pituitary apoplexy
E. Subarachnoid haemorrhage

18.55. A 33 year old man undergoes a CT scan for recurrent headaches, which reveals a 21×15 mm pituitary adenoma. On further questioning he has been feeling more tired over recent months and feeling low in his mood. He is tested for pituitary dysfunction and visual field disturbance. The secretion of which hormone is often the first to be affected due to mass effect by a pituitary macroadenoma?

A. ACTH
B. FSH
C. GH
D. LH
E. TSH

18.56. A 55 year old woman is found to have a significant pituitary mass on MRI scanning. High circulating levels of which hormone would direct treatment for a pituitary macroadenoma down a primarily medical, rather than surgical, route?

A. ACTH
B. GH
C. LH
D. Prolactin
E. TSH

18.57. 52 year old woman is referred to the clinic with a 3-month history of polyuria. She additionally complains of increased thirst, drinking up to 5 L per day. Fasting plasma glucose is normal at 4.2 mmol/L (76 mg/dL).

She attends for a water deprivation test. Which of the following confirms a diagnosis of diabetes insipidus?

A. 24-hour urine volume of 3 L
B. Plasma osmolality <280 mOsm/kg at the start of the test
C. Plasma osmolality >300 mOsm/kg and urine osmolality <600 mOsm/kg
D. Plasma sodium concentration 145 mmol/L
E. Reduction in body weight of 1% over the test period

18.58. A 32 year old man is referred having been found to have hypercalcaemia and a high PTH level. He has recently been investigated for episodes of sweating, lightheadedness and confusion, which were helped by eating sugary foods. Which of the following is associated with MEN 1?

A. Acromegaly
B. Cerebellar haemangioblastoma
C. Marfinoid habitus
D. Medullary thyroid carcinoma
E. Phaeochromocytoma

Answers

18

18.1. Answer: D.
Primary hypoadrenalism results in increased synthesis and secretion of adrenocorticotrophic hormone (ACTH) from the pituitary gland. Due to the co-secretion of melanocyte-stimulating hormone as part of the larger prohormone (pro-opiomelanocortin; POMC), hyperpigmentation occurs, classically of the palmar creases. Primary adrenal failure (Addison's disease) is usually autoimmune in aetiology and this can be confirmed with the detection of anti-adrenal autoantibodies. If diagnosed, potential coexisting autoimmune conditions should be looked for. Alternative causes of Addison's disease include tuberculous adrenalitis, which should be strongly considered in endemic areas and when autoantibodies are negative. Abdominal imaging in such cases may reveal calcification of the adrenal glands. Secondary hypoadrenalism due to pituitary pathology, with resultant low ACTH levels, is associated with skin pallor. The dexamethasone suppression test forms part of the workup for suspected Cushing's syndrome. Imaging should not be done until the biochemical diagnosis is made.

18.2. Answer: B.
High concentrations of insulin (hyperinsulinaemia) exert proliferative effects through the insulin-like growth factor-1 (IGF-1) receptors, stimulating epidermal keratinocyte and dermal fibroblast proliferation in the axillae.

18.3. Answer: A.
Hyperprolactinaemia (often due to a microprolactinoma) is a common cause of secondary amenorrhoea in this age group. Prolactin is synthesised by lactotrophs in the anterior pituitary gland. Synthesis and release of prolactin is under the tonic inhibition of dopamine, which is released from the hypothalamus and passes down capillaries surrounding the pituitary stalk to the anterior pituitary.

18.4. Answer: A.
Following overnight water deprivation, you would expect urine to be more concentrated, with an osmolality of >600 mOsm/kg, particularly given that the plasma sodium level is at the upper end of the normal range and

plasma osmolality is >300 mOsm/kg. This therefore confirms diabetes insipidus. The concentrating ability of the kidney is improved following the administration of desmopressin (DDAVP), providing evidence of a central cranial cause. In nephrogenic diabetes insipidus, urine osmolality would show little improvement following administration of DDAVP.

18.5. Answer: A.
Arginine vasopressin acts via V2 receptors in the renal collecting ducts to cause the insertion of aquaporin-2 that allows increased water permeability across the collecting ducts with subsequent reabsorption of water, leading to the production of more concentrated urine.

18.6. Answer: D.
Iodide is actively transported into follicular cells by a sodium/iodide transporter (Fig. 18.6). Pendrin is found at the apical membrane, where it transports iodide into colloid. A defect in this transporter underlies Pendred's syndrome (congenital hypothyroidism and

deafness). Thyroid peroxidase catalyses the conversion of iodide ions into organic iodine and couples it with tyrosine to form MIT and DIT. This later step is inhibited by thionamides such as carbimazole. DIT and MIT combine forming T_4 and T_3. The organification of iodide and coupling of iodinated tyrosine molecules occurs on the surface of thyroglobulin. This is subsequently cleaved, releasing thyroid hormone. Uncoupled iodinated tyrosine can be dehalogenated, allowing recycling of the iodine. The majority of T_4 circulates bound to thyroxine-binding globulin (TBG).

18.7. Answer: D.
Through a classical negative feedback loop, TSH secretion will increase with a reduction in circulating free T_4 or T_3. TSH synthesis follows a circadian rhythm with a peak at 0100 hrs and nadir at 1100 hrs. Free T_4 circulates at concentrations around three times that of free T_3, although T_3 is a more potent activator of thyroid hormone receptors. Both play a role in feeding back to the hypothalamus. Small

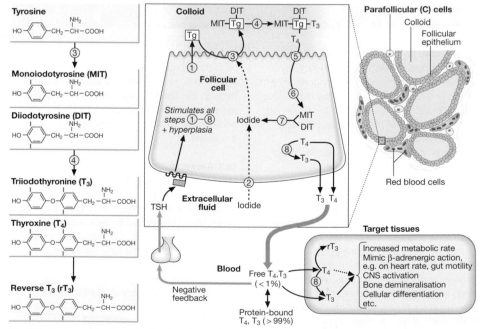

Fig. 18.6 Structure and function of the thyroid gland.
(1) Thyroglobulin (Tg) is synthesised and secreted into the colloid of the follicle. (2) Inorganic iodide (I⁻) is actively transported into the follicular cell ('trapping'). (3) Iodide is transported on to the colloidal surface by a transporter (pendrin, defective in Pendred's syndrome) and 'organified' by the thyroid peroxidase enzyme, which incorporates it into the amino acid tyrosine on the surface of Tg to form monoiodotyrosine (MIT) and diiodotyrosine (DIT). (4) Iodinated tyrosines couple to form T_3 and T_4. (5) Tg is endocytosed. (6) Tg is cleaved by proteolysis to free the iodinated tyrosine and thyroid hormones. (7) Iodinated tyrosine is dehalogenated to recycle the iodide. (8) T_4 is converted to T_3 by 5′-monodeiodinase.

changes in an individual's free T_4 will result in altered TSH secretion.

18.8. Answer: D.
This woman has subclinical hypothyroidism. There is no benefit in checking thyroglobulin antibodies as it does not change her diagnosis or management. With positive thyroid peroxidase antibodies she has a higher risk of progression to overt thyroid failure. A trial of thyroxine replacement would be advocated if her TSH was >10 mIU/L or she developed symptoms suggestive of progression to clinical disease. Reviewing her biochemistry and symptomatology is therefore necessary.

18.9. Answer: A.
This picture is in keeping with post-partum thyroiditis. This typically presents 4–8 months post-partum. Thyroid scintigraphy will show negligible uptake and can be helpful in differentiating against Graves' disease. Antithyroid drugs are ineffective. Symptomatic management with a non-selective β-adrenoceptor antagonist (β-blocker) is the most appropriate treatment at this stage. She is likely to develop hypothyroidism, and close monitoring of her thyroid function to allow identification and early treatment is advocated. Oral selenium is used for the treatment of mild to moderate dysthyroid eye disease and is not appropriate here.

18.10. Answer: E.
Exopthalmus but not lid retraction is specific to Graves' disease. Lid retraction is a consequence of adrenergic stimulation of the levator palpebrae muscles and may be seen in any form of thyrotoxicosis. Thyrotoxicosis can result in an increase in sex hormone-binding globulin (SHBG), altering the ratio of free testosterone to oestradiol and, as such, result in gynaecomastia. Females have a greater susceptibility to autoimmune disease in general, including Graves' disease. Smoking is a significant risk factor for the development of eye disease. The presence of a goitre in the setting of clinical and biochemical hyperthydroidism is common with Graves' disease but not universal or diagnostic. The presence of TRAbs or a classical picture of diffuse increased uptake on a scintigraphy scan are diagnostic.

18.11. Answer: A.
Hypothyroidism can result in impaired left ventricular contractility reducing cardiac output. Reduced circulating thyroid hormone levels can additionally cause reduced ventricular diastolic relaxation, increasing diastolic pressure with subsequent increase in vascular smooth muscle contractility and peripheral vascular resistance. Through alteration in cholesterol synthesis and metabolism, hypothyroidism results in hypercholesterolaemia.

18.12. Answer: B.
Exogenous thyroxine and transient thyroiditis will result in low uptake of ^{99m}technetium on scanning. Iodine deficiency can cause goitre and raised TSH, but thyrotoxicosis would only potentially occur following iodine supplementation. Although present in 80–95% of Graves' disease, TRAbs are not universal in all cases, necessitating additional investigation to confirm the diagnosis. A thyroid scintigraphy scan reveals uniform increased uptake in the setting of Graves' disease.

18.13. Answer: D.
This is the classic image of a toxic adenoma with increased uptake in the adenoma and suppressed uptake in the remaining gland. The presence of multiple nodules with high uptake of ^{99m}technetium would be consistent with toxic multinodular goitre. 'Cold nodules' on scintigraphy have a much greater likelihood of malignancy. Thyroglossal duct cysts are typically located in the midline and are cold, whilst thyroiditis displays widespread reduced uptake of tracer.

18.14. Answer: E.
Radioactive iodine is administered orally as a capsule or liquid. The doses used for the treatment of Graves' disease are much smaller than for the follow-up management of thyroid cancer at 400–600 MBq (approximately 10–15 mCi). There is a significant risk of hypothyroidism when using ^{131}I for the treatment of Graves' disease; this is approximately 40% after 1 year and 80% after 15 years. Failure to adjust energy consumption to the reduced metabolic rate associated with correction of hyperthyroidism may precipitate weight gain. With a potential adverse effect on developing sperm, male individuals are advised to refrain from conceiving for a minimum of 6 months post-treatment. There are reports that

18

radioactive iodine can exacerbate active Graves' ophthalmopathy and so it is best avoided in this situation if alternative treatment options carry less risk. High-dose glucocorticoids can be used to reduce the risk of potentiating eye disease.

18.15. Answer: D.

Simple diffuse goitre is a benign condition with hypertrophy of thyroid tissue. Thyroid function is normal and it will therefore not shrink significantly with radioactive iodine treatment. Surgery is a better option if there is concern about cosmetic appearance. It may enlarge in response to alterations in circulating oestrogens such as during pregnancy. The goitre usually regresses over time but may develop into a multinodular goitre with autonomous function. In areas of endemic iodine deficiency, iodine supplementation may cause some regression of the goitre.

18.16. Answer: E.

Intestinal absorption of levothyroxine is impaired by co-ingestion of iron, colestyramine and calcium supplements, but enhanced by vitamin C. Increased clearance occurs with a variety of medications, including antiepileptic medications and rifampicin. Clearance is reduced with increasing age, potentially necessitating smaller doses for replacement.

18.17. Answer: E.

After commencement of levothyroxine for hypothyroidism, symptoms of dry skin and hair can take 3–6 months to improve. Reduction in periorbital oedema occurs more rapidly. The dose of levothyroxine should be adjusted to keep TSH within the reference range, with serum T_4 in the upper reference range. Treatment with T_3 is controversial, but may be considered in selected cases. The half-life of levothyroxine is around 7 days and it therefore takes around 6 weeks following commencement of levothyroxine to see resolution of thyroid function tests. There is no indication to check the patient's TRAbs. Malabsorption can result in under-treatment of hypothyroidism, although there is nothing in this clinical scenario to suggest coeliac disease.

18.18. Answer: E.

Central hypothyroidism results in both low TSH and T_4. Amiodarone treatment usually causes a mild elevation in free T_4, with free T_3 and

TSH both at the lower end of the reference range. Thyroiditis typically causes an initial thyrotoxic phase followed on by a period of hypothyroidism, which may resolve or persist. Non-thyroidal illness results in reduced peripheral conversion of T_4 to T_3 with reduced secretion of TSH. The differential diagnosis for this pattern would include a TSH-secreting pituitary tumour or thyroid hormone resistance, but in this scenario it is most likely that the patient has not been reliably taking levothyroxine for several weeks (causing the TSH to rise) and then in the few days prior to the blood test has taken an increased dose of levothyroxine (resulting in the borderline elevated free T_4).

18.19. Answer: C.

In subacute thyroiditis, inflammation results in the release of colloid and stored thyroid hormone, resulting in thyrotoxicosis. Damage to follicular cells impairs retention of iodine, resulting in subsequent hypothyroidism and produces the classic picture of a 'cold' image on scintigraphy. Acute thyroiditis usually results from bacterial infection such as *Staphylococcus aureus* and *Streptococcus haemolyticus*, whilst subacute thyroiditis often follows a viral illness. Management of hypothyroidism resulting from thyroiditis may involve at least temporary replacement with levothyroxine and close monitoring of thyroid function tests. After 4 months of TSH being within the reference range, reduction in levothyroxine dose to 50 µg may be tried with further TSH monitoring after 6 weeks. If TSH remains within the normal range, a trial of levothyroxine can be attempted, with repeat thyroid function testing after a further 6 weeks.

18.20. Answer: E.

These results are in keeping with non-thyroidal illness or 'sick euthyroidism'. This occurs due to decreased peripheral conversion of T_4 to T_3 as well as altered circulating levels and binding of thyroid hormone to thyroxine-binding globulin, with resultant altered feedback on the hypothalamic–pituitary–thyroid axis. During recovery from the systemic illness, the TSH may increase to levels associated with hypothyroidism. Over time these will, however, normalise; hence, unless there is clinical evidence of concomitant thyroidal disease, repeated measurements and monitoring is advised.

18.21. Answer: B.

Given the history and pattern of thyroid function tests, this is likely to be amiodarone-induced thyrotoxicosis. Amiodarone has a structure analogous to that of thyroxine. Standard daily dosing of 200 mg daily contains around 600 times the recommended daily requirement of iodine. Amiodarone additionally has a direct cytotoxic effect, inhibiting the conversion of thyroxine (T_4) to thyronine (T_3). For these reasons, thyroxine production from the thyroid gland is suppressed, resulting in globally reduced uptake on a scintigraphy scan.

18.22. Answer: C.

It can be difficult to distinguish between type I and type II amiodarone-induced thyrotoxicosis. In type I, excess iodine induces increased thyroid hormone synthesis and is usually responsive to antithyroid medication. In type II, the picture is more of a thyroiditis due to cytotoxic effect of amiodarone and is usually responsive to glucocorticoid treatment. The excess iodine provided by amiodarone renders it unresponsive to treatment with radioactive iodine. Amiodarone has a long half-life of 50–60 days and interim treatment is therefore needed, even if amiodarone is withdrawn, as effects may persist for 6–9 months.

18.23. Answer: A.

Anaplastic thyroid carcinoma is rapidly progressive with a median survival of only 7 months and usually presents in those over 60 years of age. It may cause hoarseness due to recurrent laryngeal nerve compression and stridor due to tracheal compression. There is no effective treatment, although surgery and radiotherapy may be considered in some individuals. Follicular and papillary carcinoma are much more indolent, with a 10-year survival of around 95% and the majority are cured with surgery, with or without radio-iodine therapy. These usually present as a single focus with or without nodal involvement. Distant metastases, greater age at presentation, male sex and certain histological subtypes have a worse prognosis. The differential diagnosis in this case is lymphoma.

18.24. Answer: E.

With more extensive disease, levothyroxine replacement is provided with an aim of suppressing TSH, preventing stimulation of any potential residual tissue. Studies have shown equivalent efficacy for treatment with 1100 MBq and 3700 MBq (approximately 30 and 100 mCi, respectively) radioactive iodine post-thyroidectomy for relatively low-risk thyroid carcinomas, but with extensive disease the higher dose should be used. Radioactive iodine should not be given unless TSH is elevated to >20 mIU/L. This can either be achieved through discontinuation of levothyroxine or through administration of recombinant TSH. Thyroglobulin can be used as a tumour marker following completion thyroidectomy and provides a sensitive marker of recurrence. Ultrasound is a more sensitive imaging modality for local recurrence than CT scanning. Medullary thyroid cancer can be associated with multiple endocrine neoplasia (MEN) 2 (also known as MEN 2a) but there is no known genetic predisposition to date for the development of well-differentiated thyroid cancer.

18.25. Answer: D.

Regular menses imply, but do not confirm, ovulation. During a 28-day cycle, ovulation can be predicted by a surge in LH on day 14 and by measuring the responding increase in progesterone on day 21 (Fig. 18.25). Timings have to be adjusted depending on the length of the woman's menstrual cycle. Alternatively, ultrasound scanning can be used to track the growth and development of follicles, thus predicting ovulation.

18.26. Answer: E.

Functional hypothalamic amenorrhoea is characterised by abnormal hypothalamic GnRH secretion with resultant reduction in pulsation of gonadotrophins. FSH levels are often within the

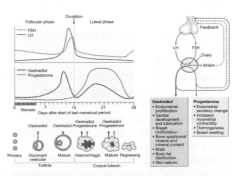

Fig. 18.25 Female reproductive physiology and the normal menstrual cycle. (FSH = follicle-stimulating hormone; LH = luteinising hormone.)

normal range and can result in a high FSH-to-LH ratio. Functional hypothalamic amenorrhoea can be caused by eating disorders, mental or physical stress or over-exercising. Circulating levels of the 'satiety' hormone leptin have been shown to be reduced in hypothalamic amenorrhoea, which may impact on the production of LH. Gonadotrophin-releasing hormone insensitivity is a rare autosomal recessive condition that would present in a similar manner but would be detected on genetic testing. Hyperprolactinaemia accounts for around 1.9% of hypogonadotrophic hypogonadism, but again would be detected through plasma measurements.

18.27. Answer: B.

High gonadotrophins in the context of low oestradiol and secondary amenorrhoea implicate premature ovarian failure. The most likely causes are acquired injury to the ovaries (e.g. previous chemotherapy), autoimmune or genetic disorders such as Turner's syndrome. Karyotype and genetic screening is therefore necessary. MRI pituitary would be the investigation of choice for hypogonadotrophic hypogonadism.

18.28. Answer: C.

Constitutional delay is observed more frequently in boys. Reduced growth velocity is observed as early as 3–6 months. Due to delay in age of pubertal growth spurt, height can drift further from the growth chart at this time but catches up once puberty is achieved. Bone age is consistent with age appropriate for height rather than chronological age. In childhood when long bones are still developing, the ratio of upper-to-lower body is >1, which is then reversed by adulthood. Constitutional delay has no effect on final height and can therefore be predicted based on mid-parental heights.

18.29. Answer: A.

Hypogonadotrophic hypogonadism in the context of small testes suggests absent, incomplete or partial pubertal development due to Kallmann's syndrome or idiopathic hypogonadotrophic hypogonadism. Individuals with Kallmann's syndrome may have either anosmia or hyposmia. This may, however, not be obvious to the individual until more formally tested. A similar biochemical pattern is seen in men in the context of central obesity, but testicular volumes are not reduced to the extent seen here. Testicular trauma would be associated with hypergonadotrophic hypogonadism. Klinefelter's syndrome due to XXY karyotype results in small under-developed testes with resultant elevation in gonadotrophins.

18.30. Answer: E.

A variety of theories exist as to the aetiology of hyperandrogenism associated with PCOS. Disordered gonadotrophin secretion has been observed with a higher ratio of LH to FSH. Androgens are synthesised by theca cells in the ovary under the influence of LH, whilst FSH stimulates aromatisation of androgens by granulosa cells. Challenging the pituitary gland with GnRH has shown a preponderance for the production of LH but no evidence exists for disruption in hypothalamic function of GnRH. Hyperinsulinaemia leads to a reduction in SHBG and resultant increase in metabolically active free androgens. Mutations in 3β-hydroxysteroid dehydrogenase cause a virilising form of congenital adrenal hyperplasia.

18.31. Answer: D.

The karyotype in this scenario is consistent with Turner's syndrome and usually presents with short stature and amenorrhoea. There is no increased risk of ovarian cancer. Excess androgen is not usually a feature. Cardiovascular malformations (especially aortic root dilatation) may go undiagnosed until later in life and present a high risk of morbidity and mortality, especially during pregnancy with increased circulatory volume. Only up to 5% of individuals with Turner's syndrome become pregnant spontaneously, with the majority requiring intervention such as egg donation. Turner's syndrome is not associated with mental retardation but is associated with degrees of learning disability later in life. As it is not heritable, Turner's syndrome cannot be passed on to future generations with unassisted pregnancies.

18.32. Answer: C.

Delayed puberty in the context of hypergonadotrophic hypogonadism in males is usually due to Klinefelter's syndrome with karyotype 47XXY, and testing for this should therefore be part of the next-line investigation. The differential diagnosis is acquired gonadal damage due to chemotherapy/radiotherapy, trauma or surgery, which should be apparent on taking a full history. Autoimmune gonadal failure or post-infection orchitis due to mumps or tuberculosis are differential diagnoses. Alternative developmental or congenital gonadal disorders include enzyme deficiency in the biosynthesis of sex steroids or anorchidism/cryptorchidism.

18.33. Answer: C.

Klinefelter's syndrome results from genotype XXY. This leads to hyalinisation and fibrosis of the seminiferous tubules. LH resistance can occur rarely due to abnormalities in LH receptor. Disordered migration of GnRH-producing neurons occurs in Kallmann's syndrome, whilst defect in the steroidogenesis pathway underlies congenital adrenal hyperplasia. TGF-β has both a stimulatory and inhibitory effect on Leydig cell steroidogenesis.

18.34. Answer: C.

Finasteride is used for the treatment of benign prostatic hypertrophy and inhibits the conversion of testosterone to its metabolically active form, dihydrotestosterone. This results in a reduced testosterone-to-oestrogen ratio, resulting in gynaecomastia. Tamoxifen and clomifene can be used in the treatment of gynaecomastia by reducing oestradiol synthesis and function, respectively, restoring a higher testosterone-to-oestrogen ratio. Potassium-sparing, but not thiazide, diuretics can cause gynaecomastia. Through aromatisation, androgen replacement can lead to gynaecomastia but this should not occur with the metabolically active form, dihydrotestosterone.

18.35. Answer: C.

This case describes secondary hyperparathyroidism secondary to chronic renal failure. A similar biochemical picture is seen with vitamin D deficiency. Parathyroid hormone aims to maintain calcium homeostasis by reabsorbing calcium from bone through altered activity of osteoblasts and osteoclasts. In the kidney, PTH activates the enzyme 1α-hydroxylase in the proximal tubules, which in turn activates 25-hydroxyvitamin D to 1,25-dihydroxyvitamin D. It is the latter that enhances absorption of calcium and phosphate from the gut. A complex relationship exists between feedback of magnesium on PTH secretion, but PTH results in reabsorption of magnesium from the distal convoluted tubule.

18.36. Answer: C.

With mild hypercalcaemia and hypermagnesaemia along with a family history of the same, the most likely underlying cause is familial hypocalciuric hypercalcaemia (FHH). This may go undiagnosed until detected incidentally when blood tests are taken for an alternative reason. Diagnosis would be confirmed by a urine calcium-to-creatinine ratio of <0.01 and urine calcium <5 mmol/24 hrs (<200 mg/24 hrs). The condition is caused by an inactivating mutation in the calcium-sensing receptor gene. MEN syndromes are associated with hyperparathyroidism, which is also inherited in an autosomal dominant manner. However, hypermagnesaemia would not be expected in this situation or in hyperparathyroidism secondary to a parathyroid adenoma. Dehydration can cause elevated serum calcium, but this man's urea is not elevated, so he does not appear dehydrated from a biochemical perspective.

18.37. Answer: D.

This woman has all the biochemical features of primary hyperparathyroidism. The indications for consideration of surgery include: 0.25 mmol/L (1 mg/dL) or above the normal reference range for serum calcium, urine calcium excretion >10 mmol/24 hrs (>400 mg/24 hrs), a 30% reduction in creatinine clearance, bone mineral density T-score below −2.5 at any site and age younger than 50 years. Prior to surgery she should have imaging (by ultrasound and/or sestamibi scanning) to try to localise a parathyroid adenoma. Given her young age, consideration should be given to screening for genetic causes of hyperparathyroidism. There is nothing to suggest vitamin D deficiency (i.e. hypocalcaemia) and thiazide diuretics may increase serum calcium concentrations. Loop diuretics may occasionally be used in the management of severe hypercalcaemia, but only under specialist supervision.

18.38. Answer: E.

These results are consistent with secondary hyperparathyroidism as a result of vitamin D deficiency. With normal renal function and given her symptoms, the underlying diagnosis is osteomalacia. Parathyroid adenoma is associated with primary hyperparathyroidism and thus hypercalcaemia. All of the other

18

answers cause hypoparathyroidism and result in hypocalcaemia.

18.39. Answer: D.
The outermost layer of the adrenal cortex, zona glomerulsoa, is the site of aldosterone synthesis, whilst glucocorticoids are produced in the middle zona fasciculata and androgens in the innermost zona reticularis. Chromaffin cells in the adrenal medulla are the source of catecholamines. This clinical picture could result from disruption of the renin–angiotension system from medications such as angiotensin-converting enzyme inhibitors or angiotensin receptor blockers or, more rarely, due to defective synthesis of angiotensin due to genetic mutations in the *CYP11B2* gene.

18.40. Answer: E.
Females with milder forms of CAH develop precocious puberty, cliteromegaly, accelerated growth or can present with oligomenorrhoea, hirsutism and infertility later in life. Up to 95% of cases are due to 21-hydroxylase deficiency. This results in reduced cortisol synthesis with resultant increase in intermediate compounds including 17-hydroxyprogesterone and an increase in androgen synthesis. Severe forms can be detected from birth due to ambiguous genitalia and can result in failure to thrive and vomiting due to salt wasting.

18.41. Answer: A.
The results of the overnight dexamethasone suppression test suggest a possible diagnosis of Cushing's syndrome. However, it is necessary to perform a second test to confirm a diagnosis of Cushing's – either a 24-hour urine collection for urine free cortisol or a late-night salivary cortisol. Once Cushing's syndrome is confirmed, further investigations are required to determine the underlying cause.

18.42. Answer: B.
This case describes classic symptoms of Cushing's syndrome, which can be associated with excess ACTH from a variety of cancers, including small cell and carcinoid tumours of the lung. Other examples include islet cell tumours of the pancreas, medullary carcinoma of the thyroid and tumours of the thymus gland.

18.43. Answer: A.
Hypercortisolaemia results in hypokalaemia as a result of increased mineralocorticoid receptor activation. Cortisol is a potent mineralocorticoid, but is usually prevented from activating mineralocorticoid receptors because it is metabolised to inactive cortisone by the enzyme 11β-hydroxysteroid dehydrogenase type 2 (11β-HSD2). In Cushing's syndrome, the presence of high levels of cortisol overwhelms the 11β-HSD2 system.

18.44. Answer: C.
Greatest risk of malignancy is seen in unilateral lesions with an irregular surface, of size >4 cm, with a lipid-poor consistency (Hounsfield units >10 HU) and retention of contrast on scanning.

18.45. Answer: E.
This presentation is in keeping with a phaeochromocytoma. At such a young age genetic screening should be performed to detect any underlying inherited disorders. Treatment is initially with an α-adrenoceptor antagonist (α-blocker) such as phenoxybenzamine. Initial prescription of β-blocker therapy may cause a hypertensive crisis. Ketoconazole may used in the treatment of Cushing's syndrome. Dexamethasone and fludrocortisone are synthetic glucocorticoids and mineralocorticoids, respectively, and have no role here.

18.46. Answer: B.
Initially considered a rarity, primary hyperaldosteronism is thought to underlie hypertension in 5–15% of cases. Diagnosis is suggested by finding an elevated aldosterone:renin ratio. Thiazide and loop diuretics increase renin levels, whilst β-blockers inhibit renin secretion. Discontinuation of these agents for at least 2 weeks is therefore necessary before measuring plasma levels. Substitution can be made with calcium channel antagonists and α-blockers to control blood pressure in the interim.

18.47. Answer: B.
Glucagon-like peptide-1 (GLP-1) and gastric inhibitory polypeptide are the two major incretin hormones secreted from the gastrointestinal tract which act on β cells within the pancreas, increasing insulin secretion. Dipeptidyl peptidase-4 is involved in the degradation of incretins, thereby reducing insulin secretion. Leptin and somatostatin additionally have an inhibitory role on insulin secretion.

18.48. Answer: C.
With high insulin concentrations and suppressed C-peptide, the likely diagnosis is exogenous insulin use. An insulinoma would result in elevated insulin and C-peptide concentrations, as would sulphonylurea ingestion. Alcohol and critical illness both result in a picture of suppressed insulin and C-peptide concentrations.

18.49. Answer: A.
The history and clinical presentation are in keeping with a neuroendocrine tumour and subsequent metastases to the liver resulting in the classical features of carcinoid syndrome. Measurement of 5-HIAA, the main breakdown product of 5-hydroxytryptamine (5-HT, serotonin), in urine allows confirmation that this is a carcinoid tumour and allows quantification of its secretory activity. Care must be taken to ensure the avoidance of certain foods and medications that can result in false-positive results when performing 24-hour urine collections for 5-HIAA. Although these tumours may be detected using imaging modalities such as CT, MRI or direct visualisation using colonoscopy or small bowel capsule endoscopy, this provides no assessment of type or hormonal activity of the tumour. There is nothing in the history to suggest excess secretion of insulin or somatostatin to necessitate their quantification.

18.50. Answer: C.
From superior to inferior, the cavernous sinus contains cranial nerves III (oculomotor), IV (trochlear), VI (abducens) as well as V1 (ophthalmic branch of trigeminal) and V2 (maxillary branch of trigeminal).

18.51. Answer: A.
Rathke's pouch separates and develops into the adenohypophysis (anterior pituitary). In contrast, the neurohypophysis (posterior pituitary) develops from the infundibulum. The pituitary gland sits within the saddle-shaped sella turcica and the superior aspect is covered by the diaphragma sellae.

Craniopharyngiomas are benign tumours and may be located in the sella turcica or suprasellar space. They are often cystic with solid components. They commonly present as the result of pressure on adjacent structures causing hypopituitarism and/or cranial diabetes insipidus. Hyperphagia, temperature dysregulation and loss of thirst sensation can be the result of hypothalamic involvement.

18.52. Answer: D.
In endocrinology, hormones are usually secreted in a pulsatile fashion. For the majority of hormones, samples taken at random times can be hard to interpret. As a result, if there is a suspicion of over-production of a hormone, then tests should be performed to suppress secretion, and if there is thought to be deficiency of a hormone, then tests should aim to enhance secretion. Growth hormone is secreted in a pulsatile manner with alterations in response to sleep, stress, exercise and circulating glucose concentrations. Elevated circulating glucose concentrations, as induced through the use of an oral glucose tolerance test, should normally result in suppression of growth hormone secretion. In the situation of a pituitary tumour with autonomous growth hormone secretion, an oral glucose tolerance test will result in minimal or no suppression. Dexamethasone suppression test and 24-hour urinary steroid profile are used in the diagnosis of Cushing's syndrome. A saline suppression test is used to diagnose hyperaldosteronism and an insulin tolerance test is used for the diagnosis of hypoadrenalism.

18.53. Answer: D.
Prolactin levels over 5000 mIU/L are usually indicative of a macroadenoma, which secretes prolactin (a macroprolactinoma). This should be confirmed with MRI imaging. Macroprolactin is a physiologically inactive form of prolactin that is complexed with immunoglobulin G (IgG) antibody and, unless accounted for on laboratory measurement, gives a false impression of clinically relevant hyperprolactinaemia. Given her symptoms and the likelihood of this being a macroadenoma, she should be commenced on dopamine agonist therapy, as described in option D. Given the risk of growth and compression on surrounding structures, monitoring without treatment is not advised. Carbimazole is an antithyroid medication used for the treatment of Graves' disease. Prolactin levels are significantly higher than would be expected simply as a result of stress. Surgical decompression is usually only necessary if a macroprolactinoma fails to respond sufficiently to dopamine agonist therapy.

18

18.54. Answer: D.

Bitemporal quadrantanopia implies the presence of a mass lesion compressing part of the optic chiasm, most commonly a pituitary macroadenoma. Pituitary apoplexy is a rare endocrine emergency characterised by a sudden-onset headache due to acute haemorrhage or infarct of a pituitary gland, resulting in headache, visual disturbance and hormonal dysfunction. Treatment involves urgent replacement of fluid, electrolytes and pituitary hormones, particularly glucocorticoids.

18.55. Answer: C.

Growth hormone (GH) secretion is usually the first affected, classically followed by LH, FSH, TSH, ACTH and prolactin, in that order. However, in practice any pattern of hormone deficiency can occur.

18.56. Answer: D.

As prolactinomas are responsive to dopamine agonist therapy, prolactin levels should always be measured prior to undertaking surgical resection of a pituitary macroadenoma. This may avoid the need for unnecessary pituitary surgery, as prolactinomas will often shrink in size following commencement of a dopamine agonist.

18.57. Answer: C.

Low plasma osmolality at the start of the test may suggest primary polydipsia as the cause of her symptoms. A plasma sodium concentration above the normal range and 24-hour urine volume greater than 3 L can be an indicator of diabetes insipidus but are not diagnostic. A water deprivation test should be discontinued if body weight falls by 3% or more and if plasma osmolality rises to >300 mOsm/kg with continued dilute urine (osmolality <300 mOsm/kg). DDAVP (2 µg intramuscularly) should subsequently be administered to assess response and determine if the underlying diagnosis is cranial or nephrogenic diabetes insipidus.

18.58. Answer: A.

MEN 1 is characterised by tumours involving the parathyroid glands (95% of cases), pancreas (neuroendocrine tumours, which may be non-functional or functioning; gastrinoma; insulinoma; glucogonoma; VIPoma; somatostatinoma) (30–80% cases), lung (neuroendocrine carcinoid) (5%), gastrointestinal tract (neuroendocrine carcinoid) (2%) and anterior pituitary tumours (commonly prolactinomas) (30%). The underlying genetic defect is the *MEN1* gene, which is on chromosome 11. MEN 2 is characterised by tumours of the parathyroid and adrenal glands along with medullary thyroid carcinoma. MEN 3 can additionally be associated with mucocutaneous neuromas and Marfanoid habitus. Hemangioblastomas are a feature of von Hippel–Lindau syndrome.

E Przybyszewski, A Shand

19

Nutritional factors in disease

Multiple Choice Questions

19.1. A 27 year old woman presents to clinic for the first time. She has no known medical history and takes no medications, but complains of lethargy and fatigue. She weighs 97 kg and has a body mass index (BMI) of 32 kg/m². She states that her weight has been climbing over the past few years, more rapidly over the past few months.

On examination, her temperature is 36.8°C, pulse is 70 beats/min, and blood pressure is 128/78 mmHg. She has no conjunctival pallor, sclera are anicteric, examination of her neck is normal, there is no lymphadenopathy, and no cardiac murmurs are heard. Her abdomen is obese without ascites and there is no peripheral oedema. Which of the following is the best next step in management?

A. Check serum thyroid-stimulating hormone (TSH)
B. Measure triceps skinfold thickness
C. Prescribe orlistat
D. Recommend a very-low-calorie diet
E. Refer for a bone densitometry (dual X-ray absorptiometry; DXA) scan

19.2. A 43 year old man with a history of hypertension, hyperlipidaemia and gout presents to his family physician for routine follow-up. The man does not smoke or drink alcohol and lives with his wife. He denies chest pain and dyspnoea on exertion. He has a BMI of 34 kg/m² and android distribution of body fat. Serum cholesterol is 6.3 mmol/L (244 mg/dL). The family physician recommends decreasing his consumption of high-fat foods. Which of the following is true regarding fat metabolism?

A. Consumption of fats should represent 15–30% of total daily energy intake
B. Energy provided per gram of fat is less than the energy provided per gram of protein
C. Fats are the main source of short-chain fatty acid production by colonic bacteria
D. Increasing consumption of saturated fats should lower circulating low-density lipoprotein (LDL) concentrations
E. *Trans* fatty acids consumption promotes anti-inflammatory effects via prostaglandin production

19.3. A 19 year old woman presents to her family physician complaining of pain in her foot when she runs. She is a competitive runner and currently trains 60 miles per week. Her menstrual periods are typically irregular, and she has not had her menstrual period in 6 months.

On examination, her pulse is 50 beats/min, blood pressure is 89/68 mmHg and her BMI is 15.7 kg/m². Beta-human chorionic gonadotrophin (hCG) testing is negative. The following features may all be due to her nutritional state, except one. Which one is NOT likely to be a consequence of her nutritional status?

A. Amenorrhoea
B. Decreased basal metabolic rate
C. Foot pain
D. High insulin state for maximal nutrient delivery to cells
E. Increased lethargy for energy conservation

19.4. A 63 year old man with a history of chronic alcohol use is admitted after being found unresponsive in a park. He required several stitches in for repair of a forehead laceration and later developed alcohol withdrawal seizures requiring diazepam for several days on the ward. After a prolonged period of delirium and inattention, the decision is made to place a nasogastric tube for enteral feeding. Three days after initiating feeding, he becomes more alert, but complains of nausea, weakness and palpitations. In addition to obtaining an electrocardiogram (ECG), which of the following is the most appropriate next step in management?

A. Check serum electrolytes
B. Obtain a computed tomography (CT) scan of his head
C. Obtain an echocardiogram
D. Reassure him that he is getting adequate nutrition via the nasogastric tube
E. Treat with calcium gluconate, insulin and dextrose

19.5. A 34 year old woman with obstructive sleep apnoea and diabetes is referred to general surgery for a Roux-en-Y gastric bypass procedure. Her BMI is 41 kg/m^2 and she has been unsuccessful in achieving weight loss with multiple attempts at lifestyle modification and pharmacological therapy. Which of the following statements would be most appropriate in counselling this patient?

A. It will likely take years to see improvement in diabetes control
B. She is at low risk for post-surgical complications such as wound infection
C. She should wait at least 2 years before considering pregnancy
D. She will likely experience amenorrhoea post-operatively
E. Although effective for weight loss, bariatric surgery is not associated with reduced mortality

19.6. A 72 year old man with a history of hypertension and hyperlipidaemia presents to his family physician complaining of fatigue and constipation. On further questioning, he admits to recently chewing ice on occasions. Physical examination reveals conjunctival pallor and koilonychia.

Initial blood tests show white cell count (WCC) 6.2×10^9/L, haemoglobin 96 g/L, mean cell volume (MCV) 72 fL, platelets 263×10^9/L, international normalised ratio (INR) 1.0. Further

evaluation with flexible sigmoidoscopy demonstrates a large tumour in the descending colon.

Which of the following is true regarding the most likely micronutrient deficiency associated with his anaemia?

A. This deficiency causes impaired wound healing through defective collagen fibrils
B. Duodenal hepcidin production is suppressed in states of this deficiency
C. Absorption of this micronutrient is enhanced by dietary calcium
D. Absorption of this micronutrient is impaired by vitamin C
E. Long-term deficiency can lead to cirrhosis

19.7. A 34 year old overweight woman with a history of mild chronic asthma presents to a gastroenterologist complaining of bloating and diarrhoea. Over the past year she has been attempting to lose weight through lifestyle modification with some success. She recently adjusted her diet to replace added sugar with sugar-free foods and artificial sweeteners.

Which of the following is the most likely reason for her gastrointestinal complaints?

A. Consumption of non-starch polysaccharides has increased
B. She is no longer producing lactase
C. Short-chain fatty acid production has increased
D. Sugar alcohols are not absorbed by the gut
E. Sugar alcohols have a high glycaemic index

19.8. A 23 year old woman from northern Scotland presents to her family physician complaining of chronic tiredness. She has a history of right fibula fracture in childhood, but is otherwise well and takes no medications or supplements. She is up to date with routine vaccinations and is currently working as a librarian. Examination is normal. A β-hCG test is negative.

Which of the following nutritional recommendations is most appropriate at this time?

A. Advise her to begin vitamin E supplementation for cardioprotection
B. Begin daily vitamin B_{12} supplementation to reduce the incidence of neural tube defects
C. Initiate supplementation with cholecalciferol (vitamin D), at least during winter months
D. Initiate supplementation with retinol now in the event that she becomes pregnant

NUTRITIONAL FACTORS IN DISEASE • 205

E. Recommend treatment with ascorbic acid for the prevention of kidney stones

19.9. A 58 year old woman from Angola is seen in clinic after recently emigrating to the UK. Her husband states that she has been confused and at times disorientated. On further questioning, the patient states that she has nausea and diarrhoea, with seven bowel movements daily. On examination, she is afebrile, anicteric, without conjunctival pallor or lymphadenopathy. Her tongue appears enlarged; no cardiac murmurs are heard; and her abdomen is soft, mildly tender and non-distended. A dry cracking rash is seen on the skin of her neck and upper extremities bilaterally.

Which of the following treatments is most likely to improve her symptoms?

A. Ascorbic acid 250 mg orally 3 times daily
B. Folate 500 µg orally once daily
C. Nicotinamide 100 mg orally 3 times daily
D. Pyridoxine hydrochloride 50 mg orally 3 times daily
E. Riboflavin 10 mg orally once daily

19.10. A 45 year old man with a history of alcoholic cirrhosis presents to the emergency department after being found unresponsive at home. On examination he is minimally responsive, disorientated, anicteric, cachectic and has restricted horizontal eye movement bilaterally. His lab results are notable for mildly elevated transaminases and low albumin. Treatment is initiated with parenteral multivitamin therapy.

Which of the following is true regarding his most clinically significant vitamin deficiency?

A. Adults have limited stores of thiamine in the liver and may manifest deficiency after a short period
B. Thiamine deficiency commonly leads to coagulopathy
C. Hepatocytes are most vulnerable to damage as a result of thiamine deficiency
D. Thiamine acts as a co-factor in folate co-enzyme recycling
E. Thiamine is fat soluble

19.11. A 41 year old previously healthy woman is brought to the hospital by her husband who states she has been febrile to 39°C for the past 2 days and jaundiced for the past 7 days. On examination she is delirious and jaundiced. Her

chest is clear to auscultation, her abdomen is soft but mildly tender to palpation in the right upper quadrant and she has no oedema. Blood tests show WCC 23×10^9/L, platelets 340×10^9/L, INR 1.5, alanine aminotransferase (ALT) 32 U/L, albumin 34 g/L. Extrahepatic biliary dilatation is seen on abdominal ultrasound.

Which of the following is the most likely factor leading to her mild coagulopathy?

A. Hepatic synthetic dysfunction
B. Intracerebral haemorrhage
C. Medication effect
D. Obstruction of the biliary tree
E. Previously undiagnosed coeliac disease

19.12. A 68 year old man is being discharged from the hospital after experiencing palpitations. An ECG has revealed new-onset atrial fibrillation and he is started on warfarin for anticoagulation and stroke prophylaxis. His cardiologist explains that warfarin works by antagonising vitamin K and that the patient should not vary his vitamin K intake while on warfarin. Which of the following foods is highest in vitamin K and should be consumed with the least amount of variation?

A. Egg yolk
B. Kale
C. Liver
D. Pork
E. Sunflower oil

19.13. A 32 year old woman gives birth to a baby boy weighing 4.2 kg. She defaulted from antenatal care and takes no medications or supplements. On examination of the child after 10 minutes, his pulse is 136 beats/min and he is crying vigorously with arms and legs held in flexion. The skin appears pink with a protuberant mass on his back in the midline at the level of L4. Treatment with a water-soluble vitamin may have prevented this birth defect through which of the following mechanisms?

A. Accepting and donating hydrogen in nicotinamide adenine dinucleotide (NAD)
B. Decarboxylation of pyruvate to acetyl-co-enzyme A to initiate the Krebs cycle
C. Donating a methyl group in DNA and protein synthesis
D. Facilitating absorption of calcium in the small intestine
E. Hydroxylation of proline and lysine in the formation of mature collagen

19

19.14. A 78 year old man presents to hospital with an acute abdomen. At laparotomy he is found to have extensive infarction of the superior mesenteric artery territory. It is noted at the time of surgery that he has 90 cm of healthy jejunum remaining, anastomosed to an intact colon.

He may need additional treatments in the future as a result of this. Which of the following treatments is he LEAST likely to need?

A. Daily oral administration of a glucose/ electrolyte solution as a substitute for free fluids
B. Oral loperamide
C. Parenteral (intravenous or subcutaneous) fluid
D. Parenteral nutrition
E. Restriction of oral free fluid intake

19.15. An 85 year old woman suffers a total anterior circulation stroke that leaves her unable to swallow safely. After a few days on intravenous fluids, her family request that she is fed intravenously. The attending multidisciplinary team explain their preference is for nasogastric feeding in the first instance. Which of the following statements is true of the enteral route of nutrition versus the parenteral route?

A. It improves quality of life
B. It is associated with fewer costs financially
C. It leads to greater preservation of hepatic and pulmonary immune function
D. It leads to reduced levels of systemic inflammatory response
E. It reduces the pathogenicity of intestinal microorganisms

19.16. A 49 year old woman with a 10-year history of terminal ileal Crohn's disease treated with mesalazine is admitted with a complex fistulating mass involving small bowel, bladder and sigmoid colon. It is not possible to fashion a primary anastomosis and a proximal small bowel stoma (jejunostomy) is brought out to skin. Post-operatively, the fluid losses from this stoma are >2000 mL/day, leading rapidly to dehydration.

Which of the following measures is likely to lead to a worsening of fluid losses from the high-output stoma?

A. Administration of oral omeprazole 20 mg once daily
B. Advice to take oral fluids ad libitum to replace stomal losses

C. Oral administration of a glucose/electrolyte solution in place of oral fluids
D. Oral administration of loperamide 2 mg 4 times daily
E. Restriction of oral fluid intake

19.17. An 89 year old woman who lives independently in her own second-storey flat presents to her family physician with a complaint of easy bruising on her forearms and hands. On examination it is noted she has extensive ecchymoses on the upper and lower limbs as well as a petechial rash. A full blood count and tests of clotting parameters are all normal and the rash and bruising disappears rapidly with oral administration of vitamin C (ascorbic acid) 250 mg 3 times daily for 7 days.

Which of the following clinical features is associated with vitamin C deficiency (scurvy)?

A. Gingival swelling and bleeding
B. Impaired cognitive function
C. Lanugo hairs
D. Nail clubbing
E. Spider naevi

19.18. Which of the following is an essential amino acid?

A. Alanine
B. Asparagine
C. Glutamine
D. Glycine
E. Tryptophan

19.19. An 83 year old man with a long history of Alzheimer's disease and progressive cognitive and functional impairment is noted to have lost interest in food and is losing weight. Thorough investigation by CT scanning and gastroscopy has failed to demonstrate another underlying physical explanation for this. Nasogastric tube feeding is suggested. In this situation, which statement below best describes the outcomes with routine use of tube feeding, as based on strong evidence?

A. Improved cognitive function
B. Improved muscle strength
C. Improved quality of life
D. Prolonged survival
E. There is little evidence for improved survival or cognitive outcomes with routine tube feeding

19.20. The long-term carers of a 40 year old man with cerebral palsy report that he is finding it increasingly difficult to chew and swallow food. The act of feeding is very tiring for him and is taking up much of the day. Increasingly, there are days when he may not eat or drink at all and there are concerns that he is losing weight and becoming dehydrated. After multidisciplinary assessment it is felt he should be fed by gastrostomy to allow adequate food and fluid to be given on a daily basis.

Which of the following is NOT a recognised risk of gastrostomy insertion or gastrostomy feeding?

A. Aspiration pneumonia
B. Colonic perforation
C. Insertion site infection
D. Laceration of the liver
E. Pulmonary embolus

Answers

19.1. Answer: A.
This is an obese patient being evaluated for the first time with a history of weight gain that has accelerated recently, along with fatigue. This history suggests an underlying disorder such as hypothyroidism or Cushing's syndrome may be related to the weight gain (Box 19.1). All obese patients should have thyroid function tests performed. Very-low-calorie diets require the supervision of an experienced physician and dietician and can be considered if short-term rapid weight loss is required.

i 19.1 Potentially reversible causes of weight gain

| Endocrine factors |
| Hypothyroidism |
| Cushing's syndrome |
| Insulinoma |
| Hypothalamic tumours or injury |
| **Drug treatments** |
| Atypical antipsychotics (e.g. olanzapine) |
| Sulphonylureas, thiazolidinediones, insulin |
| Pizotifen |
| Glucocorticoids |
| Sodium valproate |
| β-blockers |

19.2. Answer: A.
Fats have the highest energy density of the macronutrients and should represent 15–30% of daily energy intake compared to 55–75% for carbohydrates and 10–15% for proteins (Box 19.2). High saturated fat consumption is associated with higher levels of LDL cholesterol. Whereas omega-3 fatty acids promote prostaglandin production and anti-inflammatory cascade, *trans* fatty acids are associated with cardiovascular disease.

i 19.2 WHO recommended population macronutrient goals

Nutrient (% of total energy unless indicated)	Target limits for average population intakes	
	Lower	Upper
Total fat	15	30
Saturated fatty acids	0	10
Polyunsaturated fatty acids	6	10
Trans fatty acids	0	2
Dietary cholesterol (mg/day)	0	300
Total carbohydrate	55	75
Free sugars	0	10
Complex carbohydrate	50	70
Dietary fibre (g/day):		
As non-starch polysaccharides	16	24
As total dietary fibre	27	40
Protein	10	15

19.3. Answer: D.
This female runner's presentation is concerning for under-nutrition and the female athlete triad of disordered eating, amenorrhoea and decreased bone mineral density. Her foot pain may be related to osteopenia and a stress fracture. In a state of under-nutrition, her basal metabolic rate will be decreased to minimise further weight loss. In addition, she will have a low-insulin state in order to promote liberation of energy stores from tissues such as the liver, muscle, and adipose tissue for systemic utilisation (Fig. 19.3).

19.4. Answer: A.
This patient with a history of chronic alcoholism is at risk for malnutrition and refeeding syndrome due to restoration of carbohydrate metabolism, insulin secretion and electrolyte shifts into cells. Refeeding syndrome (Box 19.4) may present with nausea, vomiting, weakness, seizures, respiratory depression, and cardiac arrhythmias or arrest. Initiation of nutrition

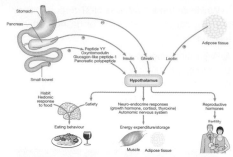

Fig. 19.3 Regulation of energy balance and its link with reproduction. ⊕ indicates factors that are stimulated by eating and induce satiety. ⊖ indicates factors that are suppressed by eating and inhibit satiety.

---

i 19.4 Complications of nasogastric tube feeding

Tube misplacement, e.g. tracheal or bronchial placement (*rarely*, intracranial placement)
Reflux of gastric contents and pulmonary aspiration
Interrupted feeding or inadequate feed volumes
Refeeding syndrome

---

should be done slowly with careful monitoring of electrolytes, especially potassium, phosphate and magnesium, with repletion as appropriate.

19.5. Answer: C.

Bariatric surgery is the only anti-obesity intervention that has been shown to reduce mortality. While diabetes control usually improves rapidly, especially with gastric bypass procedures, micronutrient deficiencies (e.g. iron, folate, vitamin B$_{12}$) may complicate the post-procedure period. As a result, pre-menopausal women should wait at least 2 years for nutritional status to stabilise before becoming pregnant.

19.6. Answer: B.

This patient is presenting with anaemia in the setting of chronic blood loss, koilonychias, and pica, consistent with iron deficiency anaemia. In a state of iron deficiency, hepcidin production decreases in order to promote the transport of iron from the enterocyte basolateral surface into circulation. Absorption of iron is facilitated by vitamin C and impaired by dietary calcium.

19.7. Answer: D.

Artificial sweeteners use sugar alcohols (e.g. sorbitol, xylitol) to provide sweet taste without caloric contribution. Sugar alcohols are not absorbed by the gut and in high quantities can act as an osmotic agent to move water

intraluminally and cause diarrhoea. Since sugar alcohols are not absorbed, they do not increase the blood glucose concentration and have a very low glycaemic index.

19.8. Answer: C.

Supplementation with vitamin D, or cholecalciferol, is recommended for this woman from northern Scotland. The combination of low dietary vitamin D intake and limited sunlight exposure in the UK has led to the UK recommendation of 10 µg of vitamin D daily. Vitamin D supplementation should be considered for everyone during winter months (October to April) and all year for certain groups: e.g. those who may not be outside much, those who tend to cover up their skin, those with darker skins.

In countries where vitamin A deficiency is endemic, pregnant women may be advised to consume foods high in vitamin A. In contrast, in countries where vitamin A deficiency is not endemic, vitamin A supplementation is avoided, as moderate doses of retinol are teratogenic. Increased vitamin E intake has been shown to be associated with lower rates of coronary artery disease; however, randomised controlled trials have not demonstrated significant benefits. Vitamin C excess is associated with the formation of renal oxalate stones. Folate supplementation is used to reduce the incidence of neural tube defects in pregnancy. In this case, the woman is of child-bearing age but clearly not pregnant at the time (β-hCG test is negative).

19.9. Answer: C.

This patient from Angola presents with dementia, diarrhoea and dermatitis consistent with pellagra, or niacin deficiency. The enlarged tongue is due to non-infective inflammation of the gastrointestinal tract leading to glossitis. Pellagra can develop in certain parts of Africa and South America where corn-based diets predominate. Treatment is with oral or parenteral nicotinamide and usually results in rapid improvement of symptoms.

19.10. Answer: A.

This malnourished alcoholic patient presents with clinical features suggestive of Wernicke's encephalopathy (delirium and ophthalmoplegia), which is a manifestation of thiamin (vitamin B$_1$) deficiency. Thiamin is a water-soluble vitamin that acts as a co-factor in aerobic metabolism of glucose. Neuronal cells are most vulnerable to damage from thiamin deficiency as they exclusively utilise glucose for energy requirements. The liver has very limited stores of thiamin, so deficiency can manifest after only 1 month of a thiamin-free diet.

19.11. Answer: D.
The patient is presenting with four features of Reynolds' pentad of ascending cholangitis (fever, right upper quadrant pain, jaundice, altered mental status), probably caused by obstruction of the biliary tree. In obstructive jaundice, bile is unable to enter the gut lumen for fat digestion. As a result, the fat-soluble vitamins, including vitamin K, are poorly absorbed (Box 19.11). Vitamin K is required in

i	**19.11 Gastrointestinal disorders that may be associated with malabsorption of fat-soluble vitamins**

Biliary obstruction
Pancreatic exocrine insufficiency
Coeliac disease
Ileal inflammation or resection

the synthesis of coagulation factors II, VII, IX and X. Deficiency can lead to coagulopathy. While cirrhosis, malabsorption and medications (e.g. warfarin) can also lead to coagulopathy, this patient is previously healthy prior to this acute episode.

19.12. Answer: B.
Vitamin K is a fat-soluble vitamin produced by intestinal bacteria. Green leafy vegetables are rich sources of vitamin K, along with soya oil. Egg yolks represent a source of biotin and vitamin D. Liver is rich in vitamin A and sunflower oil is rich in vitamin E (Box 19.12).

19.13. Answer: C.
The child was born with a neural tube defect, but is otherwise healthy. Folate deficiency in pregnancy is associated with spina bifida, anencephaly and encephalocele due to increased requirements during embryonic development. Pregnant women are advised to take folate supplements during the first trimester. Mechanistically, folate acts as a

i **19.12 Summary of clinically important vitamins**			
	Sources*		**Reference nutrient intake**
Vitamin	**Rich**	**Important**	**(RNI)**
Fat-soluble			
A (retinol)	Liver	Milk and milk products, eggs, fish oils	700 µg men 600 µg women
D (cholecalciferol)	Fish oils	Ultraviolet exposure to skin, egg yolks, margarine, fortified cereals	10 µg if >65 years or no sunlight exposure
E (tocopherol)	Sunflower oil	Vegetables, nuts, seed oils	No RNI. Safe intake: 4 mg men 3 mg women
K (phylloquinone, menaquinone)	Soya oil, menaquinones produced by intestinal bacteria	Green vegetables	No RNI. Safe intake: 1 µg/kg
Water-soluble			
B₁ (thiamin)	Pork	Cereals, grains, beans	0.8 mg per 9.68 MJ (2000 kcal) energy intake
B₂ (riboflavin)	Milk	Milk and milk products, breakfast cereals, bread	1.3 mg men 1.1 mg women
B₃ (niacin, nicotinic acid, nicotinamide)	Meat, cereals		17 mg men 13 mg women
B₆ (pyridoxine)	Meat, fish, potatoes, bananas	Vegetables, intestinal microflora synthesis	1.4 mg men 1.2 mg women
Folate	Liver	Green leafy vegetables, fortified breakfast cereals	200 µg
B₁₂ (cobalamin)	Animal products	Bacterial colonisation	1.5 µg
Biotin	Egg yolk	Intestinal flora	No RNI. Safe intake: 10–200 µg
C (ascorbic acid)	Citrus fruit	Fresh fruit, fresh and frozen vegetables	40 mg

*Rich sources contain the nutrient in high concentration but are not generally eaten in large amounts; important sources contain less but contribute most because larger amounts are eaten.

19

methyl donor in the synthesis of DNA, RNA and protein, with increased requirements during cellular division.

19.14. Answer: D.

The residual length of jejunum following massive small bowel resection or bypass is a powerful predictor of the need for parenteral fluid or nutritional support. Those left with an intact colon that can be anastomosed at the time of initial surgery or at some time subsequently tend to fare better than those where the colon is lost (due to the further capacity of the colon to absorb water and electrolytes). However, most patients with <200 cm of jejunum remaining will require oral fluid restriction and the use of a glucose/electrolyte solution (with sodium concentration of 90–120 mmol/L to minimise diarrhoea and maximise absorption of fluid and electrolytes. In addition, those with <100 cm of jejunum remaining will require a variable volume of parenterally administered sodium chloride to maintain an adequate balance between what they can absorb orally and their overall fluid requirements. Those with <75 cm of jejunum will also be unable to maintain their overall energy requirements by oral means and will require a variable amount of calories administered parenterally (parenteral nutrition) in addition to the other treatments above.

19.15. Answer: B.

Where the intestine is largely intact, functionally normally and accessible to an enteral tube, the proven benefits of enteral over parenteral nutrition are that the overall health-care costs are less, that it is associated with fewer episodes of infection, more rapid restoration of normal intestinal function and a reduced length of hospital stay.

19.16. Answer: B.

Although it may appear initially counterintuitive, it is absolutely vital in this situation that further intestinal losses are not incurred by inappropriate advice to simply drink more fluid. The jejunum is inherently 'leaky', allowing rapid fluxes of sodium (and water) across the epithelial barrier. Taking fluids with a sodium concentration of <90 mmol/L results in a net efflux of sodium and water into the intestinal lumen (and therefore greater stomal fluid losses). Drinking a larger volume of such 'dilute' fluids leads to even more stomal losses. Oral fluid intake should be restricted in such patients to 500 mL per day. A further 1000 mL of a glucose/electrolyte solution with a sodium concentration of at least 90 mmol/L should be given (e.g. St Mark's solution or Glucodrate, Nestlé) but no oral fluids over and above this limit. Any subsequent deficit between intake and output should be made up by parenteral fluid administration.

19.17. Answer: A.

Deficiency of the water-soluble vitamin C (ascorbic acid) has been shown to be prevalent in those aged >65 years living independently in the UK. Its clinical presentation may be precipitated by events such as trauma, surgery, burns or infections and it tends to be more prevalent in those who smoke or use drugs such as glucocorticoids or non-steroidal anti-inflammatory drugs. Ascorbic acid is very heat labile and many traditional cooking methods lead to its degradation.

Patients may notice poor healing of wounds. It may present with petechial or perifollicular bleeding or larger ecchymoses. Gingival swelling or haemorrhage may occur and, less commonly, haemarthrosis or gastrointestinal bleeding. Anaemia is recognised.

19.18. Answer: E.

There are nine essential amino acids (Box 19.18) that cannot be synthesised by the body (e.g. through transamination) and must therefore be obtained in the diet. They are required in order to synthesise other proteins, which have a variety of important functions. Five other amino acids can only be synthesised if there is an adequate dietary supply of their precursors. These are known as 'conditionally essential' amino acids.

i 19.18 Amino acids	
Essential amino acids	
Tryptophan	Valine
Histidine	Phenylalanine
Methionine	Lysine
Threonine	Leucine
Isoleucine	
Conditionally essential amino acids and their precursors	
Cysteine: methionine, serine	
Tyrosine: phenylalanine	
Arginine: glutamine/glutamate, aspartate	
Proline: glutamate	
Glycine: serine, choline	

19.19. Answer: E.

The evidence that tube feeding in advanced dementia improves any of these parameters is very weak and inconsistent. Patients and their families are often caught up in a vicious cycle of dementia and malnourishment (Fig. 19.19). It is important to screen patients with dementia for malnutrition, to monitor body weight, encourage an adequate intake of food and provide a pleasant home-like environment for meals. Oral nutritional supplements have been shown to be of benefit. Cases should be assessed individually. However, unless there is some acute, reversible event (e.g. further stroke, treatable infection), which may be bridged by a short period of tube feeding, there is little benefit to artificial nutritional support in advanced cases of dementia.

19.20. Answer: E.

Gastrostomy is known to be associated with risks of insertion (pain, bleeding, aspiration pneumonia, infection of the insertion site, inadvertent damage to an intra-abdominal organ or viscus, tube displacement) and longer-term risks (infection at insertion site, tube displacement, aspiration of feed). It does not offer any advantage over nasogastric feeding in terms of aspiration risk. The decision to go ahead should be taken when patients or their carers are fully aware of the risks and benefits involved.

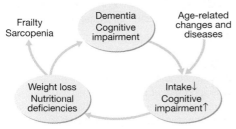

Fig. 19.19 Malnutrition in dementia – a vicious circle. *From Volkert D, Chourdakis M, Faxen-Irving G, et al. ESPEN guidelines on nutrition in dementia. Clin Nutr 2015; 34:1052–1073.*

19

CM Farrell, C Thurtell

20

Diabetes mellitus

Multiple Choice Questions

20.1. A 110-kg 57 year old man presents with 1-month history of lethargy, urinary frequency and increased thirst. He has been dieting for years but only recently has managed to lose 10 kg with little effort. What would be the simplest test that could make the diagnosis?

A. Autoantibodies to glutamic acid decarboxylase (GAD), protein tyrosine phosphatase islet antigen-2 (IA-2) and zinc transporter 8 (ZnT8)
B. Capillary blood glucose
C. Fasting venous blood glucose
D. Oral glucose tolerance test (OGTT)
E. Random venous blood glucose

20.2. A 49 year old black woman with a body mass index (BMI) of 42 kg/m^2 presents with a 6-month history of fatigue and lethargy. Over the past few days she has become increasingly thirsty, is getting up at night to pass urine and has experienced some dysuria. On admission, blood glucose was measured at 40 mmol/L (720 mg/dL) with ketones of 4 mmol/L and bicarbonate 12 mmol/L. She is treated for diabetic ketoacidosis (DKA), but what is the most likely underlying diagnosis?

A. Impaired glucose tolerance
B. Latent autoimmune diabetes of adulthood (LADA)
C. Metabolic syndrome
D. Type 1 diabetes mellitus
E. Type 2 diabetes mellitus

20.3. The most common monogenic forms of diabetes are caused by defects in insulin secretion. Maturity-onset diabetes of the young (MODY) commonly develops under the age of 25 and is dominantly inherited. One form of MODY is due to mutation in glucokinase. How should these patients be managed?

A. Basal insulin
B. Biguanide (metformin) alone
C. Diet alone
D. No treatment required
E. Sulphonylurea with meals

20.4. The diabetes team were asked to review a hyperglycaemic 37 year old man on the surgical ward who presented with abdominal pain, general lethargy, weight loss and pale loose bowel motions. He has been in hospital a number of times with upper abdominal pain with a normal abdominal ultrasound scan. He has a family history of type 2 diabetes mellitus. He recently lost his job as a taxi driver as there was concern after he came to work smelling strongly of alcohol and was found to be above the legal limit to drive. Mean corpuscular volume (MCV) was raised on blood tests from 3 years ago. On admission he had a blood glucose of 20 mmol/L (360 mg/dL) with ketones of 3 mmol/L and bicarbonate 20 mmol/L. What is the most likely diagnosis?

A. Impaired glucose tolerance
B. LADA
C. Monogenic diabetes
D. Pancreatic insufficiency
E. Type 2 diabetes mellitus

20.5. DKA is a medical emergency in people with type 1 diabetes. What is the most common mechanism of death in DKA in children and adolescents?

A. Acute respiratory distress syndrome
B. Cerebral oedema
C. Hypokalaemia
D. Pneumonia
E. Septic shock

20.6. A 57 year old woman with a 5-year history of diet-controlled diabetes is struggling to make any further changes to her lifestyle. Her HbA_{1c} is above target. What would be the best first-line pharmacological therapy?

A. Biguanide (e.g. metformin)
B. Dipeptidyl peptidase-4 (DPP-4) inhibitor (e.g. sitagliptin)
C. Insulin
D. Sodium and glucose co-transporter 2 (SGLT2) inhibitor (e.g. empagliflozin)
E. Sulphonylurea (e.g. gliclazide)

20.7. A 47 year old man with type 2 diabetes has been treated with a biguanide (metformin) and a sulphonylurea (gliclazide) for a number of years. Unfortunately his glycaemic control has deteriorated and his doctor is considering adding in a thiazolidinedione (pioglitazone). What is its mechanism of action?

A. Activation of peroxisome proliferator-activated receptor γ (PPARγ) in adipocytes
B. Delays carbohydrate absorption
C. Prevents breakdown of incretin hormones
D. Promotion of β-cell insulin secretion
E. Sensitises tissues to insulin

20.8. A 58 year old obese woman with an 8-year history of type 2 diabetes and an HbA_{1c} 80 mmol/mol (9.5%) attends the diabetes clinic. She is recommended to start a glucagon-like peptide-1 (GLP-1) agonist. What are the possible side effects?

A. Bladder cancer
B. Genital fungal infections
C. Hypoglycaemia
D. Pancreatitis
E. Weight gain

20.9. A 24 year woman with type 1 diabetes is attending the antenatal clinic. She is 16 weeks pregnant and is concerned that her baby is big for gestation. What is the most likely mechanism for this?

A. Fetal hypoinsulinaemia
B. Genetic factors
C. Hypertension

D. Maternal hyperglycaemia
E. Pregnancy-induced hyperphagia

20.10. A 38 year old man with poorly controlled type 1 diabetes suddenly develops double vision. On examination he is unable to abduct his left eye. He undergoes an urgent CT scan of his brain, which is normal. What is the most likely diagnosis?

A. Brain tumour
B. Diabetic mononeuropathy
C. Giant cell arteritis
D. Graves' eye disease
E. Stroke

20.11. A 21 year old student attends her family physician feeling generally unwell with a 3-day history of vomiting. She has been trying to lose weight and has been on a low-fat diet and started to exercise daily. She felt unwell with diarrhoea and vomiting for 3 days following a seafood meal. The family physician checked a blood glucose level, which was 5.2 mmol/L (94 mg/dL) and urine dipstick showed glucose trace and ketones 3+.
    What is the most likely cause of ketonuria?

A. Diabetic ketoacidosis
B. Fasting
C. High-carbohydrate diet
D. Repeated vomiting
E. Strenuous exercise

20.12. A 52 year old English lorry driver with type 1 diabetes returns to clinic for his annual review. HbA_{1c} is stable at 62 mmol/mol (7.8%) and he reports no hypoglycaemic episodes. He is well aware of the need to check his glucose prior to driving and does so; however, he does not keep a record of them. Which of the following is legally required in the UK for people prescribed insulin to enable them to drive a heavy goods vehicle?

A. Annual driving test
B. Annual review with 3 months' glucose meter readings
C. Biannual diabetes review
D. Continuous glucose monitoring
E. Retinal screening

20.13. A 56 year old woman has type 2 diabetes. She also has non-alcoholic fatty liver disease (NAFLD), arthritis, coeliac disease, mild visual impairment and chronic obstructive pulmonary disease (COPD). She smokes up to 20 cigarettes

20

a day. Which of the following conditions has a pathophysiological link and is more common in individuals with type 2 diabetes?

A. Coeliac disease
B. COPD
C. NAFLD
D. Optic atrophy
E. Rheumatoid arthritis

20.14. A 67 year old female has had type 1 diabetes for 50 years. She has an HbA$_{1c}$ of 42 mmol/mol (6%) and is very strict about her diet. She was admitted for an elective total hip replacement. On the day of surgery, she was found by the junior doctor to be very drowsy with a capillary blood glucose of 2.2 mmol/L (40 mg/dL). What should ideally happen next?

A. Cancel theatre
B. Intravenous (IV) access and 100 mL of 20% dextrose and repeat blood glucose in 15 minutes
C. IV access and 100 mL of 50% dextrose
D. IV access and 200 mL of 20% dextrose
E. Withhold insulin for rest of day

20.15. A woman at 20 weeks' gestation undergoes a 75-g oral glucose tolerance test with the following results: 0 minutes = 5.6 mmol/L (101 mg/dL); 120 minutes = 9.2 mmol/L (166 mg/dL). According to the National Institute for Clinical Excellence (NICE) guidelines, what should be the immediate management?

A. Dietary modification
B. GLP-1 receptor agonist
C. Insulin
D. Metformin
E. Sulphonylurea, e.g. glibenclamide

20.16. A frail 93 year old man with type 1 diabetes for 46 years attends for review. His HbA$_{1c}$ is 69 mmol/mol (8.5%). Blood pressure is 152/82 mmHg for which he is taking an angiotensin-converting enzyme (ACE) inhibitor (ramipril) and a calcium channel blocker (amlodipine). He has mild background diabetic retinopathy. Which of these treatment targets is most appropriate in this scenario?

A. Avoidance of hypoglycaemia
B. HbA$_{1c}$ of 48 mmol/mol (6.5%) or less
C. HbA$_{1c}$ of 58 mmol/mol (7.5%) or less
D. Microvascular disease prevention
E. No need to monitor blood glucose in view of his age

20.17. A 32 year old woman attends the antenatal clinic for her booking scan. She is 12 weeks pregnant with twins and has been struggling with 'morning sickness'. She has a BMI of 36 kg/m^2 and undergoes an OGTT, the results of which are: fasting plasma glucose 4.8 mmol/L (86 mg/dL); 2-hour plasma glucose 7.0 mmol/L (126 mg/dL).

As part of her routine checks the midwife dips her urine and she has 2+ ketones. What is the most likely diagnosis?

A. Diabetic ketoacidosis
B. Gestational diabetes
C. Hyperemesis gravidarum
D. Normal physiological response in pregnancy
E. Undiagnosed type 2 diabetes

20.18. A 51 year old man with type 1 diabetes returns to the foot clinic. He attends for regular review as he has an ulcer on his left heel. He has been on a walking holiday to the Amalfi coast for 2 weeks. The podiatrist asks for a medical review as he is concerned that the left foot is now warm and swollen. The ulceration looks much improved and the patient feels well. X-ray does not reveal any obvious bony abnormality. What is the most likely diagnosis?

A. Acute Charcot arthropathy
B. Deep vein thrombosis (DVT)
C. Dry gangrene
D. Gout
E. Osteomyelitis

20.19. A 47 year old woman with type 1 diabetes attends for annual review. She denies any significant hypoglycaemia. Her results are as follows: HbA$_{1c}$ 46 mmol/mol (6.4%); blood pressure (BP) 152/98 mmHg (average of 3); weight 61 kg (BMI 24 kg/m^2); urinalysis: + glucose, trace nitrites, albumin:creatinine ratio (ACR) 5 mg/mmol (previously early morning sample 6.2 mg/mmol); total cholesterol 3.8 mmol/L (147 mg/dL).

Current medication: basal analogue insulin (glargine), bolus/rapid-acting analogue insulin (NovoRapid), ACE inhibitor (lisinopril), statin (simvastatin).

Which result is it most important to act upon?

A. Blood pressure
B. Cholesterol
C. HbA$_{1c}$
D. Urinalysis
E. Weight

20.20. James is a 19 year old man from Ireland; he has a family history of diabetes. His mother developed diabetes later in life; he is unsure if she required insulin but she often attended the hospital. She died suddenly when he was young. James is an active man but has recently been hindered by general malaise, lethargy and pain in his knees. He has had a steroid injection into his left knee with little improvement. The following tests have been carried out:

Haemoglobin 145 g/L (14.5 g/dL)
White blood cell count 6.2 × 10⁹/L
Urea 5.2 mmol/L (31 mg/dL)
Creatinine 62 µmol/L (0.70 mg/dL)
Glucose 11.4 mmol/L (205 mg/dL)
HbA₁c 51 mmol/mol (6.8%)

Anti-GAD antibody: negative
Anti-IA-2 antibody: negative
Antineutrophil cytoplasmic antibody (ANCA): negative
Ferritin 1137 µg/L

What is the most likely diagnosis?

A. Hereditary haemochromatosis
B. MODY
C. Steroid-induced diabetes
D. Type 1 diabetes
E. Type 2 diabetes

20.21. Insulin is the main regulator of glucose metabolism and storage. It is secreted from pancreatic β cells. These cells regulate blood glucose concentrations by coupling glucose with insulin secretion. Glucose enters the pancreatic β cells by facilitated diffusion down its concentration gradient through cell membrane glucose transporters (GLUTs). Through which GLUT does glucose enter pancreatic β cells?

A. GLUT1
B. GLUT2
C. GLUT3
D. GLUT4
E. GLUT5

20.22. Blood glucose is tightly regulated in order to provide a constant supply of glucose to the central nervous system. Following ingestion of a meal containing carbohydrate, which of the following is most likely to occur in the normal physiological state?

A. Inhibition of GLP-1 release
B. Inhibition of insulin release
C. Stimulation of glucagon release
D. Stimulation of hepatic gluconeogenesis
E. Stimulation of hepatic glucose uptake

20.23. A 59 year old man with a BMI of 29 kg/m² is admitted to hospital with pleuritic chest pain and a productive cough and is found to have pneumonia. He has no history of diabetes and takes no regular medication. As part of his admission investigations, a plasma glucose is found to be 10.0 mmol/L (180 mg/dL). Which of the following is the most appropriate management?

A. Blood glucose monitoring with fasting plasma glucose after recovery from infection
B. Commence treatment with liraglutide
C. Commence treatment with metformin
D. No further assessment of glycaemic control
E. Variable-rate intravenous insulin infusion

20.24. A 70 year old woman attends her family physician complaining of excessive thirst and fatigue. A random venous glucose is 13.2 mmol/L (238 mg/dL), confirming a diagnosis of diabetes. She takes a number of medications for hypertension, ischaemic heart disease and polymyalgia rheumatica. Which of the following medications can precipitate hyperglycaemia?

A. ACE inhibitor (e.g. ramipril)
B. Aspirin
C. Calcium channel blocker (e.g. amlodipine)
D. Nitrate (e.g. isosorbide mononitrate)
E. Steroid (e.g. prednisolone)

20.25. An 18 year old female with type 1 diabetes is admitted with suspected pyelonephritis. She has not taken any insulin for 24 hours during her acute illness. Her initial blood tests include: plasma glucose 24 mmol/L (432 mg/dL), bicarbonate 12 mmol/L and ketones 5.5 mmol/L. Which electrolyte will most likely require regular monitoring and aggressive intravenous supplementation?

A. Bicarbonate
B. Calcium
C. Magnesium
D. Phosphate
E. Potassium

20.26. A 75 year old male with no prior diagnosis of diabetes is admitted to hospital because he has become progressively more drowsy and unwell since being started on oral amoxicillin by his family physician for a suspected chest infection 2 weeks ago. He appears clinically

20

dehydrated. His initial blood tests include: plasma glucose 55 mmol/L (991 mg/dL), ketones 0.1 mmol/L, sodium 149 mmol/L and serum osmolality 368 mmol/kg. Which of the following statements is correct with regard to the management of this patient?

A. A solution of 10% dextrose is the initial intravenous fluid of choice

B. Close monitoring of fluid balance is unnecessary

C. Intravenous insulin is not required initially in the absence of significant ketonaemia

D. Serum osmolality should normalise within 4 hours of treatment

E. Thromboprophylaxis is contraindicated

20.27. A 28 year old female has recently been found to have hepatocyte nuclear factor 1α (HNF1α) MODY. It is decided to treat her diabetes with gliclazide. Gliclazide, a sulphonylurea drug, exerts its hypoglycaemic effect by enhancing endogenous insulin secretion. By which mechanism is this achieved?

A. Activation of PPARγ

B. Activation of the GLP-1 receptor

C. Closure of the transmembrane β-cell K_{ATP} channel

D. Inhibition of DPP-4

E. Inhibition of SGLT2

20.28. A 21 year old female with type 1 diabetes since childhood attends the diabetes clinic for review. She has been symptomatic of hypoglycaemia several times since her last appointment 6 months ago. Which of the following is classed as a neuroglycopenic symptom of hypoglycaemia?

A. Anxiety

B. Confusion

C. Headache

D. Hunger

E. Sweating

20.29. A 24 year old male with type 1 diabetes of 12 years' duration presents with frequent episodes of hypoglycaemia. He goes running for up to 60 minutes 4 times per week and the hypoglycaemic episodes occur after exercise. He has good awareness of hypoglycaemia and is able to take corrective action on each occasion. He is on a basal-bolus insulin regimen and his latest HbA_1c is 62 mmol/mol (7.8%). Which of the following interventions is the most appropriate management?

A. Advise him to avoid exercise

B. Always omit the short-acting insulin dose after exercise

C. Reduce his total daily insulin dose to relax his glycaemic control

D. Refer for structured diabetes education programme

E. Refer to a tertiary centre for consideration of pancreatic islet transplantation

20.30. A 58 year old man with type 2 diabetes of 10 years' duration and a BMI of 33 kg/m^2 attends clinic for review of his diabetes management. He has a suboptimal HbA_1c of 69 mmol/mol (8.5%) on metformin monotherapy 1 g twice daily and would like to discuss the addition of a second-line agent. Which of the following options are the most appropriate if he wishes a strategy that promotes weight loss?

A. DPP-4 inhibitor (e.g. sitagliptin)

B. GLP-1 agonist (e.g. liraglutide)

C. Insulin

D. PPARγ agonist/thiazolidinedione (e.g. pioglitazone)

E. Sulphonylurea (e.g. glipizide)

20.31. A 50 year old woman with type 2 diabetes presents to her family physician complaining of genital thrush, which has not settled with topical antifungal treatment. She had been started on a new oral hypoglycaemic drug 4 months earlier. Which of the following drugs is most likely to be responsible for her presentation?

A. DPP-4 inhibitor (e.g. sitagliptin)

B. Glucosidase inhibitor (e.g. acarbose)

C. PPARγ agonist/thiazolidinedione (e.g. pioglitazone)

D. SGLT2 inhibitor (e.g. empagliflozin)

E. Sulphonylurea (e.g. glimepiride)

20.32. A 35 year old woman with type 1 diabetes of 20 years' duration presents with chronic nausea, early satiety and intermittent vomiting after meals. She has a history of poor glycaemic control, retinopathy and peripheral neuropathy. Which of the following investigations will be most helpful in establishing a diagnosis?

A. Abdominal ultrasonography

B. Anti-tissue transglutaminase (anti-tTG) antibody

C. Barium swallow

D. Gastric emptying study

E. Plain chest radiograph

20.33. A 21 year old women with type 1 diabetes of 8 years' duration with good glycaemic control – HbA$_{1c}$ 48 mmol/mol (6.5%) – on basal-bolus insulin presents to her young adult specialist clinic for routine review. She has been experiencing intermittent abdominal bloating, diarrhoea and weight loss over the last 3 months. Recent urea and electrolytes, liver function tests and thyroid function tests were all within normal limits. Which of the following is the best next investigation to perform?

A. Abdominal ultrasonography
B. Anti-tTG antibody
C. Flexible sigmoidoscopy
D. Gastric emptying study
E. Upper GI endoscopy

20.34. A 19 year old male with type 1 diabetes is admitted to hospital complaining of generalised abdominal pain and vomiting. He is apyrexial, tachycardic and clinically dehydrated. There is no peritonism in the abdomen. He has the following blood results: blood glucose 22 mmol/L (396 mg/dL), ketones 4.3 mmol/L, bicarbonate 11 mmol/L, alkaline phosphatase 250 U/L, white cell count 19 × 10^9/L and haemoglobin 182 g/L. Which of the following statements regarding interpretation of these results is correct?

A. He can safely be discharged home
B. Measurement of venous pH will be normal
C. The elevated alkaline phosphatase enzyme invariably indicates vitamin D deficiency
D. The elevated haemoglobin concentration will likely normalise after intravenous fluid administration
E. The elevated white cell count invariably indicates underlying infection

20.35. A 48 year old man with type 1 diabetes of 30 years' duration attends clinic for routine review. He is on a basal-bolus insulin regimen and has an HbA$_{1c}$ of 70 mmol/mol (8.6%). He is on no other medication. Blood pressure is 155/92 mmHg (repeated 3 times with similar results) and he has microalbuminuria with an ACR of 7.3 mg/mmol. Estimated glomerular filtration (eGFR) rate is 54 mL/min/1.73 m^2. Which of the following drugs would be most beneficial?

A. ACE inhibitor (e.g. lisinopril)
B. β-blocker (e.g. atenolol)
C. Calcium channel blocker (e.g. amlodipine)

D. Centrally acting antihypertensive (e.g. moxonidine)
E. Thiazide diuretic (e.g. bendroflumethiazide)

20.36. A 65 year old man with type 2 diabetes of 20 years' duration is referred to the specialist diabetes foot clinic by his family physician with an ulcer of the plantar surface of the right foot. The ulcer has been present for approximately 6 weeks and there is a history of peripheral diabetic neuropathy. On examination, there is a 2-cm diameter ulcer in proximity to the first metatarsal head. It has an offensive odour and discharge. The area around the ulcer is hot and erythematous. Which of the following features, if present, would most strongly indicate the presence of osteomyelitis (bone infection)?

A. A normal plain foot radiograph
B. Elevated blood white cell count
C. Increased skin temperature compared to the contralateral foot
D. Peripheral oedema
E. The ulcer probing to the depth of bone

20.37. A 72 year old man is admitted to hospital by his family physician for urgent investigation of weight loss. He has a progressive 3-month history of back pain, jaundice, dark urine and anorexia. He has lost approximately 15 kg in weight. In the last 4 weeks he has developed increased thirst and is drinking excessively. A random venous glucose is 16.0 mmol/L (288 mg/dL). Which investigation is most likely to reveal the cause of his diabetes?

A. Anti-GAD and anti-IA-2 antibodies
B. CT scan of the pancreas
C. Dexamethasone suppression test
D. Faecal elastase
E. Serum C-peptide

20.38. A 29 year old woman with type 1 diabetes for 18 years attends clinic for routine review. She has poor glycaemic control with an HbA$_{1c}$ of 90 mmol/mol (10.4%). She is keen to embark on stricter glycaemic management in advance of planning pregnancy. Which of the following complications of diabetes would be the most likely to deteriorate significantly should her glycaemic control improve suddenly?

A. Foot ulceration
B. Gastroparesis
C. Microalbuminuria
D. Peripheral vascular disease
E. Retinopathy

20

20.39. An 18 year old woman with type 1 diabetes attends her diabetes clinic to discuss the possibility of continuous subcutaneous insulin therapy (insulin pump therapy). She has a suboptimal HbA$_{1c}$ of 68 mmol/mol (8.4%) and takes multiple daily injections of insulin. Which of the following statements is correct with regard to insulin pump therapy?

A. A continuous glucose monitoring system (CGMS) is mandatory for all patients
B. DKA does not occur as insulin administration is constant
C. Patients have to inject long-acting insulin in addition to the pump-delivered insulin
D. The rate of insulin delivery can be adjusted depending on the time of day
E. There is an increased risk of microvascular disease compared to multiple daily injections

20.40. A 45 year old man with diabetes presents with a 4-week history of weight loss, polyuria and polydipsia. His blood results include: random plasma glucose 20 mmol/L (360 mg/dL), ketones 2 mmol/L and HbA$_{1c}$ 110 mmol/mol (12.2%). He was diagnosed with diabetes 6 months ago at which point his BMI was 23 kg/m^2 and HbA$_{1c}$ 65 mmol/mol (8.1%). There is no family history of diabetes. Since diagnosis he has been treated with metformin and a sulphonylurea. β-cell antibodies are checked and he is found to have a very high titre of anti-GAD antibodies. Which of the following diagnoses best fits with this scenario?

A. LADA
B. Mitochondrial diabetes
C. MODY
D. Pancreatic disease
E. Type 2 diabetes

Answers

20.1. Answer: E.
This patient has osmotic symptoms in keeping with hyperglycaemia. Given that he is symptomatic, a random venous blood glucose of ≥ 11.1 mmol/L (≥ 200 mg/dL) is sufficient to give the diagnosis of diabetes. This test will be the least burdensome to the patient and most cost-effective.

20.2. Answer: E.
This patient is correctly treated for DKA as she has elevated blood glucose in keeping with diabetes, elevated ketones and a metabolic acidosis. Given her ethnicity, BMI and prodromal illness, a diagnosis of 'ketosis-prone' diabetes (which is more common in patients of African origin) is likely with an underlying diagnosis of type 2 diabetes. This is important as initially patients require insulin treatment but as glucose levels are controlled and β cells recover, patients may be able to transfer off insulin to oral hypoglycaemic agents.

20.3. Answer: D.
MODY is defined as non-insulin-dependent diabetes that develops under the age of 25 in one family member. Glucokinase is a pancreatic glucose sensor and patients with glucokinase mutations have an altered set-point for glucose. This results in a slightly high fasting blood glucose but a normal post-prandial response. Therefore, patients with glucokinase MODY generally have stable, mild hyperglycaemia, do not require treatment or monitoring and are at very low risk of developing any diabetes complications.

20.4. Answer: D.
This patient has symptoms and signs in keeping with pancreatic insufficiency, both endocrine and exocrine. The history of alcohol excess is helpful to aid diagnosis. Alcohol excess can cause recurrent bouts of acute pancreatitis, which can lead to progressive destruction of the pancreas. Diabetes due to pancreatic insufficiency can sometimes be managed with oral therapy but often requires treatment with insulin.

20.5. Answer: B.
The average fluid loss in an adult with moderately severe DKA is 6 L. Patients are therefore aggressively fluid replaced in the first few hours. Caution is required in fluid replacement in children and young adults due to the risk of cerebral oedema (a paediatric-specific DKA protocol should be used). The osmolar gradient caused by the high blood glucose results in water shift from the intracellular fluid to extracellular fluid and

contraction of cell volume. Correction of the blood glucose with insulin and fluids can result in a rapid reduction in the osmolarity, which in turn reverses the fluid shift and development of cerebral oedema. It is thought that the cerebral oedema is related to cerebral vasoconstriction, brain ischaemia and hypoxia. As children's brains have higher oxygen requirements than adults, this may explain their unique susceptibility. Hypokalaemia-related cardiac events used to be a major cause of death but potassium monitoring and replacement is now much improved.

20.6. Answer: A.
Metformin is a potent blood glucose-lowering treatment that is weight-neutral or can lead to weight loss. It is low cost and does not cause hypoglycaemia. It is used as first line for type 2 diabetes in all patients who can tolerate it. The long-term benefits were shown in the UK Prospective Diabetes Study. It is usually maintained when other medications are added.

20.7. Answer: A.
Thiazolidinediones predominantly work in adipose tissue. They bind and activate PPARγ. This nuclear receptor regulates the expressions of many genes involved in metabolism. Thiazolidinediones enhance the action of endogenous insulin in the adipose cells but also alter the release of adipokines, which adjust insulin sensitivity in the liver.

20.8. Answer: D.
All incretin-acting drugs have been reported to be associated with an increased risk of pancreatitis. Unlike sulphonylureas they do not cause hypoglycaemia as they only promote insulin secretion when there is a glucose trigger. Sulphonylureas can lead to weight gain, as can pioglitazone and insulin, but GLP-1 agonists usually cause weight loss. Pioglitazone is associated with an increased risk of bladder cancer. SGLT2 inhibitors cause increased glycosuria, resulting in genital fungal infections and increased risk of urine tract infections.

20.9. Answer: D.
Maternal hyperglycaemia causes fetal hyperglycaemia due to transmission of glucose across the placenta. Fetal insulin levels will consequently rise. Insulin is a major fetal growth factor, and high levels of fetal insulin therefore drive fetal growth, resulting in an increased birth weight.

20.10. Answer: B.
Diabetic mononeuropathy is loss of a sensory or motor function within a single peripheral or cranial nerve, in this case the 6th cranial nerve – resulting in sudden-onset diplopia. Given that the CT brain is normal and there are no other symptoms or signs, it is unlikely to be in keeping with brain tumour or stroke. He would be unlikely to present with Graves' eye disease with no features in keeping with thyrotoxicosis. Giant cell arteritis commonly presents with temporal tenderness and amaurosis fugax not diplopia.

20.11. Answer: D.
Ketone bodies are organic acids that are formed during fat metabolism. When the body has insufficient insulin or depletes its own carbohydrate stores it will metabolise fat for energy. Ketonuria may be found in normal people who have been fasting or exercising strenuously for long periods, who have been vomiting repeatedly or who have been eating a diet high in fat and low in carbohydrate (all of these circumstances can cause glycogenic depletion). The history and glucose level in this case are not in keeping with diabetic ketosis. The history here suggests vomiting to be the most likely cause of ketonuria.

20.12. Answer: B.
In the UK, according to the Driver and Vehicle Licensing Agency (DVLA) it is a legal requirement for people on insulin who drive larger vehicles such as buses or heavy goods vehicles to have an annual examination by a diabetes specialist along with a review of 3 months of glucose meter readings. This patient should keep a record of his blood glucose readings and the team should consider advocating a blood glucose meter, which can be electronically downloaded to provide this data at his annual review.

20.13. Answer: C.
Hypertension, NAFLD and hypercholesterolaemia are associated with type 2 diabetes due to insulin resistance. This cluster of conditions has been termed the 'insulin resistance syndrome' or 'metabolic syndrome' and is much more common in obese individuals. Coeliac disease – gluten

20

intolerance – is an autoimmune condition affecting primarily the small bowel, caused by a reaction to gliadin, a gluten protein. Optic atrophy and rheumatoid arthritis may also have underlying autoimmune aetiologies. Autoimmune diseases are more commonly associated with type 1 diabetes than type 2 diabetes.

20.14. Answer: B.

Treatment of hypoglycaemia depends on the severity and whether the patient is able to swallow. Conscious patients should be treated with oral carbohydrate. If assistance is required to treat hypoglycaemia this is called 'severe hypoglycaemia'. Patients should receive 100–200 mL 20% dextrose or intramuscular glucagon. If the patient is conscious and able to swallow, GlucoGel or refined sugar drink can be used. Blood glucose should be re-checked after 15 minutes and re-treated if needed. Once conscious, an oral complex-carbohydrate snack should be given. Insulin should not be omitted. If a dosing error was made, then adjustment may be required. Fifty per cent glucose is generally discouraged due to risk of infusion vein irritation.

20.15. Answer: A.

The aim of managing gestational diabetes is to normalise the maternal blood glucose and therefore reduce excessive fetal growth. The first step is dietary modification, namely reducing the amount of fast-acting refined carbohydrate. Regular blood glucose monitoring is required. If diet alone does not achieve targets, then metformin should be started. If not tolerated or additional treatment is required, insulin should be commenced. Glibenclamide can be used if metformin and insulin are not tolerated, because it does not cross the placenta. In some countries, glibenclamide and metformin are not licensed for use in pregnancy. There is no evidence for safety of any other hypoglycaemic agents in pregnancy.

20.16. Answer: A.

The aims of treatment and target HbA_{1c} depends on the individual patient. Early in diabetes a target HbA_{1c} of 48 mmol/mol (6.5%) or less may be appropriate to try to prevent microvascular disease. An HbA_{1c} of 58 mmol/mol (7.5%) or less may be more appropriate in some older patients with cardiovascular

disease, or those treated with insulin, given risks of hypoglycaemia. The benefits of a lower target HbA_{1c} need to be weighed up against the risk of hypoglycaemia in insulin-treated patients. Longer diabetes duration and frequency of hypoglycaemic episodes are risk factors for impairment of symptomatic response to hypoglycaemia. Advanced age itself is a risk factor for hypoglycaemia. Multiple comorbidities, reduced appetite and renal function can predispose to hypoglycaemia in older age. Given this patient's age and duration of disease, the main aim of treatment should be towards safety and symptom control: i.e. to avoid hypoglycaemia.

20.17. Answer: C.

The most likely diagnosis is hyperemesis gravidarum, a complication of pregnancy characterised by severe nausea, vomiting and dehydration. The diagnosis is usually clinical but has been defined as three of more episodes of vomiting in a day such that weight loss of 5% has occurred and there is evidence of ketones in the urine. Risk factors include first pregnancy, multiple pregnancy, obesity and a family history. When vomiting is severe it can lead to dehydration and ketosis.

A diagnosis of gestational diabetes is based upon maternal blood glucose measures that are associated with increased fetal growth. Women at high risk of developing gestational diabetes include: BMI > 30 kg/m²; previous macrosomic baby; previous gestational diabetes; a first-degree relative with gestational diabetes; and high-risk ethnicity. These women should all undergo screening. This woman has a BMI of 36 kg/m², so warrants screening; however, her results did not reach the NICE criteria for gestational or any other type of diabetes.

20.18. Answer: A.

Acute Charcot arthropathy almost always presents with signs of inflammation – a hot, red, swollen foot. Initial X-ray may show bony destruction but can be normal. There is often a history of peripheral neuropathy or previous foot ulceration. As Charcot can be difficult to differentiate from osteomyelitis, MRI of the foot can be helpful. The pathophysiology is not well understood but may involve unperceived trauma with underlying neuropathy leading to progressive destruction. In this case, minor trauma may have occurred on his walking holiday and repeated 'trauma' may have led to bony destruction. In view of the recent ulcer, osteomyelitis should be excluded (MRI should be considered), but there is some reassurance that the area of ulceration has improved and the patient is systemically well. Although he has been on a flight, he has otherwise been active and has a swollen foot – not calf – making DVT less likely. The history is not in keeping with gout or gangrene.

20.19. Answer: A.
Microalbuminuria is the presence of small amounts of albumin in the urine at a concentration not detected on standard urinalysis. Early morning urine is measured for albumin:creatinine ratio. Microalbuminuria is present if ACR is 2.5–30 mg/mmol creatinine in men and 3.5–30 mg/mmol creatinine in women. False positives should be excluded and 2 out of 3 samples should be positive to confirm the diagnosis (ideally an early morning sample on repeat).

Microalbuminuria is a good predictor of progression to nephropathy in type 1 diabetes. The presence of established microalbuminuria should prompt action to reduce the risk of progression of nephropathy and of cardiovascular disease. This should be done by aggressive reduction of blood pressure, optimising glycaemic control and cardiovascular risk reduction.

This patient has good glycaemic control and has a healthy BMI with normal level of cholesterol. Blood pressure may need further validation in the first instance, but presuming it is persistently elevated, then it is diagnostic for hypertension and needs lowering for vascular and renal protection.

20.20. Answer: A.
The raised ferritin in this case points to a diagnosis of hereditary haemochromatosis, a disease characterised by excessive intestinal absorption of dietary iron, resulting in a pathological increase in total body iron stores. Excess iron accumulates in tissues and organs, disrupting their normal function. The most susceptible organs include liver, adrenal glands, heart, skin, gonads, joints and pancreas. Patients can present with cirrhosis, polyarthropathy, adrenal failure, heart failure or diabetes. The hereditary form is most common in those of Northern European and Celtic descent. The disease is inherited in an autosomal recessive pattern.

20.21. Answer: B.
GLUT2 is present in renal tubular cells, liver cells and pancreatic β cells. It is a bidirectional transporter, allowing glucose to flow in two directions. This is required in pancreatic β cells so that the intracellular environment can accurately measure the serum glucose levels. GLUT1 is expressed in erythrocytes and in the endothelial cells of the blood–brain barrier. It is responsible for the low level of basal glucose uptake needed to maintain respiration in all cells. GLUT3 is mostly expressed in neurons and in the placenta. GLUT4 is found in adipose tissue and striated muscle; it is regulated by insulin and is responsible for insulin-regulated glucose storage. GLUT5 is a fructose transporter expressed in enterocytes in the small intestine.

20.22. Answer: E.
In the post-prandial period, there are rises in portal vein glucose and insulin and a fall in glucagon. The production of glucose in the liver is suppressed and the uptake of glucose in the liver and peripheral tissues is increased. The incretin hormones – GLP-1 and gastric inhibitory polypeptide (GIP) – augment insulin secretion following oral glucose delivery.

20.23. Answer: A.
The patient most likely has 'stress hyperglycaemia' provoked by acute illness, in this case infection. Underlying impaired glycaemic control or diabetes, however, could also be present. A diagnosis of diabetes in the asymptomatic individual requires follow-up testing of plasma glucose. In this case, the patient's capillary blood glucose levels should be monitored and he ought to have a repeat assessment of his plasma glucose when recovered from the acute illness.

20.24. Answer: E.
The only medication listed that may result in hyperglycaemia and the development of drug-induced diabetes is prednisolone, a glucocorticoid. There is an increased risk of developing diabetes while taking β-adrenoceptor antagonists (β-blockers) and thiazide diuretics for blood pressure control, but not with other antihypertensive agents. Other groups of patients at risk of developing

20

diabetes are those taking atypical antipsychotic medications and transplant recipients taking calcineurin inhibitors.

20.25. Answer: E.
There is marked whole-body depletion of potassium in DKA and serum levels do not correlate with the total body deficit. Both hypokalaemia and hyperkalaemia can occur in DKA and be fatal. Hypokalaemia can be exacerbated by intravenous insulin, which moves potassium into the intracellular compartment. Therefore, in DKA management, serum potassium levels must be carefully monitored. Phosphate levels typically fall in DKA but there is no need to routinely replace in the absence of muscle weakness. Bicarbonate levels normalise with fluid resuscitation; bicarbonate infusion is not recommended and may in fact be harmful.

20.26. Answer: C.
Hyperosmolar hyperglycaemic state (HHS) is a potentially fatal complication of type 2 diabetes, which sometimes occurs in patients with no prior history of diabetes. Patients are extremely dehydrated and require fluid resuscitation, initially with a solution of 0.9% sodium chloride, with careful monitoring of fluid balance. There is a high risk of venous thromboembolism; hence low-molecular-weight heparin is indicated. IV insulin infusion is necessary only in the presence of significant (> 1.0 mmol/L) ketonaemia or metabolic acidosis (i.e. DKA/HHS overlap). Infection is a common precipitant of HHS but antibiotics are not used prophylactically in the absence of infection. It typically takes 72 hours or longer for the biochemical disturbances to correct with treatment of HHS.

20.27. Answer: C.
Hypoglycaemic drugs have varied mechanisms of action. Sulphonylureas exert their effect on pancreatic β cells by closing the K_{ATP} channel, which results in downstream effects culminating in insulin exocytosis. Gliptins inhibit DPP-4, thereby potentiating the action of endogenous incretins such as GLP-1 and GIP. Thiazolidinediones activate PPARγ in adipose tissue. GLP-1 analogues activate the GLP-1 receptor. SGLT2 inhibitors have their action in the kidney where they inhibit SGLT2, thereby reducing re-uptake of glucose from the urine.

20.28. Answer: B.
Non-specific symptoms include nausea, headache and tiredness. Autonomic symptoms result from activation of the autonomic nervous system and include sweating, hunger, trembling, anxiety and palpitation. Neuroglycopenic symptoms result from the brain being deprived of glucose and include delirium, drowsiness, speech disturbance, inability to concentrate, incoordination, irritability, visual disturbance and focal neurological deficit. Autonomic symptoms usually occur first to allow patients to recognise the hypoglycaemia and treat it, but may be absent in individuals with impaired hypoglycaemia awareness.

20.29. Answer: D.
Patient education is fundamental to the prevention and management of hypoglycaemia. Structured education can provide assistance with carbohydrate intake and insulin management around the time of exercise. He already has a suboptimal HbA_{1c} and relaxing this will put him at increased risk of microvascular complications as well as offering no genuine protection against hypoglycaemia. Exercise should not be discouraged as a means of avoiding hypoglycaemia. Reduction of insulin dose pre-exercise may be a useful strategy to avoid hypoglycaemia during exercise but structured education will equip him with a broader range of strategies for the future. Pancreatic islet transplantation is only considered in individuals who experience recurrent severe hypoglycaemia despite optimisation of glycaemic control after structured education.

20.30. Answer: B.
Liraglutide, a GLP-1 agonist, may lead to weight loss as well as improved glycaemic control. SGLT2 inhibitors are also associated with weight loss. The other options are either weight-neutral (sitagliptin, a DPP-4 inhibitor) or promote weight gain (glipizide, a sulphonylurea; pioglitazone, a thiazolidinedione; insulin).

20.31. Answer: D.
Empagliflozin, an inhibitor of the sodium and glucose co-transporter 2 (SGLT2) in the kidney, exerts its glycaemic effect by increasing the amount of glucose in the urine. This can result in fungal infection in approximately 5% of

patients taking the drug. Only if the problem becomes recurrent or unacceptable to the patient is the drug withdrawn. The other drugs do not cause genital tract infection but have their own class-specific side-effects.

20.32. Answer: D.
The most likely diagnosis is gastroparesis as a manifestation of autonomic dysfunction in diabetes. An upper gastrointestinal (GI) tract endoscopy is commonly performed as part of the diagnostic workup, but definitive diagnosis is achieved by demonstrating delayed gastric emptying by [99m]technetium scintigraphy following a solid-phase meal with imaging over 4 hours. The other investigations will not provide a definitive diagnosis.

20.33. Answer: B.
The most likely diagnosis is coeliac disease, which is strongly associated with type 1 diabetes. Up to 1 in 20 people with type 1 diabetes go on to develop coeliac disease. The best screening test for this condition is anti-tTG antibody, which is typically present in high titre in this condition, with the exception of concurrent immunoglobulin A deficiency. An upper GI endoscopy with D2 (second part of duodenum) biopsy is required to confirm the diagnosis but only after initial anti-tTG testing. Coeliac disease should be considered in those who present with weight loss, gastrointestinal symptoms, iron/folate deficiency anaemia, infertility, osteoporosis/low bone mineral density and malabsorption.

20.34. Answer: D.
The patient's clinical status and biochemical findings are consistent with DKA. He requires urgent treatment in hospital. His pH on venous or arterial blood gas would be < 7.30 (H^+ > 50.1 nmol/L) consistent with metabolic acidosis. The white cell count and alkaline phosphatase levels are often elevated in DKA and subside with treatment. Due to significant volume depletion in this condition, haemoglobin concentrations are often elevated and will reduce with expansion of the intravascular compartment following administration of intravenous fluid.

20.35. Answer: A.
ACE inhibitors such as lisinopril or angiotensin receptor blockers would be the most

appropriate antihypertensive agents in this case. These drugs confer additional benefit beyond simply lower blood pressure – they are associated with significantly reduced progression of nephropathy. Patients with microalbuminuria benefit from aggressive lowering of BP (often with multiple agents), control of cardiovascular risk factors and optimisation of glycaemic control.

20.36. Answer: E.
Features that potentially indicate osteomyelitis in the diabetic foot include: dactylitis (marked swelling of the entire digit), an ulcer that probes to the depth of bone and evidence of bony destruction on a plain radiograph (X-ray). X-ray, however, may be normal in 50% of cases. MRI is far more sensitive for osteomyelitis than a plain X-ray. The presence of oedema, increased heat and elevated inflammatory markers may occur in soft tissue infection alone and are not specific for osteomyelitis. If there is clinical or radiological evidence of osteomyelitis, the patient is typically treated with antibiotics for at least 6 weeks.

20.37. Answer: B.
The clinical scenario presented is that of pancreatic carcinoma, which may present with diabetes as a feature. Pancreatic insufficiency may also present with weight loss typically in a patient with a history of alcohol excess, but this condition is not associated with obstructive jaundice. This patient is likely to require insulin therapy to control the osmotic symptoms of his diabetes.

20.38. Answer: E.
It is well recognised that when glycaemic control improves rapidly, there can be a transient deterioration in the degree of retinopathy. This is thought to be due to loss of hyperglycaemia-induced hyperperfusion in the retinal circulation. The effect typically wears off within 18 months. Therefore, in patients with established retinopathy, it is recommended that improvement in glycaemic management should be effected gradually. Transient worsening of peripheral neuropathy symptoms can similarly be seen in this situation.

20.39. Answer: D.
Insulin pump therapy is becoming more widely used for glycaemic control in type 1 diabetes. The pump delivers a constant infusion of

20

short-acting insulin; there is no need for additional long-acting insulin. CGMS is not mandatory, although it is a useful adjunct for monitoring glucose levels while on pump therapy. As the technology becomes more sophisticated, there will be more 'closed loop' systems, whereby the glucose monitor and pump communicate with one another to optimise insulin delivery. DKA is still a possibility, for example in the case of pump failure. One of the attractions of pump therapy is the ability to alter the basal rate of insulin depending on the time of day or level of physical activity (i.e. lower basal rate at night or during exercise to reduce the risk of hypoglycaemia). The risk of microvascular complications of diabetes depends on the HbA_{1c} and glucose variability rather than the mode of insulin delivery.

20.40. Answer: A.

It is estimated that 50% of cases of type 1 diabetes present in adulthood. The patient is best described as having LADA, an insidious form of type 1 diabetes that develops in adulthood. This condition initially presents like type 2 diabetes but is characterised by a relatively rapid progression to insulin treatment and the presence of β-cell antibodies. MODY and mitochondrial diabetes typically occur where there is a strong family history of diabetes, sometimes with other clinical manifestations such as sensorineural deafness in the case of mitochondrial disease. Pancreatic exocrine disease typically occurs in those with a history of conditions that affect pancreatic function such as pancreatitis, haemochromatosis, pancreatectomy and pancreatic cancer.

E El-Omar, F Clegg, MH McLean

21

Gastroenterology

Multiple Choice Questions

21.1. A 38 year old woman, para 2+0 consults her family physician on account of new-onset painful mouth ulcers. Which statement about mouth ulcers is correct?

A. They are a common feature of inflammatory bowel disease

B. They are malignant in 10% of cases

C. They are managed with antibiotics in recurrent cases

D. They are more common in pregnancy

E. They are particularly common in patients with diverticulitis

21.2. A 19 year old female consults her family physician with recurrent oral thrush. He takes a detailed clinical history, checks a number of routine blood tests, offers her advice and starts her on an oral medication. Which statement is correct?

A. Asking about dysphagia is irrelevant because this is not caused by fungal infections

B. Oral fluconazole would be an appropriate treatment in this case

C. The correct treatment is broad-spectrum antibiotics

D. The doctor should not start any treatment before confirming the presence of *Candida albicans* on brushings or biopsies

E. The oral contraceptive pill is the commonest cause of oral thrush in young females

21.3. Which of the following statements about achalasia is correct?

A. Barrett's oesophagus is a common finding on endoscopy

B. Chest pain and heartburn are the usual presenting symptoms

C. In Europe and North America, most cases are caused by infestation with *Trypanosoma cruzi*

D. Manometry demonstrates failure of relaxation of the lower oesophageal sphincter on swallowing and absent or weak simultaneous contractions in the oesophageal body after swallowing

E. Peroral endoscopic myotomy (POEM) is the treatment of choice

21.4. A 32 year old man with a body mass index of 32 kg/m^2 consults his family physician with a long history of heartburn and frequent use of over-the-counter antacids. The family physician prescribes a 1-month course of omeprazole, which cures his symptoms but they soon return after stopping the omeprazole. The family physician refers him for an upper gastrointestinal (GI) endoscopy, which shows evidence of a small hiatus hernia and Barrett's oesophagus. Which statement is true?

A. Acid is the only refluxate that causes injury to the lower oesophageal mucosa

B. Gastro-oesophageal reflux disease (GORD) can be reliably diagnosed by symptoms

C. Most patients who develop oesophagitis, Barrett's oesophagus or peptic strictures have a hiatus hernia

D. Patients are invariably obese

E. The incidence of GORD is decreasing in most populations

21.5. The patient in Question 21.4 returns to his family physician after the endoscopy with considerable anxiety. He was alarmed by the mention of 'Barrett's oesophagus' in his endoscopy report, which his internet search classified as a 'pre-malignant' condition. His maternal uncle died of 'gullet cancer' and he is naturally very concerned about his own risks. Which statement about Barrett's oesophagus is correct?

A. Annual surveillance endoscopy in all patients with Barrett's oesophagus is mandatory

B. Barrett's oesophagus is a condition in which the normal columnar mucosa of the lower oesophagus is replaced by squamous mucosa

C. It is a pre-malignant condition with a 1000-fold increased relative risk of oesophageal cancer but with a lower absolute risk (5–10% per year)

D. It is an entirely benign condition and his family physician should reassure him that it is not associated with oesophageal cancer

E. Treatment of Barrett's oesophagus is only indicated for symptoms of reflux or complications, such as stricture

21.6. A sprightly 82 year old woman with a past history of a small hiatus hernia is recently diagnosed with osteoporosis and started on appropriate treatment. Three months later she complains to her family physician during a routine visit of progressive dysphagia to solids, especially to meat. The family physician notes that she has lost 3 kg in weight although she retains a good appetite. She has no other symptoms and clinical examination is otherwise unremarkable. What is the most likely explanation?

A. She has an early oesophageal cancer

B. She has developed eosinophilic oesophagitis, a common condition at that age

C. She has developed the Plummer–Vinson syndrome

D. She is developing early dementia and forgetting to eat her meals

E. She was started on bisphosphonates for the osteoporosis

21.7. A 28 year old male body builder consults his family physician on account of intractable heartburn, severe regurgitation and retrosternal/epigastric pain. An upper GI endoscopy 2 years previously confirmed the presence of moderate oesophagitis. He had already received multiple courses of different proton pump inhibitors (PPIs) in escalating doses and symptoms have

settled on the highest dose of esomeprazole. Although he lives a very healthy lifestyle (non-smoker, no alcohol), he is unwilling to abandon his body building and heavy exercise regime. Which statement is correct?

A. He should be referred for a POEM because of his young age

B. He should be referred for an open Heller's myotomy

C. He should be referred for oesophageal manometry and 24-hour pH studies with a view to laparoscopic fundoplication

D. His medical therapy should be optimised with the addition of calcium channel blockers

E. Long-term use of PPIs is not a concern in this young and healthy patient

21.8. A 56 year old man with no prior history of GORD presents with progressive dysphagia and weight loss of 10 kg over a 3-month period. He is a heavy smoker (40 pack years) and consumes on average 40 units of alcohol per week. He also complains of fits of coughing after swallowing. Which statement is correct?

A. He is likely suffering from a chronic food bolus obstruction

B. He is more likely to have a squamous cell carcinoma than an oesophageal adenocarcinoma

C. He likely has 'Boerhaave's syndrome'

D. He should be referred for an urgent barium swallow

E. The lack of GORD symptoms excludes oesophageal adenocarcinoma arising on a background of Barrett's oesophagus

21.9. Considering oesophageal carcinoma, which statement is correct?

A. Approximately 70% of patients have extensive disease at presentation

B. Globally, adenocarcinoma is more common than squamous cell carcinoma

C. Metastases from oesophageal carcinoma are usually localised to regional nodes adjacent to the tumour

D. Oesophageal adenocarcinoma is particularly common in the middle third of the oesophagus

E. Risk factors for squamous cell carcinoma include achalasia, radiation oesophagitis, caustic oesophageal stricture, Barrett's mucosa and Plummer–Vinson (Paterson–Brown–Kelly) syndrome

21.10. A 74 year old man with dysphagia and weight loss is diagnosed with oesophageal adenocarcinoma on upper GI endoscopy. He has a past medical history of hypertension, diet-controlled type 2 diabetes and mild asthma. Which statement concerning his investigations and management is correct?

A. Endoscopic ultrasound (EUS) is particularly useful in assessing distant metastasis

B. Invasion of the aorta, major airways or coeliac axis usually precludes surgery

C. Oesophageal adenocarcinoma is very sensitive to radiotherapy

D. Staging is futile, as his past medical history precludes any operative intervention

E. The overall 5-year survival of oesophageal adenocarcinoma is 50%

21.11. Which statement is true regarding *Helicobacter pylori* (*H. pylori*) infection?

A. Asymptomatic subjects are rarely infected by *H. pylori*

B. It is always present in patients with dyspepsia

C. It is always present in patients with peptic ulcers

D. It is usually acquired during early adulthood

E. When present, it is always associated with gastritis

21.12. A 55 year old man presents with progressive anorexia, weight loss, diarrhoea, nausea and vomiting, and profound peripheral oedema. Blood tests show evidence of anaemia and hypoalbuminaemia. Upper GI endoscopy shows enlarged, nodular and coarse gastric folds. What is the most likely diagnosis?

A. Classic NSAID gastropathy

B. Crohn's disease of the stomach

C. Cronkhite–Canada syndrome

D. GI manifestations of thyrotoxicosis

E. Ménétrier's disease

21.13. A 57 year old man who is a heavy smoker presents to his family physician with epigastric pain, occasional vomiting, tiredness and easy fatigability. Clinical examination reveals signs of anaemia and epigastric tenderness but no masses or organomegaly. Routine blood tests confirm mild iron deficiency anaemia but no other abnormalities.

Which action by the family physician is the most appropriate?

A. She should arrange for him to have an urgent barium meal

B. She should check his *H. pylori* serology and start him on eradication therapy if positive.

C. She should start him immediately on *H. pylori* eradication therapy

D. She should start him on a course of PPIs and review him in 2 months for repeat blood tests

E. She should start him on PPIs and refer him for an urgent upper GI endoscopy

21.14. The above patient undergoes upper GI endoscopy, which shows a 2-cm chronic ulcer on the lesser curve of the stomach with no stigmata of recent haemorrhage. The rest of the upper GI tract is normal. Which statement regarding his management is the most appropriate?

A. He must have biopsies of the gastric ulcer to rule out malignancy and must have a repeat endoscopy 6–8 weeks later to confirm full healing after treatment

B. He should avoid eating citrus fruits as these may delay healing of peptic ulcers

C. He should be referred to a surgeon for consideration of highly selective vagotomy

D. He should only have antral biopsies to check for presence of *H. pylori* infection, as gastric ulcers are usually benign

E. There is no strong indication to stop smoking, as this has no impact on healing rates

21.15. The patient in Question 21.14 is found to have *H. pylori* infection. Which statement about eradication therapy is correct?

A. Erythromycin is the most useful component of eradication regimens

B. If first-line eradication therapy fails, the same course should be repeated for another week

C. Metronidazole is no longer of benefit in eradication regimens due to the very high resistance rates

D. The inclusion of high-dose, twice-daily PPI therapy in eradication regimens increases efficacy of treatment

E. The rate of success of eradication therapy is strongly dependent on the rate of amoxicillin resistance in the population

21.16. A 78 year old woman with osteoarthritis and long-term indometacin therapy presents as

21

an emergency with a short history of dizziness
and passage of black stools over 2 days.
Clinically, she has signs of anaemia,
tachycardia and hypotension. Her haemoglobin
is 55 g/L and her urea is 21 mmol/L (126 mg/
dL) with a creatinine of 85 μmol/L (0.96 mg/
dL). What is the most likely diagnosis?

A. She has acute on chronic renal failure due to
long-term NSAID therapy
B. She has bled from a gastric Dieulafoy lesion
C. She has had an acute lower GI bleed from
an NSAID-induced ulcer
D. She has had an acute upper GI bleed from
an NSAID-induced ulcer
E. She has suffered a silent myocardial
infarction, which is often asymptomatic in
older patients

21.17. Considering the acute management of
the patient in Question 21.16, what is the most
important action?

A. She should be immediately referred to the
on-call surgical team
B. She should be resuscitated with colloids/
crystalloids followed by blood products
C. She should be started on octreotide to stop
the bleeding
D. She should be started on tranexamic acid to
stop the bleeding
E. She should undergo immediate endoscopy
to treat any bleeding lesions

21.18. Gastric cancer is a leading cause of
cancer-related mortality worldwide. Which
statement about this malignancy is correct?

A. Africa has the highest incidence rates due to
the poor diet
B. Diet is the most important risk factor
C. *H. pylori* infection is the most recognised
acquired risk factor
D. The incidence has been steadily rising in
most parts of the world in the past 3
decades
E. The overall 5-year survival rates are now
around 50%

21.19. A 65 year old man presents with a
3-month history of nausea, vomiting, anorexia,
7-kg weight loss and iron deficiency anaemia.
Abdominal examination shows an epigastric
mass and a bulging nodule in the umbilicus.
Upper GI endoscopy confirms the presence
of a tumour occupying most of the
proximal stomach but not involving the

gastro-oesophageal junction. Biopsies are
obtained from the tumour and from the
tumour-free distal stomach.
Which statement is correct?

A. Biopsies from the tumour-free distal gastric
mucosa will invariably show evidence of
H. pylori infection
B. Despite the large size of this tumour, it could
still be regarded as an early cancer because
the chance of metastasis to distant organs is
small
C. The bulge in the umbilicus is known as a
Krukenberg tumour
D. The bulge in the umbilicus is likely a
metastatic nodule (Sister Joseph's
nodule)
E. The most likely histology of this tumour is
squamous cell carcinoma because of its
proximity to the oesophagus

21.20. In relation to the patient in Question
21.19, consider the management options for
gastric cancer. Which of the statements below
is the most accurate?

A. Endoscopic management is still possible if
local lymph node spread is limited
B. For locally advanced tumours, partial
gastrectomy with lymphadenectomy is the
operation of choice
C. In patients with inoperable tumours,
chemotherapy is of no value in prolonging
survival
D. Proximal tumours involving the
oesophago-gastric junction also require a
distal oesophagectomy
E. The biological agent trastuzumab may
benefit some patients whose tumours
over-express TP53

21.21. Which statement regarding gastric
lymphoma is correct?

A. EUS is a poor tool in staging gastric
lymphomas
B. For lymphomas containing t(11:18)
chromosomal translocations, *H. pylori*
eradication alone is sufficient in controlling
the disease
C. *H. pylori* infection is the cause of all gastric
lymphomas
D. High-grade B-cell lymphomas should be
treated by a combination of infliximab and
radiotherapy
E. The stomach is the most common site for
extranodal non-Hodgkin lymphoma

21.22. Which statement regarding gastrointestinal stromal cell tumours (GISTs) is correct?

A. They are differentiated from other mesenchymal tumours by expression of the *c-kit* proto-oncogene
B. They are invariably benign and do not require any specific management
C. They are particularly aggressive and require resection and treatment with imatinib (a tyrosine kinase inhibitor)
D. They arise from the interstitial cells of Lieberkühn
E. They only bleed if patients also take NSAIDs

21.23. A 23 year old woman presents with 8-month history of bloating, loose stool and bowel-opening frequency of 3 times per day. There is no weight loss. Blood tests reveal a haemoglobin of 108 g/L, a ferritin of 7 µg/L and a folate of 1 µg/L and are otherwise normal. What is the next best investigation?

A. Abdominal X-ray
B. Coeliac serology with serum immunoglobulin A (IgA)
C. Colonoscopy
D. Stool calprotectin
E. Stool culture

21.24. A 42 year old man from the Indian subcontinent presents with right iliac fossa pain that has progressively increased in severity over the last few months. This is associated with weight loss and low-grade fever. Blood analysis reveals alkaline phosphatase (ALP) of 235 U/L and γ-glutamyl transferase (GGT) of 120 U/L. Chest X-ray is normal.
What is the most likely diagnosis?

A. Chronic appendicitis
B. Crohn's disease
C. Human immunodeficiency virus (HIV)
D. Ileocolonic tuberculosis (TB)
E. Whipple's disease

21.25. A 25 year old woman presents to the family physician requesting a test for coeliac disease as her sister has received a recent diagnosis of this condition. Her blood results show a mildly positive anti-tissue transglutaminase (tTG) with a low serum IgA. What is the next best investigation?

A. Check anti-endomysial antibody (anti-EMA) and immunoglobulin G (IgG)

B. Check human leucocyte antigen (HLA) status
C. Commence a gluten-free diet and monitor for symptoms
D. Endoscopy for gastric and jejunal biopsies
E. Recheck anti-tTG and IgA on a gluten-containing diet for 7 days

21.26. Of those listed below, which pathophysiological process most likely leads to coeliac disease?

A. *H. pylori* colonisation of the small bowel mucosa
B. Ingestion of gluten-containing foods in genetically susceptible individuals leading to a T-cell-mediated mucosal response in the small bowel, associated with microbial dysbiosis
C. Ingestion of gluten-containing foods in individuals with HLA-DQ2/DQ8 status
D. Ingestion of gluten-containing foods leading to microbial dysbiosis and microbial secretion of short-chain fatty acids
E. Interrupted T-cell tolerance in the colon leading to activation of Th17 immune cells that react with gluten in the proximal small bowel

21.27. A 50 year old man presents with diarrhoea, low-grade fever and joint pains. A colonoscopy is normal. Biopsies from the terminal ileum reveal the presence of foamy macrophages. What is the appropriate management?

A. Two weeks of intravenous ceftriaxone, then oral antibiotics for 1 year
B. Seven days of oral metronidazole
C. Intravenous immunoglobulin
D. No treatment is re1quired – symptoms usually settle spontaneously
E. Oral omeprazole and restriction of dietary gluten

21.28. An 82 year old man presents with persistent fresh rectal bleeding on passing stool. He has a past history of prostate cancer diagnosed 2 years ago. Flexible sigmoidoscopy reveals a 10-cm segment of mucosal erythema associated with an abnormal vessel pattern and no ulceration. What is the most appropriate management?

A. 5-Aminosalicylate suppository
B. Endoscopic argon plasma coagulation
C. Loperamide
D. Predfoam enema
E. Sucralfate enema

21

21.29. A 36 year old woman presents with an intermittent history of diarrhoea and increased bowel-opening frequency over a 2-year period. For the last 8 months, her symptoms have worsened and become persistent. She is currently passing stool 8 times per day with urgency. The consistency of stool is watery and she reports that her stool is green in colour. Her past medical history is mild asthma and cholecystectomy 12 months ago. She has no family history of note.

What investigation is most likely to lead to the diagnosis?

A. Colonoscopy
B. Endoscopy and duodenal biopsy
C. Hydrogen breath test
D. ^{75}Se-homocholic acid taurine (SeHCAT) scan
E. Thyroid function test

21.30. A 19 year old woman presents with a 6-month history of diarrhoea, right iliac fossa pain and weight loss. Blood tests show her platelet count is 721×10^9/L, haemoglobin 100 g/L and C-reactive protein (CRP) 62 mg/L. Investigation reveals a diagnosis of terminal ileal Crohn's disease and her symptoms improve with a course of oral prednisolone. What is the next most appropriate treatment?

A. A 4-week course of ciprofloxacin
B. Anti-α4β7 integrin biologic therapy
C. Azathioprine
D. Immunoglobulin
E. Methotrexate

21.31. Inflammatory bowel disease is associated with extra-intestinal manifestations of disease. Which of the following is most commonly associated with ulcerative colitis?

A. Blepharitis
B. Primary sclerosing cholangitis
C. Psoriasis
D. Pyoderma gangrenosum
E. Renal calculi

21.32. A 27 year old man with known ulcerative colitis is admitted to hospital for management of an acute severe flare in colitis. His stool frequency is 10 times per day including nocturnal bowel opening, and he has a mild fever. Blood pressure is 122/78 mmHg, pulse is 88 beats/min; CRP is 82 mg/L. What is the most appropriate initial management?

A. Intramuscular glucocorticoids for 10 days, low-molecular-weight heparin (LMWH), intravenous fluid and then reassess response
B. Intravenous glucocorticoids for 3 days, LMWH, intravenous fluid and then reassess response
C. Intravenous vedolizumab infusion and smoking cessation
D. Loperamide and metronidazole
E. Surgery with subtotal colectomy and ileostomy

21.33. A 54 year old man with ulcerative colitis is receiving hospital treatment for acute severe ulcerative colitis. He becomes acutely unwell with sweating and shortness of breath. Pulse is 110 beats/min, blood pressure is 120/68 mmHg, temperature is 37.7°C and respiratory rate is 28 breaths/min. Oxygen saturation is 94% on air. What is the most appropriate investigation to lead to the diagnosis?

A. Chest X-ray
B. CT pulmonary angiography
C. Echocardiogram
D. Electrocardiogram
E. Troponin I

21.34. A patient with inflammatory bowel disease is commenced on azathioprine for maintenance immunosuppression. What is the appropriate advice to give the patient?

A. The patient requires an annual chest X-ray and hepatitis serology
B. The patient requires blood analysis within 1 week of starting this medication to test amylase
C. The patient requires regular blood analysis to test liver and bone marrow function
D. The patient should not conceive whilst on this medication
E. This medication reduces the risk of future malignancy

21.35. Which of the following statements most accurately describes a key pathophysiological process underlying the development of Crohn's disease?

A. Activation of colonic nicotinic receptors by smoking leads to altered host handling of adherent invasive *Escherichia coli*
B. Cytokines secreted from innate lymphoid cells cause mucosal inflammation throughout the colon

C. It is caused by an autosomal recessive inherited interleukin-10 (IL-10) genetic mutation
D. The oral microbiome changes, with predominance of *Bacteroides* spp.
E. Transmural Th1 predominant adaptive mucosal immune responses occur in association with colonic microbial dysbiosis

21.36. A 30 year old woman presents with diarrhoea, associated with passing rectal mucus and blood. A diagnosis of mild rectosigmoiditis is made on flexible sigmoidoscopy. Biopsy histology shows chronic inflammatory cell infiltrate, crypt abscesses and mild architectural distortion of the crypts. What is the most appropriate initial treatment?

A. Infliximab, anti-TNF biological therapy
B. Oral 5-aminosalicylic acid (5-ASA) such as mesalazine
C. Oral glucocorticoids
D. Predfoam enema every 2 days
E. Ustekinumab, anti-p40 biological therapy

21.37. A 23 year old man has a known diagnosis of terminal ileal Crohn's disease, diagnosed 5 years previously and treated with azathioprine therapy. He presents with increasing abdominal pain, bloating and nausea after eating. He has lost 3 kg in weight in the last 4 months. What is the best investigation to assess disease activity?

A. Barium enema
B. Calprotectin
C. Capsule enteroscopy
D. Small bowel barium meal and follow through
E. Small bowel magnetic resonance imaging (MRI) enterography

21.38. A 54 year old woman presents to clinic with urgency to pass stool and daily episodes of faecal incontinence. Flexible sigmoidoscopy does not reveal any mucosal pathology. Her history includes vaginal birth of three children, two of which required assisted delivery with forceps. What is the most appropriate first management?

A. Botox injection into internal anal sphincter
B. Defunctioning colostomy
C. Fluoxetine
D. Pelvic floor exercises and biofeedback
E. Topical treatment with 2% diltiazem cream

21.39. A 68 year old man is referred with an 8-week change in bowel-opening habit with increased frequency to 4 times/day (baseline once/day) and change in consistency to looser stool. Blood analysis reveals haemoglobin 100 g/L and ferritin of 12 µg/L. What is the most appropriate investigation to lead to the diagnosis?

A. Barium enema
B. Colonoscopy
C. CT scan of abdomen and pelvis
D. Stool culture
E. Upper GI endoscopy and duodenal biopsies

21.40. Which statement is true when considering genetic aspects of colorectal cancer?

A. Colonic polyps are precursors to the development of colorectal cancer and only arise in individuals with *APC* gene mutation
B. Familial adenomatous polyposis (FAP) is most commonly an autosomal dominant condition with mutation within the *APC* gene
C. Hereditary non-polyposis colon cancer (HNPCC) occurs in up to 50% of colorectal cancer cases and is associated with mutation in mismatch repair genes
D. Sporadic colonic cancer is directed solely by epigenetic changes rather than mutations of somatic genes
E. Sporadic colorectal cancer is associated with mutation in the *TP53* gene as an early occurrence

21.41. A 46 year old woman with scleroderma presents with frequent watery diarrhoea, bloating and weight loss. Colonoscopy is normal with no abnormality found on biopsy histology. Coeliac serology is negative, thyroid function normal and stool culture negative. Bacterial overgrowth is suspected. What would you expect to see on blood analysis to support this diagnosis?

A. Increase in immunoglobulins
B. Increased ferritin and normal haemoglobin
C. Low vitamin B_{12} and increased mean cell volume
D. Positive cytomegalovirus serology
E. Reduced gastrin

21.42. A 23 year old woman presents to the clinic with an 8-month history of variable bowel-opening habit ranging from once to 4 times per day, passing soft stool in the morning and associated with bloating in the evening. She describes left-sided crampy abdominal pain, relieved by defaecation. She is a single mother to a 3 year old boy. The company she works for has declared that jobs may not be stable during a management change. Thyroid function is normal and coeliac serology is normal.

What is the next best investigation?

A. C-reactive protein
B. Platelet count
C. Small bowel MRI
D. Stool calprotectin
E. Upper GI endoscopy and duodenal biopsies

21.43. A 30 year old woman has a diagnosis of diarrhoea-predominant IBS. Her symptoms are negatively impacting her ability to work in the local supermarket and she is avoiding social functions for fear of unpredictable onset of symptoms. She has tried a variety of dietary manipulations including a wheat-exclusion diet, a dairy-free diet and avoidance of caffeinated drinks, with no improvement of her symptoms. What is the next most appropriate treatment to consider?

A. 5-HT$_4$ agonist, prucalopride
B. Nocturnal small-dose diazepam
C. Peppermint capsule
D. Probiotics
E. Referral to dietician for consideration of a low-FODMAP (fermentable oligo-, di- and monosaccharides, and polyols) diet

21.44. Which of the statements is true when considering the normal function of the colon?

A. Absorption of folic acid occurs in the colon
B. The colon absorbs 50% of ingested protein and fats
C. The colon absorbs electrolytes and water
D. The colonic microbiota is acquired at birth and is static throughout life
E. The pH of the colonic lumen is 3

21.45. The arterial blood supply to the pancreas is shared with which other organ/tissue?

A. Left kidney
B. Ovaries
C. Psoas muscle
D. Sigmoid colon
E. Terminal ileum

21.46. A 40 year old male with a diagnosis of chronic pancreatitis complains of foul-smelling pale stools, which are difficult to flush. A deficiency in which of the following hormones/enzymes is responsible?

A. Chymotrypsin
B. Glucagon
C. Lipase
D. Maltase
E. Somatostatin

21.47. A 42 year old man has recurrent duodenal ulceration with bleeding despite omeprazole therapy use. *H. pylori* serology has been negative on three occasions. An abnormality is noticed on imaging of his pancreas. What other health problems might this man have?

A. Marfan's syndrome
B. Medullary thyroid cancer
C. Phaeochromocytoma
D. Pituitary adenoma
E. Type 1 diabetes mellitus

21.48. A 56 year old man with a history of heavy alcohol use presents with abdominal bloating following a recent episode of severe central abdominal pain radiating to the back. Clinical examination reveals resolving periumbilical bruising and abdominal distension with shifting dullness. Blood tests demonstrate bilirubin 18 μmol/L (1.05 mg/dL), alanine aminotransferase (ALT) 50 U/L, ALP 200 U/L, GGT 823 U/L, international normalised ratio (INR) 1.1. What initial test is most likely to give the correct diagnosis?

A. Alpha-fetoprotein
B. Ascitic fluid albumin
C. Ascitic fluid amylase
D. Ascitic fluid cell count
E. Serum albumin

21.49. Pancreatic fluid is normally excreted via the main pancreatic duct into the duodenum. In pancreas divisum, during embryonic development the dorsal and ventral ducts fail to fuse, leading to main excretion via the dorsal duct. Which structure does pancreatic fluid bypass in pancreas divisum?

A. Ampulla of Vater
B. Duodenum
C. Gallbladder
D. Hepatic portal vein
E. Liver

21.50. Twelve hours after endoscopic retrograde cholangiopancreatography (ERCP) for stent insertion due to biliary stricture, a patient develops severe central abdominal pain. Blood tests show bilirubin 20 μmol/L, ALT 120 U/L, ALP 80 U/L, GGT 98 U/L, amylase 1400 U/L, haemoglobin 120 g/L, WCC 12.4×10⁹/L.
What complication has she developed?

A. Ascending cholangitis
B. Common bile duct perforation
C. Duodenal perforation
D. Haemorrhage
E. Pancreatitis

21.51. A 40 year old male with long-standing alcohol excess has an episode of severe central abdominal pain. Six weeks later he develops vomiting following eating. On examination he has a gastric splash. What investigation will give the diagnosis?

A. Barium meal
B. CT pancreas
C. Oesophageal manometry
D. Upper gastrointestinal endoscopy
E. Water-soluble contrast meal

21.52. The CT scan below is from an 18 year old with recurrent chest infections since childhood and chronic diarrhoea. What abnormality can you see?

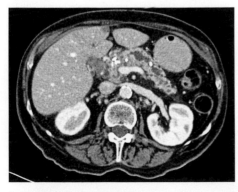

A. Calcification of pancreas
B. Colonic diverticulae
C. Common bile duct gallstones
D. Distended gallbladder
E. Small bowel stricture

21.53. A 46 year old woman with a history of gallstones presents with upper abdominal pain and is diagnosed with acute pancreatitis. Which of these features at presentation would suggest a worse prognosis?

A. Amylase 2302 U/L
B. Calcium 2.42 mmol/L
C. CRP 120 mg/L
D. Glucose 4 mmol/L (72 mg/dL)
E. PaO₂ 7.8 kPa (59 mmHg)

21.54. A 55 year old man presents with obstructive jaundice and an abnormal pancreas on CT. An elevation in which blood test would suggest this condition may respond to glucocorticoids?

A. Alpha-fetoprotein
B. Bilirubin
C. Hepatitis E IgM
D. IgG4
E. IgM

21.55. A 32 year old man with a previous pituitary adenoma has repeated admissions with duodenal ulceration despite proton pump inhibitor. What is the likely genetic mutation?

A. BRCA1
B. BRCA2
C. JAK2
D. MEN1
E. RET

21.56. A 22 year old woman presents with abdominal swelling and vomiting. Which is the diagnosis that should be excluded first?

A. Ascites
B. Bowel obstruction
C. Constipation
D. Obesity
E. Pregnancy

21.57. A 35 year old male underwent a gastric bypass 6 months ago, and now presents with fatigue and breathlessness. Blood tests demonstrate haemoglobin 58 g/L, mean cell volume 128 fL. A deficiency in which cells will lead to these test result abnormalities?

A. Chief cells
B. D cells
C. G cells
D. Oxyntic glands
E. Parietal cells

21.58. Dysbiosis within the intestinal microbiota has been associated with all of the following except one. Which of these conditions is NOT associated with dysbiosis?

21

A. Basal cell carcinoma
B. Crohn's disease
C. Depression
D. Hepatocellular carcinoma
E. Type 2 diabetes mellitus

21.59. Which of the following is a defence mechanism that is unique to the stomach?

A. Hydrochloric acid secretion
B. Immunoglobulins
C. Macrophages
D. Peyer's patches
E. T lymphocytes

21.60. A female patient with rheumatoid arthritis presents with dysphagia and is referred for oesophago-gastroduodenoscopy (OGD). However, the endoscopist would prefer a barium swallow as this patient's first investigation. Of which complication of OGD might the patient be particularly at risk given her history?

A. Acute severe colitis
B. Atlantoaxial subluxation
C. Cardiac arrhythmias
D. Respiratory distress
E. Small bowel perforation

21.61. A 60 year old man presents with a history of dysphagia. Which of the following features would suggest that the problem originates in the oesophagus?

A. A sticking sensation retrosternally in response to oral intake
B. Altered voice
C. Drooling
D. Nasal regurgitation
E. Symptoms worse with liquids

21.62. A 29 year patient with type 1 diabetes on insulin with poor glycaemic control has a 6-month history of vomiting around 1 hour following food. What is the most likely diagnosis?

A. Gastric outlet obstruction
B. Gastroparesis
C. *H. pylori* infection
D. Medication-induced vomiting
E. Raised intracranial pressure

21.63. A 24 year old man presents with fresh haematemesis the day after a night of heavy alcohol consumption, during which he had a prolonged period of vomiting. Which of the following statements is correct?

A. A Mallory–Weiss tear never causes significant bleeding
B. In the absence of melaena, upper gastrointestinal endoscopy is not indicated
C. Results showing urea 6 mmol/L (36 mg/dL), haemoglobin 131 g/L and blood pressure 112/65 mmHg mean the patient can be safely discharged
D. The likely diagnosis is oesophageal varices
E. The majority of cases like this heal completely within 2 weeks

21.64. A 60 year old with a background of non-alcoholic steatohepatitis with cirrhosis presents with fresh haematemesis, melaena and collapse. Endoscopy reveals oesophageal varices as the origin of bleeding. Which of the following is an appropriate treatment?

A. Band ligation
B. Clip placement
C. Heater probe coagulation
D. Injection of adrenaline (epinephrine)
E. Laparotomy

21.65. A 40 year old man presents with diarrhoea, weight loss, night sweats and multiple enlarged lymph nodes. He has recently had a vesicular rash on his right torso. Which one investigation would give a unifying diagnosis?

A. Coeliac serology
B. Colonoscopy
C. Faecal calprotectin
D. HIV test
E. Thyroid function tests

21.66. An individual with coeliac disease is admitted to the high dependency unit with a pneumococcal bacteraemia. What disease associated with coeliac disease is likely responsible?

A. Primary biliary cirrhosis
B. Sarcoidosis
C. Small bowel lymphoma
D. Splenic atrophy
E. Type 1 diabetes mellitus

Answers

21.1. Answer: A.
The incidence of mouth ulcers is not increased during pregnancy but it is higher in women prior to menstruation. Although mouth ulcers are very common in the general population (up to 30%), malignancy is relatively rare. Mouth ulcers are not related to diverticulitis but they are common in inflammatory bowel diseases such as Crohn's disease and ulcerative colitis. There is no evidence that antibiotic therapy is particularly useful in the management of mouth ulcers but topical (and occasionally oral) glucocorticoids are useful.

21.2. Answer: B.
Dysphagia and odynophagia should always be asked about in case there is oesophageal candidiasis. There is no convincing evidence that the oral contraceptive pill, particularly in young females, is associated with oral thrush. First-line treatment is with nystatin or amphotericin suspensions or lozenges. Resistant cases (as likely in this case with recurrent infection) or immunosuppressed patients may require oral fluconazole. Antibiotic use is associated with increased risk of oral thrush. The diagnosis is largely clinical and treatment could be started on the basis of the history and examination alone. Mycological confirmation could be sought in brushings or biopsies but is not usually necessary.

21.3. Answer: D.
In South America, infestation by the parasite *T. cruzi* causes a condition (Chagas' disease) that is clinically indistinguishable from achalasia. In Europe and North America, the cause of achalasia is largely unknown. The commonest presenting symptoms are dysphagia, regurgitation (indigested food) and weight loss. Chest pain is uncommon and heartburn is not a feature, as acid reflux does not occur against a closed sphincter. As such, patients do not develop Barrett's oesophagus. However, achalasia is regarded as a pre-malignant condition with a small risk of oesophageal cancer (squamous cell and adenocarcinoma), usually after 20 years. The classic manometric findings of achalasia are failure of relaxation of the lower oesophageal sphincter on swallowing and absent or weak simultaneous contractions in the oesophageal body after swallowing.

POEM is a new endoscopic technique that is performed in very specialised units and has not replaced the more established treatment modalities of pneumatic dilatation, endoscopic botulinum toxin injection of the lower oesophageal sphincter and surgery (Heller's myotomy).

21.4. Answer: C.
Hiatus hernia is very common in GORD and its complications, and is implicated in the pathogenesis of reflux. Symptoms are notoriously misleading in the diagnosis. Acid, bile and pepsin all cause injury, although acid is the main factor. The incidence is rising in most populations. GORD can occur in very lean individuals, although it is more common in overweight and obese individuals.

21.5. Answer: E.
Barrett's oesophagus is a pre-malignant condition in which the normal squamous lining of the lower oesophagus is replaced by columnar mucosa that may contain areas of intestinal metaplasia. The relative risk of oesophageal cancer is 40- to 120-fold increased but the absolute risk is low (0.1–0.5% per year). Surveillance is expensive and cost-effectiveness studies have been conflicting, but it is currently recommended that patients with Barrett's oesophagus with intestinal metaplasia, but without dysplasia, should undergo endoscopy at 3- to 5-yearly intervals if the length of the Barrettic segment is less than 3 cm and at 2- to 3-yearly intervals if the length is greater than 3 cm. Those with low-grade dysplasia should be endoscoped at 6-monthly intervals. Neither potent acid suppression nor anti-reflux surgery stops progression or induces regression of Barrett's oesophagus, and thus treatment is only indicated for symptoms of reflux or complications, such as stricture.

21.6. Answer: E.
Elderly patients generally have a higher prevalence of oesophageal motility disorders that affect swallowing. In this case, she is very likely to have been started on bisphosphonates for her osteoporosis. Bisphosphonates cause oesophageal ulceration and should be used with caution in patients with known

21

oesophageal disorders. Patients should be clearly instructed to always take their dose with a full glass of water on an empty stomach, and to stand or sit upright for at least 30 minutes after taking the dose. Eosinophilic oesophagitis is much more common in children. This patient is less likely to have a cancer as she retains her appetite and general well-being. The Plummer–Vinson syndrome is a rare disease characterised by dysphagia, iron deficiency anaemia, angular stomatitis, atrophic glossitis, cheilosis and oesophageal webs. She had none of these features on clinical examination.

21.7. Answer: C.
Long-term PPI therapy is associated with reduced absorption of iron, vitamin B_{12} and magnesium. The drugs also predispose to enteric infections with *Salmonella*, *Campylobacter* and possibly *Clostridium difficile* and have recently been shown to have an undesirable impact on the composition of the gut microbiota. Heller's myotomy and POEM are procedures for treatment of achalasia not GORD. In this young and healthy patient, medical therapy has clearly failed and he requires laparoscopic anti-reflux surgery. Some calcium channel blockers relax the lower oesophageal sphincter and can cause reflux and heartburn.

21.8. Answer: B.
The diagnosis here is strongly in favour of a malignant oesophageal stricture. With such a presentation, he should be referred for an urgent upper GI endoscopy with biopsies in the first instance. Barium swallow demonstrates the site and length of the stricture but adds little useful information. Food bolus obstruction presents acutely and is an endoscopic emergency. Lack of GORD symptoms is frequently noted in patients who present with oesophageal adenocarcinoma and Barrett's oesophagus, although GORD is a strong risk factor for both. In this case, the combination of lack of GORD symptoms, heavy smoking and alcohol consumption favour a diagnosis of oesophageal squamous cell cancer. Boerhaave's syndrome is spontaneous oesophageal perforation that results from forceful vomiting and retching. In this case, the fits of coughing on swallowing are likely caused by a fistula between the oesophagus and the trachea or bronchial tree. Fistulation can also lead to pneumonia and pleural effusion.

21.9. Answer: A.
The majority of oesophageal cancers worldwide are squamous cell carcinomas, but the incidence of adenocarcinoma in Western countries now exceeds that of squamous carcinoma. Unfortunately, oesophageal cancer presents late and 70% of patients present with extensive and inoperable disease. All of the listed risk factors are pre-malignant lesions but Barrett's metaplasia is associated with the development of adenocarcinoma, not squamous carcinoma. Squamous carcinoma can occur in any part of the oesophagus, and almost all tumours in the upper oesophagus are squamous cancers. Adenocarcinomas typically arise in the lower third of the oesophagus from Barrett's oesophagus or from the cardia of the stomach. Oesophageal cancer is very aggressive, invading locally and metastasising to local and distant sites quite early.

21.10. Answer: B.
His past medical history is not unusual and does not preclude surgical intervention. The patient should undergo extensive staging with thoracic and abdominal CT, often combined with positron emission tomography (CT-PET). This will identify metastatic spread and local invasion. Patients with resectable disease on imaging should undergo endoscopic ultrasound (EUS) to determine the depth of penetration of the tumour into the oesophageal wall and to detect locoregional lymph node involvement. EUS is clearly not suitable for assessing distant metastasis. The overall 5-year survival of oesophageal cancer is very poor (< 15%). Squamous carcinoma is sensitive to radiotherapy, unlike adenocarcinoma, although radiotherapy could be used to palliate obstructing tumours of both varieties.

21.11. Answer: E.
H. pylori is usually acquired during childhood; acquisition in adults is rare. Dyspeptic patients have a higher prevalence of *H. pylori* compared to asymptomatic subjects but many patients with dyspepsia do not have the infection. Around 90% of duodenal ulcer patients and 70% of gastric ulcer patients are infected with *H. pylori*. The remaining 30% of gastric ulcers are caused by non-steroidal anti-inflammatory drugs (NSAIDs)/aspirin. There are also more rare causes of ulcers such as Zollinger–Ellison syndrome and gastroduodenal Crohn's

disease. Half of the world's population is infected with *H. pylori* and the majority are asymptomatic. The hallmark of *H. pylori* infection is the induction of gastritis, which is the pathognomonic histological consequence of the infection. This histological gastritis may or may not be endoscopically visible and may or may not cause symptoms.

21.12. Answer: E.

These features are very consistent with Ménétrier's disease, which is a rare condition of unknown aetiology characterised by excessive production of transforming growth factor-alpha (TGF-α). As a result, the mucosal folds of the body and fundus are greatly enlarged. Whilst some patients have upper gastrointestinal symptoms, the majority present in middle or old age with protein-losing enteropathy due to exudation from the gastric mucosa. Endoscopy shows enlarged, nodular and coarse folds. Crohn's disease of the stomach usually presents with deep ulcers. Hyperthyroidism is associated with gastrointestinal symptoms but does not usually cause any endoscopic features. Cronkhite–Canada syndrome may present with generalised gastrointestinal polyps, cutaneous pigmentation, alopecia and onychodystrophy. NSAID gastropathy presents with gastritis, erosions or single/multiple superficial ulcers.

21.13. Answer: E.

This patient clearly requires urgent upper GI endoscopy to rule out significant pathology, particularly gastric neoplasia. The absence of weight loss and persistent vomiting is reassuring but the presence of anaemia is alarming and should trigger urgent referral for endoscopy. Barium meal is rarely used. The other options are inappropriate because urgent endoscopy is mandatory in this situation and over-rides the other suggestions.

21.14. Answer: A.

Gastric ulcers may occasionally be malignant and therefore must always be biopsied and followed up to ensure healing. He should, of course, have antral biopsies to check for *H. pylori* and this should be eradicated if positive, but he should also have the ulcer edge biopsied. Surgery is no longer an option in the management of peptic ulcer disease unless there are severe complications such as gastric outlet obstruction, uncontrollable bleeding or

perforation. Once a peptic ulcer forms, it is more likely to cause complications and less likely to heal if the patient continues to smoke. There is no specific dietary advice and citrus fruits have no relevance in this situation.

21.15. Answer: D.

The rate of success of treatment is dependent on several factors, including medication adherence and antibiotic resistance. The most important is resistance to clarithromycin. Amoxicillin resistance is very rare. Treatment is based on a PPI taken simultaneously with two antibiotics (from amoxicillin, clarithromycin and metronidazole) for at least 7 days. High-dose, twice-daily PPI therapy increases efficacy of treatment, as does extending treatment to 10–14 days. Metronidazole is still useful in eradication regimens because in vitro resistance to the antibiotic could be overcome in vivo by combination with other effective antibiotics, especially clarithromycin. If the first-line therapy fails, the same course should not be repeated but quadruple therapy, consisting of a PPI, bismuth subcitrate, metronidazole and tetracycline (OBMT) for 10–14 days, is recommended. Erythromycin is never used in eradication regimens but clarithromycin, another macrolide, is one of the most effective in use.

21.16. Answer: D.

She has a high urea but her creatinine level is within the upper range of normal for women. NSAIDs cause renal damage but the most serious abnormality in this case is the suspected GI bleed. A silent myocardial infarction is a possible complication of an acute and significant GI bleed but it is not the most likely diagnosis here. NSAIDs cause ulceration throughout the GI tract but lesions that bleed are most likely in the upper part, including gastric and duodenal ulcers. Melaena (black tarry stool) is characteristic of an upper GI bleed. Lower GI bleeds present with fresh blood. Dieulafoy lesions are rare causes of upper GI bleeding and are caused by a single tortuous small artery in the submucosa that may erode through the mucosa and cause significant bleeding. These lesions are diagnosed endoscopically.

21.17. Answer: B.

This patient is clearly haemodynamically compromised and in shock. The most

21

immediate management should focus on resuscitation. Upper GI endoscopy should not be carried out before resuscitation.

21.18. Answer: C.

The incidence of gastric cancer has, in fact, been falling steadily across the world, although it is still a global killer. *H. pylori* infection is the most important risk factor and this far outweighs all the other traditional risk factors, such as diet. *H. pylori* plays a key pathogenic role and the infection has been classified by the International Agency for Research on Cancer (IARC) as a definite human carcinogen. Despite advances in treatment, the overall 5-year survival is still low (<30%). Africa has a low incidence of gastric cancer (the so-called African enigma) despite having high rates of *H. pylori* infection.

21.19. Answer: D.

Virtually all gastric tumours are adenocarcinomas arising from mucus-secreting cells in the base of the gastric crypts. Gastric cancers are very aggressive and usually present quite late with large sizes and with distant spread. While most gastric cancers are initiated by *H. pylori* infection, the organism often disappears in the latter stages with onset of gastric atrophy and achlorhydria. Krukenberg tumours are metastatic deposits on the ovaries. Sister Joseph's nodule is a metastatic deposit in the umbilicus usually from a cancer in the pelvis or abdomen.

21.20. Answer: D.

Endoscopic management of gastric cancer is confined to very early mucosal or submucosal disease with no spread elsewhere. For the majority of patients with locally advanced disease, total gastrectomy with lymphadenectomy is the operation of choice. In the surgical management of proximal gastric cancers involving the oesophago-gastric junction, distal oesophagectomy is also required. The biological agent trastuzumab may benefit some patients whose tumours over-express HER2. In patients with inoperable tumours, survival can be improved and palliation of symptoms achieved with chemotherapy using 5-fluorouracil and cisplatin, ECF (epirubicin, cisplatin and fluorouracil) or other platinum- and taxane-based regimens.

21.21. Answer: E.

The stomach is the most common site for extranodal non-Hodgkin lymphoma and 60% of all primary gastrointestinal lymphomas occur at this site. *H. pylori* infection is closely associated with the development of a low-grade lymphoma (classified as extranodal marginal-zone lymphomas of mucosa-associated lymphoid tissue (MALT) type). EUS plays an important role in staging these lesions by accurately defining the depth of invasion into the gastric wall. High-grade B-cell lymphomas should be treated by a combination of rituximab, chemotherapy, surgery and radiotherapy. While initial treatment of low-grade lesions confined to the superficial layers of the gastric wall consists of *H. pylori* eradication and close observation, 25% contain t(11:18) chromosomal translocations. In these cases, additional radiotherapy or chemotherapy is usually necessary.

21.22. Answer: A.

GISTs arise from the interstitial cells of Cajal. They are differentiated from other mesenchymal tumours by expression of the *c-kit* proto-oncogene. They are usually benign tumours, particularly the smaller lesions <2 cm, and asymptomatic, but the larger ones may have malignant potential. Very large lesions should be treated pre-operatively with imatinib to reduce their size and make surgery easier. Imatinib can also be used for prolonged control of metastatic GISTs. They can bleed independently of NSAIDs.

21.23. Answer: B.

Given the duration of the symptoms, this is not likely to be infection. X-ray is not likely to aid diagnosis and exposes the patient to ionising radiation. Given the constellation of symptoms, mild anaemia and low folate in a patient of this age, coeliac disease should be considered initially and therefore coeliac serology is the next best investigation.

21.24. Answer: D.

Abdominal TB is a common cause of these symptoms in the Indian subcontinent and other areas of the world where TB is endemic. In the UK/US, Crohn's disease would be the most likely diagnosis. Granulomatous hepatitis resulting in cholestatic liver function tests can be present in TB. Despite the diagnosis, chest X-ray can be normal.

21.25. Answer: A.
Anti-tTG response is IgA mediated and therefore can be false negative in IgA deficiency. Therefore, IgG-mediated antibodies should be checked next. If positive, the patient should be offered an endoscopy for distal duodenal/duodenal bulb biopsies. HLA status is not exclusive and is not a reliable diagnostic test, although it can aid diagnosis in some cases where serology/histology are equivocal.

21.26. Answer: B.
The pathophysiology of coeliac disease is multifactorial. HLA status is associated but not exclusive. There is no evidence that *H. pylori* is linked to coeliac disease.

21.27. Answer: A.
These symptoms and the presence of small bowel foamy macrophages histologically lead to a diagnosis of Whipple's disease. The appropriate treatment is extended antibiotic treatment with 2 weeks of intravenous ceftriaxone, then oral antibiotics for 1 year. The other treatments discussed would not be appropriate.

21.28. Answer: E.
The diagnosis is radiation proctitis. This commonly occurs after radiotherapy for prostate cancer. The aetiology is chronic ischaemia rather than inflammation and therefore steroid/anti-inflammatory treatments are ineffective. Endoscopic argon plasma coagulation (APC) can be used for acute bleeding but can increase risk of fistula formation with repeated use. Evidence suggests sucralfate enema is the best treatment and, if this fails, hyperbaric oxygen therapy should be considered.

21.29. Answer: D.
All these investigations can be considered in this patient. Given the colour and consistency of stool and previous cholecystectomy, the most likely diagnosis is bile acid malabsorption; therefore a radionuclide SeHCAT scan is the correct answer in this scenario.

21.30. Answer: C.
There is no evidence for use of antibiotics. Immunoglobulin is used for chronic *Giardia* infection associated with immunoglobulin deficiency. Options B, C and E (all immunosuppressants) can be used in Crohn's

disease, as well as anti-tumour necrosis factor (TNF) biological therapy. Methotrexate would not be used here given toxicities that include teratogenicity in women of child-bearing age. Thiopurine immunosuppression with azathioprine is the next most appropriate medication to prevent a further flare in disease.

21.31. Answer: B.
Inflammatory bowel disease (IBD) is a multisystemic disorder with extra-intestinal manifestations (Fig. 21.31). Psoriasis is not usually associated with IBD but can be associated with anti-TNF biological therapy. Ocular manifestations are episcleritis and anterior uveitis. Blepharitis is not associated with IBD. Pyoderma gangrenosum and renal calculi are associated with Crohn's disease rather than ulcerative colitis. Ulcerative colitis with primary sclerosing cholangitis is associated with high risk of colon cancer and these patients require annual surveillance colonoscopy.

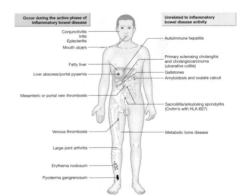

Fig. 21.31 Systemic complications of inflammatory bowel disease.

21.32. Answer: B.
Intravenous glucocorticoid therapy is indicated in this case of acute severe ulcerative colitis (>6 bloody stools/24 hrs, raised CRP). Current guidelines suggest review at day 3 and then day 5 for clinical and biochemical response. If non-response, rescue medical therapies with anti-TNF biological therapy or ciclosporin can be considered. Alternatively, non-response to intravenous (IV) steroid therapy ± rescue medical therapies require a surgical review for

21

consideration of subtotal colectomy and ileostomy. LMWH is required as these patients are at increased risk of thrombosis. Loperamide may precipitate toxic megacolon. There is no evidence for antibiotic therapy. Vedolizumab (anti-α4β7 integrin biological therapy) can be considered for maintenance treatment of IBD; it has a long onset of action and therefore has no role in the management of acute severe colitis.

21.33. Answer: B.

A complication of acute severe IBD is thrombosis. This presentation and clinical status suggest a pulmonary embolus and therefore CTPA is most likely to lead to the diagnosis. Whilst some of the other investigations may be appropriate in the acute scenario, they will not necessarily lead to the diagnosis.

21.34. Answer: C.

Regular blood monitoring is required to assess for bone marrow suppression and liver dysfunction. The interval between blood analysis increases as time passes from induction. Very rarely, azathioprine can cause acute pancreatitis; amylase should be tested if a patient presents with acute abdominal pain and vomiting soon after starting this medication. If a patient is stable on azathioprine, advice is to continue throughout pregnancy, as risk of teratogenicity is very low and a greater risk is uncontrolled IBD.

The side-effects of thiopurines include a small increased risk of malignancy with extended use, particularly lymphoma and non-melanoma skin cancer. A chest X-ray and hepatitis serology should be checked prior to anti-TNF biological therapy to avoid reactivation of latent TB or worsening of hepatitis B/C infection.

21.35. Answer: E.

The pathogenesis of IBD is complex and involves breakdown of the epithelial barrier and disordered mucosal immune responses, associated with microbial dysbiosis in genetically susceptible individuals. Genome-wide association studies have identified multiple polymorphisms in genes, including cytokine genes, but there is no one somatic mutation driver gene identified. The immune response involves both innate and adaptive aspects and the cytokines secreted

from these cells. Crohn's disease can affect the whole gastrointestinal tract and is associated with a predominant Th1 adaptive response and ulcerative colitis is associated with a Th2 response. There is ongoing research into the pathogenesis of IBD, including alterations in the oral microbiome and the role of specific bacteria, including *E. coli*.

21.36. Answer: B.

The distribution and histology features of the inflammation are in keeping with ulcerative colitis. In mild disease, a high-dose oral 5-ASA is appropriate first-line therapy, reducing to a maintenance dose when symptoms are under control. If symptoms do not settle, then addition of topical (enema) treatment with either 5-ASA or steroid, or a course of oral glucocorticoids, can be considered. Anti-TNF therapy is a treatment for moderate to severe ulcerative colitis, refractory to other immunosuppression including thiopurines (such as azathioprine). Clinical trial data suggest that ustekinumab may be a new treatment choice in severe Crohn's disease but it is still in development and is not yet used as a standard of care.

21.37. Answer: E.

This patient's symptoms are consistent with active small bowel Crohn's disease with subacute obstruction precipitated by eating and he needs investigation to assess disease activity and presence of stricturing. MRI enterography is a sensitive modality to assess mucosal inflammation and calibre of small bowel lumen. A small bowel barium meal and follow through will also show this information but is less sensitive than MRI and exposes this young patient to ionising radiation. A capsule enteroscopy is contraindicated here, given suspicion of stricturing with risk of impaction. Small bowel disease is suspected in this case and a barium enema would assess the colon. If colonic investigation is required, a colonoscopy would be first choice in a patient of this age. Stool calprotectin would likely be high, in keeping with intestinal inflammation, but would not give additional information on structural aspects of disease activity.

21.38. Answer: D.

This woman is likely to have damage to the pelvic floor/anal sphincter from previous childbirth. Exercises to strengthen the pelvic floor along with biofeedback techniques to regulate bowel-opening pattern is the first treatment to try. If unsuccessful, sacral nerve stimulators can be considered and some patients require defunctioning colostomy. Botox injection and topical diltiazem cream are used for relaxation of the anal sphincter to treat anal fissure.

21.39. Answer: B.
In a patient of this age with 'red flag' symptoms of change in bowel-opening habit to loose stool and iron deficiency anaemia, the suspicion is colorectal cancer and therefore colonoscopy is the best next investigation. CT scan will detect large mass lesions and metastatic disease but is not sensitive for smaller localised mucosal lesions. Colonoscopy allows biopsies to be taken for histological analysis.

21.40. Answer: B.
Most colorectal cancer is sporadic with no identifiable genetic predisposition. Most sporadic colorectal cancer arises from a benign pre-malignant adenoma (polyp). Aetiology is multifactorial, involving genetic and environmental risk factors. The genetic risk factors include acquired mutations of somatic genes such as *APC*, *TP53* and *SMAD4*, and these tend to occur sequentially over time, with *APC* mutations an early feature and *TP53* a late feature. Epigenetic changes can also lead to altered gene expression. These genetic changes are not mutually exclusive – not all individuals with these mutations develop colorectal cancer and not all colorectal tumours will contain all of these genetic mutations. Approximately 5% of colorectal cancers are attributable to genetic syndromes, the most common being FAP and HNPCC.

21.41. Answer: C.
Often patients with bacterial overgrowth are anaemic with a macrocytosis and low vitamin B_{12} due to bacterial utilisation of the vitamin B_{12} in the gastrointestinal lumen. The other answers are not findings you would expect with this diagnosis.

21.42. Answer: D.
The history is consistent with irritable bowel syndrome (IBS). It is important to explore social history. She is experiencing stress in her life with regard to employment and worry of loss of financial income to support her child and this may be impacting on these symptoms. In a patient of this age, the main diagnostic considerations are IBS and IBD. CRP and platelet count may be elevated in the latter but not always. A stool calprotectin is a more sensitive marker of gastrointestinal inflammation in this scenario to guide need for further investigation and appropriate treatment. Coeliac serology is negative, so there is no indication for proceeding to duodenal biopsy.

21.43. Answer: E.
There is no evidence for the use of benzodiazepines for IBS. An appropriate next-line treatment would be a low-dose nocturnal tricyclic antidepressant such as amitriptyline. There is no evidence for the use of probiotics. Peppermint capsules can often help with bloating and flatus in IBS patients. Prucalopride is used as a treatment in constipation-predominant IBS that has failed to respond to laxative therapy. There is emerging evidence that a low-FODMAP diet is effective in the treatment of IBS. This should be supervised by a dietician and is initially very restrictive, with gradual reintroduction of food groups dependent on symptom response.

21.44. Answer: C.
Protein, fat and folic acid absorption occur in the small bowel. The colonic luminal pH is mildly acidic to neutral (5.5–7). The colonic microbiota is acquired at birth, matures to that of an adult by the age of 3 years and changes over time as a natural part of ageing in the elderly years. It can also change in relation to environmental alterations such as use of antibiotics. The colon acts to absorb water and electrolytes from stool.

21.45. Answer: E.
The pancreatic body and tail receive supply from the splenic artery derived from the coeliac artery. The head of pancreas received supply from the inferior pancreaticoduodenal artery derived from the superior mesenteric artery (SMA). The SMA also supplies the ileum, alongside jejunum, ascending and transverse colon. The left kidney is supplied by the renal artery, ovaries by the gonadal artery, the sigmoid colon by the inferior mesenteric artery and the psoas muscle by the lumbar arteries.

21

21.46. Answer C.

This man gives a history of steatorrhoea, due to high lipid contents in his stools. Pancreatic lipase, in the presence of its co-factor, colipase, cleaves long-chain triglycerides, yielding fatty acids and monoglycerides, which are small enough to diffuse across enterocyte cell membranes. In chronic pancreatitis, inadequate pancreatic lipase production leads to high fat content in stools due to poor digestion. Chymotrypsin may be deficient as well, but leads to protein deficiencies. Glucagon and somatostatin are endocrine hormones secreted by the pancreas and for unclear reasons tend not to be associated with deficiency in chronic pancreatitis. Maltase is an enzyme found on small intestine brush border.

21.47. Answer: D.

In recurrent duodenal ulceration in a young patient, Zollinger–Ellison syndrome should be considered. Gastrinoma as part of multiple endocrine neoplasia (MEN) type 1 is a recognised cause of Zollinger–Ellison syndrome, of which pituitary adenoma is a common additional tumour. Phaechromocytoma and medullary thyroid cancer are associated with MEN type 2 (not type 1) and Marfan's syndrome, so are not linked to gastrinoma.

21.48. Answer C.

This man gives a history of acute pancreatitis, probably secondary to alcohol, and now presents with ascites. His liver function tests show a normal liver synthetic function (bilirubin and INR), which makes portal hypertension due to chronic liver disease an unlikely cause of the ascites. Ruptured pancreatic pseudocyst is a recognised complication of acute pancreatitis and leads to an elevated ascitic fluid amylase.

21.49. Answer: A.

In a normal pancreas the pancreatic duct meets the common bile duct at the ampulla of Vater, where it enters the duodenum. The pancreatic duct does not communicate directly with the liver, hepatic portal vein or gallbladder in a normal pancreas. In pancreas divisum, two pancreatic ducts remain present, the dominant dorsal duct draining directly into the duodenum rather than joining the common bile duct at the sphincter of Oddi, bypassing this.

21.50. Answer: E.

All the options listed are recognised complications of ERCP, but an extremely high amylase would point to pancreatitis. The complication rate following ERCP is 5–10% with a 30-day mortality of 0.5–1%, depending on the procedure complexity, underlying condition and comorbidities. Acute pancreatitis is the most common complication.

21.51. Answer: B.

This man had alcohol-related acute pancreatitis and has developed a pancreatic pseudocyst. Large pancreatic pseudocysts can cause compression of surrounding structures and in this case gastric outlet obstruction. Endoscopy, barium and water-soluble contrast meals will all demonstrate dilatation of the stomach, but not the cause. Oesophageal manometry would be expected to be normal in this case.

21.52. Answer: A.

The diagnosis here is that of cystic fibrosis, of which chronic pancreatitis is a common complication. Calcification of the pancreas is highly suggestive of chronic pancreatitis.

21.53. Answer: E.

Significant hypoxia, low serum calcium, elevated serum glucose and very high CRP over 150 mg/L are associated with a poor prognosis in acute pancreatitis. Amylase level alone has not been proven to be prognostic. Other adverse factors are given in Boxes 21.53A and 21.53B.

---

i   **21.53A Glasgow criteria for prognosis in acute pancreatitis***

Age > 55 years
PO_2 < 8 kPa (60 mmHg)
White blood cell count > 15×10^9/L
Albumin < 32 g/L (3.2 g/dL)
Serum calcium < 2 mmol/L (8 mg/dL) (corrected)
Glucose > 10 mmol/L (180 mg/dL)
Urea > 16 mmol/L (45 mg/dL) (after rehydration)
Alanine aminotransferase > 200 U/L
Lactate dehydrogenase > 600 U/L

Severity and prognosis worsen as the number of these factors increases. More than three implies severe disease.

i	21.53B Features that predict severe pancreatitis
Initial assessment	
Clinical impression of severity	
Body mass index > 30 kg/m²	
Pleural effusion on chest X-ray	
APACHE II score > 8	
24 hours after admission	
Clinical impression of severity	
APACHE II score > 8	
Glasgow score > 3	
Persisting organ failure, especially if multiple	
CRP > 150 mg/L	
48 hours after admission	
Clinical impression of severity	
Glasgow score > 3	
CRP > 150 mg/L	
Persisting organ failure for 48 hours	
Multiple or progressive organ failure	

(CRP = C-reactive protein)

21.54. Answer: D.

IgG4 is elevated in autoimmune pancreatitis, which responds well to glucocorticoids. Autoimmune pancreatitis often mimics pancreatic cancers with an elevated bilirubin, but bilirubin is not specific to the disease as it would be elevated in the main differential diagnosis of carcinoma of head of pancreas. Alpha-fetoprotein is elevated in hepatocellular carcinoma, germ cell tumours and pregnancy, none of which would be expected to respond to glucocorticoids. Hepatitis E IgM is elevated in acute infection and is not steroid responsive. Serum IgM levels are not affected by autoimmune hepatitis.

21.55. Answer: D.

If there is recurrent duodenal ulceration in a young patient, Zollinger–Ellison syndrome should be considered. Gastrinoma as part of multiple endocrine neoplasia (MEN) type 1 is a recognised cause of Zollinger–Ellison syndrome, of which pituitary adenoma is a common additional tumour. *MEN1* is a tumour suppressor gene, mutations of which are seen in MEN type 1. Mutations in *BRCA1* and *BRCA2* are associated with breast cancer. *RET* is a proto-oncogene, where mutations to increase activity lead to MEN types 2 and 3 (also known as MEN types 2a and 2b). *JAK2* mutations are associated with polycythaemia vera and myeloproliferative disorders.

21.56. Answer: E.

In any young female, it is essential to consider pregnancy as a cause of abdominal symptoms or vomiting. This will dictate what further investigations and medications can be given safely.

21.57. Answer: A.

The removal of a large portion of the stomach leads to a significant reduction in chief cells responsible for production of intrinsic factor, required to absorb vitamin B_{12} in the terminal ileum. They also have a role in pepsinogen production, although protein absorption tends to be affected less.

21.58. Answer: A.

Basal cell carcinoma has not been demonstrated to be associated with the intestinal microbiome. All the others have been shown to be associated with dysbiosis.

21.59. Answer: A.

Hydrochloric acid secretion is unique to the stomach. The others' main contributions occur in the small intestine.

21.60. Answer: B.

Rheumatoid arthritis may be associated with atlantoaxial subluxation due to flexion of the neck during endoscopy. This can lead to high spinal cord injury. Rheumatoid arthritis is the most common cause of this complication in adults.

21.61. Answer: A.

A sticking sensation retrosternally suggests an oesophageal problem. All other features listed suggest oropharygeal origin.

21.62. Answer: B.

Gastroparesis is an autonomic complication of poorly controlled diabetes, which presents with persistent vomiting. Symptoms may improve after a period of sustained improved glycaemic control. There are no features in the history that suggest *H. pylori* infection or a cause for gastric outlet obstruction, e.g. ulcers, nor raised intracranial pressure (positional headache worse on lying flat). Insulin is not associated with vomiting as a side-effect.

21.63. Answer: C.

The Blatchford scoring system (Box 21.63) risk stratifies upper gastrointestinal bleeding

21

according to clinical features, initial blood tests and comorbidities, giving a score of 0 in this case. This history is typical of a Mallory–Weiss tear. In the presence of a low Blatchford score, Mallory–Weiss tear can often be managed without endoscopy. Whilst the majority of cases stop bleeding without intervention, those with elevated Blatchford scores and evidence of ongoing bleeding require endoscopy and around 10% require endoscopic therapy due to life-threatening bleeding.

21.63 Modified Blatchford score: risk stratification in acute upper gastrointestinal bleeding

Admission risk marker	Score component value
Blood urea	
≥25 mmol/L (70 mg/dL)	6
10–25 mmol/L (28–70 mg/dL)	4
8–10 mmol/L (22.4–28 mg/dL)	3
6.5–8 mmol/L (18.2–22.4 mg/dL)	2
<6.5 mmol/L (18.2 mg/dL)	0
Haemoglobin for men	
<100 g/L (10 g/dL)	6
100–119 g/L (10–11.9 g/dL)	3
120–129 g/L (12–12.9 g/dL)	1
≥130 g/L (13 g/dL)	0
Haemoglobin for women	
<100 g/L (10 g/dL)	6
100–119 g/L (10–11.9 g/dL)	1
≥120 g/L (12 g/dL)	0
Systolic blood pressure	
<90 mmHg	3
90–99 mmHg	2
100–109 mmHg	1
>109 mmHg	0
Other markers	
Presentation with syncope	2
Hepatic disease	2
Cardiac failure	2
Pulse ≥100 beats/min	1
Presentation with melaena	1
None of the above	0

21.64. Answer: A.
Band ligation is the endoscopic management of choice for bleeding oesophageal varices. Options B–E are used in the management of bleeding peptic ulcers or mucosal defects, but are likely to worsen bleeding secondary to varices.

21.65. Answer: D.
Diarrhoea is one of the most common symptoms associated with HIV and should be considered in all individuals with unexplained symptoms. A recent opportunistic herpes zoster infection, alongside his other symptoms, would support HIV as the unifying diagnosis.

21.66. Answer: D.
All these conditions are associated with coeliac disease (Box 21.66). However, splenic atrophy leads to a functional hyposplenism and leaves the individual at risk of encapsulated organisms such as *Streptococcus pneumoniae*. Consequently, vaccination is now routinely recommended.

21.66 Disease associations of coeliac disease

Type 1 diabetes mellitus (2–8%)
Thyroid disease (5%)
Primary biliary cirrhosis (3%)
Sjögren's syndrome (3%)
Immunoglobulin A deficiency (2%)
Pernicious anaemia
Sarcoidosis
Neurological complications:
    Encephalopathy
    Cerebellar atrophy
    Peripheral neuropathy
    Epilepsy
Myasthenia gravis
Dermatitis herpetiformis
Down's syndrome
Enteropathy-associated T-cell lymphoma
Small bowel carcinoma
Squamous carcinoma of oesophagus
Ulcerative jejunitis
Pancreatic insufficiency
Microscopic colitis
Splenic atrophy

22

Hepatology

Multiple Choice Questions

22.1. Which of the following is correct about the anatomy of the liver?

A. A fibrous capsule surrounds the liver lobule in humans

B. The hepatic vein radicles accompany the arteries in the portal tract

C. The liver has significant regenerative capacity

D. The liver is on the left side of the upper abdomen crossing the midline

E. The liver weighs around 0.75–1 kg in typical adults

22.2. Which of the following is a marker of the function of the liver that is in widespread clinical use?

A. Alanine transaminase

B. Fibroscan

C. Monoethylglycinexylidide (MEGX) test

D. Platelet count

E. Prothrombin time

22.3. A 63 year old man presents with yellowing of the skin and sclerae, dark urine and pale stools. He has no significant past medical history, other than appendicectomy as a teenager. What is the most likely diagnosis?

A. Autoimmune hepatitis

B. Gilbert's syndrome

C. Haemolysis

D. Hypothyroidism

E. Pancreatic carcinoma

22.4. An 18 year old woman presents to the emergency department having taken an overdose of an unknown quantity of paracetamol. Which of the following statements regarding the clinical presentation and progress of paracetamol overdose is true?

A. Deterioration from grade 1 to grade 4 encephalopathy typically takes place over several days

B. It has a worse outcome than acute liver failure of other aetiologies

C. If the patient recovers from acute liver failure, cirrhosis development is almost inevitable

D. Jaundice typically occurs before prothrombin time (PT) prolongation

E. Pancreatitis can be an accompanying complication

22.5. In the course of a 'well-woman' check offered by her employer, a 50 year old woman was found to have an antinuclear antibody with a multiple nuclear dot pattern and mildly abnormal liver function tests (LFTs). What is the most likely diagnosis?

A. Autoimmune hepatitis (AIH)

B. Lupus

C. Non-alcoholic steatohepatitis (NASH)

D. Primary biliary cirrhosis (PBC)

E. Primary sclerosing cholangitis (PSC)

22.6. A 70 year old woman is admitted to hospital and develops abnormal LFTs. She has been on several different medications over the last few days. Which of the following statements about drug-induced liver injury (DILI) is true?

A. Amoxicillin is a common cause of acute liver injury

B. DILI can be difficult to distinguish clinically from autoimmune hepatitis

C. In unexplained jaundice, recently started medications can be safely continued provided there have been no reports of DILI associated with them

D. It is seen with opiate use

E. The risk of co-amoxiclav-induced liver injury goes down with each repeat exposure

22.7. A 35 year old man is being considered for liver transplantation. Which of the following is true?

A. Acute cellular rejection most commonly occurs between days 2 and 5

B. At least partial human leucocyte antigen (HLA) matching is essential for a good outcome

C. Hepatorenal failure will typically improve following liver transplantation

D. Immunosuppression can be safely stopped in most patients at 5 years

E. Mycophenolate mofetil (MMF) monotherapy is a useful immunosuppression regime

22.8. A 42 year old man is in hospital with acute liver failure. The team are considering his prognosis. In this situation, which of the following liver functions, when deranged, has an important impact on outcome?

A. Glucose regulation

B. Innate immune response

C. Oxalate metabolism

D. Red cell breakdown

E. Steroid hormone clearance

22.9. A 28 year old woman presents to her family physician with fatigue and itch. She has obstructive LFTs. Which of the following is true about the autoimmune cholestatic liver disease primary biliary cholangitis?

A. It is a different condition to primary biliary cirrhosis

B. It is commoner in men than in women

C. Patients usually show elevation of PT

D. The disease is more aggressive in younger patients

E. Ursodeoxycholic acid (UDCA) is first-line therapy and should be used once the patient is symptomatic

22.10. A 20 year old student with no significant past medical history presents with a 1-week history of acute lethargy and jaundice 2 weeks after returning from a week-long holiday in Turkey. His alanine aminotransferase (ALT) is found to be over 10000 U/L. What is the most likely diagnosis?

A. Alcoholic hepatitis

B. Hepatitis B virus

C. Hepatitis C virus

D. Hepatitis E virus

E. Wilson's disease

22.11. A 25 year old woman with well-controlled, non-cirrhotic AIH attends your clinic to say she is pregnant. She is currently maintained on azathioprine monotherapy. What advice would you give her?

A. Disease flare-ups can occur following delivery

B. Her child runs a significant risk of developing AIH

C. Her disease will deteriorate during pregnancy

D. She should immediately swap to MMF maintenance therapy

E. She should undergo endoscopy

22.12. A 53 year old man with known oesophageal varices presents with a large gastrointestinal (GI) bleed. You are the first attending clinician. What is the first step you should take?

A. Alert interventional radiology in case transjugular intrahepatic portosystemic stent shunt (TIPSS) is required

B. Arrange urgent cross-match

C. Arrange urgent endoscopy and banding

D. Insert large-bore cannula and give fluid

E. Organise bedside ultrasound to assess for portal vein thrombosis

22.13. A patient with suspected variceal bleeding cannot have an endoscopy because of lack of an available trained endoscopist. She is becoming increasingly unstable. Which of the following is a medical therapy appropriate for use in the first instance to establish haemodynamic control?

A. Glypressin

B. Noradrenaline (norephinephrine)

C. Propranolol

D. Subcutaneous octreotide

E. Tranexamic acid

22.14. A computed tomography (CT) scan performed in a patient with chronic liver disease has identified a mass lesion suspicious of a hepatocellular carcinoma. What is the next investigation you should consider?

A. A magnetic resonance imaging (MRI) scan
B. Blood alpha-fetoprotein (AFP) measurement
C. Laparoscopy
D. Liver biopsy
E. Positron emission tomography (PET) scan

22.15. A 45 year old woman presents with painful hepatomegaly and ascites. What imaging findings would you predict when investigating?

A. An irregular liver on CT
B. Hepatic artery thrombosis
C. Hepatic venous thrombosis on triple-phase CT
D. Isolated gastric varies
E. Reversal of portal blood flow on ultrasound

22.16. Twenty-four hours following liver transplantation for autoimmune hepatitis, a patient's ALT is climbing rapidly. What diagnosis is the most likely?

A. Acute cellular rejection
B. Cytomegalovirus (CMV) infection
C. Delayed graft function
D. Hepatic artery thrombosis
E. Recurrent AIH

22.17. A patient with primary biliary cholangitis is concerned about the prognosis of her disease. Which of the following is predictive of a poor outcome?

A. Alkaline phosphatase (ALP) level
B. AMA titre
C. Large liver size on ultrasound
D. Older age at disease onset
E. Presence of intercurrent autoimmune disease

22.18. A 38 year old woman presents in the third trimester of pregnancy with itch. She is found to have a rise in liver enzymes and serum bile acids. Which of the following statements is correct?

A. Acute viral hepatitis is a likely cause
B. Fatty liver of pregnancy is the most likely diagnosis
C. It is likely that the mother has underlying chronic liver disease
D. There is a risk of intrauterine fetal death, meaning that consideration should be given to early delivery
E. There is no effective drug treatment

22.19. A 76 year old man is referred to the outpatient clinic. His family physician has

suspected that he has primary sclerosing cholangitis. Which of the following statements about diagnosis and treatment is correct?

A. First-line imaging technique for the bile ducts is endoscopic retrograde cholangiopancreatography (ERCP)
B. HCC is the characteristic complication
C. The diagnosis is unlikely as the patient is male
D. There is no proven therapy able to improve prognosis
E. UDCA is proven to reduce mortality

22.20. A 60 year old woman is being treated for cellulitis and has developed abnormal LFTs. Her family physician calls you for advice as she suspects that the patient has flucloxacillin-induced liver injury. Which of the following statements is correct?

A. Characteristic blood test abnormalities are elevation in ALT and eosinophil count
B. Loss of the small intrahepatic bile ducts can occur
C. Glucocorticoid therapy increases speed of recovery
D. The patient is safe to take the drug again in the future as the risk falls with repeat exposure
E. The patient should avoid all penicillin-based drugs in the future

22.21 An 18 year old medical student has his hepatitis B and C status checked as part of his occupational health screening for entrance to medical school. His results are as follows:

LFTs:
Bilirubin 12 µmol/L (0.70 mg/dL)
ALT 19 U/L
HCV antibody not detected
Hepatitis B surface antigen (HBsAg) positive
Antibody to HBsAg (anti-HBs) negative
Antibody to hepatitis B core antigen (anti-HBc) IgM negative
Anti-HBc IgG positive
What is the next step in his management?

A. Check hepatitis B e antigen (HBeAg) and HBV DNA
B. Liver biopsy
C. Repeat blood tests in 6 months
D. Tenofovir
E. Vaccinate for hepatitis B

21.22. A 42 year old female with a new diagnosis of chronic hepatitis B has recently

22

had fluctuations in her LFTs with an abnormal ALT despite a low viral load. Her delta serology is checked and is positive with a high titre. Which of the following statements is true about the hepatitis D virus (HDV)?

A. All patients with HBV have HDV co-infection

B. HBV–HDV co-infection has the same annual rate of cirrhosis and HCC as HBV mono-infection

C. HDV can infect individuals simultaneously with any acute hepatitis

D. HDV contains a single antigen to which infected individuals make an antibody (anti-HDV)

E. HDV is a DNA virus like HBV

22.23. A 25 year old female who has chronic hepatitis B and is under long-term follow-up in the hepatology clinic is 27 weeks pregnant, about to enter her third trimester. She is worried she will give her baby hepatitis B and would like you to reassure her. You review her blood tests from this clinic appointment at 27 weeks' gestation.

LFTs:
Bilirubin 18 µmol/L (1.05 mg/dL)
ALT 14 U/L
ALP 84 U/L
HBsAg positive
HBeAg negative
HBV DNA 48 U/mL (low titre)

What is the most appropriate next step in her management plan?

A. Advise elective caesarean delivery

B. Interferon-alfa in third trimester

C. Observe

D. Tenofovir in third trimester

E. Vaccinate infant at birth

22.24. A 52 year old male ex-intravenous drug user with liver cirrhosis from hepatitis C virus has complications of diuretic-resistant ascites and previous episodes of encephalopathy. He has been waiting for treatment. Whilst he waits for treatment to be initiated, what is the most appropriate management plan?

A. AFP and ultrasound in 12 months for HCC surveillance

B. Assessment for liver transplantation

C. Liver biopsy

D. Tenofovir

E. Trial of interferon for 4 weeks

22.25. A 37 year old male prisoner is newly diagnosed with HCV. He has no significant past medical history or drug history. His results are as follows:

Full blood count:
Haemoglobin 130 g/L
White cell count (WCC) 4.2×10^9/L
Platelets 98×10^9/L

LFTs:
Bilirubin 42 µmol/L (2.46 mg/dL)
ALT 60 U/L
ALP 64 U/L

Ultrasound liver: irregular, shrunken liver with no focal lesion and no free fluid. Splenomegaly. HCV genotype 1a. HCV RNA 750000 U/mL. Elastography 25 kPa (2–7 kPa).

What is the next appropriate management step?

A. Genotype 1a is more difficult to treat and therefore he should have interferon therapy

B. He does not have advanced fibrosis and therefore can be discharged from the clinic

C. He needs a liver biopsy to accurately stage his liver disease

D. He should be offered oral antiviral therapy

E. No treatment; patient should be observed with continued outpatient follow-up

22.26. A 64 year old man has been admitted to hospital feeling tired and unwell, suffering from nausea and itching. A careful history elicits that he recently celebrated his wedding anniversary on a cruise ship from which they returned a few weeks ago. He has recently noted dark urine and pale stool. His wife is not unwell but she is vegetarian and he mentions he ate large amounts from the seafood buffet. He has no other risk factors for jaundice. His LFTs confirm he is jaundiced with an acute hepatitis. Which of the following is most likely to test positive?

A. Delta antibody

B. Hepatitis A virus (HAV) RNA in sweat

C. Hepatitis B surface antigen

D. Hepatitis C antibody

E. Hepatitis E virus RNA in stool

22.27. There has been an outbreak of hepatitis A virus (HAV) at a local nursery. The head teacher of a primary school in the same area would like some advice on prevention of secondary cases of hepatitis A infection. Of note, no one at the primary school (child or adult member of staff) has been identified as unwell or an index case. What advice do you give to her?

A. Everyone in her primary school should be vaccinated
B. Good hygiene practice is the cornerstone of prevention
C. HAV is not highly infectious
D. Infected individuals will always have symptoms
E. There is a risk of becoming a chronic carrier

22.28. A 49 year old male with chronic hepatitis B who has cirrhosis and developed hepatocellular carcinoma has a liver transplant. What treatment should be prescribed in the post-operative period?

A. Hepatitis B immunoglobulin
B. Hepatitis B immunoglobulin and oral nucleoside
C. Hepatitis B vaccination
D. Interferon-alfa
E. Ribavirin

22.29. A 79 year old male is admitted to the emergency department with rigors and abdominal pain. He has a past medical history of hypertension with no history of travel abroad. On examination he is febrile with a temperature of 40°C and tachycardic. He is tender in the right upper quadrant but without guarding or rebound.

His inflammatory markers are raised with WCC 24×10⁹/L and C-reactive protein (CRP) of 300 mg/L. He has deranged LFTs with bilirubin 64 μmol/L (3.74 mg/dL), ALT 74 U/L, ALP 320 U/L. A liver screen was sent. An ultrasound abdomen showed three cystic lesions in the right lobe of the liver with a dilated common bile duct and associated filling defect suggestive of gallstones and inflamed gallbladder.

Intravenous antibiotics and fluids are started. Stool microscopy for ova/cysts and parasites was negative. Blood cultures were positive for *Escherichia coli* and subsequent aspirate of cyst was positive for the same bacteria. Which of the following is the most likely diagnosis?

A. Amoebic liver abscess
B. Hepatocellular carcinoma
C. Hydatid cyst
D. Polycystic liver disease
E. Pyogenic liver abscess

22.30. A 62 year old male with cirrhosis from non-alcoholic fatty liver disease (NAFLD) undergoes 6-monthly ultrasound for HCC surveillance and AFP. His AFP is normal but ultrasound shows a 3.5-cm lesion in the liver. What is the next appropriate management step?

A. Carcinoembryonic antigen
B. PET scan
C. Repeat ultrasound liver by consultant radiologist
D. Repeat ultrasound liver in 3 months
E. Triple-phase CT scan

22.31. A 52 year old male is referred to hepatology clinic due to an abnormal ultrasound scan. He was originally referred to haematology to be investigated for thrombocytopenia. He has a past medical history of type 2 diabetes, hypertension and body mass index (BMI) 33 kg/m². He has mildly deranged LFTs (which prompted the ultrasound scan request). Below are his results from clinic:

Full blood count:
Haemoglobin 106 g/L
WCC 5.3×10⁹/L
Platelets 89×10⁹/L
LFTs:
Bilirubin 33 μmol/L (1.93 mg/dL)
ALT 54 U/L
ALP 72 U/L
AFP 892 kU/L
Ultrasound: 5-cm lesion in liver. Liver is shrunken and nodular. Further imaging is requested.
What is the likely description of the lesion on a CT scan?

A. Enhances in arterial phase with portal venous washout
B. Fluid-filled cystic lesion
C. Focal central scar
D. Low-density lesion with delayed arterial filling
E. Thick-walled cyst with calcification

22.32. A 37 year old female presents to the emergency department with colicky right upper quadrant pain and nausea. This is her fourth presentation in 6 months. Ultrasound confirms gallstones and she is referred to the surgeons for elective cholecystectomy. Which of the following dietary recommendations do you advise her to adopt?

A. Fermentable, oligo-, di-, monosaccharides and polyols (FODMAP) diet

B. Gluten-free diet
C. High-fat diet
D. Low-fat diet
E. Low-oxalate diet

22.33. A 64 year old male with a background of ulcerative colitis and primary sclerosing cholangitis has upper abdominal pain and complains of dark urine and pale stool for a month. On further questioning he reveals recent weight loss. On examination he is afebrile, cachexic with a soft abdomen with no palpable abdominal mass. Further investigations are as follows.
    LFTs:
        Bilirubin 240 μmol/L (14.03 mg/dL)
        ALT 140 U/L
        ALP 880 U/L
    Ultrasound: dilated intrahepatic bile ducts with poorly demarcated echogenic tissue in hepatic hilum.
        Which is the next best investigation?

A. Carcinoembryonic antigen
B. Colonoscopy
C. CT abdomen
D. ERCP
E. Liver biopsy

22.34. A 42 year old female has attended the emergency department numerous times with intermittent episodes of epigastric pain. She has been investigated as an outpatient with normal upper GI endoscopy. On this attendance, her results are as below:
    Amylase 400 U/L
    Bilirubin 45 μmol/L (2.63 mg/dL)
    ALT 56 U/L
    ALP 142 U/L
    CRP 2 mg/L
    Abdominal ultrasound: normal liver, slightly dilated intrahepatic ducts and common bile duct. No stones or masses. MRCP: pancreas normal but, as on ultrasound, dilated common bile duct with no stones or masses.
    You diagnose her with sphincter of Oddi dysfunction (SOD). What is the next best appropriate management step.

A. Advise regular non-steroidal anti-inflammatory drugs and no other intervention
B. Cholecystectomy
C. Nifedipine
D. Observe
E. Sphincter of Oddi manometry

22.35. A 47 year old male with a BMI of 35 kg/m^2 presents with jaundice, loss of appetite with abdominal pain and increasing abdominal girth over 3–4 weeks. He is teetotal with no other past medical history. He does not take any regular medication. On examination he has hepatosplenomegaly and ascites, with no peripheral oedema.
    Full blood count:
        Haemoglobin 190 g/L
        WCC 13×10^9/L
        Platelets 690×10^9/L
    LFTs:
        Bilirubin 72 μmol/L (4.21 mg/dL)
        ALT 500 U/L
        ALP 460 U/L
        Albumin 31 g/L
        Ascitic fluid albumin 22 g/L
    What is the most likely cause of his presentation?

A. Alcoholic liver disease
B. Congestive cardiac failure
C. Haemochromatosis
D. Hepatic vein thrombosis
E. NAFLD

22.36. A 45 year old patient with alcoholic liver disease is accompanied by his daughter to clinic. He has been abstinent of alcohol for 4 years but developed diuretic-resistant ascites and mild encephalopathy. Which of the following scoring systems should be used to identify and prioritise whether he should be assessed for liver transplantation?

A. King's College criteria
B. Maddrey score
C. MELD (Model for End-Stage Liver Disease)
D. Rockall score
E. Serum–ascites albumin gradient

22.37. A 21 year old female is diagnosed with fibrolamellar hepatocellular carcinoma of 3 cm with no underlying cirrhosis. Her AFP is normal. Which is the best treatment option for her?

A. Chemotherapy
B. Do nothing and observe
C. Radiofrequency ablation (RFA)
D. Surgical resection
E. Transarterial chemoembolisation (TACE)

22.38. A 64 year old female with recent change in bowel habit and rectal bleeding who is awaiting lower GI investigation presents to the emergency department with dark urine and pale stool. On examination she is jaundiced with hepatomegaly and moderate-volume ascites.

LFTs:

Bilirubin 240 µmol/L (14.03 mg/dL)
ALT 84 U/L
ALP 1400 U/L
Albumin 31 g/L
Carcinoembryonic antigen (CEA) 230 µg/L
Ascitic fluid: blood-stained

Ultrasound: multiple liver lesions compressing bile ducts

Which of the following is the most likely diagnosis?

A. Cholangiocarcinoma
B. Colorectal cancer
C. Focal nodular hyperplasia
D. Hepatic adenoma
E. HCC

22.39. A hospital porter is seen in the occupational health clinic following a needlestick injury. Investigations taken in the clinic show that the patient is HBsAg negative, anti-HBc negative and anti-HBs positive. What is the correct interpretation of these results?

A. Acute infection with hepatitis B
B. Chronic dual infection with hepatitis B and delta virus
C. Chronic mono-infection with hepatitis B
D. Previous immunisation against hepatitis B without prior infection
E. Previous infection to hepatitis B but the patient has cleared the virus

22.40. When assessing the severity of NAFLD in an overweight 65 year old type 2 diabetic patient with hypertension, which of the following statements is correct?

A. A normal ALT level indicates that the disease is mild and that there is unlikely to be significant scarring of the liver
B. A raised γ-glutamyl transferase (GGT) indicates that the patient is probably dependent on alcohol
C. The AST:ALT ratio is a useful indicator of progressive liver fibrosis towards cirrhosis
D. The presence of obesity, hypertension and type 2 diabetes is not associated with a greater likelihood of steatohepatitis and liver fibrosis
E. The use of routine ultrasound can distinguish between simple steatosis and steatohepatitis

22.41. A patient has suspected NAFLD. Which of the following statements about diagnosis and treatment is correct?

A. Statins should be discontinued due to the risk of drug-induced liver injury
B. Testing for the *PNPLA3* rs738409 genetic variant is part of the routine clinical testing of patients
C. The FIB-4 Score distinguishes between alcoholic liver disease and NAFLD
D. The presence of individual features of the metabolic syndrome should be sought and treated to reduce cardiovascular risk
E. Venesection should be commenced immediately if ferritin levels are raised, as this indicates haemochromatosis

22.42. A 57 year old man is admitted with presumed alcoholic hepatitis. Which of the following statements about diagnosis and treatment is correct?

A. A Maddrey 'discriminate function' of less than 32 is indicative of a poor prognosis
B. Alcohol consumption may safely continue
C. Patients should be fasted to avoid stressing the liver
D. The Steroids or Pentoxifylline for Alcoholic Hepatitis (STOPAH) trial showed that pentoxyfilline should be the first-line treatment for alcoholic hepatitis
E. The STOPAH trial showed that prednisolone 40 mg daily for 28 days leads to a modest reduction in short-term mortality

22.43. A 54 year old male patient with alcohol-related cirrhosis is admitted with a 3-week history of increasing abdominal swelling and discomfort. He is mildly jaundiced and has a low-grade pyrexia but is haemodynamically stable. Routine blood tests and a chest X-ray have been requested. What test would you perform next?

A. Diagnostic paracentesis
B. Electroencephalogram
C. ERCP
D. Triple-phase CT liver
E. Upper GI endoscopy

22.44. An otherwise healthy 35 year old nurse and part-time tattoo artist is referred with a persistent, fluctuating transaminitis (ALT 40–120 U/L) that has been present for several years. What viral infection would you consider most likely?

22

A. Epstein–Barr virus (EBV)
B. Hepatitis A
C. Hepatitis B
D. Hepatitis C
E. Hepatitis E

22.45. A 38-year old man is referred by his family physician to the outpatient clinic. His father had haemochromatosis and he is about to get married, so he is wondering whether he is likely to be affected. What would be the best first-line screening test in this case?

A. CT liver
B. Ferritin
C. HFE genetic analysis
D. Liver biopsy
E. Transferrin saturation

22.46. A 45 year old woman presents with a 5-day history of pale stools and dark urine associated with cramping epigastric and right upper quadrant pains. Blood tests show bilirubin 120 µmol/L (7.02 mg/dL), ALT 65 U/L, ALP 580 U/L, GGT 640 U/L. What would be your first-line imaging investigation?

A. CT pancreas
B. Endoscopic ultrasound
C. ERCP
D. PET-CT
E. Ultrasound abdomen

22.47. A 54 year old man with alcoholic cirrhosis presents with haematemesis. The patient is commenced on terlipressin and emergency upper GI endoscopy is performed, which demonstrates large oesophageal varices with active bleeding. The varices are banded with good haemostatic effect. What medicine would you start as secondary prophylaxis to reduce the chance of further variceal haemorrhage in the future?

A. Atenolol
B. Isosorbide mononitrate
C. Losartan
D. Propranolol
E. Ramipril

22.48. A 48 year old male has recently been diagnosed with hemochromatosis with homozygous mutation of the *HFE* C282Y gene. His blood tests show a ferritin of 1950 µg/L and a transferrin saturation of 88%. What treatment would be the most appropriate to commence?

A. Ferrous sulphate 200 mg 3 times daily
B. Fortnightly venosection
C. Propranolol 20 mg 3 times daily
D. Spironolactone 100 mg once daily
E. Vitamin C supplement twice daily

22.49. A patient with NAFLD cirrhosis undergoes screening upper endoscopy and is noted to have moderate (grade 2) oesophageal varices with no signs of recent bleeding. What would be the best next step?

A. Admit for TIPSS placement
B. Admit to intensive care unit and place Sengstaken–Blakemore tube immediately
C. Repeat upper GI endoscopy in 6 months
D. Start non-selective β-blocker (propranolol 20 mg 3 times daily)
E. Variceal banding

22.50. A 53 year old bank employee in the UK is found at a routine check-up to have abnormal LFTs. What is the most common aetiology for abnormal liver biochemistry in developed countries?

A. Alcoholic liver disease
B. Autoimmune hepatitis
C. Hepatitis C
D. NAFLD
E. Primary biliary cholangitis

22.51. A 60 year old man is found to have hepatitis C and undergoes a liver biopsy that confirms stage 4 fibrosis (cirrhosis). He is asymptomatic and subsequently receives antiviral therapy and successfully clears the virus (a sustained viral response). What further test will he need?

A. Cardiac angiogram
B. Chest X-ray
C. Electrocardiogram (ECG)
D. HCV RNA annually to check for recurrence
E. Ultrasound every 6 months as part of routine HCC surveillance

Answers

22.1. Answer: C.
The liver has significant regenerative capacity, with stem cells within the canals of Hering playing a key role. This regenerative capacity plays an important role in recovery from liver failure and from liver resection. It also contributes to the phenotype of cirrhosis. The liver is on the right side of the upper abdomen crossing the midline and weighs 1–2 kg, depending on body size. Although drawings can give the impression that the liver lobule is encapsulated, this is not the case in humans (although it is in pigs). The portal tracts contain portal vein radicles and arterioles, together with small bile ducts. Sinusoids cross the liver lobule to the hepatic vein radicle.

22.2. Answer: E.
Synthesis of clotting factors by the liver makes prothrombin time (PT) a useful and easily available marker of hepatocyte function (although watch for vitamin K deficiency and patients on warfarin). Alanine transaminase is a marker of hepatocyte injury not function. Platelet count lowering and elevation of Fibroscan values are markers of fibrosis/ cirrhosis (through hypersplenism and liver fibrosis, respectively). MEGX, a dynamic test of lidocaine metabolism, is a direct, active test of hepatocyte function but toxicity can be an issue and it is not in widespread clinical use.

22.3. Answer: E.
Yellowing of the sclera and skin are features suggestive of jaundice. The presence of dark urine and pale stools suggest a post-hepatic or obstructive jaundice (conjugated bilirubin is leaking back into the circulation and being excreted through the kidney, causing urine darkening, whilst bilirubin metabolites are not reaching the bowel, causing stools to be pale). Pancreatic carcinoma is a common cause of this form of jaundice. Haemolysis is a cause of pre-hepatic jaundice through increased red blood cell breakdown and bilirubin generation in the spleen and thus would not give an obstructive pattern. Gilbert's syndrome is an inherited abnormality of bilirubin transport that gives rise to clinically non-significant elevation of bilirubin (other liver biochemistry is typically normal), particularly in times of physiological stress such as intercurrent illness, which would

again not have an obstructive pattern. Autoimmune hepatitis causes hepatocellular jaundice in aggressive forms, but not obstructive jaundice. Hypothyroidism can cause skin pigmentation that can be mistaken for jaundice (although characteristically the sclerae remain normal colour, in contrast to jaundice where yellowing is characteristic).

22.4. Answer: E.
Pancreatitis can be a rare complication of paracetamol overdose and typically has a very poor outcome (also frequently preventing liver transplantation). Paracetamol overdose causes acute liver injury, but if the acute event is survived, the liver typically returns to normal. Once encephalopathy develops, deterioration is typically very rapid (hours or even minutes). Encephalopathy typically occurs after PT prolongation and prior to the onset of jaundice. The outcome of acute liver failure in paracetamol is typically better than other causes of acute liver failure.

22.5. Answer: D.
The commonest autoantibody in PBC is antimitochondrial antibody (AMA; present in over 95% of patients). A minority of patients (around 20%) have characteristic antinuclear antibodies that are reactive with either nuclear dot or nuclear rim antibodies. Where present, these carry the same degree of diagnostic value as AMA (and may suggest a worse prognosis). Both AIH and lupus are associated with antinuclear antibodies but with a diffuse nuclear staining pattern. Low-titre diffuse nuclear antibodies are seen frequently in NASH. The 'characteristic' autoantibody in PSC is perinuclear antineutrophil cytoplasmic antibody (pANCA), although this is seen in only around 30% of patients.

22.6. Answer: B.
DILI can be difficult to distinguish on liver biopsy from autoimmune hepatitis due to a number of shared features, including parenchymal inflammation and eosinophilia. Clinical context needs to be considered (e.g. autoimmune disease history and drug exposure) and other immunological features of AIH (elevated IgG and autoantibodies) sought. Opiates are not reported to cause DILI; in

22

terms of drugs of abuse, the major risk is ecstasy. When approaching a patient with possible DILI, the precautionary principle should apply and any potential risk therapy should be stopped until the causality becomes clearer.

22.7. Answer: C.

Hepatorenal failure complicating chronic liver disease is best regarded as a vascular consequence of cirrhosis and it typically improves when liver function returns to normal. HLA matching is unnecessary in liver transplantation (ABO and weight matching, in contrast, are important). Immunosuppression regimes differ between centres but most centres continue life-long immunosuppression. Research into safe discontinuation of immunosuppression has not translated into clinical practice. MMF monotherapy can be associated with very resistant cellular rejection. The most common time window for acute cellular rejection is days 7–10.

22.8. Answer: B.

The Kupffer cells play a key role in innate immunity, in particular acting as a barrier for gut bacteria/bacterial products entering the portal vein. Sepsis is one of the major causes of death in acute liver failure. Steroid hormone clearance is a liver function and loss of clearance function contributes to fluid retention/ ascites (aldosterone) and feminisation in men (oestrogen) with chronic liver failure. There is no impact in the acute setting. The liver plays a critical role in glucose homeostasis, buffering portal venous blood through glycogen synthesis/breakdown. Hepatocytes are also key in gluconeogenesis. Acute liver failure is frequently characterised by hypoglycaemia but this is relatively easy to manage with intravenous (IV) glucose in practice, and it is only rarely so profound as to impact on outcomes. Breakdown of red cells at the end of their life span is a function of the spleen not the liver. Hyperoxaluria is an inborn error of oxalic acid metabolism, expressed in the liver but manifest as renal failure. Transplantation of the kidney without the liver simply results in rapid renal failure in the graft. Combined transplant, in contrast, is highly effective. Oxalic acid plays no role in acute liver failure.

22.9. Answer: D.

Primary biliary cholangitis is the new name for primary biliary cirrhosis, so it is the same condition. The name was changed following a patient campaign in 2015. Typically thought of as a disease of middle-aged and older women (it is 10 times commoner in women than men), recent large cohort studies have identified an important group of younger patients (aged 20–50) who are more symptomatic and less likely to respond to UDCA. Younger patients should be monitored closely and treated aggressively. UDCA is first line-therapy and should be used at a dose of 13–15 mg/kg in all patients, regardless of symptom status or disease severity. The most characteristic blood test change is elevation of the alkaline phosphatase value, which reflects the cholestatic nature of the disease. Transaminase elevation can be a feature of aggressive disease and overlap with AIH. PT, as well as bilirubin and albumin levels, tend to be normal until late in the disease, as hepatocellular function is typically well preserved in this cholestatic disease.

22.10. Answer: D.

The clinical scenario is strongly suggestive of an acute viral hepatitis infection and the timing of onset would be most compatible with hepatitis E virus (HEV). The prodrome and onset in hepatitis B virus (HBV) are much more prolonged than those described here (although clearly infection prior to the holiday is possible). Hepatitis C virus (HCV) almost exclusively causes chronic liver injury with no recognised acute infection event. Wilson's disease can present with an acute hepatitis episode but is a rare condition and the acute presentation even rarer. There is an almost automatic assumption in some quarters that a hepatitis in a young man returning from abroad will be alcohol-related. In this case this is very unlikely, as an ALT of 10 000 U/L would be very atypical (normal or even low ALT is characteristic of alcoholic hepatitis).

22.11. Answer: A.

AIH typically improves in terms of disease activity during pregnancy. It can, however, flare up during the early post-partum period. If patients have cirrhosis, then portal hypertension can worsen during the third trimester, so consideration should be given to endoscopy as they enter the third trimester. This only applies to cirrhosis patients. MMF is teratogenic and is contraindicated in pregnancy, so azathioprine should be continued. The offspring of mothers with AIH run a slightly increased risk of AIH later in life (because of the genetic contribution to pathogenesis). This small risk should not impact on plans for pregnancy.

22.12. Answer: D.

Variceal bleeding can be high pressure and can lead to the patient exsanguinating rapidly. It is therefore essential to secure venous access early and commence fluid resuscitation. Delay can lead to later failure to gain access. Cross-matching is clearly urgent but should be done once access is secured. However, the acute intervention of choice is endoscopy and banding; this should only be undertaken once the patient is haemodynamically stable. TIPSS is a radiological intervention that is appropriate after failed endoscopy or early rebleed. Ultrasound scan is a part of the workup to explore triggers for bleeding – portal venous thrombosis or occult hepatocellular carcinoma (HCC) being potential factors – but should be undertaken once the acute bleeding state is under control.

22.13. Answer: A.

Glypressin is recognised to reduce the severity of acute variceal bleeding and can act as a bridge to endoscopy and an adjunct to endoscopy (helping a clearer endoscopic field). Noradrenaline (norepinephrine) may be required in the critical care setting to maintain cardiovascular status but is not primarily an agent to reduce bleeding risk. Octreotide has benefits in variceal bleeding but its use has been superseded by Glypressin: where used, it has to be intravenous. Propranolol should never be used in acute bleeding but is an important agent in the treatment of chronic portal hypertension. There is no clear evidence to support the use of tranexamic acid in GI bleeding (including variceal bleeding) although trials are ongoing.

22.14. Answer: A.

A second imaging modality is the key next investigation in a case of suspected HCC. AFP has some use as a screening test in at-risk patients but it can be normal in patients with HCC, meaning it has no use in diagnosis. Laparoscopy and liver biopsy can be of use in staging and planning therapy in specific cases, once the diagnosis is supported by dual imaging. PET scan has utility in specific

situations, in particular to explore for the presence of metastasis.

22.15. Answer: C.

This clinical presentation is typical of Budd–Chiari syndrome (hepatic venous thrombosis). Cirrhosis is typically associated with a small, painless shrunken liver and reversal of portal venous flow; pain would be very unusual. Hepatic artery thrombus is a specific complication of liver transplantation.

22.16. Answer: D.

ALT elevation following liver transplantation is, as in other settings, a marker of liver injury. The commonest aetiology is dependent on the time point post-transplant. Immediately post-surgery, the commonest causes are thrombosis of the hepatic artery (a specific complication of liver transplant) and primary graft dysfunction (typically a consequence of preservation injury). Acute cellular rejection would typically not be seen until days 5–10. CMV infection is another characteristic post-transplant challenge, typically when there is a mismatch between the CMV status of the donor and recipient. Prophylactic regimes in at-risk individuals are effective. AIH recurrence post-liver transplant is described but is typically a late phenomenon.

22.17. Answer: A.

Alkaline phosphatase level at presentation and in particular after therapy with ursodeoxycholic acid is predictive of outcome, with clinically relevant cut-offs identified and now in widespread clinical use. AMA is an important diagnostic feature but titre is not predictive of outcome. Intercurrent autoimmune disease is common and requires management but has no impact of liver disease risk. Liver size is typically increased in early PBC. Small liver size is a feature of cirrhosis with a worse outcome. Younger age is associated with a lower likelihood of response to UDCA and thus increased risk. PBC is typically benign in older patients.

22.18. Answer: D.

The combination of abnormal biochemistry, pregnancy stage and, in particular, elevation of serum bile acids all point to cholestasis of pregnancy. The bile acid elevation makes fatty liver of pregnancy unlikely. UDCA therapy is effective and rifampicin has been used in severe cases. There is no association with

22

pre-existing maternal liver disease. Cholestasis pruritus can be very severe. The major clinical concern is sudden intrauterine death due, it is thought, to a toxic effect of bile acids on the fetal cardiac conducting apparatus. The risk rises exponentially from 36 weeks' gestation onwards and there is a strong case for early delivery to avoid this risk.

22.19. Answer: D.

PSC is a fibrotic cholestatic liver disease of presumed autoimmune aetiology, which has a male predominance. Although UDCA is widely used, and typically improves the cholestatic liver function tests seen in PSC, there is no evidence that it reduces mortality and there is no evidence to support any drug therapy. HCC can complicate cirrhosis PSC (as with cirrhosis of any cause) but the specific associated cancers are cholangiocarcinoma and colonic carcinoma, both of which should be screened for. Imaging of the bile ducts is a key part of the diagnostic workup but should be through magnetic resonance cholangiopancreatography (MRCP) in the first instance because of the risks associated with ERCP. The latter should be reserved for therapeutic, rather than diagnostic, procedures.

22.20. Answer: B.

Flucloxacillin-induced liver injury is one of the commoner forms of drug-induced liver injury. It is thought to have an immune pathogenesis (there is a strong HLA association) and there is no crossover with other penicillins, which can be used safely. The immune element probably underpins the characteristic pattern of worsening injury with repeat exposure – a phenomenon that means that repeat use is absolutely contraindicated in patients suspected of the reaction. The process is principally cholestatic, with elevation of alkaline phosphatase being the characteristic biochemical change (eosinophilia can be seen as in all drug reactions). In severe cases, intrahepatic bile duct loss can be seen and UDCA therapy is advocated by some (although the evidence basis is limited). Glucocorticoid therapy has no role.

22.21. Answer: A.

This medical student has chronic hepatitis B. Hepatitis B surface antigen is the hallmark of chronic HBV infection if present for more than 6 months. This patient is unlikely to have acute infection with normal transaminases and negative anti-HBc IgM. Further management of the patient will depend on HBeAg status and HBV DNA to distinguish disease phase.

21.22. Answer: D.

HDV is an RNA-defective virus that requires the simultaneous presence of HBV for replication and has the same sources and modes of spread. HBV replication is usually suppressed by HDV. Liver damage is believed to be due to HDV and persistent HDV replication in co-infected patients leads to higher annual rates of cirrhosis and HCC. Interferon-alfa is the only effective drug against HDV but the optimal duration of therapy is not well defined.

22.23. Answer: E.

Pregnant women with chronic hepatitis B are most infectious when markers of continuing viral replication, such as HBeAg, and high levels of HBV-DNA are present in the blood. Tenofovir can be given if there are high levels of HBV-DNA in the last trimester of pregnancy; however, in this clinical scenario, the patient has very low titres. Interferon-alfa is contraindicated in pregnancy. Neonates born to hepatitis B-infected mothers should be immunised at birth. In addition, to prevent vertical transmission, hepatitis B immunoglobulin (HBIg) is given to newborns of highly viraemic HBeAg-positive mothers. Guidelines do not recommend elective caesarean delivery for mothers with chronic hepatitis B infection.

22.24. Answer: B.

Liver transplantation should be considered when complications of cirrhosis occur. He should be undergoing 6-monthly interval AFP and ultrasound for HCC surveillance. This surveillance will be ongoing even after his HCV is cured, as he will still have cirrhosis. Interferon is contraindicated in decompensated cirrhosis, and tenofovir is a treatment used in hepatitis B.

22.25. Answer: D.

This patient is cirrhotic as evident by thrombocytopenia, ultrasound imaging and high elastography score. He does not need a liver biopsy. He should be treated for his hepatitis C with new all-oral direct-acting antiviral therapy. Combinations of these drugs have been targeted to be pan-genotypic with sustained viral response (SVR) rates >90%. Once treated, he will require life-long follow-up in clinic for HCC surveillance, and as he has only been recently diagnosed with cirrhosis he should also have an endoscopy to screen for varices.

22.26. Answer: E.

The clinical presentation of hepatitis E is similar to that of hepatitis A with the likely source as shellfish in this clinical scenario. However, this question focuses on detection methods. Hepatitis A virus is excreted in faeces or diagnosis is made by detection of HAV IgM antibodies in the blood, which persists for up to 14 weeks after initial infection. Alternative samples such as serum and saliva can be used but assays are expensive and sensitivities vary. Therefore, answer E is the correct option.

22.27. Answer: B.

HAV belongs to the picornavirus group of enteroviruses. HAV is highly infectious and is spread by the faecal–oral route, but a chronic carrier state does not occur. Infected individuals may be asymptomatic. Health departments will investigate outbreaks and advise regarding vaccination. In this scenario vaccinating everyone is not necessary, as no one has been identified as the index case or close contact at the primary school.

22.28. Answer: B.

The use of post-liver transplant prophylaxis with direct-acting antiviral agents and hepatitis B immunoglobulins has reduced the reinfection rate to 10% and increased 5-year survival to 80%, making transplantation an acceptable treatment option. Hepatitis B vaccination is ineffective in those already infected by HBV. Ribavirin is a treatment used in hepatitis C infection.

22.29. Answer: E.

Hepatic abscesses are rare and clinical features of pyogenic and amoebic liver abscesses can be similar. However, pyogenic abscesses are most common in older patients and usually result from ascending infection due to biliary obstruction (cholangitis). They are often described as more aggressive. *E. coli* and various streptococci, particularly *Strep. milleri*, are the most common organisms. Any associated biliary obstruction and cholangitis require biliary drainage. Hepatic hydatid disease is a parasitic zoonosis caused by the *Echinococcus* tapeworm.

22.30. Answer: E.

AFP is produced by 60% of HCCs; therefore a negative AFP does not exclude HCC. Carcinoembryonic antigen is a tumour marker that can be raised in colorectal cancer. Combination of imaging modalities more accurately diagnoses and stages the extent of disease, and using at least two modalities (typically, CT or MRI following initial screening ultrasound identification of a mass lesion) is recommended.

22.31. Answer: A.

In this clinical scenario, the patient has cirrhosis as evidenced by thrombocytopenia and ultrasound imaging of liver. In this case, the likely aetiology is NAFLD with risk factors of diabetes, hypertension and obesity. The high AFP is diagnostic for HCC. HCC are hypervascular in the arterial phase, followed by washout in the portal venous phase. Option E is typical of a hydatid cyst and daughter cysts may be present. Option C is the appearance of a hepatic adenoma and focal nodular hyperplasia can be differentiated from adenoma because of a focal central scar.

22.32. Answer: D.

This patient has biliary colic. Gallstones are conventionally classified into cholesterol or pigment stones, although the majority are of mixed composition. Patients are generally advised a low-fat diet to help reduce symptoms as fat releases cholecystokinin, which precipitates gallbladder contraction and might result in biliary pain. Low-oxalate diet is associated with renal stones. A FODMAP diet is a treatment option for patients with irritable bowel syndrome and gluten-free diets are for patients with coeliac disease.

22.33. Answer: C.

Primary sclerosing cholangitis carries a lifetime risk of cholangiocarcinoma of approximately 20%. It can arise from anywhere in the biliary tree. Often the diagnosis is made by a combination of CT and MRI. A liver biopsy may cause tumour seeding. The patient will need an ERCP due to biliary obstruction but is not currently septic and therefore the best next investigation would be further imaging. Patients with ulcerative colitis and PSC should undergo yearly colonoscopy as they are at high risk of colorectal cancer, but this is not the focus of this scenario.

22

22.34. Answer: E.
The patient has SOD type I. The gold standard for diagnosis is sphincter of Oddi manometry. All biliary SOD patients with type I disease are treated with endoscopic sphincterotomy. Medical therapies can be tried in SOD type II patients.

22.35. Answer: D.
The patient has polycythaemia vera causing Budd–Chiari syndrome. The ascitic fluid is an exudate with a serum–ascites albumin gradient (SAAG) of <11 g/L. The other causes listed would have a high SAAG.

22.36. Answer: C.
The MELD score is used to identify and prioritise patients for liver transplantation. The Maddrey score enables the clinician to assess prognosis in alcoholic hepatitis. The King's College criteria identify indices associated with poor prognosis in patients with acute liver failure. The Rockall score identifies patients needing intervention in upper GI bleeds.

22.37. Answer: D.
Fibrolamellar HCC occurs in young adults in the absence of cirrhosis. The treatment of choice is surgical resection. The tumour biology is different to standard HCC and, in the absence of cirrhosis, surgical resection is less likely to cause liver failure. TACE and RFA are treatment options for HCC.

22.38. Answer: B.
This patient has secondary liver disease. Given the recent change in bowel habit and raised CEA, the primary is likely to be colorectal cancer. She has biliary obstruction from tumour burden in liver. Options D and E are benign lesions that would not present this way. Serum levels of the tumour marker CA19-9 are elevated in cholangiocarcinoma.

22.39. Answer: D.
HBV surface antigen (HBsAg) is a marker of current infection. HBV surface antibody (anti-HBs) may be positive following previous infection with HBV or if the patient has been immunised against HBV but immunisation against HBV does not induce HBV anti-core (anti-HBc) antibody production. As this patient is HBsAg negative, he is not currently infected. The absence of anti-HBc despite the presence of anti-HBs indicates he has not been exposed to the virus in the past but has been immunised to the virus.

22.40. Answer: C.
NAFLD is an increasingly common liver disease that is associated with features of the metabolic syndrome; the more features that an individual possesses, the more likely they are to have progressive disease. NAFLD is often asymptomatic and may be associated with normal liver biochemistry, even when disease is advanced. AST rises and ALT falls as disease progresses towards cirrhosis. The AST:ALT ratio is included in calculated scores such as the NAFLD fibrosis score and FIB-4 score that are used to risk-stratify patients for presence of advanced fibrosis. GGT levels may be raised in NAFLD and so cannot be used to discriminate between alcoholic and non-alcoholic liver disease. Routine imaging modalities cannot distinguish between steatosis and steatohepatitis; at present this can only be reliably performed histologically.

22.41. Answer: D.
NAFLD is a common, progressive liver disease that is also associated with an increased risk of cardiovascular disease. In patients with NAFLD, liver-related mortality is the third most common cause of death, after cardiovascular disease and extrahepatic malignancy. If a patient is found to have NAFLD, other features of the metabolic syndrome (including type 2 diabetes, hypertension, dyslipidaemia) should be sought and treated. NAFLD is not associated with an increased risk of statin-related liver injury and so statins are generally considered safe. Raised ferritin levels may be seen in patients with NAFLD and do not necessarily indicate the presence of haemochromatosis, which can be excluded by checking transferrin saturation. Although carriage of the *PNPLA3* gene rs738409 variant is associated with more severe NAFLD, it is not currently used as part of routine clinical testing. The FIB-4 score is used to risk-stratify patients for presence of advanced fibrosis in NAFLD; it should not be used in patients with alcoholic liver disease.

22.42. Answer: E.
A Maddrey discriminate function greater than 32 is indicative of severe disease. Cessation of all alcohol consumption is essential. Good nutrition is very important, and enteral feeding via a fine-bore nasogastric tube may be needed

in severely ill patients. The STOPAH study was a large multicentre double-blind randomised trial to evaluate the relative merits of steroids and/or a weak anti-tumour necrosis factor (anti-TNF) agent (pentoxifylline), alone or in combination. In a cohort of 1103 patients, no significant benefit from pentoxifylline treatment was identified; however, treatment with prednisolone 40 mg daily for 28 days led to a modest reduction in short-term mortality, from 17% in placebo-treated patients to 14% in the prednisolone group. These findings were consistent with earlier studies, where an improvement in 28-day survival from 52% to 78% was seen when steroids were given to those with a Glasgow score of more than 9. However, neither steroids nor pentoxifylline improved survival at 90 days or 1 year. Sepsis is the main side-effect of steroids, and existing sepsis and variceal haemorrhage are the main contraindications to their use.

22.43. Answer: A.

The most likely diagnosis would be spontaneous bacterial peritonitis. Diagnostic paracentesis (ascetic tap) may show cloudy fluid, and an ascites neutrophil count above 250×10^6/L almost invariably indicates infection. The source of infection cannot usually be determined, but most organisms isolated are of enteric origin and *E. coli* is most frequently found. Ascitic culture in blood culture bottles gives the highest yield of organisms. Spontaneous bacterial peritonitis (SBP) needs to be differentiated from other intra-abdominal emergencies, and the finding of multiple organisms on culture should arouse suspicion of a perforated viscus.

22.44. Answer: D.

Hepatitis A, hepatitis E and EBV infections usually cause only a short-lived, acute hepatitis, with the exception that HEV may become chronic in patients that are immunocompromised. Health-care workers are routinely immunised against HBV, making chronic HBV infection less likely in this situation. HCV is caused by an RNA flavivirus. Acute symptomatic infection with hepatitis C is rare. Most individuals are unaware of when they became infected and are only identified when they develop chronic liver disease. Eighty per cent of individuals exposed to the virus become chronically infected and late spontaneous viral clearance is rare. Unlike HBV, there is no active

or passive protection against HCV. HCV is usually identified in asymptomatic individuals screened because they have risk factors for infection, such as previous injecting drug use, tattoos, needlestick injury, etc.

22.45. Answer: E.

In hereditary haemochromatosis, iron is deposited throughout the body and causes damage to several organs, including the liver. Serum iron studies show a greatly increased ferritin, a raised plasma iron and saturated plasma iron-binding capacity. The differential diagnoses for elevated ferritin includes inflammatory disease, NAFLD or excess ethanol consumption for modest elevations (<1000 μg/L). Transferrin saturation of more than 45% is highly suggestive of iron overload and not affected by inflammatory state and so is more specific than ferritin. Genetic testing can be considered later, but in the first instance tests for iron overload would be first line and best value.

22.46. Answer: E.

The patient presents with a painful obstructive jaundice. The blood tests represent a typical cholestatic picture with elevated ALP and GGT, making viral hepatitis unlikely. In this setting, ultrasound would be the first-line investigation to seek evidence of biliary obstruction with dilated common bile duct due to, for example, gallstone disease. Depending on the findings, it may then be necessary to proceed to MRCP or endoscopic ultrasound prior to ERCP if an obstruction is identified. Pancreatic cancer is more classically associated with a painless obstructive jaundice.

22.47. Answer: D.

Non-selective β-adrenoceptor antagonists (β-blockers; e.g. propranolol) are used as a secondary measure to prevent recurrent variceal bleeding. Following successful treatment by endoscopic therapy, patients should also be entered into an oesophageal banding programme with repeated sessions of therapy at intervals until the varices are obliterated. In selected individuals, TIPSS may also be considered in this setting.

22.48. Answer: B.

The patient carries two copies of the most common *HFE* variant, C282Y, and has evidence of iron overload. Venesection would

22

be the most appropriate treatment with frequency adjusted according to fall in ferritin and transferrin saturation. Vitamin C supplementation increases absorption of iron from the diet and so should be avoided.

22.49. Answer: D.

TIPSS is used in the management of refractory variceal bleeding that has not responded to other therapies. Placement of a Sengstaken–Blakemore tube is an emergency holding measure used when there is an uncontrollable variceal haemorrhage – for example, while plans are made for a TIPSS – and so is not necessary in this situation.

If non-bleeding varices are identified at endoscopy, β-blocker therapy with propranolol (80–160 mg/day) or nadolol is effective in reducing portal venous pressure. Administration of these drugs at doses that reduce the heart rate by 25% has been shown to be effective in the primary prevention of variceal bleeding. In patients with cirrhosis, treatment with propranolol reduces variceal bleeding by 47% (number needed to treat for benefit (NNT_B) 10), death from bleeding by 45% (NNT_B 25) and overall mortality by 22% (NNT_B 16). The efficacy of β-blockers in primary prevention is similar to that of prophylactic banding, which may also be considered, particularly in patients unable to tolerate β-blocker therapy. Carvedilol, a non-cardioselective vasodilating β-blocker, is also effective.

22.50. Answer: D.

Increasingly sedentary lifestyles and changing dietary patterns mean that the prevalence of obesity and insulin resistance has increased worldwide; thus, fat accumulation in the liver is a common finding during abdominal imaging studies and on liver biopsy. In the absence of high alcohol consumption (typically a threshold of <20 g/day for women and <30 g/day for men is adopted), this is called non-alcoholic fatty liver disease. Non-alcoholic fatty liver disease (NAFLD) is the most common cause for abnormal LFTs worldwide, estimated to affect 20–30% of the general population in Western countries and 5–18% in Asia, with about 1 in 10 NAFLD cases exhibiting non-alcoholic steatohepatitis (NASH). NAFLD is the leading cause of liver dysfunction in the non-alcoholic, viral hepatitis-negative population in Europe and North America and is predicted to become the main aetiology in patients undergoing liver transplantation during the next 5 years.

22.51. Answer: E.

Although the virus has been successfully cleared, the patient was found to have cirrhosis and so remains at risk of developing hepatocellular carcinoma (HCC). He will require follow-up and management to check for risks associated with cirrhosis, including HCC and portal hypertension/varices.

HG Watson, DJ Culligan,
LM Manson

23

Haematology and transfusion medicine

Multiple Choice Questions

23.1. In a patient with a vague history of weight loss but little else on examination you find lymphadenopathy confined to the right axilla. Which of the following conditions is most likely?

A. Chronic lymphocytic leukaemia
B. Follicular lymphoma
C. Glandular fever
D. Human immunodeficiency virus (HIV) seroconversion illness
E. Metastatic breast cancer

23.2. In the investigation of a patient with suspected essential thrombocythaemia, in which of the following genes may you find abnormalities?

A. *BCL-2*
B. *BCR*
C. *c-MYC*
D. *CAL-R*
E. *MYH-9*

23.3. Having made a new diagnosis of polycythaemia rubra vera (PRV) you are consulting with the patient regarding prognosis and complications of the condition. He has read the information booklet and wishes to know about common vascular complications of the condition. Which of the following is the most common vascular complication?

A. Budd–Chiari syndrome
B. Ischaemic stroke
C. Livedo reticularis
D. Mesenteric vein thrombosis
E. Pulmonary embolism

23.4. A 65 year old man presents with an immune-mediated thrombocytopenia. He has been treated with antibiotics during a recent hospital admission. Which of the following is most likely implicated in the new development?

A. Amoxicillin
B. Ciprofloxacin
C. Gentamicin
D. Metronidazole
E. Vancomycin

23.5. A patient with systemic lupus erythematosus (SLE) and immune thrombocytopenia (ITP) presents with a platelet count of 5×10^9/L. Which of these is the most likely presenting symptom?

A. Haemarthrosis
B. Intracranial haemorrhage
C. Muscular haematoma
D. Oral mucosal bleeding
E. Retroperitoneal haematoma

23.6. Which of the following anticoagulants has a mechanism of action involving antithrombin-dependent inhibition of thrombin and factor Xa?

A. Apixaban
B. Bivalirudin
C. Dabigatran
D. Dalteparin
E. Edoxaban

23.7. A 72 year old woman who is on warfarin consults to ask if she can change to an alternative oral anticoagulant. You review her clinical case. In which of the following clinical circumstances would the answer be that she should stay on warfarin?

A. Atrial fibrillation in a patient with a prosthetic mitral valve
B. Distal deep vein thrombosis (DVT) following plaster cast immobilisation
C. Lone atrial fibrillation with a CHA_2DS_2-VASc score of 2
D. Proximal DVT following total knee replacement
E. Unprovoked pulmonary embolism

23.8. A patient who is admitted to the intensive care unit (ICU) with multi-organ failure and sepsis is suspected of having heparin-induced thrombocytopenia (HIT). Which of the following pieces of clinical information is most likely to suggest an alternative diagnosis?

A. The heparin treatment commenced 16 days ago
B. The patient has been receiving treatment with unfractionated heparin (UFH)
C. The patient has had complex cardiac surgery with cardiopulmonary bypass
D. The patient has sustained a post-operative pulmonary embolus
E. The platelet count has dropped from normal to a level of 53×10^9/L

23.9. What is the most likely diagnosis in a 2 year old boy who presents with an apparently unprovoked knee haemarthrosis?

Initial investigations show that he has a normal platelet count and a normal prothrombin time (PT). His activated partial thromboplastin time (APTT) is prolonged at 76 seconds.

A. Lupus anticoagulant
B. Severe factor XI deficiency
C. Severe factor XII deficiency
D. Severe haemophilia A (factor VIII deficiency)
E. Severe haemophilia B (factor IX deficiency)

23.10. A 13 year old girl with significant menorrhagia is investigated to see if there is an underlying bleeding disorder. Her investigations show a normal platelet count, PT and fibrinogen. Her APTT is prolonged and her factor VIII level is 0.2 U/mL, her von Willebrand factor ristocetin co-factor (vWF:RiCO) level is 0.05 U/mL and her von Willebrand factor antigen (vWF:Ag) is 0.14 U/mL. What is the most likely diagnosis?

A. Haemophilia A carrier with low VIII levels
B. Type 1 von Willebrand disease
C. Type 2A von Willebrand disease
D. Type 2N von Willebrand disease
E. Type 3 von Willebrand disease

23.11. In the context of routine clerking of a pre-surgical patient, which of the following is the most informative question in detecting an underlying bleeding disorder in a patient who reports a 'problem with bleeding'?

A. Bleeding after shaving
B. Easy bruising
C. Epistaxis as a child
D. Post-partum haemorrhage
E. Previous post-surgical bleeding

23.12. A Dutch woman is referred following the development of a pulmonary embolism without obvious provoking factors. If she were investigated further, which form of inherited thrombophilia would you be most likely to find in this case?

A. Antithrombin deficiency
B. Factor V Leiden
C. Protein C deficiency
D. Protein S deficiency
E. Prothrombin gene mutation

23.13. A 65 year old man is admitted as a medical emergency. A diagnosis of pulmonary embolism is made. Which of the following features in his clinical history is most likely to have contributed most to his thrombosis risk?

A. He had a total knee replacement (TKR) 9 months previously
B. He had just flown back to the UK from a weekend break in Paris
C. He has recently started quinine for night cramps
D. He was discharged from hospital 4 weeks ago following treatment for congestive cardiac failure (CCF)
E. His 64 year old cousin has recently suffered from a pulmonary embolism following bowel surgery

23.14. You are asked to see a 59 year old man following 3 months of anticoagulation for an episode of proximal DVT that occurred without any identifiable risk factor. You are trying to decide whether you think he would benefit from long-term anticoagulation or not. Of the following, which is the strongest risk factor for predicting recurrence following discontinuation of the treatment?

A. Age over 50 years
B. D-dimer level after stopping treatment
C. Hormone replacement therapy use
D. Male sex
E. Unprovoked episode

23.15. A 32 year old woman who has been previously well presents with apparent loss of consciousness. You suspect a diagnosis of thrombotic thrombocytopenic purpura (TTP). Which of the following observations would be LEAST common in fitting with that diagnosis?

A. Confusion
B. Fever
C. Microangiopathic haemolytic anaemia
D. Purpura
E. Thrombocytopenia

23.16. Thrombin is generated as part of the process of activation of coagulation. Thrombin has many actions. Which of these actions directly results in the cross-linking of fibrin clot?

A. Activation of factor VIII
B. Binding of endothelial cell-bound thrombomodulin
C. Binding of the platelet thrombin receptor
D. Cleavage of factor XIII
E. Cleavage of the fibrinopeptides on fibrinogen

23.17. A 36 year old man presents with night-time cough and wheezing over the previous 2 months. He has a previous history of eczema. What finding in his full blood count would be in fitting with the scenario and help towards the diagnosis?

A. Basophilia
B. Eosinophilia
C. Lymphocytosis
D. Monocytosis
E. Neutrophilia

23.18. A junior doctor phones you about a patient who is unwell after an episode of post-cholecystectomy pancreatitis. The patient has a normochromic normocytic anaemia, a leucocytosis and a mild thrombocytosis. The prothrombin time is 55 seconds, the APTT is 46 seconds and the fibrinogen is normal (4 g/L). What is the most likely diagnosis?

A. Anticoagulation with LMWH
B. Disseminated intravascular coagulation
C. Factor XIII deficiency

D. Liver failure
E. Vitamin K deficiency

23.19. The blood film of a 67 year old man is reported to show target cells, acanthocytes, Howell–Jolly bodies, a leucocytosis and a mild thrombocytosis. What is the most likely cause of this picture?

A. Alcoholic liver disease
B. Essential thrombocythaemia
C. *Falciparum* malaria
D. Hyposplenism
E. Myelofibrosis

23.20. Consider the haemoglobin–oxygen dissociation curve, below. Which condition results in increased oxygen release to hypoxic tissue, i.e. moves the dissociation curve to the right?

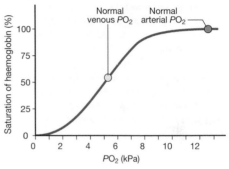

A. Haemoglobin S (HbS)
B. Hypothermia
C. Low levels of 2,3-bisphosphoglycerate (2,3-BPG)
D. Low levels of CO_2
E. Reduced pH

23.21. Which of the following changes is commonly seen in normal pregnancy?

A. Low protein C levels
B. Low vitamin B_{12} levels
C. Lupus anticoagulant
D. Polycythaemia
E. Reducing fibrinogen level with advancing gestation

23.22. When examining the abdomen for the presence of splenomegaly, which of the following statements is true?

A. A palpable spleen moves downwards on expiration
B. A palpable spleen moves upwards on inspiration

23

C. A splenic rub is frequently heard following acute infarction of massive splenomegaly

D. If you can get above a mass in the left upper quadrant, then it is likely to be a spleen

E. The spleen is usually palpable in small people

23.23. Which of the following statements relating to normal haematopoietic stem cells is true?

A. Daughter cells of stem cells are always destined to become mature blood cells

B. Stem cells are easily identified when examining the bone marrow down the microscope

C. Stem cells can only give rise to daughter cells of a particular lineage

D. Stem cells circulate in the blood and can be mobilised into the blood in increased numbers by growth factors such as granulocyte colony-stimulating factor (G-CSF)

E. They are the commonest cell found in the bone marrow

23.24. A patient is referred after being found unexpectedly to have anaemia. Which of the following statements is in keeping with a diagnosis of acute myeloid leukaemia?

A. Bleeding into a knee joint in a 6 month old boy

B. Splenomegaly is frequently massive

C. The leukaemic blasts proliferate excessively but differentiate normally

D. The platelet count is most likely to be increased

E. The presence of a high white cell count but very low neutrophil count in an elderly man

23.25. A 65 year old man presents to his doctor with increasing shortness of breath and is found to have an abnormal full blood count. With regard to the myelodysplastic syndromes (MDS), which of the following statements is true?

A. Anaemia is the most frequent presenting abnormality and is commonly macrocytic

B. Erythropoietin (EPO) is not a useful therapy if the renal function is normal

C. Ring sideroblasts are dysplastic white cells and associated with mutations in the gene *SF3B1*

D. The median age of presentation is about 50 years

E. Transformation to acute myeloid leukaemia (AML) is diagnosed when the blast count rises to >30%

23.26. Which of the following situations would be in keeping with a diagnosis of monoclonal gammopathy of uncertain significance (MGUS)?

A. A light chain only paraprotein with immunoparesis for immunoglobulin G (IgG) and immunoglobulin A (IgA)

B. A low-level IgG paraprotein associated with a single lytic lesion in the femur

C. A low-level IgG paraprotein with normal serum free light chain ratio

D. An IgA paraprotein in someone presenting with acute renal failure

E. An immunoglobulin M (IgM) paraprotein in someone presenting with mild anaemia and splenomegaly

23.27. Which of the following clinical situations represents a likely diagnosis of multiple myeloma?

A. A 10 year old child with acute renal failure and a positive urine test for Bence Jones protein

B. Acute renal failure in a 65 year old woman with hypercalcaemia, rib pain, immunoparesis for IgG and IgA but no intact paraprotein

C. An IgG paraprotein of 10 g/L in a young woman with widespread joint pains and neutropenia

D. Hypercalcaemia in an elderly man with a high alkaline phosphatase and sclerotic bone lesions

E. Pneumonia in a middle-aged man with lymphopenia, increased polyclonal plasma cells in the bone marrow and a polyclonal rise in immunoglobulins

23.28. A 56 year old man presents to hospital with abdominal discomfort and is found to have splenomegaly and an abnormal full blood count. In CML, which of the following statements is correct?

A. Allogeneic stem cell transplantation remains the first-choice therapy in chronic phase

B. At presentation a majority of white cells are blast cells

C. The disease arises from a mutated stem cell containing the t(15;17) translocation

D. The Philadelphia (Ph) chromosome is a small chromosome 22 resulting from the translocation t(9;22)

E. The platelet count is usually reduced

23.29. Which of the following cases most likely represents a case of Hodgkin lymphoma (HL) rather than non-Hodgkin lymphoma (NHL)?

A. A 19 year old man with pancytopenia and a large mediastinal mass with pleural and pericardial effusions

B. A 21 year old woman with painless, rubbery, cervical lymphadenopathy increasing over 3 months and an asymptomatic mediastinal mass on chest X-ray

C. A 25 year old woman with symptoms of mediastinal obstruction and massive mediastinal lymphadenopathy; the biopsy shows sheets of centroblasts that are CD20 positive

D. A 50 year old woman with new-onset epilepsy and a mass in the right cerebral hemisphere surrounded by oedema

E. A 60 year old man with widespread, asymptomatic, painless lymphadenopathy and splenomegaly

23.30. A 68 year old man presents to his family physician with fever, night sweats and unexplained weight loss. Which one of the following is defined by low-grade, mature-looking lymphocytes that are CD5 and cyclin D1 positive but CD23 negative.

A. B-cell acute lymphoblastic leukaemia (B-ALL)

B. Chronic lymphocytic leukaemia (CLL)

C. Diffuse large B-cell NHL (DLBL)

D. Follicular lymphoma

E. Mantle cell lymphoma

23.31. A 73 year old man is found to have some abnormalities in a full blood count taken to investigate a symptom of fatigue. In patients with chronic lymphocytic leukaemia (CLL), which one of the following features is true?

A. Most patients are symptomatic and require treatment at presentation

B. Patients with mutated immunoglobulin genes have a poorer prognosis than those with unmutated immunoglobulin genes

C. Signalling through the B-cell receptor complex (BCR) is not a useful target for treatment

D. The peripheral blood lymphocyte count is persistently above 5×10^9/L

E. The presence of a *TP53* mutation predicts for a good response to chemotherapy

23.32. A 48 year old woman with general malaise is found to have acute myeloid leukaemia (AML). With regard to allogeneic stem cell transplantation for patients with this condition, which of the following statements is true?

A. Complications of the procedure lead to a treatment-related mortality (TRM) of about 1–5% by 2 years after transplantation

B. Older female donors are a better source of stem cells than younger male donors

C. Patients with chronic graft-versus-host disease (GVHD) are more likely to relapse from AML after the transplant

D. Reduced-intensity conditioning (RIC) is used for very young, fit patients

E. The anti-leukaemic effect originates predominantly from transplanted donor T lymphocytes (graft versus leukaemia; GvL)

23.33. Which of the following best describes the action of the anthracycline group of chemotherapy drugs?

A. They act as small-molecule inhibitors of tyrosine kinases and include nilotinib

B. They act as antimetabolites and include methotrexate

C. They act as inhibitors of topoisomerase II and include etoposide

D. They act as inhibitors of tubulin polymerisation and include vincristine

E. They act to intercalate between double-stranded DNA base pairs and include daunorubicin

23.34. The first-line therapy for a 50 year old man with severe aplastic anaemia is best described as follows?

A. A myeloablative allogeneic stem cell transplant from an unrelated donor

B. Immunosuppressive therapy with high-dose glucocorticoids

C. Immunosuppressive therapy with horse anti-thymocyte globulin (ATG) followed by ciclosporin

D. Immunosuppressive therapy with rabbit ATG

E. Supportive care only with red cells, platelets and G-CSF

23

23.35. A 68 year old woman has been found to have a low haemoglobin in the context of long-term rheumatoid arthritis and chronic kidney disease. What does the mechanism of the anaemia of chronic disease include?

A. Chronic gastrointestinal (GI) tract bleeding
B. High hepcidin levels inhibiting iron export from macrophages
C. Iron toxicity to the bone marrow
D. Poor iron absorption because of achlorhydria
E. Red cell sequestration in a chronically enlarged spleen

23.36. A 4 year old girl is brought to her doctor with fever and is found to have acute leukaemia. Which of the following is considered the most important prognostic feature for childhood acute lymphoblastic leukaemia?

A. T-cell rather than B-cell phenotype
B. The age and sex of the child
C. The chromosomal abnormalities acquired by the leukaemic cells
D. The height of the white cell count at presentation
E. The presence of minimal residual disease (MRD) post induction therapy

23.37. A 6 year old patient has had severe neutropenia ($<0.2\times10^9$/L) lasting for more than 7 days following initial treatment for AML. Which of the following is true?

A. Azole prophylaxis against fungal infection with posaconazole is not recommended
B. Gram-negative sepsis is more common than Gram-positive sepsis
C. Indwelling Hickman lines are more commonly infected with Gram-negative organisms than Gram-positive ones
D. Neutropenic fever should be treated empirically prior to receiving the results of blood cultures
E. Quinolone prophylaxis is not recommended to prevent sepsis

23.38. A 42 year old woman with alcoholic liver disease presents as an emergency to hospital with massive haematemesis. Her temperature is 37°C, pulse rate 130 beats/min and blood pressure is 70/40 mmHg. She is cool peripherally. She has stigmata of chronic liver disease with a palpable spleen at 3 cm below the left costal margin. She is initially resuscitated with intravenous fluids.

Investigations show: haemoglobin 61 g/L; white cell count (WCC) 5.2×10^9/L; platelet count 84×10^9/L.

You request 4 units of packed red cells urgently. Group and screen 2 years previously showed group B Rhesus D (RhD)-positive with a negative antibody screen.

There is insufficient time to do compatibility testing. What is the most appropriate blood to transfuse?

A. AB RhD-negative
B. B RhD-negative
C. B RhD-positive
D. O RhD-negative
E. O RhD-positive

23.39. A 28 year old female, para 1+0, presents to obstetric triage at 27 weeks. All was well at booking. She reports intermittent vaginal bleeding for the past 2 weeks. Other than requiring a 3-unit red cell transfusion following a road traffic accident 3 years ago she has been well.

Investigations show: haemoglobin 121 g/L; WCC 8.4×10^9/L; platelet count 238×10^9/L.

Group and screen: group A RhD-negative with a positive antibody screen.

Antibodies: anti-D (titre 1/32)

What is the most likely reason for the development of the antibody?

A. Fetal maternal haemorrhage during this pregnancy
B. Physiological increase in naturally occurring antibody
C. Previous pregnancy
D. Routine antenatal anti-D prophylaxis
E. Transfusion

23.40. A patient receives a blood transfusion and has developed complications. Which of the following combinations will result in least insult to the patient?

A. Group AB red cells into a group O adult
B. Group B red cells into a group A adult
C. Group B red cells into a group A neonate
D. Group O fresh frozen plasma (FFP) into a group A adult
E. Group O FFP into a group B adult

23.41. A 28 year old female, para 1+1, presents to obstetric triage at 22 weeks. She reports intermittent vaginal bleeding for the past 24 hours and thinks it is likely implantation bleeding. There has been no preceding trauma.

On examination she appears comfortable at rest. Her temperature is 36.7°C, pulse rate is 88 beats/min and blood pressure is 98/68 mmHg. Fundal height measures 22 cm.

There are no concerns about the baby.

Investigations: haemoglobin 101 g/L; WCC 8.4×10⁹/L; platelet count 238×10⁹/L.

Group and screen: group O RhD-negative with a negative antibody screen.

What is the most appropriate initial management for this patient?

A. Arrange a 2-unit red cell transfusion
B. Arrange an urgent abdominal ultrasound to exclude placental issues
C. Commence her on oral iron
D. Reassure her that baby is well and bloods are normal for this stage of pregnancy
E. Take blood for a Kleihauer test and give anti-D

23.42. A 72 year old man with NHL attends the oncology assessment area post-chemotherapy with chest discomfort and shortness of breath at rest. His temperature is 37.4°C, pulse rate is 110 beats/min and blood pressure is 90/64 mmHg.

Investigations: haemoglobin 81 g/L; WCC 1.1×10⁹/L; platelet count 40×10⁹/L. Troponin: awaited. ECG shows T-wave flattening.

The patient agrees to a 2-unit red cell transfusion. Which of the following actions is the most important one in ensuring a safe transfusion without patient harm?

A. He confirms his name and date of birth to the person taking his pre-transfusion sample
B. He is provided with written patient information
C. He provides written consent
D. The reason for the transfusion is clearly documented in the notes
E. Transfusion is delayed until troponin is available

23.43. A 78 year old man with stable ischaemic heart disease is admitted with a traumatic hip fracture. He undergoes a right hemi-arthroplasty. Twenty-four hours post-operatively, investigations reveal a haemoglobin of 65 g/L. Fifteen minutes into transfusion of the first unit of red cells, his observations are: temperature 38.4°C; pulse rate 88 beats/min; blood pressure 100/60 mmHg.

He is flushed but otherwise well. Observations were normal before transfusion was started. How would you manage this clinical situation?

A. Do nothing
B. Stop the transfusion, give chlorphenamine and, provided well, restart in 15 minutes
C. Stop the transfusion, give paracetamol and, provided well, restart in 15 minutes
D. Stop the transfusion, initiate fluid resuscitation and inform the hospital transfusion team
E. Stop the transfusion, take blood cultures, give antibiotics and return unit to blood bank as concern about bacterial contamination

23.44. A 22 year old man is admitted following a severe road traffic accident. He suffered significant blood loss at the scene. He is resuscitated with Gelofusine plasma expander and group O negative packed red cells. Intra-operatively the anaesthetist phones you for advice.

Bloods show: haemoglobin 66 g/L; WCC 11.2×10⁹/L; platelet count 83×10⁹/L; PT 28 seconds; APTT 72 seconds; fibrinogen: 1.9 g/L.

What is most appropriate to use to reduce his bleeding risk?

A. Cryoprecipitate
B. Fresh frozen plasma
C. Platelets
D. Prothrombin complex concentrate
E. Vitamin K

23.45. A 69 year old man with myelodysplasia is admitted with haematuria. He is transfused with 2 units of packed red cells. Eight hours following his transfusion you are called to review him as he is now acutely unwell with breathlessness and chest tightness. Observations reveal: temperature 37.8°C, pulse rate 130 beats/min, blood pressure 88/60 mmHg, respiratory rate 34 breaths/min and oxygen saturation 82%. He is distressed with bilateral chest crepitations, R>L. Heart sounds are normal. Jugular venous pressure (JVP) is normal. Chest X-ray shows normal heart size, Kerley B lines and bilateral nodular infiltrates. Electrocardiography (ECG) shows sinus tachycardia.

What is the most likely cause of the patient's deterioration?

23

A. Myocardial infarction
B. Pulmonary embolus
C. Sepsis
D. Transfusion-associated circulatory overload
E. Transfusion-related acute lung injury

23.46. A 21 year old female medical student presents to her family physician with fatigue, shortness of breath and a sore mouth. On examination she is pale with a yellow tinge with a palpable splenic tip on inspiration. Bloods are checked.

Investigations show: haemoglobin 68 g/L; mean cell volume (MCV) 118 fL; mean cell haemoglobin (MCH) 35 pg; WCC 1.9×10^9/L; platelet count 92×10^9/L.

A blood film report reads: macrocytosis with macro-ovalocytes and hypersegmented neutrophils (see below).

What is the most likely diagnosis?

A. Acute myeloid leukaemia
B. Alcohol excess
C. Vitamin B_{12} deficiency
D. Hyperthyroidism
E. Iron deficiency

23.47. A 19 year old student presents to the emergency department feeling sweaty and unwell over the last 24 hours. Her initial observations show a temperature of 39.4°C, pulse 120 beats/min, blood pressure 94/64 mmHg, respiratory rate 22 breaths/min and oxygen saturations 99% on room air.

Investigations reveal: haemoglobin 118 g/L; MCV 84 fL; MCH 29 pg; WCC 33.0×10^9/L; neutrophils 26×10^9/L; monocytes 4×10^9/L; lymphocytes 3×10^9/L; platelet count 580×10^9/L; blood glucose 6.9 mmol/L (124 mg/dL).

Blood film: neutrophilia with toxic granulation (see below).

What is the most likely cause of her leucocytosis?

A. Acute bacterial infection
B. Acute myeloid leukaemia
C. Diabetic ketoacidosis
D. Infectious mononucleosis
E. Systemic autoimmune disease

23.48. A 56 year old Scottish woman, previously fit and well, presents to her family physician with a 2-week history of increasing tiredness. On examination she is pale and jaundiced. Bloods are checked.

Investigations: haemoglobin 68 g/L; MCV 109 fL; WCC 5.3×10^9/L; platelet count 152×10^9/L; reticulocyte count 280×10^9/L; alkaline phosphatase (ALP) 100 U/L; alanine aminotransferase (ALT) 54 U/L; bilirubin 32 μmol/L (1.87 mg/dL).

Blood film: polychromasia with spherocytes; no red cell fragments (see below).

What is the most appropriate next investigation?

A. Bone marrow aspiration and trephine biopsy
B. Direct antiglobulin (Coombs) test
C. Hepatitis screen
D. Serum vitamin B_{12} and folate
E. Thyroid function tests

23.49. A 38 year old woman with known sickle-cell disease presents to the emergency department on Christmas Eve with severe back pain. Observations reveal: temperature 37.8°C, pulse rate 90 beats/min, blood pressure 118/80 mmHg, respiratory rate 18 breaths/min and oxygen saturation 96%. On examination she is distressed. Radiological examination is unremarkable.

Investigations: haemoglobin 52 g/L; MCV 70 fL; WCC 12×10^9/L; platelet count 384×10^9/L; C-reactive protein (CRP) 18 mg/L.

She is commenced on oxygen, broad-spectrum antibiotics, intravenous fluids and analgesia, but fails to improve. What is the most important next step in her management?

A. Exchange transfusion
B. Folic acid
C. LMWH
D. Oral iron replacement
E. Red cell transfusion

23.50. A couple attends for pregnancy counselling. They both have beta-thalassaemia trait.

Which of the following is correct?

A. 1 in 2 chance the baby will be normal
B. 1 in 4 chance the baby will develop hydrops fetalis
C. 1 in 4 chance the baby will have beta-thalassaemia trait
D. 1 in 4 chance the baby will have beta-thalassaemia major
E. Pregnancy is unlikely to be successful

23.51. A 16 year old boy with known sickle-cell disease is brought to the emergency department profoundly unwell. He has a reduced conscious level, temperature 39°C, pulse rate 160 beats/min and blood pressure 70/40 mmHg.

Investigations: haemoglobin 78 g/L; MCV 68 fL; WCC 17×10⁹/L; platelet count 480×10⁹/L; reticulocyte count 120×10⁹/L; CRP 41 mg/L.

Blood film: neutrophilia with toxic granulation; red cell changes consistent with sickle cell disease and hyposplenism (see below).

What is the most likely clinical diagnosis?

A. Aplastic crisis
B. Infectious mononucleosis
C. Meningococcal sepsis
D. Painful vaso-occlusive crisis
E. Sickle chest syndrome

23.52. A pale and lethargic 2 year old boy is brought to the emergency department by his parents. He recently started nursery. His temperature is 36.9°C, pulse rate is 110 beats/min and blood pressure is 90/40 mmHg. His urine is dark brown in colour.

Investigations: haemoglobin 60 g/L; MCV 68 fL; MCH 31 pg; WCC 9.3×10⁹/L; platelet count 330×10⁹/L; reticulocyte count 240×10⁹/L; ALT 61 U/L; ALP 108 U/L; bilirubin 60 µmol/L (3.5 mg/dL).

Blood film shows polychromasia with bite and blister cells.

What is the most appropriate next investigation?

A. Direct antiglobulin test
B. Donath–Landsteiner assay
C. Glucose-6-phosphate dehydrogenase (G6PD) assay
D. Mid-stream urine (MSU)
E. Parvovirus serology

23.53. A previously well 26 year old woman presents at term, after an uneventful pregnancy, in the late stages of labour. This is her first pregnancy. Delivery is uneventful; the baby is well but is noted to have a widespread petechial rash.

Investigations: haemoglobin 168 g/L; MCV 90 fL; WCC 12×10⁹/L; platelet count 7×10⁹/L; PT 12 seconds; APTT 30 seconds; fibrinogen 4.0 g/L.

Blood film: true thrombocytopenia.

What is the most likely cause of the low platelets?

A. Disseminated intravascular coagulation
B. Immune thrombocytopenic purpura

C. Infection
D. Intrauterine growth retardation
E. Neonatal alloimmune thrombocytopenia

23.54. A 25 year old man wishes to be a blood donor. Which of the following will his blood not be screened for evidence of exposure to?

A. Hepatitis A
B. Hepatitis B
C. Hepatitis C
D. Human T-lymphotrophic virus (HTLV)
E. Syphilis

23.55. A 68 year old woman with ischaemic heart disease and rheumatoid arthritis presents with worsening angina.

Bloods show: haemoglobin 98 g/L; MCV 80 fL; MCH 29 pg; WCC 7×10⁹/L; platelets 300×10⁹/L; iron 6 µmol/L (33.5 µg/dL); transferrin saturation 12%; total iron-binding capacity 33 µmol/L; vitamin B₁₂ 400 ng/L; folate 8 µg/L.

What is the most likely cause of her anaemia?

A. Anaemia of chronic disease
B. Autoimmune haemolysis
C. Folate deficiency
D. Iron deficiency
E. Myelodysplasia

23.56. A 57 year old woman has just started a blood transfusion following coronary bypass grafting yesterday. What may happen 30 minutes later as a result of the transfusion?

A. She becomes hypothermic
B. She becomes iron overloaded
C. She becomes thrombocythaemic
D. She develops an urticarial rash
E. She develops hypokalaemia

23.57. A 36 year old man receives a platelet transfusion prior to Hickman line removal following a stem cell transplantation for acute myeloid leukaemia. Ten minutes after the transfusion starts, he becomes acutely breathless, hypotensive and febrile. Despite intensive resuscitation he dies.

What is the most likely cause for his death?

A. Bacterial contamination
B. Metabolic-induced cardiac arrhythmia
C. Pulmonary embolism
D. Transfusion-associated circulatory overload
E. Transfusion of an ABO-incompatible unit

23

Answers

23.1. Answer: E.

Follicular lymphoma and chronic lymphocytic leukaemia (CLL) are systemic malignancies with involvement of lymphoid tissue in many sites. HIV and Epstein–Barr virus (EBV) infection produce generalised lymphadenopathy and systemic illness. Cancers tend to metastasise to local regional nodes draining a specific tissue and so breast cancer tends to present with localised unilateral axillary lymphadenopathy.

23.2. Answer: D.

All of these mutated genes are associated with haematological conditions: *BCR* with chronic myeloid leukaemia (CML), *c-MYC* and *BCL-2* with lymphoma, and *MYH-9* with congenital thrombocytopathy. Only *CAL-R*, calreticulin, is associated with the myeloproliferative neoplasm essential thrombocythaemia.

23.3. Answer: B.

The most common complications of PRV involve vascular occlusion. All of the conditions listed are associated with PRV, but the most common is ischaemic stroke.

23.4. Answer: E.

Vancomycin is associated with immune-mediated thrombocytopenia – the others are not.

23.5. Answer: D.

Haemarthrosis, muscular haematoma and retroperitoneal haemorrhage more commonly complicate bleeding disorders associated with reduced levels of coagulation factors. Intracranial haemorrhage can complicate severe thrombocytopenia or severe coagulation factor deficiency but oral mucosal bleeding is by far the most common feature of severe thrombocytopenia along with skin purpura.

23.6. Answer: D.

Dalteparin is a low-molecular-weight heparin (LMWH), the effect of which is mediated by enhanced avidity of antithrombin for its natural substrates, thrombin and factor Xa. Apixaban and edoxaban are direct-acting inhibitors of factor Xa, while dabigatran and bivalirudin are direct thrombin inhibitors.

23.7. Answer: A.

All of the other circumstances are licensed indications for the use of rivaroxaban except for the management of patients with prosthetic heart valves. CHA_2DS_2-VASc is a well-known scoring system to evaluate risk of thrombosis in a patient with atrial fibrillation.

23.8. Answer: A.

HIT is most commonly seen in surgical patients, especially following major orthopaedic and cardiac surgery. HIT is more commonly seen when UFH is used compared with low-molecular-weight heparin (LMWH); it is commonly associated with moderate as opposed to severe thrombocytopenia and it is associated, somewhat paradoxically, with thrombotic events. The key period for developing HIT is after 5–10 days of exposure, with longer exposures less likely to be associated.

23.9. Answer: D.

All of these conditions can present with a normal PT and a prolonged APTT. Lupus anticoagulant is very rarely associated with a bleeding diathesis. Factor XII deficiency causes a very marked prolongation of the APTT but is never associated with bleeding. Severe XI deficiency is associated with variable severity of bleeding and is rare. Factor VIII and IX deficiencies present with identical phenotypes but severe haemophilia A is 5 times more common than severe haemophilia B. The scenario is classical of the first presentation of severe haemophilia A or B.

23.10. Answer: C.

She has a low factor VIII level, which is compatible with all the diagnoses given. However, she has a level of functional vWF (RiCO) that is out of keeping with her vWF antigen level (ratio is 0.35). This suggests a dysfunctional molecule and therefore type 2 vWD. Type 2N vWD is associated with isolated low factor VIII and so the most likely diagnosis here is type 2A vWD. This is a common presentation in affected young women.

23.11. Answer: E.

Epistaxis, easy bruising and bleeding after shaving are all symptoms commonly reported in patients without a bleeding disorder and so are very non-specific indicators of a bleeding disorder. Post-partum haemorrhage is usually associated with other pregnancy-associated illness, uterine atony or vaginal trauma.

23.12. Answer: B.
Factor V Leiden is a gain-of-function mutation found in around 5% of northern Europeans. The others are all less commonly found abnormalities associated with venous thromboembolic (VTE) risk.

23.13. Answer: D.
The TKR is too remote in time to be relevant; however, it is a strong risk factor for VTE in the 35 days post-surgery. Quinine can result in the development of thrombocytopenia and a systemic reaction but is not associated with VTE. Travel is a common but weak risk factor for thrombosis and only journeys of >3 hours of continuous travel are relevant. A cousin is not a first-degree relative and the event suffered by this man's cousin was provoked. CCF, or indeed any significant hospitalisation, is a strong risk factor for subsequent VTE – The Million Women Study suggests the period of attributable risk is about 12 weeks.

23.14. Answer: E.
The background to the event is the strongest predicting factor for recurrence. Unprovoked events have a far higher rate of recurrence than provoked events where the provoking factor has been removed. In predicting recurrence after an unprovoked event, male sex and elevated D-dimer are predictive of recurrence.

23.15. Answer: D.
Purpura is rare in TTP despite the name of the disorder. In conditions where prothrombotic states are associated with thrombocytopenia, it is often the case that there is a lack of purpura: e.g. in haemolytic uraemic syndrome (HUS) and heparin-induced thrombocytopenia.

23.16. Answer: D.
Factor XIII is cleaved and the A subunit then cross-links fibrin to form stable clot. Thrombomodulin binding results in activation of the protein C pathway, which has an anticoagulant effect. Activation of factor VIII amplifies coagulation activation and the cleavage of fibrinopeptides results in production of fibrin monomers.

23.17. Answer: B.
Eosinophilia is often seen in association with atopic and allergic conditions. It can also be seen in pulmonary vasculitis. Other causes of reactive eosinophilia include drug reactions and parasitic infections.

23.18. Answer: E.
Anticoagulation with LMWH produces minor prolongation of APTT only. Disseminated intravascular coagulation can complicate pancreatitis but would be expected to be associated with reduced platelet count and fibrinogen. Liver failure, again, can result in prolonged APTT and PT, but in advanced disease you would expect the fibrinogen level to fall. Vitamin K deficiency results in prolongation of PT and APTT with a normal fibrinogen level and is a common complication of hepatobiliary surgery.

23.19. Answer: D.
The described appearances are all part of a hyposplenic picture. Irrespective of the cause of the hyposplenism or splenectomy. Liver disease is associated with target cells but not with a hyposplenic picture. Myelofibrosis is associated with target cells, teardrop poikilocytes, polychromasia and a leucoerythroblastic appearance but not with the features of hyposplenism.

23.20. Answer: E.
The oxygen dissociation curve shifts to the right – i.e. improves the release of oxygen to tissues – in conditions where the pH is decreased (Fig. 23.20). The other changes would tend to move the dissociation curve to the left, making

23

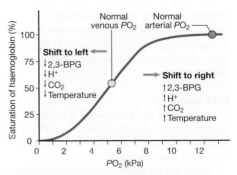

Fig. 23.20 The haemoglobin–oxygen dissociation curve. Factors are listed that shift the curve to the right (more oxygen released from blood) and to the left (less oxygen released) at given PO_2. To convert kPa to mmHg, multiply by 7.5. (2,3-BPG = 2,3-bisphosphoglycerate)

oxygen release to tissues less readily. HbS does not have any affect on oxygen dissociation.

23.21. Answer: B.
Low measured vitamin B_{12} level is common in pregnancy although vitamin B_{12} deficiency is rare – indeed decreased fertility is associated with vitamin B_{12} deficiency. Protein C levels rise in pregnancy, protein S levels fall. Procoagulant factors like factor VIII and fibrinogen increase as pregnancy progresses. Pregnant patients tend to have increased plasma volume and, if anything, tend to be anaemic rather than polycythaemic. Lupus anticoagulant is never a normal finding.

23.22. Answer: C.
The normal spleen is rarely if ever felt and a palpable spleen has the clinical features of moving down on inspiration as the diaphragm contracts and upwards (away from the hand) on expiration. The examining hand cannot get above the spleen and under the left costal margin. Inflammation of the splenic capsule following infarction leads to an audible rub over an acutely painful spleen.

23.23. Answer: D.
Stem cells are rare, accounting for about 0.1% of marrow cells. They cannot be identified on routine morphology and require immunological staining for identification. They have the important characteristics of self-renewal (daughter cells can remain as stem cells rather than differentiating into mature blood cells) and pluripotency (they give rise to cells of different lineages depending on requirements). Stem cells circulate in the blood in small numbers normally and these can be increased up to 1000-fold by mobilisation procedures following chemotherapy, G-CSF or plerixafor. In this way, stem cells can be harvested from the blood for transplantation.

23.24. Answer: E.
The hallmark of acute leukaemia is bone marrow failure: the presence of one or more of anaemia, thrombocytopenia and neutropenia. This is because the leukaemic blast cells proliferate but fail to differentiate normally. The disease is most common in older adults. The total white cell count can be low, normal or high, depending on how many of the blasts escape the marrow into the blood.

Splenomegaly is hardly ever massive, which is a feature of chronic myeloid leukaemia (CML). Bleeding is into skin and mucous membranes because of thrombocytopenia, not joints as in haemophilia.

23.25. Answer: A.
MDS are diseases of the elderly, with a median age of over 70 years. Anaemia is the commonest abnormality, occurring in 80% of patients at some point, and is usually macrocytic. Patients with anaemia and low transfusion requirement and a baseline EPO level of <200 U/L have a 70% chance of responding to EPO therapy, independent of renal function. Dysplasia is present in more than 10% of an affected bone marrow lineage and ring sideroblasts are one form of dysplastic red cell. Mutations in *SF3B1* (a splicing factor) are very strongly associated with the presence of ring sideroblasts. Progression to AML is diagnosed when the blasts are over 20%.

23.26. Answer: C.
In MGUS, the paraprotein is at a low level and with no evidence of end-organ damage, i.e. no evidence of anaemia, bone disease or renal disease. IgM paraproteins are associated with low-grade lymphomas, most notably lymphoplasmacytic lymphoma, but can present as MGUS if there is no clinical evidence of lymphoma. A normal serum free light chain ratio in MGUS carries a very good prognosis.

23.27. Answer: B.
Myeloma is a disease of middle to old age. It is never seen in children and extremely rare under the age of 30 years. The diagnosis requires a paraprotein (including light chain only as in option B) with signs of end-organ damage and usually with an increase in bone marrow monoclonal plasma cells. Option D is most likely metastatic prostate cancer; option C is autoimmune disease, e.g. rheumatoid arthritis; and option E would fit with HIV infection. Normal light chains can appear in the urine in acute renal failure because of failed reabsorption by the renal tubules, as in option A.

23.28. Answer: D.
CML arises from a mutated stem cell containing the Ph chromosome, which results from the translocation t(9;22) and the resulting fusion gene *BCR–ABL*. The leukaemic clone

proliferates and differentiates so in chronic phase the blast count is low and platelets tend to be high (sometimes very high: >2000×10⁹/L). First-choice therapy for all patients in chronic phase is tyrosine kinase inhibition (TKI), e.g. imatinib, nilotinib or dasatinib, with allogeneic stem cell transplantation reserved for TKI failure. The translocation t(15;17) occurs in acute promyelocytic leukaemia (APL).

23.29. Answer: B.

HL most commonly starts in the cervical region and spreads contiguously along the lymphatic channels. Young women with the nodular sclerosing subtype of HL typically present with cervical and mediastinal lymphadenopathy. The nodes are typically painless and rubbery or sometimes firm or hard if there is lots of sclerosis. All the other answers are more in keeping with forms of NHL: option C, primary mediastinal large B-cell lymphoma; option E, follicular lymphoma; option D, primary central nervous system lymphoma; option A, T-lymphoblastic lymphoma.

23.30. Answer: E.

Mantle cell lymphoma tends to present with morphologically low-grade looking mature lymphocytes that are positive for CD5 but negative for CD23. Mantle cell lymphoma harbours the translocation t(11;14), which leads to overexpression of cyclin D1. CLL tends to be CD5 and CD23 positive, whilst all the other conditions tend to be CD5 negative. ALL will have blast cells, not mature lymphocytes, and DLBL is also a high-grade lymphoma with centroblasts.

23.31. Answer: D.

This is a requirement for CLL diagnosis. Patients with lower CLL lymphocyte counts are termed monoclonal B-cell lymphocytosis of uncertain significance. Some patients present with lymphadenopathy and lymphocyte counts <5×10⁹/L and are called small cell lymphocytic lymphoma. Most patients are asymptomatic at presentation and undergo watch and wait. Mutated immunoglobulin genes carry a good prognosis and *TP53* mutations carry a poor prognosis and a tendency to chemotherapy resistance. Targeting the BCR complex with drugs such as ibrutinib (Bruton's tyrosine kinase inhibitor) is a successful new form of therapy.

23.32. Answer: E.

The donor-derived T cells provide a new cell-mediated immune system that attacks residual leukaemic cells – GvL. Maintaining full (100%) donor chimerism in the T-cell population promotes long-term remission of AML and other haematological malignancies. The T cells also cause acute and chronic GVHD, which for similar reasons is associated with lower relapse rates. Older females are more likely to have been pregnant and to be sensitised to human leucocyte antigens (HLAs) and therefore younger male donors are preferable, all other criteria such as HLA matching and cytomegalovirus (CMV) status being equal. RIC is less tissue damaging and safer for older patients; however, younger and fitter patients benefit from full conditioning. The TRM for allogeneic transplants after 2 years is about 20%, mainly from infection and GVHD. The figure of 1–5% would apply to autologous stem cell transplantation.

23.33. Answer: E.

Anthracyclines lead to the inhibition of DNA and RNA synthesis by intercalating between base pairs of the DNA/RNA strand, thus preventing the replication of cancer cells. Some anthracyclines also inhibit topoisomerase II, but etoposide is not an anthracycline class of topoisomerase II inhibitor. All other answers describe a different class of chemotherapy drug.

23.34. Answer: C.

The treatment of choice is immunosuppression with horse ATG, which is safer than currently available rabbit ATG. Horse ATG should be followed by ciclosporin as longer-term immunosuppression. Allogeneic stem cell transplantation is reserved as first-line treatment for young patients (<30 years), ideally with a fully matched sibling donor. Supportive care is important but not as sole therapy and there is no proven useful role for G-CSF. Long-term glucocorticoids dramatically increase the risk of fatal fungal infection in neutropenic patients.

23.35. Answer: B.

The anaemia of chronic disease largely results from induced hepcidin production from the liver. This occurs secondary to increased interleukin-6 (IL-6) levels in inflammation. Iron is trapped in iron-exporting cells, including duodenal enterocytes and macrophages. Iron

23

does not cause direct marrow toxicity. Chronic GI tract bleeding leads to iron deficiency anaemia, as does achlorhydria, e.g. post-gastrectomy. Option E describes hypersplenism.

23.36. Answer: E.
All have been recognised prognostic factors at one time or another but the presence of MRD is now recognised as the most significant prognostic factor and used to modify therapy accordingly.

23.37. Answer: D.
Nowadays the use of indwelling lines and antibiotic prophylaxis with quinolone antibiotics (e.g. levofloxacin, ciprofloxacin) leads to more identified Gram-positive infections than Gram-negative, although Gram-negative infections are still more life-threatening. Quinolone prophylaxis and posaconazole prophylaxis have both been shown to be beneficial and to reduce mortality during induction therapy for AML. Indwelling plastic lines are more commonly infected with Gram-positive organisms, e.g. *Staphylococcus epidermidis*. Neutropenic sepsis is a medical emergency and must be treated empirically, e.g. with piperacillin/tazobactam with or without aminoglycosides, whilst waiting for culture results. Positive cultures only occur in about 30% of episodes of neutropenic sepsis.

23.38. Answer: D.
In an emergency, group O red cells can be given safely to any patient as the group O red cells lack surface antigens against which the patient's isohaemoglutinins can react (Box 23.38). There is a historic ABO and Rhesus D type available; however, group-specific units can only be issued when the group has been confirmed from a current sample. As this woman has child-bearing potential, she should receive RhD-negative. Plasma of group AB RhD-negative can safely be given to any patient as it lacks isohaemoglutinins that can react against the patient's red cell surface antigens.

23.39. Answer: A.
A female of child-bearing age would have received RhD- and Kell-negative units. Routine antenatal anti-D prophylaxis is administered at 28 weeks. Anti-D only occurs in RhD-negative individuals exposed to exogenous D antigen, and has clinical implications. She has not been pregnant before. It is most likely that her partner is D antigen positive and the fetus has inherited this antigen causing maternal allo-anti-D to form.

23.40. Answer: C.
Group O FFP contains both anti-A and anti-B, which will react with the recipient's red cells expressing A or B antigens. Group O patients have anti-A and anti-B that will react with A and or B antigens expressed on transfused cells. Group A patients have anti-B, which will react with B antigens expressed on transfused cells. The neonate immune system does not produce antibodies when exposed to exogenous antigens and so neonates tolerate ABO incompatibility better than adults.

23.41. Answer: E.
A Kleihauer test or acid elution test is a blood test used to measure the amount of fetal haemoglobin transferred from a fetus to a mother's blood stream. It is vital not to miss this sensitising event. Implantation bleeds occur in the first trimester. Although exclusion of placental abnormality is required, the priority is to minimise the likelihood of RhD sensitisation occurring. Normal pregnancy causes a fall in the haemoglobin through haemodilution for which transfusion is not indicated. Red cell parameters will guide the need for iron replacement.

23.42. Answer: A.
It is good practice to explain and document the reason for transfusion to the patient and to obtain the patient's consent but this may not always be possible. Key steps in the transfusion process are to positively identify the patient at the bedside prior to taking a blood sample and before administering a blood component. As he has evidence of cardiorespiratory compromise, transfusion should not be withheld.

i	**23.38 ABO blood group antigens and antibodies**		
ABO blood group	Red cell A or B antigens	Antibodies in plasma	UK frequency (%)
0	None	Anti-A and anti-B	46
A	A	Anti-B	42
B	B	Anti-A	9
AB	A and B	None	3

23.43. Answer: C.

All symptoms and signs of a possible transfusion reaction require rapid clinical assessment of the patient after the transfusion has been stopped (Fig. 23.43). His symptoms are consistent with a febrile non-haemolytic transfusion reaction.

23.44. Answer: B.

His PT and APTT are significantly prolonged; therefore, FFP is indicated at a dose of 15 mL/ kg. He will likely require platelets; however, at present, they are greater than the recommended threshold of 50×10^9/L. Cryoprecipitate is primarily used to replace fibrinogen when below 1.5 g/L. Prothrombin complex concentrate is used to reverse warfarin. Vitamin K has a 4- to 6-hour onset of action.

23.45. Answer: E.

Transfusion-related acute lung injury is characterised by the sudden onset of breathlessness within 6–24 hours of transfusion with bilateral nodular infiltrates on X-ray. This condition results in pulmonary oedema but is non-cardiac in origin. Temperature, JVP and ECG are normal. There is no history of pleuritic chest pain. Although the other conditions should be considered, the pattern is most consistent with transfusion-related acute lung injury.

23.46. Answer: C.

Vitamin B_{12} deficiency results in ineffective haematopoiesis with nucleocytoplasmic asynchrony. Iron deficiency results in anaemia with small, pale red cells. Acute myeloid leukaemia can cause a pancytopenia but is associated with circulating immature blast cells. Alcohol excess can result in a macrocytosis and poor diet, usually leading to folate deficiency. Hypothyroidism can cause a macrocytosis and fatigue with normal neutrophil appearances on film.

23.47. Answer: A.

The blood film shows an increase in neutrophils with heavily staining granules consistent with bacterial infection. There are no immature blast cells. Infectious mononucleosis is associated with a lymphocytosis. Whilst diabetic ketoacidosis can cause a neutrophilia, the blood glucose is normal. Autoimmune disease is associated with a neutropenia.

23.48. Answer: B.

Investigations are in keeping with haemolysis. A positive direct antiglobulin (Coombs) test would support an autoimmune aetiology, the most likely cause of this woman's haemolysis. A bone marrow aspirate is not indicated. Spherocytes are not associated with hepatitis, vitamin B_{12} or folate deficiency, or hypothyroidism.

23.49. Answer: E.

This patient is experiencing a vaso-occlusive crisis with compromised blood flow to the small vessels. A red cell transfusion will facilitate oxygenation and reverse the sickling process. Exchange is reserved for life-threatening crises. Folic acid and LMWH are indicated but not the most important next step. Sickle-cell disease is associated with small cells and normal iron metabolism.

23.50. Answer: D.

Beta-thalassaemia trait is not associated with reduced fertility. With appropriate antenatal care, pregnancy outcome is successful. Hydrops fetalis is associated with alpha-chain abnormalities. The baby has a 1 in 4 chance it will not inherit the beta-thalassaemia gene, a 1 in 2 chance it will inherit one beta-thalassaemia gene and a 1 in 4 chance it will inherit two beta-thalassaemia genes and develop beta-thalassaemia major.

23.51. Answer: C.

Patients with sickle-cell disease have compromised splenic function resulting from microvascular occlusion. This puts them at risk of life-threatening infections from capsulated organisms. Aplastic crises produce a very low haemoglobin with a reticulocytopenia. There is no history of joint pain or shortness of breath to suggest a vaso-occlusive painful crisis or sickle chest syndrome.

23.52. Answer: C.

This child has non-spherocytic haemolysis. G6PD deficiency is the most common cause in this age group. The Donath–Landsteiner antibody is found in paroxysmal cold haemoglobinuria. The direct antiglobulin test detects antibody-coated red cells found in autoimmune haemolysis. Parvovirus is associated with anaemia and reticulocytopenia. The urine discolouration is caused by haemosiderinuria.

23

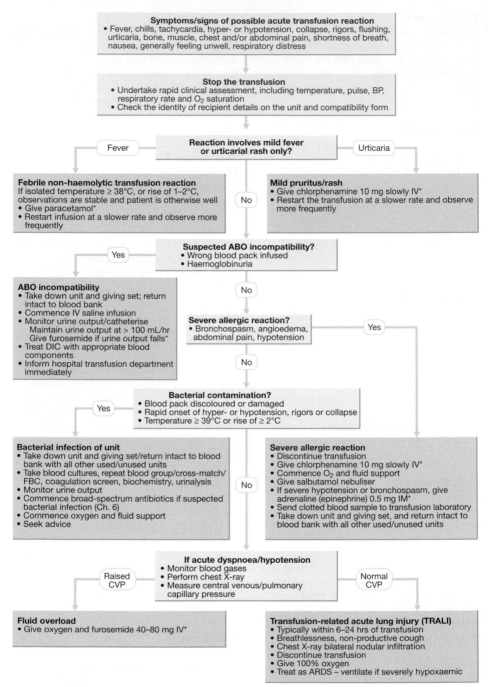

Fig. 23.43 Investigation and management of acute transfusion reactions. *Use size-appropriate dose in children. (ARDS = acute respiratory distress syndrome; BP = blood pressure; CVP = central venous pressure; DIC = disseminated intravascular coagulation; FBC = full blood count; IV = intravenous)

23.53. Answer: E.
Neonatal alloimmune thrombocytopenia occurs when maternal alloantibodies form against fetal platelet antigens inherited from the father. This can result in severe life-threatening thrombocytopenia in utero or at delivery, and in first pregnancy. Immune thrombocytopenic purpura is unlikely given the absence of a history of maternal immune thrombocytopenia. The coagulation is normal. Aside from the petechial rash, there are no concerns regarding the baby. The platelet count will recover spontaneously.

23.54. Answer: A.
Hepatitis A is transmitted through the faeco-oral route. All the other infective agents are transmitted through direct contact with infected blood or bodily fluids. The rate of transfusion-transmitted infection is monitored through national haemovigilance schemes. The UK Serious Hazards of Transfusion (SHOT) scheme has reported on proven or suspected cases of infection transmission arising from blood and component use in the UK since 1996.

23.55. Answer: A.
She has a normochromic, normocytic anaemia with low iron, iron-binding capacity and transferrin saturation in keeping with anaemia of chronic disease. Anaemia of chronic disease results from impaired iron handling. In iron deficiency anaemia, the patient is iron depleted, leading to a raised iron-binding capacity in the context of low iron and transferrin saturation. Folate deficiency, myelodysplasia and autoimmune haemolysis are associated with an elevated MCV.

23.56. Answer: D.
Non-specific allergic reactions can occur during a transfusion. Iron overload is associated with repeated red cell transfusion. Massive transfusion is associated with hyperkalaemia, hypothermia and thrombocytopenia.

23.57. Answer: A.
Bacterial contamination of platelets can result in rapid onset of acute circulatory compromise. It is thought to occur secondary to exposure to significant bacterial toxin within the contaminated platelet unit rather than the bacterial load itself. Transfusion-associated circulatory overload is associated with transfusion of large volumes relative to the patient. Whilst transfusion can cause hyperkalaemia, this is in the context of massive transfusion. Pulmonary emboli are not generally associated with fever. ABO incompatibility resulting in catastrophic circulatory collapse is most often associated with red cell transfusion.

23

24

Rheumatology and bone disease

Multiple Choice Questions

24.1. Which cell in the bone microenvironment is primarily responsible for coordinating the regulation of bone remodelling?

A. Bone lining cells
B. Bone marrow stromal cells
C. Osteoblasts
D. Osteoclasts
E. Osteocytes

24.2. Within the bone microenvironment, which of the following receptors are responsible for activation of bone resorption and bone formation, respectively?

A. Osteoprotegerin and Wnt
B. Osteoprotegerin and sclerostin
C. Receptor activator of nuclear factor kappa B ligand (RANKL) and osteoprotegerin
D. Receptor activator of nuclear factor kappa B (RANK) and lipoprotein receptor-related protein 5 (LRP5)
E. RANKL and sclerostin

24.3. A 75 year old man presents with pain of moderate severity affecting the base of both thumbs. Hand X-rays shows evidence of osteoarthritis at both first carpometacarpal (CMC) joints. Local application of gel containing diclofenac has not helped his symptoms. What would be the next most appropriate drug treatment for his pain?

A. Co-codamol
B. Diclofenac

C. Gabapentin
D. Paracetamol
E. Tramadol

24.4. A 65 year old woman with osteoarthritis attends her family physician because of knee pain worse on going up- and downstairs. She is a non-smoker, does not drink alcohol, but is taking simvastatin 20 mg daily for high cholesterol and lisinopril 10 mg daily for hypertension. On examination her height is 154 cm and weight is 95 kg. What would be the most appropriate treatment for her knee pain?

A. Arthroplasty
B. Cognitive behavioural therapy (CBT)
C. Regular weight-bearing exercise
D. Surgical synovectomy
E. Weight loss

24.5. Which of the following disease-modifying antirheumatic drugs (DMARDs) does NOT require any monitoring of full blood count or liver function tests?

A. Azathioprine
B. Hydroxychloroquine
C. Leflunomide
D. Methotrexate
E. Myocrisin

24.6. A previously healthy 45 year old man is woken up at 0400 hrs with acute pain, swelling and redness of the right ankle with no obvious trigger factor. Height is 168 cm, weight 104 kg.

He has a history hypertension treated with bendroflumethazide 2.5 mg daily. He drinks 2–3 pints of beer each night and consumes 26 units of alcohol per week. What is the most likely diagnosis?

A. Gout
B. Osteoarthritis
C. Psoriatic arthritis
D. Rheumatoid arthritis
E. Septic arthritis

24.7. A 77 year old woman with a history of generalised osteoarthritis (OA) is admitted to hospital with a delirious episode associated with dehydration and a urinary tract infection. During the admission, she develops pain, swelling and redness of the left wrist gradually worsening over a period of 4–6 hours. Blood tests reveal a neutrophilia (white cell count 12.5×10^9/L), a raised erythrocyte sedimentation rate (ESR; 65 mm/hr) and a raised C-reactive protein (CRP; 154 mg/L).

What would be the most likely diagnosis?

A. Calcium pyrophosphate deposition disease
B. Gout
C. Reactive arthritis
D. Septic arthritis
E. Vasculitis

24.8. A 63 year old woman with a 10-year history of rheumatoid arthritis presents with gradually worsening pain and swelling of the left knee joint over a period of 2–3 days. Her arthritis has generally been under good control with methotrexate 20 mg weekly and the tumour necrosis factor alpha (TNF-α) inhibitor etanercept 50 mg weekly. On examination the knee is warm and swollen, with signs of an effusion. What would be the most appropriate course of action?

A. Aspirate the knee and inject with 80 mg methylprednisolone?
B. Aspirate the knee and send the synovial fluid for culture and microscopy
C. Commence treatment with a broad-spectrum antibiotic
D. Commence treatment with diclofenac 75 mg twice daily
E. Increase the dose of methotrexate to 25 mg weekly

24.9. A 66 year old woman presents with pain and stiffness affecting the wrists, proximal interphalangeal (PIP) and metacarpophalangeal

(MCP) joints of the hands, gradually worsening over a period of 6–8 weeks. On examination, there is symmetrical swelling and tenderness of both wrists and the MCP and PIP joints of the hands. Investigations show that anti-citrullinated peptide antibodies (ACPAs) and rheumatoid factor are negative, but that she has an elevated ESR (25 mm/hr) and a raised CRP (65 mg/L). X-rays of the hands are normal. Which of the following statements is correct?

A. Magnetic resonance imaging (MRI) of the hands should be done to clarify the diagnosis
B. Rheumatoid arthritis is excluded by the negative ACPA test and normal radiographs
C. The joint pain and swelling is most likely due to generalised osteoarthritis
D. The presentation is consistent with polymyalgia rheumatica (PMR)
E. The presentation is typical of seronegative rheumatoid arthritis

24.10. Which of the following is a common complication of seronegative (ACPA and rheumatoid factor negative) rheumatoid arthritis?

A. Felty's syndrome
B. Osteoporosis
C. Rheumatoid nodules
D. Uveitis
E. Vasculitis

24.11. A 36 year old woman presents with 3-month history of joint pain and swelling affecting the wrists, MCPJs and proximal interphalangeal joints (PIPJs) of the hands, both shoulders, both knees and the MCPJs of both feet. Laboratory investigations reveal an ACPA level of 145, an ESR of 68 mm/hr and a CRP of 84 mg/L. On examination she has 22 tender and 16 swollen joints and rates the activity of her arthritis as 65/100, giving a Disease Activity Score 28 (DAS28) of 7.54. What would be the most appropriate initial treatment?

A. Adalimumab 40 mg every 2 weeks and prednisolone 5 mg daily
B. Hydroxychloroquine 200 mg twice daily and ibuprofen 400 mg 3 times daily
C. Methotrexate 15 mg weekly, folic acid 5 mg weekly and prednisolone 30 mg daily
D. Prednisolone 30 mg daily, ibuprofen 400 mg 3 times daily and omeprazole 30 mg daily
E. Rituximab 1000 mg on two occasions a fortnight apart combined with prednisolone 5 mg daily

24

24.12. Which one of the following statements is true with respect to post-menopausal osteoporosis?

A. Bone pain is the most common presenting feature
B. Calcium and vitamin D supplements can prevent its development
C. It is a rare complication of polymyalgia rheumatica
D. Obesity is an important risk factor
E. Patients are usually asymptomatic until a fracture occurs

24.13. A 73 year old woman presents to her family physician with sudden onset of pain in the lower back region that developed after removing weeds in her garden. She has a history of breast cancer treated 10 years previously with surgery and radiotherapy followed by tamoxifen for 5 years. She has a history of hypertension controlled with bendroflumethazide 2.5 mg daily. Her height is 154 cm, weight 53 kg and physical examination is unremarkable. A spine radiograph is shown below.

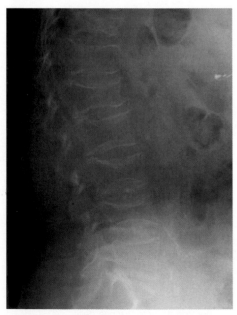

What is the most likely cause of the back pain?

A. Diffuse interstitial skeletal hyperostosis
B. Metastatic bone disease
C. Osteoarthritis of the spine
D. Osteoporotic vertebral fractures
E. Spondylolisthesis

24.14. A 60 year old woman suffers a low trauma fracture of the right wrist after a fall. She is a non-smoker and drinks 8 units of alcohol per week. Her menopause occurred at aged 52. She is on no current medication and has no significant medical history but reports that her mother, aged 79, has recently suffered a hip fracture.

What would be the most appropriate course of action?

A. Advise her to stop drinking alcohol completely
B. Commence treatment with alendronic acid
C. Commence treatment with calcium and vitamin D supplements
D. Request a dual X-ray absorptiometry (DXA) scan
E. Request a spine radiograph

24.15. Which one of the following is a common adverse effect of oral bisphosphonate therapy in patients with osteoporosis?

A. Atypical subtrochanteric fractures
B. Iritis
C. Leucopenia
D. Osteonecrosis of the jaw
E. Upper gastrointestinal upset

24.16. A 48 year old woman with seropositive rheumatoid arthritis (RA) has persistent pain and swelling of the wrists, elbows, shoulders and MCP joints of both hands despite 12 months' therapy with methotrexate 25 mg weekly, folic acid 5 mg weekly, sulfasalazine 3 g daily and hydroxychloroquine 400 mg daily. Examination reveals tenderness and swelling of 10 affected joints, and a raised ESR (45 mm/hr). She rates the activity of her arthritis as 80/100 on a visual analogue scale yielding a DAS28 of 6.45.

What would be the most appropriate next course of action?

A. Commence treatment with apremilast 30 mg twice daily
B. Commence treatment with the interleukin (IL)-17 blocker secukinumab 150 mg monthly
C. Commence treatment with the TNFα inhibitor etanercept 50 mg weekly
D. Increase the frequency of methotrexate to 3 times weekly
E. Stop sulfasalazine and substitute leflunomide 10 mg daily

24.17. A 56 year old man presents with acute pain, redness and swelling of the first metatarsophalangeal (MTP) joint of the right foot. Investigations show an elevated ESR (35 mm/hr), CRP of 56 mg/L, a mild neutrophilia (12.1×10⁹/L), serum creatinine 75 μmol/L (0.85 mg/dL), estimated glomerular filtration rate (eGFR) >60 mL/min/1.73 m² and a serum uric acid level of 450 μmol/L (7.6 mg/dL). Radiographs reveal evidence of erosions in the affected joint.

What would be the most appropriate treatment?

A. Allopurinol 100 mg daily initially gradually increasing in dose until uric acid falls below 360 μmol/L (6.1 mg/dL)
B. Colchicine 500 mg 3 times daily until symptoms settle followed by colchicine 500 mg daily on a long-term basis
C. Colchicine 500 mg 3 times daily until symptoms settle followed by long-term diclofenac 75 mg twice daily
D. Diclofenac 75 mg twice daily followed by long-term low-dose aspirin 75 mg/day
E. Etoricoxib 60 mg daily followed by allopurinol starting at 100 mg daily, gradually increasing in dose until uric acid falls below 360 μmol/L (6.1 mg/dL)

24.18. A 35 year old woman with well-controlled RA states that she wishes to become pregnant. Her medication consists of methotrexate 20 mg weekly, folic acid 5 mg weekly and ibuprofen 400 mg 3 times daily. What advice would you give with regard to her plans to conceive and her medication?

A. She can go ahead and try to conceive so long as she reduces the dose of methotrexate to 10 mg weekly and ibuprofen to 200 mg 3 times daily
B. She should stop the ibuprofen for at least 3 months before trying to conceive but can continue the methotrexate
C. She should stop the methotrexate and the ibuprofen and then go ahead and try to conceive
D. She should stop the methotrexate for at least 12 months before trying to conceive but can continue the ibuprofen
E. She should stop the methotrexate for at least 3 months before trying to conceive but can continue the ibuprofen

24.19. A 75 year old woman is referred to the rheumatology clinic complaining of pain and swelling affecting the proximal interphalangeal joints (PIPJs) and distal interphalangeal joints

(DIPJs) of both hands. Investigations show a haemoglobin of 118 g/L, white cell count 6.3×10⁹/L, platelets 355 × 10⁹/L and ESR 20 mm/hr. An X-ray of the hands and wrists is performed.

Which radiological features are typical of osteoarthritis?

A. Irregularity and fusion of the sacroiliac joints
B. Joint space narrowing and subchondral sclerosis of the PIPJ and DIPJ of the hands
C. Marginal erosions affecting the MCPJ of the hands
D. Periarticular osteoporosis affecting the PIPJs and DIPJs in the hands
E. Punched-out erosions of the first MTP joint of the feet

24.20. A 65 year old man presents to his family physician complaining of pain in the left knee, worse on ascending and descending stairs. He smokes 15 cigarettes a day, and drinks about 4 units of alcohol daily (28 units per week). He is a former amateur soccer player who suffered a cruciate ligament tear in his 30s. He has lived alone since his wife died 5 years previously. He has been avoiding dairy products since he thinks they cause gastrointestinal upset.

Which of the following risk factors predispose to the development of osteoarthritis?

A. Alcohol intake >21 units per week
B. Cigarette smoking
C. Immobilisation
D. Low dietary calcium intake
E. Previous anterior cruciate ligament tear

24.21. A 66 year old woman is referred to the rheumatology clinic with pain in the right hip of gradual onset over the past 2 years, worse on weight-bearing. Examination reveals limitation and pain on internal rotation of the right hip. Her height is 154 cm and weight is 82 kg (body mass index (BMI) 34.6 kg/m²). A pelvic X-ray shows joint space narrowing and osteophytes of the right hip joint, consistent with osteoarthritis.

Which one of the following statements is true with regard to the treatment of osteoarthritis of the hip?

A. A cyclo-oxygenase 2 (COX-2) selective NSAID is more likely to be effective than a non-selective NSAID in the treatment of pain
B. Joint replacement surgery is indicated if the response to paracetamol is inadequate
C. Long-term prophylactic NSAID therapy has a disease-modifying effect

24

D. Oral glucosamine is an effective treatment

E. Oral NSAIDs are more effective than paracetamol in controlling symptoms

24.22. A 67 year old woman attends her family physician complaining of generalised aches and pains and feeling tired all the time. She has been under a lot of stress at work and has also been concerned that her son is unemployed and unable to get a job. Physical examination is unremarkable.

Routine biochemistry and haematology tests are completely normal with the exception of the serum 25-hydroxyvitamin D (25(OH)D) value, which is 30 nmol/L (12 ng/mL). This is reported by the biochemistry laboratory as showing evidence of vitamin D insufficiency.

Which of the following statements is true?

A. Circulating serum 25(OH)D levels are highest in the spring and lowest in the autumn

B. Circulating serum 25(OH)D levels remain constant in most people throughout the year

C. Circulating vitamin D is mainly derived from dietary intake of fish and meat

D. Circulating vitamin D is mainly derived from synthesis from 7-dehydrocholesterol in the skin by the action of ultraviolet (UV) light

E. It is likely that her symptoms will respond well to supplementation with vitamin D, so long as the circulating levels are restored to above 50 nmol/L (20 ng/mL)

24.23. Which of the following statements is correct with regard to metabolism of vitamin D?

A. The biologically active form 25(OH) vitamin D is hydroxylated in the kidney by the enzyme CYP27B1 to generate the inactive metabolite 1,25(OH)$_2$D

B. The biologically active form 25(OH) vitamin D is inactivated by the enzyme CYP24A1 in the kidney

C. The biologically inactive form 25(OH) vitamin D is hydroxylated in the kidney by the enzyme CYP24A1 to give the active metabolite 1,25(OH)$_2$D

D. The biologically inactive form 25(OH) vitamin D is hydroxylated in the kidney by the enzyme CYP27B1 to give the active metabolite 1,25(OH)$_2$D

E. The vitamin D metabolite 24,25(OH)$_2$D is biologically inactive and stimulates intestinal calcium absorption and bone resorption

24.24. A 66 year old Muslim woman of Middle Eastern origin presents with a 2-month history of gradually worsening pain, weakness and stiffness affecting the muscles of the shoulder and pelvic girdle. She has a past medical history of type 2 diabetes controlled with diet and metformin 500 mg twice daily. She is also taking atorvastatin 40 mg daily and has been recently prescribed trimethoprim for a urinary tract infection.

Investigations show a normal full blood count, ESR 13 mm/hr, normal urea and electrolytes, serum creatine kinase 100 U/L, serum adjusted calcium 2.25 mmol/L (9.0 mg/dL), serum 25(OH)D <20 nmol/L (8 ng/mL), phosphate 0.70 mmol/L (2.17 mg/dL); bilirubin 10 µmol/L (0.58 mg/dL), aspartate aminotransferase (AST) 20 U/L, alkaline phosphatase (ALP) 275 U/L, parathyroid hormone (PTH) 35 pmol/L (330 pg/mL).

What is the most likely diagnosis?

A. Osteomalacia

B. Osteoporosis

C. Polymyalgia rheumatica

D. Statin-induced myopathy

E. Vitamin D insufficiency

24.25. A 56 year old woman presents with generalised musculoskeletal pain associated with multiple focal tender spots on local pressure of the muscle on the trunk and upper arms and is diagnosed as having probable fibromyalgia. Investigations reveal normal urea and electrolytes, normal full blood count, ESR 10 mm/hr, and normal bilirubin, AST and ALP. Serum 25(OH)D level is 25 nmol/L (10 ng/mL), serum calcium is 2.41 mmol/L (9.7 mg/dL), phosphate 1.2 mmol/L (3.72 mg/dL) and PTH is 5.2 pmol/L (49 pg/mL). Which of the following statements is true?

A. Fibromyalgia is associated with vitamin D deficiency

B. High-dose vitamin D supplements (25 000 units per week) are likely to be an effective treatment for the musculoskeletal pain

C. Low-dose vitamin D supplements (800 units daily) are likely to be an effective treatment for the musculoskeletal pain

D. The low vitamin D levels are likely to be secondary to the fibromyalgia

E. The muscle pain and tenderness are likely to be due to osteomalacia

24.26. A 25 year old man is referred to the clinic because of focal bone pain affecting the mid-shaft of the left femur. On examination he has short stature and bilateral bowing deformities of the lower limbs. He was diagnosed as having childhood rickets and treated with vitamin D metabolites but stopped treatment aged 16 years and was lost to follow-up. There is a family history of rickets affecting his mother and brother.

Investigations reveal a serum calcium of 2.25 mmol/L (9.0 mg/dL), phosphate 0.60 mmol/L (1.86 mg/dL), PTH 12.5 pmol/L (118 pg/mL), ALP 160 U/L and serum 25(OH)D 54 nmol/L (22 ng/mL).

What is the most likely diagnosis?

A. Tumour-induced osteomalacia
B. Vitamin D-deficient rickets
C. Vitamin D-resistant rickets type I
D. Vitamin D-resistant rickets type II
E. X-linked hypophosphataemic rickets

24.27. Which of the following statements is true with regard to Paget's disease of bone?

A. Dietary calcium deficiency and smoking are recognised risk factors
B. It can be inherited in families in association with mutations in the *SQSTM1* gene
C. It is a focal skeletal disorder characterised by inhibition of bone formation and an increased risk of fracture
D. It is a systemic skeletal disorder characterised by a generalised increase in bone turnover
E. There is a strong genetic component mediated by variants at the human leucocyte antigen (HLA) locus on chromosome 6

24.28. A 68 year old man presents with gradually worsening pain in the right hip region, which is present at rest and worsens slightly on weight-bearing. Investigations reveal a creatinine of 140 μmol/L (1.58 mg/dL) and an eGFR of 35 mL/min/1.73 m² but otherwise normal urea and electrolytes, normal serum calcium and phosphate, but an ALP of 350 U/L. The full blood count is normal. A pelvic radiograph is performed and is shown below.

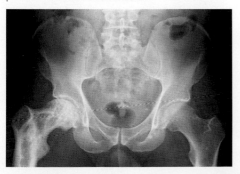

What is the most likely cause of the pain?

A. Osteoarthritis
B. Osteomalacia
C. Osteoporosis
D. Paget's disease
E. Renal osteodystrophy

24.29. Which of the following clinical or radiographic features is consistent with a diagnosis of Scheuermann's disease?

A. At least two wedge deformities in the thoracic spine with a T-score of <−2.5 at either spine or hip on DXA examination
B. Crush deformity affecting at least three vertebrae in the lumbar spine
C. Disc space narrowing in the lumbar spine with marked osteophyte formation
D. Two vertebral crush deformities in the thoracic spine and one in the lumbar spine with evidence of osteopenia on radiographs
E. Wedge deformity affecting several adjacent vertebrae in the thoracic spine with disc space narrowing

24.30. A 32 year old man is referred to the rheumatology clinic having sustained a fracture of the right femur after falling when he tripped over an uneven pavement. Examination is unremarkable apart from the fact that he has blue sclerae. He is known to have osteogenesis imperfecta (OI) and has a history of low trauma fractures dating back to childhood.

Which of the following statements is true with regard to this condition?

A. Bisphosphonates are highly effective at preventing fractures in adults with OI
B. Fractures of the vertebrae are an uncommon complication
C. The diagnosis can be excluded if the sclerae are of normal colour
D. The incidence of fractures increases progressively with age
E. The incidence of fractures is highest in childhood

24.31. A 23 year old woman presents with pain, swelling and deformity affecting the distal tibia of the right leg. On examination she has areas of café-au-lait pigmentation on her right shoulder and left forearm. The past medical history is unremarkable and she is on no medication apart from the oral contraceptive pill. Radiographs reveal expansion of the left tibia with alternating areas of osteolysis and osteosclerosis.

24

What is the most likely diagnosis?

A. Camurati–Engelmann disease
B. Fibrous dysplasia
C. Osteomyelitis
D. Osteopetrosis
E. Paget's disease of the tibia

24.32. A 58 year old man with haemochromatosis is referred to the rheumatology clinic with a 3-year history of pain mainly affecting the small joints of the hands and wrists. Four weeks previously he had developed acute pain, swelling and redness of the right wrist, which had responded to treatment with naproxen 500 mg 3 times daily. He has a history of type 2 diabetes treated with diet and metformin and has been treated with regular venesection for the previous 3 years.

Clinical examination of his hands is unremarkable with no evidence of synovitis. Laboratory investigations are as follows: haemoglobin 115 g/L, white cell count 8.2×10^9/L, platelets 345×10^9/L, ESR 20 mm/hr, serum iron 100 μmol/L (558 μg/dL), AST 35 U/L, bilirubin 15 μmol/L (0.88 mg/dL) and ALP 150 U/L.

Radiographs of the hands and wrists show joint space narrowing and subchondral cysts affecting the MCP and the radiocarpal joints with no osteophyte formation.

Which of the following statements is true?

A. The arthritis is an incidental finding unrelated to the diagnosis of haemochromatosis
B. The clinical picture is consistent with rheumatoid arthritis
C. The most likely cause for his joint symptoms is diabetic cheiroarthropathy
D. The most likely explanation for the acute flare in his joint symptoms is calcium pyrophosphate deposition disease
E. The risk of further flares in symptoms can be reduced by continued venesection and restoration of serum iron levels to normal

24.33. A 64 year old woman with a 10-year history of rheumatoid arthritis affecting the hands and wrists, which is controlled with sulfasalazine 3 g daily and hydroxychloroquine 200 mg twice daily, presents with a disturbance of sensation and tingling affecting the thumb and anterior aspects of the index and second fingers of the right hand.

On examination there is no evidence of active synovitis but there is altered perception of fine touch on examination of the affected digits in the right hand. Investigations are as follows: haemoglobin 120 g/L, white cell count 6.5×10^9/L, platelets 456×10^9/L, ESR 20 mm/hr, CRP 6 mg/L.

What is the most likely cause of the symptoms?

A. Bone erosions secondary to the long-standing RA
B. Median nerve compression
C. Mononeuritis associated with rheumatoid vasculitis
D. Osteoarthritis of the first CMC joint
E. Ulnar nerve compression

24.34. Which one of the following statements is true with regard to joint hypermobility?

A. Affected patients may experience episodes of postural hypotension accompanied by tachycardia
B. It is a rare complication of osteogenesis imperfecta
C. Mutations in the *FBN1* gene are the most common cause
D. The diagnosis can be confirmed by a Beighton score of more than 4 in patents who have dislocated at least one joint
E. Treatment with NSAIDs is highly effective in controlling ligament and joint pain in affected patients

24.35. A 67 year old woman with a 15-year history of type 2 diabetes treated with diet, metformin and sitagliptin presents with gradual onset of pain and deformity affecting the right ankle and foot.

On general examination, blood pressure is 145/85 mmHg, pulse 85 beats/min, height 153 cm and weight 89 kg. Neurological examination reveals absent ankle jerks and impairment of fine touch and proprioception in both feet. Peripheral pulses are absent below the femoral arteries. Examination of the ankle joint reveals swelling and deformity of the ankle joint and a severe valgus deformity.

Investigations show moderate renal dysfunction with a serum creatinine of 165 μmol/L (1.87 mg/dL) and eGFR of 25 mL/min/1.73 m^2. Serum AST is 20 U/L, ALT 85 U/L, bilirubin 12 μmol/L (0.70 mg/dL) and serum uric acid 400 μmol/L (6.7 mg/dL). Full blood count shows mild anaemia with a haemoglobin of 110 g/L and an ESR of 25 mm/hr.

Radiographs show severe destruction of the ankle and the mid-foot joints with bony fragments within the joint.

What is the most likely cause of the ankle pain?

A. Calcium pyrophosphate deposition disease
B. Charcot joint
C. Diabetic cheiroarthropathy
D. Gout
E. Osteoarthritis

24.36. A 17 year old male presents with pain and swelling of the middle of the right tibia that has been gradually increasing in severity over a period of 6–8 weeks. An X-ray shows expansion of the bone and a soft tissue mass containing islands of calcification.

What is the most likely diagnosis?

A. Fibrous dysplasia
B. Hypertrophic pulmonary osteoarthropathy
C. Metastatic bone disease
D. Osteosarcoma
E. Paget's disease

24.37. Which physiological process is primarily responsible for the development of osteoporosis in patients on long-term glucocorticoid therapy?

A. Increased degradation of 25(OH)D
B. Increased osteoclastic bone resorption
C. Inhibition of 25(OH)D production
D. Inhibition of bone formation
E. Secondary hyperparathyroidism

24.38. Which of the following environmental exposures has been associated with susceptibility to, and severity of, rheumatoid arthritis?

A. Cigarette smoking
B. Excessive alcohol intake (>21 units per week)
C. Human immunodeficiency virus (HIV) infection
D. Obesity (BMI >30)
E. Vitamin D insufficiency

24.39. In investigating the cause of an acute monoarthritis in a 50 year old man in a non-tuberculosis (TB) endemic region, synovial fluid from the swollen joint is sent for Gram stain, culture and polarised microscopy. The laboratory staff call with the results: they say 'Gram stain negative; culture results are not available for another 48 hours. There are many

neutrophils and there are negatively birefringent crystals in the fluid.' What is the correct management?

A. Antibiotics and steroids should be used together
B. Intra-articular steroids can be given straight away because the diagnosis is reactive arthritis
C. The patient can be treated for gout because infection has been excluded
D. The joint should be drained and analgesia given but steroids should be withheld until the culture result is available
E. The results favour a diagnosis of pseudogout

24.40. Psoriatic arthopathy contains a number of the radiographic signs in the answers below. Which one of the following radiographic signs is NOT typically recognised in psoriatic arthritis (PsA)?

A. Bone sclerosis
B. Calcification of peri-odontoid ligaments
C. Juxta-articular new bone formation
D. Sacroiliac erosions
E. Syndesmophytes

24.41. A young man has a history of chronic low back pain and stiffness, which disturbs his sleep and takes time to wear off in the morning after waking. In making a diagnosis, which is the most appropriate combination of tests to do after clinical assessment?

A. HLA-B27 and ESR
B. MRI lumbar spine and sacroiliac joints and bone scintigraphy
C. MRI SIJs and ESR
D. Pelvis radiograph and HLA-B27
E. Pelvis radiograph, whole-spine and SIJs MRI, and HLA-B27

24.42. Which one of the following is a recognised use of ultrasound in rheumatology practice?

A. Adding information to the diagnostic workup of patients with polymyalgia rheumatica
B. Detection of the vascularity of synovitis in MCP joints
C. Diagnosing sacroiliac inflammation
D. Discrimination of hip adductor tendonitis from symphysitis
E. Guiding needle placement to a lumbar spine facet joint in treating facet joint arthritis with injectable steroid

24

24.43. A woman, aged 51 years, has never had a fracture but has been on intermittent steroids (5 × 4-week courses) for her Crohn's disease over the last 2 years. Her DXA scan results are: lumbar spine bone mineral density (BMD) T-score −2.0; femoral neck BMD T-score −1.5; and total hip BMD T-score −2.2.

Which is the correct statement?

A. Calcium and vitamin D should be the only therapy considered
B. FRAX assessment will be useful in this case
C. Lateral spinal X-rays should NOT be obtained
D. Nothing should be done as T-scores are >−2.5, except DXA to be arranged in 5 years time
E. Steroids should NOT be used to treat her Crohn's disease

24.44. Blood is taken from a pre-menopausal woman with joint pains, xerostomia and fatigue. Antinuclear antibody (ANA) is positive; anti-DNA antibody titre 1 U/L, anti-Ro(SSA) positive, anti-La(SSB) positive, complement C3 and C4 normal, rheumatoid factor positive, ACPA negative. Based on the following immunology results, which is the most likely diagnosis?

A. Primary Sjögren's syndrome (PSS)
B. RA
C. RA and systemic lupus erythematosus (SLE) together
D. SLE
E. Systemic sclerosis (SScl)

24.45. In discriminating causes of inflammatory polyarthritis, which statement is most likely to be true?

A. An absence of joint synovitis on examination rules out RA
B. Enthesitis occurring in PsA always causes pain or local tenderness
C. Polyarticular joint involvement may be a typical presentation of gout in an older woman
D. Pseudogout/calcium pyrophosphate deposition disease affects only peripheral joints
E. Synovitis in PIP and some MCP joints rules out OA

24.46. A woman aged 34 years presents with a 24-month fluctuating history of fatigue, widespread pains, poor appetite, non-specific bowel symptoms, non-specific skin rashes, mild weight loss and some altered cognitive function.

Which one of the following diagnoses is least likely?

A. Autoimmune connective tissue disease
B. Fibromyalgia
C. Inflammatory bowel disease
D. Malignancy
F. Sarcoidosis

24.47. A 65 year old man presents with low thoracic back pain for the first time. It has been present for about 3 months, starting initially over the course of a week and now at a constant level (no worsening, but no improvement). His sleep is disturbed. There are no systemic symptoms and no leg pains.

Of the following, which is the most likely diagnosis?

A. Axial spondyloarthritis
B. Intervertebral disc prolapse
C. Osteoporotic fracture
D. Septic discitis
E. Spondylolisthesis

24.48. A 13 year old girl presents with limp and examination evidence of left knee swelling. There are no systemic symptoms, sore throat or rash. Blood tests show normal full blood count, CRP of 10 mg/L, ESR of 10 mm/hr, negative rheumatoid factor, ACPA and ANA autoantibodies.

Which is most likely to be correct?

A. As there is no psoriasis, the condition is unlikely to be PsA
B. Methotrexate should be started immediately
C. Screening for uveitis is not necessary
D. The condition is best classified as oligoarticular juvenile idiopathic arthritis (JIA)
E. The girl has juvenile RA

24.49. Which of the following statements about JIA is most likely to be correct?

A. Oligoarthritis in the presence of high acute phase response measures is not a presenting feature of leukaemia or inflammatory bowel disease (IBD)
B. Only ANA-positive JIA patients need an ophthalmological examination
C. Systemic JIA is associated with haemophagocytic syndrome
D. Systemic JIA is usually associated with a positive ANA
E. The prevalence of JIA is about 1 in 10 000

24.50. Which of the following treatments has NOT shown efficacy in either ankylosing spondylitis or psoriatic arthritis?

A. Anti-IL-17A monoclonal (secukinumab)
B. Anti-IL-23/12 monoclonal (ustekinumab)
C. Anti-TNF-α
D. Apremilast (phosphodiesterase-4 inhibitor)
E. Rituximab (anti-CD20/anti-B-cell therapy)

24.51. A 35 year old man develops low back, posterior heel pain and a swollen knee and has a pustular skin rash on the soles of his feet. There are no preceding illnesses, no previous psoriasis or family history of it. What is the most likely diagnosis?

A. Ankylosing spondylitis
B. Gout
C. Post-streptococcal arthritis
D. Psoriatic arthritis
E. Sexually acquired reactive arthritis

24.52. Most of the genes below are implicated in influencing either susceptibility for, or severity of, ankylosing spondylitis. However, which of these genes below has NOT been implicated?

A. *ERAP-1*
B. *HLA-B27*
C. *ANK-H*
D. *IL-23* receptor
E. *STAT-3*

24.53. Which combination of features below is most likely to be relevant to a diagnosis of axSpA?

A. Achilles tendon enthesitis, anterior uveitis and pubic symphysitis
B. An aunt who has psoriasis, rheumatoid factor and fatigue
C. Back pain, joint swelling and stiffness, scleritis, fatigue and positive ACPA
D. High ESR, anterior uveitis, ankle swelling, raised serum angiotensin-converting enzyme (ACE)
E. Low back pain, rosacea, prostatism and diarrhoea

24.54. Enthesitis is the hallmark musculoskeletal lesion of all spondyloarthritides (SpAs). Which one of the following is characteristic of enthesitis in the context of an SpA condition?

A. Enthesitis can occur in PsA without causing any symptoms
B. Enthesitis cannot be detected by US

C. Enthesitis does not improve with secukinumab (anti-IL-17 DMARD)
D. Enthesitis only occurs in SpA patients who are HLA-B27
E. Enthesitis only occurs in lower limbs

24.55. Apremilast – a treatment developed for psoriatic arthritis – is a small molecule that directly inhibits which of the following?

A. Mitogen-activated protein (MAP) kinases
B. Phosphodiesterase 4 (PDE4)
C. RANK ligand
D. Signal transducer and activator of transcription 3 (STAT3)
E. T-cell CD80/86 binding

24.56. Which of the following interventions lack evidence of efficacy in the treatment of any components of fibromyalgia (pain, fatigue, physical functioning)?

A. Cannabis
B. Cognitive behavioural therapy (CBT)
C. Gabapentin
D. Supervised aerobic exercise training
E. The serotonin and noradrenaline reuptake inhibitor (SNRI) duloxetine

24.57. Which of the following is thought to be a consequence of, or associated with, constitutive substantial connective tissue laxity (hypermobility syndrome (HMS)/hypermobile-type Ehlers–Danlos)?

A. Enthesitis
B. Fibromyalgia
C. Hypertension
D. Plantar fasciitis
E. Uterine fibroids

24.58. The autoantibody profile: ANA positive, DNA/Sm/Ro(SSA)/La(SSB) negative, ribonucleoprotein (RNP) positive, is most likely to be associated with which autoimmune connective tissue disease?

A. Mixed connective tissue disease (MCTD)
B. Polymyositis
C. Primary Sjögren's syndrome (PSS)
D. Systemic lupus erythematosus (SLE)
E. Systemic sclerosis (SScl)

24.59. A 34 year old woman (currently mid-menstrual cycle) presents with small joint pain and stiffness, a UV-sensitive erythematous skin rash on exposed skin surfaces, fatigue, mouth ulcers, some ankle swelling and a

24

normal examination otherwise, apart from 3+ protein on urine dipstick and blood pressure of 145/90 mmHg.

Which is the most appropriate immediate course of action?

A. Check routine lab tests including autoimmune serology and complement and arrange routine review in a few weeks

B. Check routine lab tests including autoimmune serology and complement and start steroids immediately

C. Check routine lab tests including autoimmune serology and complement, start hydroxychloroquine and review progress in 3 months

D. Check routine lab tests including autoimmune serology and complement, arrange Gram stain and culture of urine, quantify urinary protein and arrange renal ultrasound

E. Discharge her from your care with reassurance and no follow-up

24.60. In addition to obtaining routine haematology, renal and liver laboratory tests with autoimmune serology (including myositis-specific antibodies) and muscle creatine kinase, which is the most appropriate combination of tests when investigating for polymyositis?

A. Muscle and cardiac MRI, open muscle biopsy, barium swallow

B. Muscle electromyogram (EMG), needle muscle biopsy, whole-body CT

C. Muscle MRI and EMG, chest X-ray, open muscle biopsy

D. Muscle MRI and EMG, needle muscle biopsy, whole-body CT scan, cardiac transthoracic echocardiogram, barium swallow

E. Muscle MRI and EMG, open muscle biopsy, whole-body CT scan, cardiac transthoracic echocardiogram, barium swallow

24.61. Of the following, what proactive investigational monitoring of internal organ function, despite the absence of symptoms, is essential in managing autoimmune connective tissue disease?

A. Respiratory function tests (RFTs) and chest X-ray in dermatomyositis

B. RFTs in SLE

C. Slit lamp ocular examination in SLE

D. Transthoracic echocardiogram and RFTs in SScl

E. Yearly whole-body CT in polymyositis

24.62. Which of the following is most likely to be true in relation to primary Sjögren's syndrome?

A. Overall anti-TNF-α therapy has been shown to be useful

B. PSS is not associated with malignancy

C. Severe oral dryness results from immunological destruction of the salivary glands

D. The environment does NOT play a role in influencing a patient's symptoms

E. Topical steroids should never be used for xerophthalmia

24.63. A 52 year old non-smoking man presents with a 6-week history of arthralgia and a palpable purpuric rash appearing on his limbs. He has a year-long history of recurrent fevers, sinusitis, cough and sore throats treated with repeated courses of antibiotics and steroids.

What is the most likely diagnosis?

A. Adult-onset Still's disease

B. Malignancy

C. Post-streptococcal reactive arthritis

D. Microscopic polyangiitis (MPA)

E. Rheumatic fever

24.64. Which one of the following diseases is NOT typically associated with autoantibody production?

A. Antiphospholipid syndrome

B. Giant cell arteritis (GCA)

C. Granulomatosis with polyangiitis (GPA; formerly known as Wegener's granulomatosis)

D. Microscopic polyangiitis (MPA)

E. Polymyositis

24.65. A 40 year old Armenian woman presents with recurrent bouts of fatigue, arthralgia (oligoarticular: elbow, wrists and a knee), headaches and crops of painful mouth ulcers, occasional bluish-red raised tender blotchy skin lesions and a single sore erythematous eye. She does not have diarrhoea.

ESR is 25 mm/hr but CRP is normal; full blood count shows slight lymphopenia, normal neutrophil and platelet counts. Serum adjusted calcium and PTH are in the reference range.

Which is the most likely diagnosis?

A. Behçet's disease
B. Crohn's disease
C. Sarcoidosis
D. Tuberculosis
E. Viral infection

24.66. Which of the following has NOT been implicated in contributing to the pathogenesis of vasculitis?

A. Cannabis use
B. Hepatitis C
C. HIV infection
D. HLA-B51
E. IgA

24.67. Which association between a microorganism and an autoinflammatory or autoimmune condition is speculative and LEAST well proven?

A. *Chlamydia trachomatis* and sexually acquired reactive arthritis
B. Group A streptococci and rheumatic fever
C. Hepatitis C and cryoglobulinaemic vasculitis
D. *Propionibacterium acnes* and SAPHO (synovitis–acne–pustulosis-hyperostosis–osteitis) syndrome
E. *Staphylococcus* and septic arthritis

24.68. Which of the following conditions is most likely to lead to development of an associated malignancy?

A. Diffuse idiopathic skeletal hyperostosis (DISH)
B. Giant cell arteritis
C. Primary Sjögren's syndrome
D. Relapsing polychondritis
E. Rheumatoid arthritis

24.69. The abnormality on the wrist radiograph below (arrowed) suggests which condition?

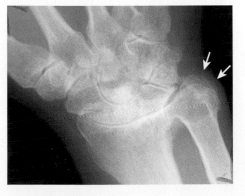

A. Calcium pyrophosphate disorder disease/arthritis
B. Gout
C. Osteoarthritis
D. Psoriatic arthritis
E. Rheumatoid arthritis

24.70. A 75 year old woman with established osteoporosis, with previous forearm fracture, known stable chronic kidney disease (CKD) stage 3 (eGFR approx. 48 mL/min/1.73 m^2) and no history of TB (she was immunised against TB as a child and has had no recent TB contacts), presents with an acutely swollen very painful knee. She feels generally unwell, had dysuria a month previously treated with antibiotics but has had no rash or diarrhoea.

Investigations show haemoglobin 122 g/L, white cell count/neutrophils slightly raised, platelet count 450×10^9/L and normal lymphocytes with ESR 45 mm/hr. Liver and thyroid function tests are normal.

Which of the following statements is correct?

A. Background renal impairment has no relevance to the current presentation
B. Blood cultures are likely to give the diagnosis
C. Septic arthritis is unlikely
D. The dysuria has no relevance to the current presentation
E. Uric acid should be tested

24.71. Conditions and their therapies have been matched, below; all are correct except one. Which therapy is NOT appropriate for its listed condition?

A. Barbotage for cutaneous calcinosis in dermatomyositis
B. Local glucocorticoid injection for chronic plantar fasciitis
C. Oral pilocarpine for primary Sjögren's syndrome
D. Rituximab (anti-CD20 monoclonal) for ANCA-associated vasculitis
E. Thalidomide for Behçet's disease

24.72. A 22 year old man presents with a 6-week history of persistent back pain and stiffness occurring with and after immobility, and heel pains. In interpreting investigations, which of the following is most likely to be true?

24

A. A negative HLA-B27 rules out axSpA
B. A normal CRP rules out ankylosing spondylitis
C. A previous diagnosis of sterile urethritis is irrelevant information to making a diagnosis

D. He may have sexually acquired reactive arthritis
E. SIJ radiographs will reveal the diagnosis

Answers

24.1. Answer: E.
Osteoclasts are responsible for resorbing bone and osteoblasts for bone formation but osteocytes are responsible for coordinating osteoblast and osteoclast activity.

24.2. Answer: D.
RANK and LRP5 are key receptors involved in the activation of osteoclastic bone resorption and bone formation, respectively. Osteoprotegerin inhibits bone resorption. Wnt stimulates bone formation but is a ligand, not a receptor. RANKL is a ligand that stimulates bone resorption.

24.3. Answer: D.
Paracetamol is the first-line systemic analgesic for mild to moderate pain. Non-steroidal anti-inflammatory drugs (NSAIDs) such as diclofenac should be used with great caution in the elderly and there would be a higher risk of adverse effects with co-codamol, gabapentin and tramadol.

24.4. Answer: E.
Obesity aggravates joint pain in osteoarthritis and weight loss is one of the most effective therapies for osteoarthritis (OA) of the lower limbs. Weight-bearing exercise is unlikely to help and may worsen symptoms. Surgical synovectomy is not indicated in OA and arthroplasty would only be indicated for advanced OA resistant to medical therapy. Cognitive behavioural therapy would be unlikely to help.

24.5. Answer. B.
Blood monitoring is not required for hydroxychloroquine but is required for all the other drugs to screen for blood dyscrasias and abnormal liver function tests.

24.6. Answer: A.
The clinical presentation is typical of gout, given the acute onset, involvement of a single joint and risk factors of obesity, thiazide therapy and excessive alcohol intake. The pattern of involvement and acute onset is not consistent with rheumatoid arthritis, psoriatic arthritis or OA. Septic arthritis is possible but unlikely in the absence of a previous history of joint disease or site of infection.

24.7. Answer: A.
Calcium pyrophosphate deposition disease is strongly associated with OA and typically affects those aged >65 years, affecting women more commonly than men. The onset is sudden with join pain and swelling developing over a period of 4–6 hours. Dehydration is a common precipitating factor, and investigations typically reveal a neutrophilia and a raised ESR and CRP. Gout and reactive arthritis can present in a similar manner but would be less likely in a woman of this age. Septic arthritis is possible but usually has a subacute onset and tends to develop more slowly, over a period of 24–48 hours.

24.8. Answer: B.
The history is suggesting of septic arthritis given the history of rheumatoid arthritis (RA) and immunosuppressive therapy with methotrexate and a TNF-α inhibitor. Options A, D and E would not be appropriate until infection had been excluded, nor would option C.

24.9. Answer: E.
The negative ACPA and normal radiograph does not exclude RA since ACPA and rheumatoid factor are negative in about one-third of patients and radiographs are normal in early RA. The presentation would not be consistent with PMR and the distribution of involvement (wrists, metacarpophalangeal joint; MCPJ) excludes OA. MRI would not be necessary since the patient has typical signs of synovitis.

24.10. Answer: B.
Osteoporosis is a common complication of RA whether seropositive or seronegative. Felty's syndrome, vasculitis and nodules can occur in RA but they are rare complications and occur in seropositive RA. Uveitis is a feature of axial spondyloarthritis (axSpA), not RA.

24.11. Answer: C.
Methotrexate is the core disease-modifying antirheumatic drug (DMARD) in the management of RA and it is often combined with prednisolone therapy at first presentation to gain disease control. Option B would be inappropriate in view of the very active disease given that hydroxychloroquine has relatively weak immunosuppressive effects. Options A and E would not be indicated as first-line treatments. Option D would not give adequate disease control.

24.12. Answer: E.
Obesity is protective against osteoporosis and osteoporosis does not cause bone pain unless a fracture has occurred. Calcium and vitamin D supplements are used in the treatment of osteoporosis, mainly as an adjunct to other treatments, but alone they are ineffective in the prevention of osteoporosis. Osteoporosis is a common complication of PMR, not a rare complication.

24.13. Answer: D.
The radiograph shows typical features of osteoporotic vertebral fractures with biconcave deformities of L4, L3 and L2, and a wedge deformity of L1.

24.14. Answer: D.
The patient is at increased risk of osteoporosis because of the low trauma fracture and family history of hip fracture. If DXA shows osteoporosis, treatment would be indicated. There is no indication at present to start treatment with either alendronate or calcium and vitamin D supplements, nor is there a reason to advise her to stop alcohol since she has a moderate intake.

24.15. Answer: E.
Options A, B and D are rare adverse effects. Leucopenia is not a recognised adverse effect of oral bisphosphonates.

24.16. Answer: C.
The patient has failed to respond adequately to triple therapy and progression to biologic treatment would be indicated. Neither secukinumab nor apremilast is effective in RA and would not be appropriate choices. Substitution of sulfasalazine with leflunomide is unlikely to be effective. Increasing the frequency of methotrexate would not be indicated since the patient is already on the maximum recommended dose.

24.17. Answer: E.
Acute gout can be managed with either NSAID therapy or colchicine, but urate-lowering therapy with allopurinol is indicated to control hyperuricaemia in the long term, to reduce the risk of recurrence and prevent long-term joint damage. Allopurinol alone would not be appropriate since it may cause a further flare in acute gout due to the change in uric acid levels.

24.18. Answer: E.
Methotrexate is teratogenic and must be stopped completely at least 3 months before attempting to become pregnant. It is not necessary to stop ibuprofen before becoming pregnant but NSAIDs are contraindicated after 20 weeks.

24.19. Answer: B.
Osteoarthritis is characterised by joint space narrowing due to cartilage erosion and subchondral sclerosis. Erosions at all MCPJs and periarticular osteoporosis are more typical of RA (though inflammatory OA typically causes inflammation at index and middle finger MCPJs) whereas punched-out erosions of the first MTP joint of the feet suggest gout. Irregularity and fusion of the sacroiliac joint (SIJ) suggests axial spondyloarthritis (axSpA) or psoriatic arthritis (PsA).

24.20. Answer: E.
Previous joint injury is a strong risk factor for osteoarthritis due to destabilisation of the joint. None of the other factors significantly influences the development of osteoarthritis.

24.21. Answer: E.
Systemic NSAIDs are more effective that paracetamol in controlling pain in OA. There is no evidence that COX-2 selective and non-selective NSAIDs differ in efficacy. There is

24

some evidence that glucosamine has a weak beneficial effect in knee OA but it has not been studied in hip OA. Joint replacement surgery is a recognised treatment for OA, but would only be indicated when optimal medical therapy was ineffective.

24.22. Answer: D.
Although diet accounts for a proportion of circulating vitamin D, sunlight exposure is the most important source in most people. Synthesis of 25(OH)D in the skin under the influence of UV light accounts for the fact that circulating levels are highest in the summer and lowest in the winter. It is very unlikely that this patient's symptoms are related to the level of vitamin D.

24.23. Answer: D.
The inactive metabolite 25(OH) vitamin D (25(OH)D) is hydroxylated in the kidney at the 1α position by the enzyme CYP27B1 to give the active metabolite $1,25(OH)_2D$. Although 25(OH)D is hydroxylated at the 1 and 24 positions, the $24,25(OH)_2D$ metabolite is not biologically active.

24.24. Answer: A.
Osteomalacia is suggested by the symptoms, the patient's ethnic background, the low 25(OH)D, high PTH, low phosphate and high ALP. Vitamin D insufficiency is a biochemical diagnosis in patients with serum 25(OH)D levels of 25–50 nmol/L (10–20 ng/mL). Polymyalgia is unlikely in view of the normal ESR, and statin-induced myopathy is unlikely in view of the normal creatine kinase. The symptoms and biochemical abnormalities are not consistent with osteoporosis.

24.25. Answer: D.
It is likely that the low 25(OH)D levels are secondary to fibromyalgia since vitamin D deficiency is common as a secondary feature of many diseases due to lack of sunlight exposure and a poor diet. There is no evidence that vitamin D supplements help in fibromyalgia or that fibromyalgia is a complication of vitamin D deficiency.

24.26. Answer: E.
Option A is unlikely in view of the positive family history. Vitamin D-deficiency rickets is unlikely in view of the positive family history and the normal 25(OH)D level. Options C and D are

recessive disorders, which would be inconsistent with the family history of an affected mother and brother.

24.27. Answer: B.
In about 10–15% of cases the disease is inherited in families due to mutations in the *SQSTM1* gene. There is no proven association with the HLA locus. Paget's is a focal skeletal disorder characterised by increased bone resorption and formation (not reduced bone formation). Although environmental factors play a role in Paget's disease of bone, the triggers are unclear and there is no evidence that alcohol intake or smoking predispose to the disease.

24.28. Answer: D.
The radiograph shows changes typical of Paget's disease with alternating areas of osteosclerosis and osteolysis and expansion of the femur. There is also a pseudofracture on the lateral femoral cortex. The site of Paget's corresponds with the location of the pain, and the elevated ALP level indicates increased metabolic activity, suggesting that the pain may be caused by Paget's disease of bone. There is no evidence of OA, which makes this unlikely as the cause of the pain. The biochemistry does not support a diagnosis of osteomalacia and renal osteodystrophy would not be expected in a patient with mild renal impairment.

24.29. Answer: E.
Scheuermann's is characteristically accompanied by wedge deformities of several adjacent thoracic vertebrae with disc space narrowing. It typically results in contiguous vertebral paramarginal syndesmophytes. Options B, D and E would be consistent with osteoporosis. Option C would be consistent with osteoarthritis.

24.30. Answer: E.
Fractures occur most commonly in childhood, decrease during adolescence and adulthood but increase again with ageing. Option A is incorrect: it is unknown whether bisphosphonates reduce fracture risk in adults with OI. Option B is incorrect: vertebral fractures occur commonly. Option C is incorrect: blue sclerae are typical of type I OI but normal sclerae do not exclude other subtypes.

24.31. Answer: B.
The presentation is typical of fibrous dysplasia, which is caused by a somatic mutation in *GNAS1*, which activates signalling through the PTH receptor causing a focal increase in bone turnover and osteolytic lesions. It is also associated with café-au-lait pigmentation due to activation of signalling through the melanocyte-stimulating hormone receptor and endocrine abnormalities. Paget's disease can also present with focal bone deformity but would be extremely unusual in a patient of this age. Osteomyelitis is unlikely in the absence of a previous history of infection. Camurati–Engelmann disease can present similarly but is bilateral rather than unilateral. The diagnosis is not consistent with osteopetrosis, which is a systemic rather than local disorder characterised by high bone mass.

24.32. Answer: D.
Calcium pyrophosphate deposition disease (CPPD) is a common feature of the arthropathy associated with haemochromatosis and the presentation with acute pain and swelling that settles with NSAID treatment is consistent with CPPD-associated arthropathy (pseudogout). Diabetes can cause an arthropathy but has different features and RA is unlikely as symptoms have settled and there is no synovitis. Although venesection should be continued as treatment for the haemochromatosis, there is no evidence that this will improve the arthritis. Option A is incorrect since an arthropathy is associated with haemochromatosis in up to 50% of cases.

24.33. Answer: B.
The symptoms are typical of median nerve compression syndrome, which is a recognised complication of RA. Mononeuritis can occur secondary to vasculitis in RA but this is unlikely since the disease is under good control. Osteoarthritis of the CMC joint presents with local pain rather than neurological symptoms. Bone erosions are a cause of pain in RA but not neurological symptoms.

24.34. Answer: A.
Postural orthostatic hypotension syndrome (POTS) is a recognised complication of hypermobility. Option C is incorrect. Although *FBN1* mutations cause hypermobility as part of Marfan's syndrome, this is a rare cause of hypermobility – the most common cause is Ehlers–Danlos syndrome type III, which is a polygenic disorder. Option B is incorrect since hypermobility is common in osteogenesis imperfecta. Option D is incorrect. Hypermobility is diagnosed with a Beighton score of 4 or above in the presence of arthralgia. Joint dislocations are not a prerequisite to make the diagnosis.

24.35. Answer: B.
The presentation is typical of a Charcot joint secondary to peripheral neuropathy associated with the diabetes. Although the patient has hyperuricaemia, the history does not suggest gout. The history is also inconsistent with calcium pyrophosphate deposition disease. Diabetic cheiroarthropathy affects the hands, not the ankle. The clinical picture is not consistent with OA, which in the lower limbs typically affects the hips and knees.

24.36. Answer: D.
Osteosarcoma is a rare tumour that predominantly affects people under 30 years of age, presenting with pain and a soft tissue mass, often with islands of calcification within the lesion. Fibrous dysplasia can cause an expansile bone lesion but is not associated with a soft tissue mass, The patient is too young for Paget's disease. Metastatic bone disease presents differently. Although hypertrophic pulmonary osteoarthropathy can present with pain and a periosteal reaction in the limbs, it does not cause a soft tissue mass.

24.37. Answer: D.
The main mechanism is inhibition of bone formation due to osteoblast and osteocyte apoptosis. Osteoclastic bone resorption can be increased due to secondary hyperparathyroidism but this is not the main mechanism of bone loss. Options A, C and E are all incorrect; glucocorticoids do not affect vitamin D metabolism or cause hypoparathyroidism.

24.38. Answer: A.
Smoking has been associated with severity and susceptibility to RA as well as response to treatment. There is no evidence that alcohol, body weight or HIV infection predispose to RA. Although vitamin D insufficiency is common in RA, there is no evidence that it plays a causal role or influences disease activity.

24

24.39. Answer: D.
The available results are consistent with acute gout (urate crystals are negatively birefringent) but do not exclude the possibility that infection may also be present. In sepsis, often bacterial identification is not possible until culture is available. A negative Gram stain suggests there might not be infection but does not rule it out. The cause of pseudogout is calcium-containing crystals (usually pyrophosphate) and these crystals are positively birefringent. Reactive arthritis is certainly possible but intervention should be delayed until it is clear it is not septic arthritis.

24.40. Answer: B.
Calcification of peri-odontoid ligaments is a feature of crowned dens syndrome, which is a lesion seen in CPPD. Syndesmophytes are the hallmark radiographic sign in advanced ankylosing spondylitis. Bone sclerosis is a recognised feature of PsA; juxta-articular new bone formation is very common in PsA and is included in the diagnostic (CASPAR) classification. Sacroiliac disease is a common feature in all spondyloarthritides (SpA).

24.41. Answer: E.
The history suggests inflammatory back pain and hence either axSpA or ankylosing spondylitis (AS) is possible. AS and axSpA can be associated with normal ESR. Diagnosis of AS requires an abnormality of SIJs on x-ray to be present but a diagnosis of axSpA can be made before SIJ X-ray changes are present using axial skeletal MRI. Although HLA-B27 does not diagnose either disease, its presence increases the likelihood of either axSpA or AS in the appropriate clinical context.

24.42. Answer: B.
Ultrasound has poor ability to detect soft tissue abnormalities if there is extensive bone (which appears as an interface linear high signal with a reflectance void beyond it, i.e. black!). There are no characteristic features of PMR-related lesions on ultrasound. With Doppler, ultrasound is useful for gauging the vascularity of joint and tendon synovitis.

24.43. Answer: B.
Her osteoporosis risk may be quite high given her age (likely peri-menopausal), steroids and systemic inflammatory disease, and despite just an osteopenia-level BMD. Mild but definite

spinal fractures can be relatively clinically silent – causing few symptoms – so often need pro-action 'ruling out' with imaging. If present, a fragility spine fracture will elevate her further fracture risk considerably.

FRAX (www.shef.ac.uk/FRAX) allows an overall quantification of fracture risk using the main BMD-independent risk factors for fracture. It is well established that the level of BMD at which fragility fractures are likely is higher than would otherwise be expected if steroids were not being taken.

Patients with Crohn's disease, and patients on steroids, can be calcium and/or vitamin D deficient and supplements should be considered but *antiresorptive* therapies should also be considered if overall risk warrants. Whilst steroids should be minimised, there may be no other option for treatment of her acute Crohn's flare-ups.

24.44. Answer: A.
Autoimmune serology results interpreted alone out of clinical context are rarely, if ever, diagnostic. The serology is typical of PSS. Positive anti-DNA antibodies are typically associated with SLE. Anti-Ro can be present in both SLE and PSS but if both Ro and La are positive, PSS is more likely. Although patients with SScl can be ANA positive, antibodies more specific for SScl are anti-centromere or anti-topoisomerase (Scl-70). Rheumatoid factor is not specific for RA and in the context of these other serology results and negative ACPA, the rheumatoid factor is far more likely to represent PSS.

24.45. Answer: C.
The presentation of gout in men and women is typically different; particularly in post-menopausal women, the first presentation may be polyarticular. Synovitis in RA can be subtle and is not always clinically obvious – MRI and ultrasound (US) are useful in confirming early synovial disease. Axial skeletal forms of CPPD include crowned dens syndrome, intervertebral disc inflammation and ligament flavum inflammation/thickening. Studies using US have shown subclinical inflammation at entheses in PsA.

Generalised OA can present as an inflammatory 'storm' of symptoms in small joints with synovial inflammation. Involvement of PIPJs and DIPJs is more common than MCPJs, but often the index and sometimes third finger MCPJs are involved (RA often picks out the fifth MCPJ early on in the course of the disease).

24.46. Answer: D.

The features are not unusual for a rheumatology referral! The differential diagnosis can be wide and includes inflammatory and autoimmune disease. Also, significant somatic and functional effects from psychosocial triggers in a vulnerable person can provide such a symptom complex. Rheumatology assessment requires a broad approach and judicious use of investigations based on a stratified differential diagnosis based on clinical assessment. A 2-year history of an illness due to malignancy would be expected to cause progressive clinical deterioration.

24.47. Answer: C.

Men do get osteoporosis and the commonest vertebral fracture sites are low thoracic spine or L1 or L2. Fracture pain can be mild to severe but often starts acutely or subacutely, and persists. It would be rare for axSpA to present at this age for the first time. Disc prolapse lesions occur mainly in younger people and are rare in the thoracic spine – the commonest levels being L5/S1, L4/L5, L3/L4. The absence of systemic features is chiefly against this being sepsis – patients with this diagnosis are often generally quite unwell. Like prolapsed discs, the main sites of spondylolistheses are lumbar spine and sometimes in the neck, but very rarely in the thoracic spine. Malignancy is not on the list but should be considered in anyone this age presenting with non-trivial/self-limiting back pain for the first time.

24.48. Answer: D.

Oligoarthritis is the most common form of JIA, accounting for 60% of cases. Monoarthritis is an unusual presentation of RA, especially if both rheumatoid factor and ACPA antibodies are negative. Ophthalmological screening is recommended in all cases of JIA, regardless of whether ANA is positive or negative. As in adults, PsA may be the cause of monoarthritis/ oligoarthritis, whether or not psoriasis is present, i.e. PsA has to be considered possible. Initial management should be with an NSAID and consider intra-articular steroid injection (under light general anaesthetic).

24.49. Answer: C.

All JIA patients should be referred for ophthalmological examination to rule out uveitis. Both IBD and leukaemia can present with oligoarthritis. Systemic JIA is regarded as an antibody-negative condition and is analogous to adult-onset Still's disease. The prevalence of JIA (1:1000) is similar to the prevalence of diabetes in children and adolescents (1:700).

24.50. Answer: E.

Rituximab is 'B-cell depletion' therapy. B-cell proliferation and B-cell antigen presentation are not a major part of the pathophysiology of either AS or PsA. Other therapies mentioned have alternatively been shown to have some clinical effectiveness in one or both conditions.

24.51. Answer: E.

A pustular plantar foot rash occurring simultaneously with inflammatory back pain, enthesitis and synovitis does suggest reactive arthritis. A sexual history may not be volunteered but should be sought – with direct questions about new recent sexual encounters, penile discharge, dysuria and other genital symptoms, if necessary.

24.52. Answer: C.

Ankylosing spondylitis (AS) and all spondyloarthropathies are generally autoinflammatory conditions characterised by abnormalities in antigen processing (HLA-B27, ERAP-1), antigen presentation (ERAP-1, HLA-B27) and the stimulation and activity of type 17 T cells (IL-23r, STAT-3). ANK-H is associated with calcium pyrophosphate deposition disease (CPPD). ANK-H codes for a transmembrane protein important in transporting inorganic pyrophosphate.

24.53. Answer: A.

Scleritis and ACPAs are features of RA. Uveitis, ankle swelling and raised ACE are typical of sarcoid. Fatigue is a feature of all autoinflammatory and autoimmune conditions. A small minority of PsA patients may have a positive rheumatoid factor. Achilles insertional tendonitis (enthesitis) and symphysitis are recognised axSpA lesions.

24.54. Answer: A.

Direct evidence from randomised controlled trial data suggest TNF-α inhibitors ustekinumab (anti-IL-12/23 monoclonal) and secukinumab

24

(anti-IL-17) treat enthesitis successfully, although evidence that non-biologic immunotherapies do is scant. Ultrasound studies have shown inflammation at painful and at symptomless entheses in PsA. MRI and US can detect enthesitis. Enthesitis can occur at any site of entheseal tissue – which includes any soft tissue structure attachment to bone and at the nail bed–distal interphalangeal joint tissue complex. Enthesitis occurs in both HLA-B27 positive and negative individuals with spondyloarthritis.

24.55. Answer: B.
Apremilast inhibits PDE4, which then secondarily reduces pro-inflammatory cytokine production including IL-17 and TNF-α but also increases production of the anti-inflammatory cytokine IL-10. Inhibition of RANK ligand is achieved by denosumab monoclonal antibody, used in treating osteoporosis. CD80/86 binding (T-cell co-stimulatory signalling) by abatacept (CTLA–Ig), blocks T-cell function, and is licensed for use in treating RA. STAT3 is a potential therapy target in a number of autoinflammatory and autoimmune diseases given its role in promoting differentiation of Th17 cells.

24.56. Answer: A.
There is no evidence that cannabinoids improve any aspect of fibromyalgia. The quality of evidence (see http://www.cochranelibrary.com/topic/Rheumatology/Fibromyalgia/) for all treatments in fibromyalgia is generally poor, perhaps with the exception of supervised aerobic exercise. However, some evidence exists showing responses in a minority of studied patient populations for a wide range of interventions.

24.57. Answer: B.
Tenderness at entheses can occur, as there will be tenderness elsewhere, if there is pain sensitisation (as seen in fibromyalgia, which is associated); however, inflammation at entheses is not a recognised feature of HMS. Lax internal supportive connective tissue can result in uterine, vaginal or rectal prolapse. Hypertension does not occur but postural hypotension may be part of a syndrome of autonomic dysfunction (postural orthostatic tachycardia syndrome; POTS) associated with HMS.

24.58. Answer: A.
Antibodies to RNP antigens (e.g. U1RNP) are suggestive – in the appropriate clinical context

– of MCTD. Patients with MCTD have some features of SScl, SLE and myositis but the sclerodactyly differs in appearance to the sclerodactyly of SScl. Antibodies to DNA and Sm ('Smith') are characteristic of SLE and positivity to Ro(SSA) and La(SSB) together suggests PSS.

24.59. Answer: D.
The patient may well have SLE and an associated glomerulonephritis needs to be promptly identified/ruled out. Steroids may be indicated but more initial information is needed – and that may include kidney biopsy to grade glomerulonephritis and guide therapy choices. Any delay in obtaining information in a potential case of lupus nephritis can be dangerous.

24.60. Answer: E.
Investigation of patients with polymyositis necessarily needs to be comprehensive. *Skeletal muscle* (MRI and then open biopsy at MRI-identified abnormal muscle site), *cardiac muscle* (echocardiogram but not cardiac MRI initially) and *gastrointestinal tract muscle* (barium swallow) need investigating for disease involvement. Insufficient skeletal muscle may be obtained for all required analyses from needle biopsy. In a minority of cases, polymyositis is associated with malignancy, so whole-body CT may screen for deep-organ malignancy and lymph gland enlargement. DXA scan is required to guide steroid-induced osteoporosis risk management – most cases of adult polymyositis require high-dose and persistent steroid therapy.

24.61. Answer: D.
Echocardiography and RFTs in SScl screen for features of pulmonary hypertension (PHT), which in SScl may not present with dyspnoea until the lesion is quite advanced. Proactive screening identifies early right heart effects and pre-symptomatic reduced lung gas transfer. PHT is life-threatening but can be treated with a prostacyclin analogue (e.g. iloprost), sildenafil (inhibits cGMP-specific phosphodiesterase type 5) or bosentan (endothelin-1 mediated vasoconstriction blocking). Respiratory lesions should be investigated in SLE and dermatomyositis if there are any relevant symptoms and on the basis of examination signs (i.e. of interstitial lung disease). Uveitis is not a common feature of lupus in adults. The presentation of polymyositis is associated with

malignancy so initially CT screening is helpful; however, the merit of regular yearly CT monitoring in the absence of detecting malignancy thereafter has not been substantiated.

24.62. Answer: C.
Even in severe disease, structurally normal parts of salivary glands can be seen. Their sub-function may be a consequence of cytokine inhibition of neurotransmitter function. Humidity, blink rate (and therefore tasks being undertaken) and air conditioning all affect the degree to which surface moisture from eyes and mucous membranes evaporates, and therefore affects symptoms. Patients who have previously failed to benefit from eye lubricants managed to do so after a trial of topical eye drop steroids. PSS is significantly associated with the development of lymphoma.

24.63. Answer: D.
In theory, all the features can conceivably occur in all the conditions but the likelihood of a subacute, relapsing/remitting condition involving different tissues arising at different times supports the diagnosis of granulomatosis with polyangiitis (GPA; formerly Wegener's) here. Fever and rash are generally temporally related in post-streptococcal reactive arthritis, adult-onset Still's disease and rheumatic fever. Lung malignancy would not be common in a non-smoker and features of it unlikely to remit over time.

24.64. Answer: B.
The diagnostic terminology for GPA and MPA have been subsumed under the new diagnostic classification 'ANCA-associated vasculitis (AAV)', partly owing to their association with autoantibodies to neutrophil antigens (antineutrophil cytoplasmic antibody (ANCA) vs. intracellular antigens proteinase-3 (PR3) and myeloperoxidase (MPO) for GPA and MPA, respectively). A substantial number of patients with polymyositis have antinuclear antibodies (ANAs) and myositis-specific antibodies. GCA is not associated with autoantibodies.

24.65. Answer: A.
The features are suggestive of Behçet's disease (BD). A history of genital lesions may not be volunteered. Various inflammatory eye lesions can occur in BD and cerebral venous sinus thrombosis as a cause of non-specific

headache and other cranial symptoms is not uncommon in the disease. Sarcoid is possible – as the rash may be erythema nodosum, which is common to sarcoid and BD – but there is no hypercalcaemia or ankle joint involvement here, which would be more typical in sarcoid. Sinus thrombosis in BD can be detected by either head CT or MRI but sarcoid in the brain often affects meninges at the base of the brain and ideally requires gadolinium-enhanced sequences on MRI to disclose lesions adequately.

24.66. Answer: A.
Cannabis use has been linked to causing an *occlusive vasculopathy* similar to thromboarteritis obliterans. Hepatitis C is associated most commonly with cryoglobulinaemic vasculitis. HIV and indeed many viruses are considered potential triggers of vasculitis. HLA-B51 is associated with Behçet's disease – the main manifestation of which is a vasculitis. IgA production and deposition in vasculitis lesions is a characteristic of Henoch–Schönlein purpura vasculitis.

24.67. Answer: D.
Case examples and rationale exist to support an association of *Propionibacterium acnes* and SAPHO syndrome but the level of proof that the organism is responsible for, or associated with, a substantial number of cases of SAPHO is not high. SAPHO is thought to represent a spectrum of pathophysiological features possibly contiguous with features seen in childhood chronic relapsing multifocal osteomyelitis (CRMO). Associations between the other microorganisms and their autoinflammatory or autoimmune condition are more robust, based on good epidemiological, clinical and immunological data or pathogenetic principles.

24.68. Answer: C.
PSS is associated with about a 15% risk of lymphoma (PSS with mucosa-associated lymphoid tissue lymphoma; 'MALToma'). RA is associated with malignancy with a standardised incidence ratio (SIR) of 1.1. The risk is greatest for Hodgkin lymphoma (SIR 3.21) and lung cancer (SIR 1.64). Relapsing polychondritis can be associated with coincident hematological malignancy (particularly myelodysplasia) in a small minority of cases. DISH is associated with diabetes and possibly with CPPD disease, but

24

not with malignancy. Giant cell arteritis occurs in the elderly, a population in which malignancy is not unusual but there is no known association.

24.69. Answer: D.

There is new bone formation at ligament attachments at the distal ulna (this is a non-articular part of the carpus) typical of PsA. The feature of juxta-articular ('fluffy') new bone adjacent to joints is highlighted in the CASPAR classification criteria for PsA (Box 24.69). The radiocarpal joint space is reduced here from PsA also. There is an absence of subchondral cysts or sclerosis and osteophytes (thus unlikely to be primary OA or CPPD), and no RA or gout erosions present, nor periarticular osteopenia, as seen in active RA.

---

i   **24.69 The CASPAR criteria for psoriatic arthritis**

Inflammatory articular disease (joint, spine or enthesis) with ≥ 3 points from the following (1 point each unless stated):
Current psoriasis (scores 2 points)
History of psoriasis in first- or second-degree relative
Psoriatic nail dystrophy
Negative IgM rheumatoid factor*
Current dactylitis
History of dactylitis
Juxta-articular new bone[†]

*Established by any method except latex. [†]Ill-defined ossification near joint margins (excluding osteophytes) on X-rays of hands or feet.
(CASPAR = ClASsification for Psoriatic ARthritis)

24.70. Answer: E.

The clinical features are fairly non-specific and gout, septic arthritis and pseudogout are possible diagnoses. Indeed, severe gout or pseudogout can cause systemic symptoms identical to those caused by infection. The diagnosis is made on knee fluid aspiration and then Gram stain and culture of the fluid, but also polarised light microscopy of joint fluid

examining for crystals (urate-causing gout or calcium-containing causing pseudogout). CKD stage 3b–5 is associated with urate and calcium-containing crystal-induced musculoskeletal disease. Secondary joint infection following incompletely treated urine infection is possible but also previous infection can trigger subsequent bouts of crystal arthritis.

24.71. Answer: A.

Barbotage is a procedure usually done under ultrasound guidance whereby needle disruption of calcific deposits in tendons is undertaken (e.g. calcific supraspinatus tendonitis). The technique usually involves repeated high-pressure fluid injection and aspiration. It has not been shown beneficial for calcinosis cutis. Thalidomide is an extremely effective treatment for the severe mucosal ulcers in Behçet's disease. Local glucocorticoid injection is useful for treating a number of non-inflammatory enthesopathic lesions (such as plantar fasciitis and elbow epicondylitis). Rituximab has now been shown useful in some patients with AAV, inducing as well as maintaining remission. Oral pilocarpine can improve salivary and other glandular secretion in all but late PSS. A trial of therapy 5–10 mg 3 times daily can be attempted over a month.

24.72. Answer: D.

Reactive arthritis can present like axSpA or AS with low back axial symptoms. Radiographs are frequently normal in early SpA conditions. HLA-B27 is positive in 95% of people with an old (modified New York criteria) definition of AS but is less prevalent in cohorts of patients diagnosed with axSpA. In axSpA (and AS) and all SpA conditions, the acute phase response may be normal and associated clinical problems (current or previous) include anterior uveitis, psoriasis, inflammatory bowel disease, enthesitis and sterile urethritis.

JP Leach, RJ Davenport

25

Neurology

Multiple Choice Questions

25.1. A 44 year old woman is admitted with abrupt onset of neurological deficit. The referring physician suspects a brainstem stroke. Which of the following combinations of signs and symptoms would be most likely to originate from a brainstem lesion?

A. Bilateral optic neuropathy
B. Cranial nerve signs with sensory and upper motor neuron signs in all four limbs
C. Horner's syndrome with ipsilateral arm pain
D. Lower motor signs in both arms only
E. Upper motor neuron signs in both legs only

25.2. A 34 year old man is admitted with worsening weakness in both legs. Over the course of 3 days he has found it increasingly difficult to walk upstairs. In the last 12 hours he complains of feeling mildly breathless.

The referring physician finds weakness in all four limbs and cannot elicit reflexes. He can find no sensory problems.

Which diagnosis is most likely?

A. Guillain–Barré syndrome (GBS)
B. Inflammatory myopathy
C. Myasthenia gravis
D. Peripheral neuropathy
E. Spinal stroke

25.3. A 38 year old man presents with sensory changes in both legs, which he finds difficult to characterise. The referring physician asks you to review him 'to assess him for a dissociated sensory loss'.

Which of the following statements is true about dissociated sensory loss?

A. Dissociated sensory loss is a sign of peripheral nerve disease

B. Dissociated sensory loss is always associated with reflex changes
C. Dissociated sensory loss is usually a sign of brainstem pathology
D. Dissociated sensory loss means loss of sensation over one-half of the body
E. Dissociated sensory loss requires testing of pin-prick, light touch, proprioception and vibration in all four limbs

25.4. A 25 year old woman presents to the emergency department with a rapidly evolving severe headache. She has a family history of cerebral neoplasm and is worried that this is the cause of her headaches.

Which of these accompanying features would suggest a diagnosis other than migraine?

A. Asymmetrical reflexes
B. Exacerbation by exercise
C. Photophobia
D. Unilateral site
E. Vomiting

25.5. An 18 year old male presents with numbness in both legs evolving over a few weeks. He reports some variable sensory alteration and is worried that this might represent multiple sclerosis. Gait is slower than usual but there is no reported weakness.

Which of the following would suggest a lesion outside the spinal cord?

A. Band of hyperaesthesia across the trunk
B. Loss of reflexes
C. Preserved vibration but loss of pin-prick sensation over both legs

D. Sphincter disturbance
E. Wasting of both quadriceps

25.6. A 23 year old man complains of some excessive daytime sleepiness. Which clinical features may suggest an underlying diagnosis of narcolepsy.

A. Hypnic jerks
B. Myoclonus on awakening
C. Periodic limbs movements in sleep
D. Restless legs
E. Sleep paralysis

25.7. A 58 year old man presents having had three unprovoked generalised tonic–clonic seizures in the last 3 weeks. He has a history of severe head injury with frontal contusions some years before. His wife reports some blank episodes lasting a few minutes with some manual automatisms and lip smacking for 1–2 minutes. He has no history of any other medical problems.
   Which antiepileptic drug would be recommended as first line?

A. Clobazam
B. Lamotrigine
C. Levetiracetam
D. Pregabalin
E. Sodium valproate

25.8. A 19 year old woman presents having had three unprovoked generalised tonic–clonic seizures on awakening in the last 3 weeks. She has a history of some brief twitching movements occurring in the mornings after some sleep deprivation but no other episodes of altered awareness. She has no history of any other medical problems.
   Which antiepileptic drug would be recommended as first line?

A. Carbamazepine
B. Levetiracetam
C. Phenytoin
D. Sodium valproate
E. Topiramate

25.9. A 44 year old woman presents with a history of neck pain and some tingling in the upper limbs. Which of the following features would make you keen to carry out magnetic resonance imaging (MRI)?

A. Awakening with tingling in one or both hands
B. History of her hearing 'clunking' on neck movements

C. Long duration of symptoms (more than 2 years)
D. Loss of biceps reflex on the symptomatic left side
E. Restriction of lateral neck flexion

25.10. A 78 year old male presents with a year-long history of lower back pain occasionally radiating down one or both legs. What feature would suggest that MRI of the lumbosacral spine is indicated?

A. A band of altered sensation across the costal margin
B. Impaired vibration sense in both legs
C. Localised tenderness over the lower back
D. Loss of both ankle jerks
E. Recent onset of urinary incontinence

25.11. A 64 year old woman presents to hospital with a 3-day history of worsening 'confusion' and disorientation. She has no past medical history other than hypertension. She has had no recent foreign travel.
   Examination shows her to be drowsy, but even when awakened she is unable to answer questions, although she can follow direction and complies with the examination. Her temperature is 38.5°C. She has some neck stiffness but no rash.
   Cranial nerve examination is normal. She has bilaterally upgoing plantar reflexes but no apparent other neurological signs.
   What is the likely causative organism?

A. *Borrelia burgdorferi*
B. Herpes simplex
C. Herpes zoster
D. *Neisseria meningitides*
E. *Streptococcus pneumoniae*

25.12. An 18 year old male student has been home from university for 3 days, during which time he has become increasingly drowsy. He is able to be roused but is disorientated.
   He has a temperature of 39°C, has marked neck stiffness and a positive Kernig's sign. He has developed a spotting, non-blanching rash over his anterior chest wall. He has no focal neurological deficit.
   What is the most appropriate next course of action?

A. Administer intravenous (IV) benzylpenicillin
B. Arrange for a computed tomography (CT) brain scan
C. Carry out a lumbar puncture

D. Puncture one of the purpuric lesions for microscopic analysis
E. Take blood for viral polymerase chain reaction (PCR) test

25.13. With regard to the patient in Question 25.12, IV benzylpenicillin has now been administered and his cerebral imaging has been shown to be normal. A lumbar puncture has been carried out.

What is the most likely pattern of abnormality to emerge in cerebrospinal fluid (CSF)?

A. Normal white cells, normal protein, low glucose
B. Normal white cells, raised protein, normal glucose
C. Raised white cells (90% lymphocytes), raised protein, low glucose
D. Raised white cells (90% neutrophils), normal protein, normal glucose
E. Raised white cells (90% neutrophils), raised protein, low glucose

25.14. A 38 year old man presents to his family physician with a 3-month history of a change in sensation in both arms. His wife has been trying to get him to seek help for worsening hand weakness and progressive gait difficulties.

Examination shows him to have no cranial nerve signs. He has marked wasting of intrinsic muscles of both hands and brisk leg reflexes with upgoing plantar responses. Sensory examination shows him to have lost pin-prick sensation over both arms and the upper half of his trunk. Vibration and proprioception are normal.

What is the likely pathology?

A. Metastatic lesion in the upper spinal cord
B. Motor neuron disease
C. Peripheral neuropathy
D. Spinal cord stroke
E. Syringomyelia

25.15. A 64 year old man is referred to the emergency department by his family physician. He has been undergoing radiotherapy for a small cell carcinoma of lung for the last 2 months.

He sought help this morning for some back pain and gait difficulty evolving over the last day. He has no symptoms in the arms. He reports some recent difficulty in initiating urination.

Examination shows motor signs in the legs only with increased reflexes and upgoing plantars. All modalities of sensation are reduced below the costal margin.

What is the likely underlying process?

A. Cerebral metastasis
B. Metastatic spinal cord compression
C. Paraneoplastic encephalopathy
D. Paraneoplastic Guillain–Barré syndrome
E. Paraneoplastic neuropathy

25.16. A 33 year old female has had a severe pain over her left shoulder, which increased gradually over the initial 24 hours, coming on 2 weeks after an influenza vaccination. It is a dull unremitting ache for which she was given opiate analgesia for several weeks.

Since the pain subsided she has had some weakness of hand movements – most particularly in holding and turning a door key. She has reduced reflexes in the left arm, with some subjective decrease in pin-prick sensation over all dermatomes in the left arm.

What is the most likely diagnosis?

A. Brachial neuralgia
B. Cervical radiculopathy
C. Guillain-Barré syndrome
D. Herpes zoster-related neuralgia
E. Transverse myelitis

25.17. An 18 year old female is referred by her optician after an abnormal visual field test. She had her vision checked after complaining of headaches and formal perimetry has shown enlargement of both blind spots.

Further clarification of her symptoms has revealed a 6-month history of worsening daily headaches, increased on bending and coughing, sometimes accompanied by transient flashing lights lasting seconds at a time.

Neurological examination confirms the enlargement of blind spots with some accompanying papilloedema. No other focal deficit was found.

What is the likely diagnosis?

A. Cerebral venous sinus thrombosis
B. Idiopathic intracranial hypertension (IIH)
C. Intracranial neoplasm
D. Migraine with aura
E. Optic neuritis

25.18. A 21 year old man was involved in a clash of heads while playing football. He was unconscious for about a minute but recovered

25

and was able to play on for the remaining half hour. He did not report any concussive symptoms and was able to go out for a meal with a few friends where he consumed two pints of beer.

The next morning his friends cannot rouse him from sleep. An ambulance is called and takes him immediately to hospital. On admission he is apyrexial and has a Glasgow Coma Scale (GCS) score of E2 V3 M2. His pupils are symmetrical and reacting to light. Plantar response is upgoing on the right.

What is the likely diagnosis?

A. Alcoholic coma
B. Extradural haematoma
C. Post-traumatic tonic–clonic seizure
D. Subdural haematoma
E. Viral encephalitis

25.19. A 75 year old woman had a diagnosis of Alzheimer's disease made 3 years ago. Recently her mobility has begun to deteriorate and she has had a number of falls, twice having her skull X-rayed in the emergency department as a result of her injuries.

She has a history of hypertension and transient ischaemic attacks and is on aspirin and ramipril. Her daughter says that her memory and concentration are much worse over the last 2 weeks and she can go for long spells where she is difficult to rouse.

On examination she is apyrexial and drowsy, and she is disorientated in time and place. Her GCS score is E5 V4 M5. There are no cranial nerve abnormalities, but she is weaker on the left, with generally brisk reflexes and upgoing plantar reflexes. She has some frontal release signs (pout and grasp reflexes) bilaterally.

What is the most likely explanation for her decline?

A. Alzheimer's disease
B. Extradural haematoma
C. Ischaemic stroke
D. Metabolic encephalopathy
E. Subdural haematoma

25.20. A 34 year old woman has a long history of migraine with aura happening three or four times per year. After a recent episode where she had visual aura, typical severe headache, recurrent vomiting with photophobia and an intolerance of noise, she is left with a different character of headache over the subsequent 10 days. This is a severe pounding headache

precipitated by rising from a lying position, building up over 4–5 minutes each time and necessitating that she lie back down.

She is distressed and cannot sit up for any length of time. Examination shows no change in cranial nerves. Her reflexes are generally brisk but plantar responses are downgoing, and there is no other deficit in the limbs.

She has normal blood tests and a normal CT of brain but no other investigation.

What is the likely cause of her headache?

A. Cerebral venous sinus thrombosis
B. Cluster migraine
C. Intracranial tumour
D. Spontaneous intracranial hypotension
E. Subarachnoid haemorrhage

25.21. A 44 year old man has been in hospital for 3 weeks for management of decompensated alcoholic liver disease. He awakens with an inability to dorsiflex the right ankle.

Examination shows normal movements otherwise bilaterally. There is no wasting and reflexes are intact. Sensory examination shows reduced pin-prick sensation of the right lateral shin. He has slight tenderness over the lower back bilaterally but no other findings.

What is the likely cause of his weakness?

A. Alcoholic neuropathy
B. Cerebral infarct
C. Common peroneal nerve lesion
D. Sciatic nerve lesion
E. Tibial nerve lesion

25.22. A 23 year old woman presents having had three generalised tonic–clonic seizures in the previous 3 weeks. Which of the following would suggest a focal origin to her epilepsy?

A. History of 'blank spells' in childhood
B. History of morning myoclonus
C. Prolonged post-ictal dysphasia
D. Prolonged seizure (lasting 2–3 hours)
E. Seizures on awakening

25.23. A 56 year old right-handed man is admitted with an abrupt onset of loss of speech. Comprehension appears to be preserved and he can follow direction with no difficulties. He cannot repeat words or phrases.

Where is the abnormality most likely to be situated on imaging?

A. Left and right frontal lobes
B. Left frontal lobe

C. Left temporal lobe
D. Right frontal lobe
E. Right temporal lobe

25.24. A 78 year old man presents with speech difficulty. His response to speech is intact, but the words are poorly formed and at times difficult to understand. The clinical diagnosis of a dysarthria is made.

Which of the following would suggest a cerebellar cause of his dysarthria?

A. Associated pseudobulbar features
B. Fatiguability (worsening as the day goes on)
C. Nasal regurgitation when swallowing fluids
D. Scanning speech (lack of variation in cadence)
E. Stammering rapid speech

25.25. A 38 year old man has come to see you because of some progressive gait difficulties. He has had several falls at home. On calling him through to your consulting room you notice that his walk is abnormal. (Note: it is always good practice to watch your patients as they make their way in.)

Which of these features would be most likely to suggest a peripheral nerve problem as the cause of his walking difficulties?

A. Broad-based shuffling gait
B. Circumduction of one foot
C. Inability to turn quickly
D. Rapid small steps with no festination
E. Slapping one foot

25.26. A 38 year old woman presents to her optician with a history of blurred vision over several months. Computerised visual field testing shows that she has bilaterally enlarged blind spots.

Where will the pathological process occur that will cause this selective change?

A. Macula
B. Optic chiasm
C. Optic discs
D. Optic nerves
E. Peripheral retina

25.27. A 42 year old man presents with a history of two nocturnal and one daytime generalised tonic–clonic seizures over the previous 3 months. He is reluctant to start treatment because of the risk of side-effects and his uncertainty of efficacy.

What are his chances of being rendered seizure-free by a single antiepileptic drug?

A. 1%
B. 10%
C. 40%
D. 60%
E. 80%

25.28. A 30 year old woman presents having had a single generalised tonic–clonic seizure on awakening a week ago. She exhibits no neurological deficit and initial investigation with CT brain and electrocardiogram (ECG) have been normal.

She volunteers some other symptoms. Which of these would be considered physiological rather than epileptiform?

A. Bitten tongue on awakening
B. Episodes of lost time with automatic behaviour
C. Episodes of lost time with no automatisms
D. Jerking of whole body on falling asleep
E. Jerks of both arms on awakening

25.29. A 22 year old man presents with a history of fatigue and muscle cramps. He now feels unable to take part in 10 km runs with his friends.

Which of these symptoms or signs is most likely to suggest an underlying muscular problem?

A. Dark urine after prolonged exertion
B. History of 'dropping things'
C. Intermittent focal fasciculations over 5 years
D. Nocturnal leg cramps
E. Strong family history of diabetes mellitus

25.30. A 28 year old woman complains of excessive daytime sleepiness. She often finds herself falling asleep in lectures during the day. She is worried that she might have a diagnosis of narcolepsy/cataplexy.

Which of the following features is a normal phenomenon and would help you to reassure her?

A. Family history of excessive daytime sleepiness
B. Hallucinations – experiencing visions of intimidating people on awakening
C. Sleep paralysis – awakening unable to move for 45 seconds
D. Sudden collapses related to fright
E. Sudden whole-body jerking on falling asleep

25

25.31. A 35 year old female presents with a 6-day history of delirium and disorientation. She is pyrexial but aside from being unable to answer questions or follow direction, exhibits no neurological deficit.

After normal imaging has been carried out, a lumbar puncture is done, which shows the following results: white cell count 35×10^9/L; blood film – 90% lymphocytes; CSF protein 0.65 g/L; CSF glucose 4.2 mmol/L (76 mg/dL); serum glucose 6.0 mmol/L (108 mg/dL) (normal CSF glucose is >60% of contemporary serum glucose).

Which process would be a likely cause of this picture?

A. Brainstem encephalitis
B. Meningococcal meningitis
C. Subarachnoid haemorrhage
D. Tuberculous meningitis
E. Viral encephalitis

25.32. A 76 year old man presents with a left-sided facial weakness of rapid onset. He has no past medical history of note.

Which feature would suggest that the deficit is caused by an upper motor neuron lesion?

A. Deviation of the tongue to the left on protrusion
B. Hyperacusis on the left
C. Loss of taste in the anterior two-thirds of the tongue on the left
D. Preservation of eyebrow elevation on the affected side
E. Weakness of eyebrow elevation on the opposite side

25.33. A 64 year old woman presents with a left foot drop of gradual onset.

Which of the following would suggest that the responsible lesion is in the common peroneal nerve rather than a more proximal lesion?

A. Reduced left ankle jerk
B. Reduced pin-prick in lateral shin
C. Reduced pin-prick sensation in the medial shin
D. Tinel's sign over the fibular neck
E. Weakness of ankle inversion

25.34. A 57 year old man is referred to the clinic because of some difficulty with unsteadiness on walking.

Which feature would suggest a lesion within the spinal cord as the cause of his problems?

A. Bilateral lower limb hypertonicity, hyper-reflexia, and upgoing plantar reflexes
B. Circumduction of the left foot
C. Difficulty with heel-toe waking
D. High-stepping gait
E. Slapping of the feet against the ground

25.35. A 35 year old patient presents with weeks of progressively worsening left-sided facial pain. Which of the following would suggest that the cause is outside the superior orbital fissure?

A. Diplopia on gaze to the left
B. Diplopia on gaze to the right
C. Left proptosis
D. Reduced visual acuity in the left eye
E. Sensory alteration over the left eye

25.36. A 43 year old woman presents with a history of vertigo and vomiting.

Which of the following features would be most in keeping with a diagnosis of acute labyrinthitis?

A. Evolving symptoms over weeks
B. Improvement in symptoms following an Epley manoeuvre
C. Ipsilateral sensorineural hearing loss
D. Nystagmus worsened by change in position
E. Precipitation by minor head injury

25.37. A 28 year old right-handed man complains of visual disturbance after sustaining a significant head injury in a road traffic accident. CT scan shows a fracture in the left parietal region with an underlying cerebral contusion and extradural haematoma.

What visual symptoms would you expect to result from this injury?

A. Diplopia on looking to the right
B. Left-sided neglect
C. Left superior quadrantanopia
D. Reduced visual acuity on the left
E. Right inferior quadrantanopia

25.38. A 54 year old female presents with a 6-month history of recurrent headaches. They affect the right periorbital region, with a throbbing quality, and make her feel sick. Sometimes the right eyelid appears droopy with the pain, and she prefers to go to bed and sleep it off. It usually lasts a few hours. When younger, she recalled headaches with her periods for which she would take analgesia, but these were different from the current symptoms. In between attacks, she is well and on no medication.

Which of the following is the most likely diagnosis?

A. Carotid artery dissection
B. Cluster headache
C. Migraine
D. Temporal arteritis
E. Tension-type headache

25.39. A 66 year old man presented with 6 weeks of intermittent diplopia, improved by closing one eye. His family physician has checked a variety of blood tests – all were normal except antibodies to the acetylcholine receptor (AChR), which returned strongly positive with a high titre of antibodies.

What is the next most relevant test?

A. Antibodies to muscle-specific kinase (MuSK)
B. CT chest
C. Electromyography (EMG)
D. MRI head
E. Tensilon test

25.40. A 70 year old female presents with variable weakness of her legs; she has lost a significant amount of weight recently, complains of a dry mouth and, more recently, a cough, occasionally with blood. There is little to find on examination, and there is uncertainty about whether her leg reflexes are present. There are no other signs, although she looks unwell and thin.

Antibodies to which of the following are most likely to be present?

A. Acetylcholine receptor (AChR)
B. Muscle-specific kinase (MuSK)
C. N-methyl-D-aspartate (NMDA) receptor
D. Thyroid peroxidase
E. Voltage-gated calcium channel (VGCC)

25.41. A 28 year old woman presents in the sixth month of her first pregnancy with unpleasant tingling affecting the ring and little fingers, mainly on the left hand and to a lesser extent the right, which keeps her awake at night. She has developed gestational diabetes, but is otherwise well, with no previous problems. She is on no medication.

What is the most likely diagnosis?

A. Carpal tunnel syndrome (CTS)
B. Cervical spondylosis

C. Functional sensory symptoms
D. Multiple sclerosis
E. Ulnar entrapment neuropathy

25.42. An 18 year old male presents to a remote hospital 3 hours after being felled by a single punch. He was briefly knocked out, seemed to recover, before becoming increasingly drowsy, then losing consciousness.

On arrival in the emergency department, his neurological examination shows: no eye opening, incomprehensible sounds, flexing to pain on the right, extending on the left. His pulse is 50 beats/min, regular; blood pressure is 210/115 mmHg. His right pupil is fixed and dilated. His airway is compromised and he is intubated and ventilated. The nearest hospital with a neurosurgeon and scanner is 6 hours away by ambulance.

What is the best course of action?

A. Burr hole on the left side of the head
B. Burr hole on the right side of the head
C. Palliative care
D. Transfer him to the nearest hospital as soon as possible
E. Treat him with mannitol and intensive care

25.43. A 74 year old woman presents with a 12-month history of tremor affecting her right arm only.

Which feature is the most supportive of a diagnosis of Parkinson's disease?

A. Family history of learning disabilities
B. Her father had a tremor
C. Her husband reports that for the last few years she has occasionally lashed out or grabbed him while asleep
D. Tremor improves with small amounts of alcohol
E. Tremor is most apparent when using the arm

25.44. A 65 year old man has been diagnosed with Parkinson's disease. He is reluctant to start treatment, as he has heard that such treatment only lasts a short time before he will become immune to it.

Which statement is most correct?

A. He should avoid treatment as long as he can, as there is a short therapeutic window once he has started it
B. He should delay treatment until his symptoms are interfering with everyday life

noticed that his right eye waters and goes red with the pain. Occasionally he gets an attack during the day. He thinks he had something similar about 2 years ago but it disappeared after a week or so. He is otherwise well, but terrified that he has a brain tumour such is the severity of the pain.

What is the likely diagnosis?

A. Cluster headache
B. Hypnic headache
C. Migraine
D. Paroxysmal hemicrania
E. Temporal arteritis

25.55. A 50 year old male describes a 3-week history of dizziness, often occurring in bed. Shortly before the dizziness started, he had walked into a glass door, 'seen stars' but not lost consciousness. On closer questioning, he has noted that getting into or out of bed and rolling over to the left can trigger his symptoms, which is brief vertigo lasting a few seconds. He has fallen on two occasions as he got out of bed as a result. He occasionally gets it during the day, usually when getting into his sports car, but otherwise he is generally well. He is on no medication, but drinks about 60 units of alcohol per week.

What is the appropriate management?

A. Alcohol abstention
B. Betahistine
C. Low-salt diet
D. Short course of glucocorticoids
E. Vestibular repositioning (e.g. Epley manoeuvre)

25.56. A 36 year old female presents with progressive difficulty walking over the previous week, and now has difficulty passing urine. One year previously she had an episode of monocular visual loss which lasted about 2 weeks. She was abroad at the time, and by the time she returned, her vision was recovering so she did not seek attention. On examination she has an upper motor neuron pattern weakness in both legs, with brisk reflexes and upgoing plantar responses, and a palpable bladder; her right optic disc is pale. Her non-contrast MRI head is normal, but there is a long lesion seen in the thoracic spine, stretching over several spinal segments, thought to be inflammatory.

Which investigation is most likely to make confirm a diagnosis?

A. Aquaporin-4 antibody
B. Lumbar puncture for oligoclonal bands
C. Paraneoplastic antibodies
D. Repeat imaging with contrast
E. Visual evoked potentials

25.57. A 21 year old female was diagnosed with MS 2 years ago after presenting with ataxia, from which she recovered fully; she declined further treatment at the time as she was considering starting a family. She has now developed numbness of her left arm, which has alarmed her but is not compromising her function. She has no other symptoms.

What is the most appropriate immediate management?

A. Broad-spectrum antibiotic
B. Conservative
C. High-dose oral glucocorticoids
D. Physiotherapy
E. Start a disease-modifying drug of high efficacy such as natalizumab

25.58. A 30 year old female presents to her family physician. Her identical twin sister was diagnosed with MS last year, and she has read that her own risk of MS is therefore increased, and she is enquiring about this.

Approximately what is her risk of developing MS?

A. 5%
B. 20%
C. 35%
D. 50%
E. 85%

25.59. Which of the following scenarios would represent a reasonable case for requesting an electroencephalogram (EEG)?

A. A 15 year old female with a single unwitnessed blackout thought to be syncope but with associated urinary incontinence
B. A 24 year old male in a psychiatric unit on multiple antipsychotics and consistently drowsy in the mornings
C. A 64 year old female having had a single generalised tonic–clonic seizure
D. A 68 year old female with two witnessed generalised tonic–clonic seizures
E. A 68 year old male with a previous left hemisphere stroke and recent episodes of unwitnessed collapse

25.60. A 28 year old man describes evolving weakness of all four limbs over 8 weeks, and most recently some dyspnoea.

Blood tests are normal and lumbar puncture shows a raised CSF protein but no cells. A diagnosis is made of chronic inflammatory demyelinating polyneuropathy (CIDP).

Which of the following patterns of abnormality on nerve conduction studies and EMG is likely to be present at the time of diagnosis?

A. Delayed conduction in motor and sensory nerves with denervation on EMG
B. Delayed conduction in sensory and motor nerves with normal EMG
C. Normal nerve conduction and EMG studies
D. Normal nerve conduction studies but denervation changes on EMG
E. Small sensory nerve and compound motor action potentials but normal EMG

25.61. A 68 year old woman presents to her family physician with a 3-day history of 'dizziness', by which she means extreme vertigo, with a sensation of the room spinning to the right, made worse with any movement. She has vomited on occasions and has been bed-bound but reports no focal neurological deficit. Things have improved slightly in the last 24 hours and she can now make her way round the house with some assistance.

What is the likely explanation for her symptoms?

A. Acute labyrinthitis
B. Benign paroxysmal positional vertigo
C. Brainstem stroke
D. Ménière's disease
E. Migraine

25.62. A 26 year old woman saw her optician because of recent headaches. These are present on stooping or coughing and often associated with visual symptoms (small flashing dots or brief loss of vision). She has no history of vomiting or other neurological symptoms. She has no cognitive or depressive symptoms.

Examination shows her body mass index to be 40 kg/m². She has bilateral papilloedema and no venous pulsation on fundoscopy. Blind spots are enlarged in both eyes. Neurological examination is otherwise normal.

What is the likely cause of her fundal abnormalities?

A. Bilateral optic neuropathy
B. Diabetic retinopathy
C. Idiopathic intracranial hypertension
D. Intracranial space occupying lesion
E. Neuromyelitis optica

25.63. A 32 year old man has a 3-month history of slowly worsening headaches after sustaining a minor head injury while playing football. These headaches were worse if he exercises or coughs and are sometimes associated with vomiting and nausea. He has no other systemic symptoms.

Neurological examination shows him to have bilateral papilloedema but no focal neurological deficit. MRI is reported as showing dilated lateral and third ventricles but no increase in size of the fourth ventricle.

What is the likely diagnosis?

A. Cerebral venous sinus thrombosis
B. Idiopathic intracranial hypertension
C. Intracranial space-occupying lesion
D. Normal pressure hydrocephalus
E. Stenosis of the aqueduct of Sylvius

25.64. A 44 year old woman is referred to see you because of worsening headaches. These have been present for around 4 years and have increased in frequency and severity such that she is now self-medicating with doses of paracetamol and codeine tablets 3–4 times daily.

Her headaches fall into two types: a constant underlying 'throbbing, aching' pain present every moment of every day, and episodes of severe pulsating headache with photophobia, phonophobia and nausea. She has been off work for the last 3 months and has now become withdrawn, depressed and weepy. Neurological examination is normal.

What is the likely diagnosis?

A. Chronic Daily Headache
B. Chronic migraine
C. Functional headache disorder
D. Intracranial space occupying lesion
E. Subarachnoid haemorrhage

25.65. A 28 year old man presents with episodes of unsteadiness lasting days to hours at a time on around 3–4 occasions per year. These are not be worsened by changes in position, and he is not aware of any precipitants. There is no accompanying pain or visual symptoms and in

25

between these bouts he reports no symptoms.

His father had similar symptoms in later life, and his younger brother has started to display similarly intermittent symptoms. Neurological examination is normal.

What is the likely diagnosis?

A. Benign paroxysmal positional vertigo
B. Diabetic neuropathy
C. Episodic ataxia
D. Migraine
E. Spinocerebellar ataxia

25.66. A 62 year old man has a 3-month history of worsening unsteadiness, causing him to fall on several occasions. He has not sustained any serious injury but now requires more help to cook and look after himself in his home.

He has multiple medical conditions and requires a range of regular medications, which he supervises himself.

Neurological examination reveals nystagmus on lateral gaze with jerky pursuit movements and diplopia on lateral gaze (both directions). His speech is slurred but he has no other neurological deficit. Power and reflexes are normal in all four limbs. He has an intention tremor, past-pointing in both arms and cannot heel-toe walk because he is so unsteady.

Which of his medications is most likely to be contributing to his unsteadiness?

A. Diazepam
B. Digoxin
C. Phenytoin
D. Prochlorperazine
E. Salbutamol

25.67. A 68 year old female presents with a witnessed sleep-onset convulsion, with typical post-event confusion, lateral tongue biting and subsequent myalgia. She reports a single collapse at the age of 16, and remembers having a 'brain wave' test, which was normal, apparently. She is desperate not to lose her driving licence, and believes this was related to dehydration caused by the hot weather that day.

In the emergency department on the day of presentation, her ECG and routine blood tests are all normal except for a neutrophilia (total white cell count 19.8×10^9/L) and sodium of 133 mmol/L.

What is the next most appropriate investigation?

A. Brain imaging
B. Further investigation of neutrophilia and hyponatraemia
C. No further investigations necessary
D. Sleep-deprived EEG
E. Standard EEG

25.68. A 29 year old male presents 8 weeks after being hit on the head by a golf ball. He fell to the ground but it was unclear whether he lost consciousness or not (if he did, it must have been very brief). He went to hospital that day, and had a minor laceration to his scalp glued. He has since been troubled by gradually worsening headache, poor concentration, irritability and poor sleep, and now he is very miserable and low. He is off work, and spending much of his time asleep on the couch during the day.

He has returned to the emergency department on several occasions due to his symptoms, and had a CT head 2 weeks ago which was normal. Yesterday he saw an acupuncturist who recommended he seek an MRI head scan.

What is the appropriate management?

A. Explanation of the 'post-concussion syndrome'
B. MRI head
C. Neurosurgical referral
D. Psychiatric referral
E. Tramadol for his headache

25.69. A 24 year old woman had first seen her family physician a year ago with a history of anxiety and panic attacks. In the subsequent 6 months she and her family had begun to notice some cognitive difficulties and short-term memory problems (losing the ability to carry out complex tasks at work, not recognising family members).

When you see her in the clinic, she is orientated in time and person but is hesitant in her answers, being also disorientated in place. She exhibits difficulties in all domains of cognitive testing, especially in tasks requiring working memory and concentration.

On examination she has frequent twitching movements involving all four limbs (her family have noticed these over the last 2 weeks). Concentration difficulties limit the usefulness of visual examination, but otherwise she has generally brisk reflexes and upgoing plantars.

What is the most likely cause of her cognitive problems?

A. Alzheimer's disease
B. Anxiety disorder
C. Hyperthyroidism
D. Sporadic Creutzfeldt–Jakob disease (CJD)
E. Variant CJD

25.70. A 40 year old right-handed man presents after a single generalised tonic–clonic seizure. He has no risk factors for development of epilepsy but on closer questioning has had spontaneous bursts of altered sensation ('like a burning') in the left arm lasting seconds at a time.

Examination is normal except for an asymptomatic homonymous left lower temporal quadrantanopia. He has had a CT head which shows a non-enhancing abnormality in the substance of the brain.

What is the likely nature of the lesion?

A. Basal skull meningioma
B. Glioblastoma multiforme in right parietal lobe
C. Low-grade glioma in right parietal lobe
D. Medulloblastoma in the right parietal lobe
E. Optic nerve glioma

25.71. A 26 year old woman presents to the emergency department with a rapid onset of headache. There had been a slowly evolving scotoma in the right side of her vision, which had spread over around 35 minutes with some associated flickering in the vision. The headache afterwards had been severe, and she retired to bed where she vomited on several occasions. Her family had noted that her speech had been slurred during the headache phase and she felt that she had some associated altered sensation in the right hand.

You see her 24 hours later, at which point she feels drained but otherwise back to normal. Neurological examination is normal.

What is the most likely cause of her symptoms?

A. Cerebral venous sinus thrombosis
B. Focal seizure arising in the occipital region
C. Migraine with aura
D. Subarachnoid haemorrhage
E. Transient ischaemic attack

25.72. A 21 year old male has been working on a farm for the summer. He has been on treatment with flucloxacillin for jaw stiffness that had been diagnosed as an early dental abscess. Over 5 days, he has become more

unwell, with some agitation and anxiety, with a marked startle response to sound or touch.

He is apyrexial and shows no signs of localised infection. Blood pressure is 165/110 mmHg but cardiovascular examination is otherwise normal. Neurological examination is difficult but shows generalised stiffness when he is moved or but no other focal neurological deficit.

What is the likely cause of his symptoms?

A. Botulism
B. Dental abscess with extension into the basal skull
C. Functional illness
D. Juvenile myoclonic epilepsy
E. Tetanus

25.73. A 44 year old woman returned from a holiday with her German cousins 1 week ago. In the last 5 days she has begun to notice worsening diplopia in all directions of gaze. She has had some difficulty in swallowing (fluid sometimes coming up through the nose) over the last 3 days and has had worsening weakness in legs and arms over the last 24 hours. She has noticed that she is becoming breathless, even at rest. The cousin with whom she was staying has begun to notice the same symptoms in the last 3 days.

Examination shows her to be apyrexial with normal pulse and blood pressure. Forced vital capacity and forced expiratory volume in 1 second (FEV_1) are reduced. She exhibits bilateral ptosis with reduced eye movements in all directions. Pupils are equal and reactive, and palatal movement is reduced. There is weakness with preserved reflexes in all limbs.

What is the likely cause of her symptoms?

A. Botulism
B. Brainstem stroke
C. Miller Fisher syndrome
D. Multiple sclerosis
E. Myasthenia gravis

25.74. A 34 year old woman was involved in a minor road traffic accident 24 hours previously. Her car had been hit from behind but she had not lost consciousness and had not suffered a direct blow to the head. On awakening the next day she was aware of a right-sided headache with associated neck pain. She had no diplopia or visual symptoms and no other focal neurological symptoms.

25

i	25.24 Causes of dysarthria			
Type	Site	Characteristics	Associated features	
Myopathic	Muscles of speech	Indistinct, poor articulation	Weakness of face, tongue and neck	
Myasthenic	Motor end plate	Indistinct with fatigue and dysphonia. Fluctuating severity	Ptosis, diplopia, facial and neck weakness	
Bulbar	Brainstem	Indistinct, slurred, often nasal	Dysphagia, diplopia, ataxia	
'Scanning'	Cerebellum	Slurred, impaired timing and cadence, 'sing-song'	Ataxia of limbs and gait, tremor of head/limbs. Nystagmus	
Spastic ('pseudobulbar')	Pyramidal tracts	Indistinct, nasal tone, mumbling	Poor rapid tongue movements, increased reflexes and jaw jerk	
Parkinsonian	Basal ganglia	Indistinct, rapid, stammering, quiet	Tremor, rigidity, slow shuffling gait	
Dystonic	Basal ganglia	Strained, slow, high-pitched	Dystonia, athetosis	

Fatiguability of speech is characteristic of myasthenia gravis, while pseudobulbar features would be most commonly accompanying multi-infarct states. Stammering rapid speech is a feature of parkinsonian syndromes, while nasal regurgitation is a sign of palatal weakness of whatever cause.

25.25. Answer: E.

Slapping one foot while walking (often after lifting the affected leg higher than the other) is a sign of a foot drop, which is most commonly related to common peroneal nerve damage.

Circumduction is a compensatory movement to avoid tripping over a plantar-flexed foot (most usually related to upper motor neuron effects), while inability or difficulty in turning is most likely with parkinsonian disorders. Rapid small steps (marche à petits pas) is a sign of generalised cortical problems (most usually vascular), while a broad base is a compensation for the impaired coordination of cerebellar disease.

25.26. Answer: C.

The physiological blind spot corresponds to the area of the retina where the optic nerve passes through and spreads fibres radially (the optic disc). Any process that swells the optic disc will cause papilloedema and an increased blind spot.

Macular lesions will cause a reduction in visual acuity (as noted on the Snellen chart) while optic chiasm lesions (most usually a pituitary problem) will cause a bitemporal hemianopia. Optic nerve lesions can cause blindness when severe but may show only reduction in colour vision on the affected side(s). Peripheral retinal problems will cause scotomata in the corresponding area of the visual field.

25.27. Answer: D.

Most patients will be rendered completely seizure-free by the first or second drug they are prescribed. Some will have a brief relapse (perhaps related to reduced adherence) while others will require long-term treatment with two or more antiepileptic drugs in combination. Where there is incomplete or inadequate response, steps should be taken to ensure the diagnosis and classification are correct, that the patient is taking the treatment, and that there are no other confounding factors (e.g. evolving lesion, use of alcohol or epileptogenic drugs). In cases where there is an established single focus, surgical workup may be indicated.

25.28. Answer: D.

A crucial part of the assessment of patients after a single seizure is to clinically assess whether there has been any other seizure activity experienced by the patient.

Nocturnal seizures may only be signalled by some tongue biting or enuresis (often associated with some myalgia or headache). Daytime seizures of absence epilepsy or focal onset with altered consciousness will usually have the patient sitting still or fidgeting, respectively. Morning myoclonus is characteristic of genetic generalised epilepsy (particularly juvenile myoclonic epilepsy), while hypnic jerks are, of course, an entirely normal phenomenon and not indicative of any pathology (other than fatigue).

25.29. Answer: A.

A metabolic muscular problem means that prolonged exercise is liable to cause muscle damage resulting in myoglobinuria: presence of myoglobin causing the black urine.

Diabetes mellitus can occur in mitochondrial conditions, but it is common and unlikely to be directly relevant unless there are other clues (accompanying systemic disease, maternal transmission and deafness). Nocturnal leg cramps are common and history of dropping things is non-specific for muscular problems.

25.30. Answer: E.

The occurrence of daytime sleepiness in narcolepsy is usually accompanied by some of the other three components of the narcolepsy tetrad: namely, cataplexy (collapses with fright or laughter), hypnagogic hallucinations (visual hallucinations often with an emotional content) and sleep paralysis (loss of voluntary movement on awakening). The genetic basis for this condition means that a family history of excessive sleepiness may help diagnosis. Of the tetrad components, sleep paralysis is the one that is most likely to be physiological, and isolated sleep paralysis should not in itself trigger invasive or prolonged testing.

Hypnic jerks on falling asleep are a normal phenomenon. The important treatable cause of daytime sleepiness is lack of night-time sleep – exclusion of obstructive sleep apnoea may be required.

25.31. Answer: E.

A raised neutrophil count in CSF is strongly associated with a bacterial infection, although the very earliest stages of a viral encephalitis may cause neutrophils to rise.

Infections by mycobacteria, viruses, or partially treated bacterial meningitis may be associated with lymphocytic CSF. Where there has been a large subarachnoid haemorrhage, the irritant effect of blood on the meninges may cause a lymphocytic CSF, but would more likely have an abrupt onset and mild (or no) pyrexia.

25.32. Answer: D.

Supply of the upper face is bilateral (from both cerebral cortices), so a unilateral facial weakness caused by an upper motor lesion will be modified by the residual supply from the ipsilateral cortex.

Hyperacusis and dysguesia (altered taste) originate from lesion of the facial nerve and would not be prominent with an upper motor neuron facial weakness.

Bilateral facial weakness should raise the suspicion of either myasthenia or Guillain-Barré syndrome, while ipsilateral protrusion of the tongue occurs often with a facial palsy and without other signs would not imply involvement of any other cranial nerves.

25.33. Answer: D.

The common peroneal nerve supplies tibialis anterior, the toe extensors and sensation to the lateral aspect of the shin. The nerve runs round the fibular neck and irritation at that point can produce a Tinel's sign (localised tenderness of dysaesthesia over a site of nerve damage) in a nerve that is affected early. The common peroneal nerve is mostly derived from L5 roots, so clinical differentiation can be difficult.

An L5 lesion will cause a foot drop alongside reduced pin-prick in the lateral shin, as well as weakness of ankle inversion (as it supplies tibialis posterior).

The ankle jerk depends on contraction of soleus and gastrocnemius, which are supplied by tibial nerve and S1 root.

25.34. Answer: A.

A lesion of the spinal cord is likely to affect both legs equally in provoking upper motor neuron signs, leading to a spastic paraparesis with increased tone, increased reflexes and extensor plantar reflexes.

Selective or particular difficulty with heel-toe walking results from cerebellar dysfunction, while a high-stepping gait and slapping gait will, respectively, compensate for or result from impaired ankle dorsiflexion (i.e. a foot drop), which results most usually from a common peroneal or radicular lesion.

Unilateral circumduction is a sign of a unilateral upper motor neuron lesion, where the leg has to drift sideways while walking to compensate for the partial plantar flexion caused by increased tone in soleus and gastrocnemius.

25.35. Answer: D.

The superior orbital fissure is formed by the cleft between the lesser and greater wings of the sphenoid bone. Lesions in this will affect the structures that pass through, including cranial nerves III, IV and VI, which, if affected, will cause diplopia on gaze to either side or on downgaze. Compression of the orbital vein would lead to proptosis, and any effect on the

25

fifth nerve will cause sensory alteration over the upper face.

Pathology of the optic nerve will cause a reduction in acuity in one eye, but this does not pass through the superior orbital fissure. Any effect on acuity alongside some disturbance of ocular motility would suggest pathology in the cavernous sinus.

25.36. Answer: D.

Labyrinthitis (also known as acute vestibular failure) presents with abrupt onset of vertigo that tends to be most severe for a few days, severe enough to cause the patient to be bed-bound.

Ménière's disease is an idiopathic chronically recurring disorder involving episodic vertigo with tinnitus and a progressive deafness. Benign paroxysmal positional vertigo can be precipitated by minor head injury and results in vertigo that is typically precipitated by specific head positions (as in the Hallpike Test). This responds well in most cases to the Epley manoeuvre or more chronic rehabilitation.

25.37. Answer: E.

A lesion in the parietal region will cause a quadrantanopia – due to its effect on the superior fibres, the quadrantanopia will be in the contralateral inferior visual field.

Neglect will result from a parietal lesion but this is contralateral to the lesion. Reduced acuity results from a reduction in macular function and may be a manifestation of an optic neuropathy.

Diplopia results from a disturbance of ocular motility – this is unlikely to be caused by a cortical abnormality.

25.38. Answer: C.

This is a typical scenario for migraine without aura. The additional non-headache symptoms would not occur in tension-type headache, and neither temporal arteritis nor dissection behave in such a paroxysmal manner. (She is also too young for temporal arteritis.) Although she gets occasional ptosis, the other autonomic features of cluster are absent and the headache lasts too long; patients are usually very agitated with cluster and usually male.

25.39. Answer: B.

The story of variable binocular diplopia is suggestive of myasthenia gravis, and the positive AChR antibody confirms this

(false-positive tests are very rare – the antibody is very specific). Imaging his head will add nothing, as this is an autoimmune disease of the neuromuscular junction. Antibodies to MuSK are much less commonly found in myasthenia gravis, and never when the AChR antibody is positive. Whilst he may have an abnormal single-fibre EMG, the diagnosis is already made with the antibody result, so the EMG will add little or nothing; similarly, a Tensilon test may well be positive, but adds nothing to what we already know. Myasthenia gravis is, however, associated with thymic abnormalities and in older men thymomas are not uncommon; hence, he requires imaging of his chest for this reason (either CT or MRI).

25.40. Answer: E.

Whilst the differential on this limited history is wide, there are clues to suggest Lambert–Eaton myasthenic syndrome (LEMS). The weakness is variable, in keeping with a mysathenic syndrome, there are no sensory features, and the dry mouth suggests autonomic involvement, which is common in LEMS. LEMS may be paraneoplastic, and there are alarm bells for cancer, with weight loss, unwellness and haemoptysis (lung cancer is the commonest malignancy seen with LEMS). The reflex uncertainty reflects the classic reflex potentiation seen in LEMS, whereby reflexes appear absent, but may return (potentiate) with exercise. The diagnosis is supported by the presence of VGCC antibodies.

25.41. Answer: E.

The symptoms conform to the distribution of the ulnar nerve and, although carpal tunnel syndrome (median nerve) is common in pregnancy, in this case the distribution suggests ulnar not median. The most likely site of entrapment is at the elbow (as opposed to the wrist in CTS).

25.42. Answer: B.

This is very suggestive of an extradural haematoma, localising to the right side of his head. He is coning, and will not survive 6 hours in ambulance. The immediate life-saving procedure is a burr hole to evacuate the clot.

25.43. Answer: C.

The sleep disturbance is very suggestive of an REM sleep behavioural disturbance, now a well-recognised pre-motor symptom of Parkinson's disease (PD), often preceding the motor features by years. A tremor that responds to alcohol and is mainly with action suggests essential tremor (ET; usual bilateral), and whilst PD can be familial, the family history of a tremor would also fit ET better. Family history of learning disabilities suggests possible fragile X tremor ataxia syndromes, which can manifest sometimes in women.

25.44. Answer: B.
There remains some controversy about when best to start treatment in PD, although there is consensus that presently we have no proven disease-modifying therapies. Anticholinergics are no longer favoured due to their adverse effect profile and poor efficacy. Whilst the response to dopaminergic therapies becomes both attenuated and complicated as PD progresses, people do not become 'immune' to it. Whilst DBS is a very effective treatment for tremor (where drugs often fail), few would advocate this approach prior to a trial of medication. Most would recommend dopaminergic therapy sooner or later, and in the UK we would be inclined to wait until his symptoms trouble him, although there is greater enthusiasm for earlier treatment elsewhere.

25.45. Answer: C.
Parkinson's disease is a clinical diagnosis, and tests are rarely helpful. This is unlikely to be Wilson's disease (caeruloplasmin) with this age at presentation, and the scenario is not suggestive of a genetic cause (in any case, one would need to undertake genetic counselling first before any genetic testing). Structural imaging is rarely indicated in a typical story such as this, and, similarly, functional imaging with either SPECT or positron emission tomography (PET) is unnecessary when the diagnosis is clear clinically.

25.46. Answer: A.
This is likely to be secondary to long-term metoclopramide use, even though many doctors and patients think of it as an innocuous drug. Chorea can occur with stroke, but is usually unilateral and acute. Such dyskinesias may complicate Parkinson's disease when treated with levodopa, but are not a presenting feature in patients not on treatment. Huntington's disease can present this late,

although usually there is a family history, which may be suppressed.

25.47. Answer: C.
This is a very typical Essential tremor (ET) history – both arms involved, postural and kinetic components, autosomal dominant pattern of inheritance and an alcohol response in some members (only about 50% note such a response). Parkinson's tremor is more typically asymmetrical, and at rest. It can be difficult to distinguish an enhanced physiological tremor from a mild ET, as they look similar, although the other features help (family history, alcohol responsiveness). Whilst sensible to check his thyroid status, it is unlikely to explain a 10-year history.

25.48. Answer: D.
This is a typical story for TGA, with a profound anterograde amnesia lasting several hours leading to repetitive (and irritating) questions, and retrograde amnesia stretching back at least 2 years, but not so long that she had forgotten her friends or husband. Psychogenic amnesia often involves loss of self-identity (functional fugue state); the post-ictal state is usually confusion, rather than this very specific isolated amnestic syndrome. Isolated amnesia is almost never due to a TIA, and Alzheimer's presents in a much more insidious way.

25.49. Answer: C.
In general, people who worry about their memory, which no one else has noticed, rarely have an underlying disease; clinicians should worry much more about the family who bring a patient who seems blithely unaware of any problem. Minimal cognitive impairment (MCI) is a controversial entity, although some will progress to dementia. Depression can present with a pseudo-dementia, but there are no specific features of depression here. Sleep apnoea can disturb memory but is usually associated with excessive daytime sleepiness, and a sleep history of snoring and apnoeic spells.

25.50. Answer: E.
He has developed acute hemiballism, which usually localises to the contralateral subthalamic nucleus in the basal ganglia. In this case, it is almost certainly due to a stroke, but is often not recognised as such as the symptoms are unusual and may be missed by inexperienced

25

clinicians. Lesions in the motor strip would cause weakness, and lesions affecting the angular gyrus in the dominant parietal lobe are associated with Gerstmann's syndrome (agraphia, acalculia, finger agnosia and inability to differentiate left from right).

25.51. Answer: B.

The symptoms and signs suggest a pseudobulbar palsy, but the progression over several months excludes a stroke; a structural lesion could potentially cause this, but not in the frontal region. Polymyositis may affect swallowing but not speech, and would not cause these signs or emotional incontinence. Whilst myasthenia gravis can present with bulbar symptoms, the upper motor neuron signs and emotionalism do not fit. Unfortunately, this sounds very likely to be a pseudobulbar presentation of motor neuron disease.

25.52. Answer: D.

Disturbance of sense of smell (and taste, which is crucially dependent upon smell) is common after minor head injury, most typically to the occipital region, as the shearing forces cause disruption to the olfactory fibres as they pass through the cribriform plate in the anterior cranial fossa. (Patients are often mystified as to why a bang to the back of their head might affect their nose.) It would be an unusual malingering symptom, and malingering is a forensic rather than medical diagnosis. Parkinson's disease is often preceded by hyposmia, although patients rarely, if ever, present at this stage. Whilst smokers often have less acute senses of smell and taste, they rarely notice this. For most patients presenting with reduced sense of smell and no apparent triggers, the causes are either ENT related or idiopathic.

25.53. Answer: C.

The scan confirms that she is retaining urine, with incomplete bladder emptying. Thus the optimal treatment would be regular intermittent self-catheterisation, providing that her arm/hand function is not compromised by her MS. Antibiotics would not affect her bladder function, and anticholinergic drugs would exacerbate the problem. A long-term catheter would ideally be avoided.

25.54. Answer: A.

This is a typical scenario for cluster headache, one of the trigeminal autonomic cephalalgias

(TACs). The pain is always severe, lasting between 30 and 180 minutes, associated with autonomic activation and agitation. Cluster headaches typically awaken people from sleep, clusters last weeks, with months to years of remission in between. They are more common in male smokers. Migraine can awaken people from sleep, but usually patients want to lie quietly in a dark room, the opposite of cluster patients, and autonomic activation is rare. Hypnic headache also awakens people from sleep, but usually affects older women, and is not associated with agitation or autonomic activation. Temporal arteritis does not occur under the age of 50 years and does not produce such a paroxysmal history. Paroxysmal hemicrania is another form of TAC, but the symptoms are much shorter and affect women more commonly.

25.55. Answer: E.

This is a typical story for benign paroxysmal positional vertigo (BPPV), the clues being the short-lasting vertigo induced by changes in posture, typically in bed. About half of cases are triggered by minor head trauma (there is no indication for brain imaging). Treatment with an Epley manoeuvre or similar is easy (there are plenty of examples on You Tube!) and highly likely to be successful, unlike drug treatment. Although he should be advised to reduce his alcohol intake, which might perhaps have explained the initial accident, this is not directly an alcohol-related problem.

25.56. Answer: A.

The story of an episode of optic neuritis, followed by a spinal cord syndrome, with an extensive longitudinal inflammatory lesion in the spinal cord is very suggestive of neuromyelitis optica (NMO), which is commonly associated with the aquaporin-4 antibody. This does not sound like a paraneoplastic syndrome, and whilst the other tests may add further information, they are unlikely to be diagnostic. NMO is different from MS, and requires a different approach to treatment. Indeed some MS treatments can make NMO worse, so distinction is important.

25.57. Answer: B.

This is a non-disabling relapse, and thus there is no immediate indication for treatment, although it should trigger reconsideration of disease-modifying drugs. Although infection can trigger relapses, you should only treat a proven, symptomatic infection. Physiotherapy will not help sensory symptoms.

25.58. Answer: C.
The risk of developing MS is increased by 10- to 25-fold in first-degree relatives of people with MS, but varies depending upon the kinship. The highest risk is in female monozygotic (MZ) twins (in male MZ twins it is about a 6% risk of occurring).

25.59. Answer: C.
Of course in an adult with new onset seizures imaging is the important investigation, but EEG can have a role in some cases. In someone with a single seizure, a timely EEG (within 4 weeks) can help inform the risk of recurrence, and so will be worthwhile after a single generalised tonic–clonic seizure at any age.

In patients under the age of about 30 years with new-onset epilepsy (either multiple seizures or single seizure with high risk of recurrence), the EEG can help with classification of epilepsy and so will carry therapeutic implications.

In elderly patients with multiple seizures, epilepsy is almost certainly going to have a focal origin and the EEG is unlikely to be useful.

In anyone of any age with unwitnessed or indeterminate transient loss of consciousness, the inter-ictal EEG may not only fail to show abnormalities but also any resultant 'abnormalities' may be red herrings; this applies especially to patients with focal injury or to younger females who have a higher chance of displaying epileptiform features on EEG such as photosensitivity.

25.60. Answer: B.
CIDP is a condition that causes loss of myelin in peripheral nerves. Nerve conduction studies can demonstrate demyelination of peripheral nerves (via slowed conduction) or axonal damage to sensory or motor nerves (with reduced numbers of functioning axons leading to reduced amplitude of response). EMG shows spontaneous activity in muscle (fasciculation or positive sharp waves) when nerve supply to muscle is lost due to axonal damage, but not as a consequence of demyelination. The peripheral demyelination therefore would be expected to cause only abnormal nerve conduction velocities and not EMG changes.

25.61. Answer: A.
An acute onset of vertigo that begins to resolve over days is likely to be related to an acute vestibular syndrome.

BPPV is a chronic condition precipitated usually by a specific movement in each individual, and would merit treatment with the Epley manoeuvre. A brainstem stroke would usually cause more widespread neurological changes, while Ménière's disease is a chronic condition causing vertigo with associated deafness and tinnitus.

Vertigo associated with migraine is a recurring condition of relatively short-lived vertigo most usually associated with headache and/or other migrainous symptoms.

25.62. Answer: C.
The coexistence of headache and papilloedema will always merit imaging to exclude an intracranial lesion, but the patient's age and morphology, intermittent nature of the symptoms and lack of other findings would make IIH most likely. Transient loss of vision on bending (or other manoeuvres that transiently raise intracranial pressure; ICP) are characteristic, and called visual obscurations. Optic neuropathy would cause disc pallor and reduced colour vision, while retinopathy would cause field defects or, if affecting the maculae, reduced visual acuity. Neuromyelitis optica is an inflammatory condition causing neurological deficit but not headache.

25.63. Answer: E.
The aqueduct of Sylvius is the small channel that allows CSF to travel from the third to the fourth ventricle. Stenosis can become apparent in adult life and lead to symptoms of raised ICP. Imaging will show that the ventricles 'upstream' (lateral and third ventricles) will be dilated, but the fourth will be small or of normal size.

IIH is associated with normal or small ventricular size, while space-occupying lesions will be apparent on imaging, and if severe enough to cause raised intracranial pressure will often cause other neurological deficits. Venous sinus thrombosis will usually be apparent on imaging (often resulting in haemorrhage). Normal pressure hydrocephalus usually occurs in older patients, and will have no features of acutely raised ICP, but rather a triad of reduced cognition, urinary incontinence and gait abnormalities, resulting in dilation of all ventricles apparent on imaging.

25

25.64. Answer: A.
Chronic Daily Headache (sometimes known as medication overuse headache) is an increasingly common condition, made worse by ease of access to paracetamol and compound analgesics. The unrelenting nature of the slowly progressive pain with no neurological or systemic features and associated high intake of analgesia will give good clues to the diagnosis.

While migraine headache syndromes can transform with time, many of this patient's painful episodes have no other migrainous features. It would be an unusual person who was not rendered weepy or low by such severe headaches, and the concurrence of a mood disorder should not allow the physician to make a hasty attribution of symptoms to psychological causes, particularly in the presence of other diagnostic features. Subarachnoid haemorrhage would cause an abrupt-onset acute headache rather than a relentless one.

25.65. Answer: C.
The episodic ataxias are inherited channelopathies that result in prolonged paroxysms of ataxia in affected individuals, usually with normal intervening neurological examination (although some patients can develop a slowly progressive ataxia). The family history is key in this case, suggesting an autosomal dominant disorder.

Peripheral neuropathies are unlikely to be paroxysmal and would not cause an ataxia, while migraine can cause episodic vertigo, but usually alongside other migrainous phenomena. BPPV would usually have direct positional precipitants.

25.66. Answer: C.
Cerebellar function can be acutely affected by a number of medications including the older antiepileptic drugs (phenytoin, carbamazepine and valproate), lithium and amiodarone.

Digoxin and diazepam at higher doses can be associated with sedation and drowsiness but not cerebellar ataxia. Antiemetics and antipsychotics can be associated with movement disorders such as chorea and athetosis but not usually ataxia; β_2-agonists will cause tremor in acute stage.

25.67. Answer: A.
At this age, the key investigation is brain imaging (ideally MRI) to exclude a structural cause for her seizure. The event at the age of 16 is removed enough to have little relevance, while the borderline hyponatraemia is not severe enough to cause seizures. A neutrophilia is common after a seizure. While an EEG may provide some prognostic information, the most important role of investigation is to exclude a primary intracerebral lesion.

25.68. Answer: A.
People may develop a constellation of symptoms after head injury, including headache, fatigue, dizziness, poor concentration/memory, emotionalism and numerous other symptoms. These are not specific to head injury. They are often persistent and may get worse, especially if the diagnosis is not explained. The management requires a careful explanation of the diagnosis, as well as reassurance that they have not suffered any irreversible brain damage (http://www .headinjurysymptoms.org/). Unfortunately, in such scenarios, many (well-meaning) health-care workers and other professionals may exacerbate the situation by recommending more intervention, as in this case. Neither a psychiatric nor neurosurgical consult will be of any value, and tramadol is a poor choice in this situation.

25.69. Answer: E.
The history is of a progressive degenerative disorder and, in this age, with evolution of choreiform movements, variant CJD would be most likely. Myoclonus tends to be more prominent in sporadic CJD, but this involves an older population, as does Alzheimer's disease (which has a slower course and only shows neurological signs at a late stage).

The presence of significant cognitive decline and upgoing plantars would not be in keeping with a psychological cause. While age and gender would be in keeping with hyperthyroidism, the presence of neurological signs and severity of the cognitive dysfunction would make this less likely.

25.70. Answer: C.
The only localising features here are the symptoms of left sensory change and the quadrantanopia, which would both suggest a right parietal lesion. Seizures are more likely with low-grade gliomas, while highly malignant lesions such as glioblastomas will often have a

rapid onset of neurological symptoms with, for reasons that are not entirely clear, a lower risk of seizures than low-grade lesions.

Meningiomata, by definition, are situated outside the brain, while medulloblastomas are tumours more common in childhood, most likely to be situated in the posterior fossa (cerebellum). Visual changes related to optic nerve problems will be monocular rather than homonymous.

25.71. Answer: C.
Migraine is a common disorder, and preceding visual symptoms that disappear with onset of headache are characteristic of migraine with aura. Somatic sensations and dysarthria are common with migraine, but on a first occurrence would justify imaging to exclude a primary structural cause.

Subarachnoid haemorrhage will not usually have focal signs but may need excluding in abrupt-onset headache as a first or worst occurrence. TIAs are not usually associated with headache, while the prominent headache and widespread other symptoms would not be in keeping with focal seizure. Cerebral venous sinus thrombosis would not usually recover completely so quickly, and any focal signs or symptoms would tend to evolve with the headache rather than precede it.

25.72. Answer: E.
The occurrence of jaw stiffness in advance of generalised stiffness and spasms would be characteristic of tetanus, in this case most likely as the result of an infected wound. Diagnosis and adequate treatment is paramount as this disease can still be fatal even if treated.

Dental abscesses are usually very painful, and would be vanishingly unlikely to extend intracranially. While the anxiety may make doctors think of a functional illness, the characteristic pattern of intermittent jaw symptoms followed by generalised symptoms would be unlikely in functional disorders. Botulism is also caused by a bacterial toxin (from *Clostridium botulinum*) but more usually causes ocular and bulbar weakness rather than spasms.

25.73. Answer: A.
The rapidly progressive generalised weakness preceded by ocular and bulbar paralysis is characteristic of weakness caused by

botulinum toxin from *Clostridium botulinum*. (Her cousin had obviously eaten the same poorly prepared food!)

Brainstem stroke would not arrive in such a progressive manner, and Miller Fisher syndrome would cause ataxia and areflexia along with any ophthalmoplegia (nor is it contagious). Myasthenia gravis would have an onset with some fatigability. Multiple sclerosis would be unlikely to cause isolated weakness in such a progressive manner (although this can be increased in family members, the simultaneous onset is a clue to a recent infection as the cause).

25.74. Answer: E.
Carotid dissection can be precipitated by a surprisingly minor trauma. Association of unilateral pain with Horner's syndrome is characteristic of this disorder.

Signs are too focal and would be expected to be more severe with subarachnoid haemorrhage. Subdural and extradural haematomas would be unlikely to cause an isolated Horner's syndrome. A brachial plexopathy would also be expected to cause symptoms and signs in the ipsilateral arm.

25.75. Answer: A.
Acoustic neuromas may be discovered incidentally on imaging or on investigation of sensorineural deafness. If uncovered late, there may be compression of the brainstem, sometimes with compression of the fourth ventricle causing hydrocephalus and raised ICP.

Brainstem stroke would have a much more abrupt onset, and deafness is a very rare feature of multiple sclerosis. Migraine would have a more episodic course, with no neurological deficit (and normal fundi). Most acoustic neuromas are spontaneous and not related to neurofibromatosis.

25.76. Answer: E.
The symptoms of a rapidly progressive distal sensorimotor loss would be most in keeping with a neuropathy. The levels of alcohol intake and random glucose are too modest to account for an alcoholic or diabetic neuropathy, respectively. A raised ESR would highlight an immune-related cause and, with no rash or arthropathy, such a raised level would be most in keeping with myeloma.

25

There are no features to suggest a myelopathy (no upper motor neuron symptoms or sphincter deficit) and the presence of sensory symptoms and signs would not be suggestive of motor neuron disease.

25.77. Answer: B.

The symptoms and signs suggest a lower motor neuron facial palsy on the affected side. Recurrent facial palsy in someone at high risk of *Borrelia burgdorferi* infection makes Lyme disease the likely cause here. The onset and relapse would be unusual for a vascular cause, and multiple sclerosis causes upper motor neuron problems, being unlikely to cause an isolated facial palsy. Syphilis can cause some vasculitic central nervous system problems, but the typical pattern would involve a myelopathy and some brainstem signs. Even with the recent rise in incidence, it remains rarer than that other spirochete, *Borrelia*.

25.78. Answer: B.

Spinal cord problems will often cause motor, sensory and sphincter problems. Any sensory problems caused by spinal cord lesions may relate to dissociated sensory loss, which may be asymmetrical if only half of the cord is affected. Motor deficit caused by spinal cord problems are upper motor neuron lesion in character below the lesion and may be lower motor neuron character at the level of the lesion, rather than a widespread mixture of upper motor neuron and lower motor neuron signs.

Distal sensory loss is usually caused by a peripheral neuropathy, and cranial nerve deficits (e.g. diplopia) will require involvement superior to the spinal cord.

Timing of the evolution of the symptoms tends to give information on the nature rather than the site of the lesion.

P Langhorne

26

Stroke medicine

Multiple Choice Questions

26.1. A patient is referred by his doctor to the hospital stroke service. Which of the following transient symptoms would allow you to make a clinical diagnosis of transient ischaemic attack (TIA)?

A. Dizziness
B. Expressive dysphasia
C. Loss of consciousness
D. Slurred speech (dysarthria)
E. Transient confusion

26.2. A 70 year old man is admitted overnight with a 24-hour history of left hemiparesis. Which one of these drug therapies would mandate urgent computed tomography (CT) head scanning?

A. Aspirin
B. Clopidogrel
C. Ramipril
D. Simvastatin
E. Warfarin

26.3. A 43 year old woman attends the hospital accident and emergency department with a 1-hour history of sudden-onset severe occipital headache. On examination she is photophobic with neck stiffness. What is the most appropriate first-line investigation?

A. Carotid Doppler ultrasound (duplex) scan
B. CT cerebral angiography
C. CT head scan
D. Lumbar puncture
E. Skull X-ray

26.4. Which of the following ischaemic stroke patients who have undergone carotid duplex scanning would be most likely to benefit from left carotid endarterectomy?

A. Left cerebellar hemisphere infarct with good functional recovery, 80% left carotid artery stenosis
B. Left middle cerebral artery territory infarct with good functional recovery, 60% left carotid artery stenosis
C. Left middle cerebral artery territory infarct with good functional recovery, 80% left carotid artery stenosis
D. Left middle cerebral artery territory infarct with persistent dense right hemiparesis and profound dysphasia, 90% left carotid artery stenosis
E. Right middle cerebral artery territory infarct with good functional recovery, 75% left carotid artery stenosis

26.5. A 73 year old man presents with a right hemiparesis and expressive dysphasia secondary to an infarct in the territory of the left middle cerebral artery. Blood pressure is 153/82 mmHg, serum cholesterol is 4.4 mmol/L (170 mg/dL) and the electrocardiogram (ECG) shows sinus rhythm with no abnormalities. Which of the following secondary prevention medications is usually avoided in such a patient?

A. Amlodipine
B. Aspirin
C. Ramipril
D. Simvastatin
E. Warfarin

26.6. The ROSIER (Rule Out Stroke In the Emergency Room) clinical stroke tool can be used to triage patients with clinical suspicion of stroke. Which of the following features are given a *negative score* on the ROSIER scale (i.e. are not thought to be consistent with a clinical diagnosis of stroke)?

A. Leg weakness
B. Loss of speech
C. Seizure
D. Unilateral arm weakness
E. Visual field defect

26.7. A patient is admitted with a clinical picture of acute stroke. You request a plain CT scan as initial emergency brain imaging. What information can you get from plain (non-contrast) CT brain scanning in acute stroke patients?

A. Distinguishes acute stroke from TIA
B. Reliably detects intracerebral blood
C. Reliably detects subtle acute ischaemic changes
D. Shows brain function (functional imaging)
E. Shows blood flow in vessels

26.8. A 65 year old woman with a previous history of diabetes and breast carcinoma is found collapsed at home with drowsiness and a left hemiparesis. Which of the following should be carried out first?

A. Check blood glucose level
B. Check temperature
C. Clarify breast carcinoma history
D. Examine for peripheral neuropathy
E. Examine for symmetrical plantar responses

26.9. An 83 year old woman is brought to the emergency department after becoming unwell at home. Which of the following is true of total anterior circulation stroke?

A. It is caused by occlusion of small perforating arteries
B. It includes higher cerebral dysfunction and motor loss
C. It involves isolated homonymous hemianopia
D. It is not caused by cerebral embolism
E. It is a pure motor stroke

26.10. A patient with an acute stroke is admitted to the specialist stroke unit. Which of the following currently apply to mechanical clot retrieval (thrombectomy)?

A. It can be offered to most stroke patients
B. It is effective in intracerebral haemorrhage
C. It is effective in large-vessel occlusion
D. It requires less technological support than intravenous thrombolysis
E. It is a treatment that is widely available

26.11. A 38 year old man is brought to the emergency department with a suspected intracerebral haemorrhage. Which of the following are recognised risk factors for intracerebral haemorrhage?

A. Antiphospholipid abnormality
B. Cardiac embolism
C. Carotid artery stenosis
D. Cocaine use
E. Raised cholesterol

26.12. A 70 year old man with recent minor stroke is found to be in atrial fibrillation. When advising him on anticoagulant therapy, which of the following features would make you favour warfarin over a direct oral anticoagulant (DOAC)?

A. Fewer drug interactions
B. Lower drug costs
C. Lower risk of intracerebral haemorrhage
D. More effective at preventing embolism
E. Simpler dosing regimes

26.13. A 45 year old woman is admitted to hospital with symptoms of raised intracranial pressure, seizures and focal neurological symptoms. Which of the following is correct about the suspected diagnosis of cerebral vein thrombosis?

A. CT brain scanning is the definitive imaging
B. It can include an associated haemorrhage
C. It is never caused by infection
D. It is rarely treated with anticoagulation
E. It usually presents like arterial stroke

26.14. A 62 year old man with a stroke is being considered for thrombolysis therapy. Which of the following is true of intravenous thrombolysis with recombinant tissue plasminogen activator (rt-PA)?

A. It can be given up to 12 hours after symptom onset
B. It can be offered to most stroke patients
C. It improves the chance of recovery of independence

D. It reduces the risk of early death

E. It reduces the risk of early intracerebral haemorrhage

26.15. An 81 year old woman with diabetes, hypertension and a minor left hemisphere ischaemic stroke 1 week ago is found to have a right carotid artery stenosis of 70%. Which of the following features would cause you to

advise best medical therapy rather than carotid endarterectomy?

A. Her age – she is too old to benefit

B. She has a history of diabetes

C. The carotid stenosis is on the asymptomatic side

D. The stroke impact is only minor

E. There has been too long a delay since her stroke onset

Answers

26.1. Answer: B.
The definition of a TIA is the rapid onset of a focal neurological deficit, of presumed vascular origin, that resolves within 24 hours. It also includes transient monocular blindness due to vascular occlusion in the retina (amaurosis fugax). Dysphasia is caused by a deficit in the dominant cerebral hemisphere. Delirium, dizziness, lone dysarthria and loss of consciousness are not focal deficits when present on their own. Loss of consciousness can very rarely be caused by basilar ischaemia but is rarely transient. As a general rule, the diagnosis of TIA should not be made in patients who present with episodes of syncope, dizziness or delirium, as these do not reflect focal cerebral dysfunction.

26.2. Answer: E.
Early CT scanning is the ideal for all patients with suspected stroke to help plan acute therapies and plan secondary prevention. This man is beyond the time window for acute therapies. Patients who are anticoagulated with warfarin or who have a non-iatrogenic coagulopathy require urgent imaging of the brain to rule out the possibility of an intracerebral haemorrhage.

26.3. Answer: C.
The clinical signs and symptoms in this patient are suggestive of a subarachnoid haemorrhage. An emergency head CT scan is essential. About 5–10% of patients with a subarachnoid

haemorrhage will have a normal CT scan; in these cases, a lumbar puncture should be performed 12 hours following the onset of headache to look for xanthochromia (breakdown products of red blood cells).

26.4. Answer: C.
Carotid endarterectomy reduces the risk of stroke in patients with severe stenosis of the internal carotid artery but carries a significant risk of perioperative mortality and stroke. Decisions on whether to operate must, therefore, be based on a careful benefit/risk analysis. The absolute reduction in risk of future stroke is greatest for symptomatic patients with 70–99% stenosis and, in general, outweighs the risk of surgical complications. Importantly, symptomatic patients are defined as patients with a TIA or non-disabling stroke in the territory of the carotid artery on the same side as the stenosis in the preceding 6 months. The evidence to support surgery in symptomatic patients with moderate (50–69%) stenosis and asymptomatic patients with severe stenosis is less conclusive, as these patients have a smaller benefit/risk ratio than patients with severe symptomatic stenosis. Patients with stenosis of less than 50% do not benefit from carotid endarterectomy, irrespective of symptoms. Finally, a patient with severe residual disability would gain little benefit from preventing a further stroke within the same territory and may have a greater risk of surgical complications.

26

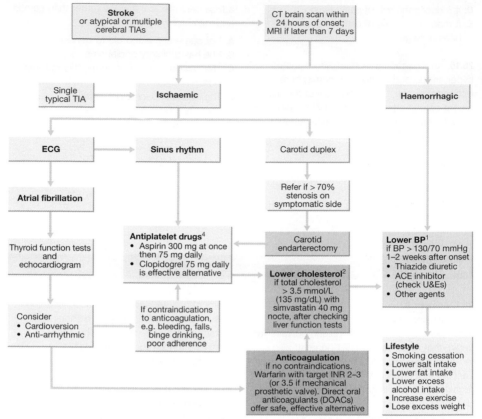

Fig. 26.5 Strategies for secondary prevention of stroke. (1) Lower blood pressure with caution in patients with postural hypotension, renal impairment or bilateral carotid stenosis. (2) Other statins can be used as an alternative to simvastatin in patients on warfarin or digoxin. (3) Warfarin and aspirin have been used in combination in patients with prosthetic heart valves. (4) The combination of aspirin and clopidogrel is indicated only in patients with unstable angina or those with a temporary high risk of recurrence (e.g. carotid stenosis). (ACE = angiotensin-converting enzyme; BP = blood pressure; CT = computed tomography; ECG = electrocardiogram; INR = international normalised ratio; MRI = magnetic resonance imaging; TIA = transient ischaemic attack; U&Es = urea and electrolytes)

26.5. Answer: E.

In addition to lifestyle modifications, antiplatelet, lipid-lowering and antihypertensive therapy form the cornerstone of secondary prevention for most patients with an ischaemic stroke (Fig. 26.5). Recent large-scale randomised trials have demonstrated the benefit of statins and antihypertensive medication in these patients, even with blood pressure and cholesterol levels within the 'normal' range. Patients in atrial fibrillation benefit from anticoagulation with warfarin following ischaemic stroke, but there is no such benefit in those who are in sinus rhythm.

26.6. Answer: C.

Although seizure does occur in <5% of acute stroke patients, seizure (with post-seizure paresis) is more commonly recognised as a

mimic of stroke. For that reason, it scores −1 on the ROSIER clinical stroke tool (Box 26.6), as does loss of consciousness, whereas all the other options score +1.

26.7. Answer: B.

The main advantages of plain CT scanning are its speed and tolerability and it can rapidly detect intracranial bleeding plus some stroke mimics. Magnetic resonance imaging (MRI) is often needed to show more subtle ischaemia, while MR angiography or CT angiography are usually required to show vessel occlusion.

26.8. Answer: A.

Hypoglycaemia can mimic stroke, is a medical emergency and is easily corrected. Although we do not know what drugs this patient takes,

i	**26.6 Rapid assessment of suspected stroke**

ROSIER scale

Can be used by emergency staff to indicate probability of a stroke in acute presentations:

Unilateral facial weakness	+1
Unilateral grip weakness	+1
Unilateral arm weakness	+1
Unilateral leg weakness	+1
Speech loss	+1
Visual field defect	+1
Loss of consciousness	−1
Seizure	−1

Total (−2 to +6); score of > 0 indicates stroke is possible cause

Exclusion of hypoglycaemia

Bedside blood glucose testing with BMstix

Language deficit

History and examination may indicate a language deficit
Check comprehension ('lift your arms, close your eyes') to identify a receptive dysphasia
Ask patient to name people/objects (e.g. nurse, watch, pen) to identify a nominal dysphasia
Check articulation (ask patient to repeat phrases after you) for dysarthria

Motor deficit

Subtle pyramidal signs:
Check for pronator drift: ask patient to hold out arms and maintain their position with eyes closed
Check for clumsiness of fine finger movements

Sensory and visual inattention

Establish that sensation/visual field is intact on testing one side at a time
Retest sensation/visual fields on simultaneous testing of both sides; the affected side will no longer be felt/seen
Perform clock drawing test

Truncal ataxia

Check if patient can sit up or stand without support

---

hypoglycaemia must be excluded. While important, the other actions do not take priority over checking the blood glucose.

26.9. Answer: B.

Classification of a stroke is helpful for both clinical and research purposes. A total anterior circulation stroke results in a mix of motor deficit, higher cerebral dysfunction and homonymous hemianopia caused by occlusion of a major cerebral artery. An embolic cause is often found.

26.10. Answer: C.

Mechanical clot retrieval (thrombectomy) appears to be particularly effective in cerebral ischaemia caused by large-vessel occlusion. However, it requires careful patient selection and considerable support from imaging investigations and catheter laboratories.

26.11. Answer: D.

The main recognised risk factors for intracerebral haemorrhage include high blood pressure, smoking, excess alcohol intake, structural abnormalities, coagulopathies and drugs such as cocaine and amphetamines. Raised cholesterol, antiphospholipid abnormality, cardiac embolism and carotid artery stenosis are recognised risk factors for ischaemic stroke.

26.12. Answer: B.

Warfarin is a less expensive drug option but does require regular monitoring. Also, at present we cannot easily monitor and reverse anticoagulation levels with DOACs (although new agents are being developed). DOACs have simpler dosing regimes with fewer drug interactions and appear to have a better balance of effectiveness and safety than warfarin.

26.13. Answer: B.

Cerebral venous sinus thrombosis usually presents with symptoms of raised intracranial pressure, seizures and focal neurological symptoms. It often includes associated haemorrhage. MR venography demonstrates a filling defect in the affected vessel. About 10% of cerebral venous sinus thrombosis is associated with infection requiring antibiotic treatment. Otherwise, the treatment of choice is usually anticoagulation.

26.14. Answer: C.

Intravenous thrombolysis with rt-PA increases the risk of early haemorrhagic transformation of the cerebral infarct with potentially fatal results. However, if it is given within 4.5 hours of symptom onset to carefully selected patients (about 20% of ischaemic stroke patients), the haemorrhagic risk is more than offset by an improvement in overall outcome The earlier the treatment is given, the greater the benefit.

26.15. Answer: C.

To benefit from carotid artery surgery, the patient needs to have an expectation of several years of reasonable quality of life to offset the risks of surgery. The stroke impact being minor and her age and other risk factors would not influence this decision. The key contraindication is that the carotid artery stenosis is on the opposite side from the patient's symptoms and so this is a lower-risk asymptomatic carotid stenosis.

26

R Darbyshire, J Olson

27

Medical ophthalmology

Multiple Choice Questions

27.1. A 23 year old male presents to the emergency department following an alleged assault. He is intoxicated, his nose is bleeding and he has a large left periorbital haematoma that prevents spontaneous eyelid opening. Alongside assessment for traumatic brain injury, which of the following ocular conditions is it most important to exclude?

A. Hyphaema
B. Medial orbital wall fracture
C. Orbital floor fracture
D. Retinal detachment
E. Retrobulbar haemorrhage

27.2. A 36 year old male primary school teacher presents with a 3-day history of bilateral red, watery, painful eyes. His vision is 6/7.5 in both eyes. He is usually fit and well with no past ocular history. He mentions one of the children in his class had a similar condition a week ago. What is the most likely diagnosis?

A. Allergic conjunctivitis
B. Bacterial conjunctivitis
C. Episcleritis
D. Microbial keratitis
E. Viral conjunctivitis

27.3. An 18 year old female presents with a 24-hour history of a severely photophobic, watery and injected right eye. Her visual acuity is reduced to 6/18 in the affected eye. Which feature of the clinical history will most affect immediate management?

A. Contact lens wear
B. Foreign travel
C. Other unwell contacts
D. Previous cold sores around the nose or mouth
E. Previous ocular history

27.4. A 53 year old man attends his family physician for ongoing neck pain, which has occurred since he was involved in a road traffic accident 6 months ago. During the consultation his wife mentions his left eyelid is drooping. On examination, the pupil on this side is 1–2 mm smaller. Which is the most appropriate investigation?

A. Chest X-ray
B. Computed tomography (CT) angiogram of the aortic arch, carotid arteries and intracranial vessels
C. CT head
D. Doppler ultrasound of the carotid artery
E. Magnetic resonance imaging (MRI) head

27.5. A 34 year old female is admitted with a life-threatening attack of asthma. After stabilisation she is transferred to the intensive care unit where she remains intubated and ventilated. The admitting doctor notices the left pupil is dilated and minimally responsive to light. There is no other neurological abnormality. What is the most likely cause?

A. An Adie's pupil
B. Argyll Robertson syndrome
C. Horner's syndrome
D. Pharmacological mydriasis
E. Physiological anisocoria

27.6. An 18 year old female has been referred following a routine visit to her optician, who noted anisocoria. Pupil measurements are as follows:

The direct and consensual reflex in the left pupil is sluggish and the pupil constricts slowly in response to accommodation. There is no

Conditions	Right pupil diameter (mm)	Left pupil diameter (mm)
Light	3	7
Dark	7	8

abnormality noted on examination of extraocular movements and no evidence of ptosis. Slit-lamp examination reveals vermiform movements at the pupillary border in the left eye. What diagnosis is this consistent with?

A. Adie's pupil
B. Episodic mydriasis
C. Horner's syndrome
D. Pharmacological mydriasis
E. Physiological anisocoria

27.7. An anxious 53 year old with high myopia has a 1-day history of new-onset large central floater in her right eye and temporal photopsia, most noticeable in low light conditions. Her visual acuity is 6/9 in the affected eye and visual fields are full to confrontation.
What is the most likely diagnosis?

A. Asteroid hyalosis
B. Posterior vitreous detachment
C. Visual snow
D. Vitreous haemorrhage
E. Vitritis

27.8. A 73 year old male attends his family physician having had cataract surgery performed on his left eye 4 days ago. He was very pleased with the vision initially, but it seems to be worsening over the past 48 hours and he has noticed some new floaters. The eye is becoming more painful. His visual acuity is 6/60 and on his last clinic letter from ophthalmology it was 6/12. A same-day ophthalmological referral is needed to exclude which of the following conditions?

A. Corneal oedema
B. Endophthalmitis
C. Post-operative acute anterior uveitis
D. Raised intraocular pressure
E. Retinal detachment

27.9. A 34 year old woman presents with a 1-week history of progressive blurring of central vision in the right eye, flashing lights and an aching pain behind the eye

exacerbated by eye movement. Her visual acuity is 6/24 in the right eye and 6/6 in the left. Examination of the right eye reveals reduction in colour vision, a relative afferent pupillary defect (RAPD) and the optic nerve appears normal. Visual fields show a central scotoma. What is this is a typical case of?

A. Demyelinating optic neuritis
B. Infectious optic neuritis
C. Leber's hereditary optic neuropathy
D. Neuroretinitis
E. Non-arteritic anterior ischaemic optic neuropathy

27.10. A 78 year old woman visits her family physician with a 3-week history of a severe right-sided headache. The area over her right forehead and scalp is so tender she cannot bear to brush her hair and is unable to sleep on that side. She reports numerous episodes where the vision in her right eye has become very blurred and then spontaneously recovered. Which investigation is considered the definitive diagnostic test for this condition?

A. C-reactive protein
B. Erythrocyte sedimentation rate
C. Plasma viscosity
D. Temporal artery biopsy
E. Temporal artery Doppler ultrasound

27.11. An 18 year old is referred from her optician querying papilloedema. She has a 3-month history of headaches. All of the following are causes of papilloedema except one. Which one is NOT a cause of papilloedema?

A. A space-occupying lesion
B. Accelerated hypertension
C. Idiopathic intracranial hypertension
D. Obstructive hydrocephalus
E. Venous sinus thrombosis

27.12. A 78 year old man attends for consideration of cataract surgery, describing gradual visual deterioration over the past few years. Past medical history includes hypertension and diabetes. He is also a smoker. Dilated fundal examination is shown below. Which of the following would have the greatest impact in managing his condition?

27

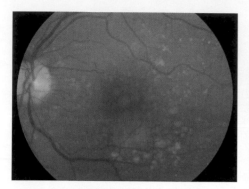

A. Control of hypertension
B. Intravitreal anti-vascular endothelial growth factor (anti-VEGF) therapy
C. Smoking cessation
D. Tighter glycaemic control
E. Vitamin supplementation with high-dose antioxidants and zinc

27.13. A 69 year old male presents with a 2-day history of sudden-onset, painless blurred vision in his left eye. His visual acuity is 6/18 in the affected eye. His past medical history includes hypercholesterolaemia, chronic obstructive pulmonary disease (COPD), osteoarthritis and gastro-oesophageal reflux disease (GORD). He has no past ocular history of note. The fundal image is shown below.

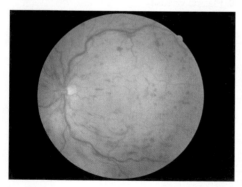

What is the most common aetiology of this condition?

A. Arteriosclerosis
B. Glaucoma
C. Hyperviscosity
D. Inflammation
E. Thrombophilia

27.14. A 62 year old female was diagnosed with type 2 diabetes mellitus 5 years ago. Her current medications include metformin and sitagliptin.

She attends the diabetic retinal screening programme for annual retinal photographs. The latest image is show below.

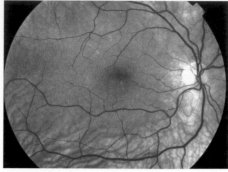

What is the earliest feature of diabetic retinopathy visible on fundus fluorescein angiography (FFA)?

A. Capillary occlusion
B. Intraretinal microvascular anomalies
C. Microaneurysms
D. Venous beading
E. Venous reduplication

27.15. A 31 year old patient with poorly controlled type 1 diabetes attends the eye casualty department complaining of blurred vision and floaters in the left eye. She manages her diabetes on a basal-bolus injection regime with insulin Lantus and NovoRapid, but admits her blood sugar levels have been high recently. Her left fundus is shown in the image below.

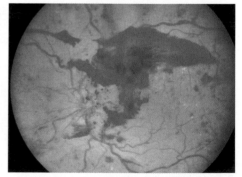

Adequate treatment with which of the following will induce a permanent regression of this condition?

A. Diffuse macular laser
B. Focal macular laser
C. Intravitreal anti-VEGF therapy
D. Pan-retinal laser therapy (photocoagulation)
E. Photodynamic therapy (PDT) with verteporfin

Answers

27.1. Answer: E.
All of the above conditions may have occurred following the inciting injury. Retrobulbar haemorrhage is a sight-threatening emergency. Bleeding behind the globe, in the absence of any decompressing fracture, raises intraorbital pressure, which irreversibly damages the optic nerve. Typical clinical features include: severe pain, progressive proptosis, reducing visual acuity, ophthalmoplegia, diplopia and an unreactive pupil. Emergency decompression surgery is required to preserve optic nerve function.

27.2. Answer: E.
Viral conjunctivitis is most commonly caused by adenovirus, a non-enveloped double-stranded DNA virus. The clinical presentation varies from subclinical to severe inflammation. The condition is highly contagious. Classic features include prominent conjunctival hyperaemia and follicles, petechial haemorrhage and pseudomembranes. Corneal involvement is characterised by epithelial microcysts, punctate epithelial keratitis and focal subepithelial infiltrates.

27.3. Answer: A.
A presentation of red eye in a known contact lens wearer should prompt a same-day referral for ophthalmological assessment including slit-lamp biomicroscopy. The cornea must be examined in detail for any features of microbial keratitis.

27.4. Answer: B.
This patient has Horner's syndrome. Horner's syndrome is a triad of ptosis, miosis and anhydrosis of the affected side of the face and neck. It can be caused by interruption of the sympathetic fibres at any point along their protracted course from their origin in the posterior hypothalamus through to their synapse in the superior cervical ganglion and then to the eye. This patient has a history of significant trauma; therefore a dissection of the internal carotid artery must be excluded by CT or MR angiography in the first instance.

27.5. Answer: D.
Nebulised salbutamol and ipratropium are involved in the management of a life-threatening asthma attack. Ipratropium is an antimuscarinic agent. This may therefore cause dilation of the pupil if vaporised drug leaks from the mask. The effect may last up to 24 hours. The diagnosis of a pharmacological mydriasis can be confirmed if there is little or no pupillary constriction following instillation of 1% pilocarpine. The other answers would be less likely given the timing and clinical scenario.

27.6. Answer: A.
An Adie's tonic pupil is caused by loss of the parasympathetic innervation to the sphincter pupillae muscle in the iris and ciliary body. The direct and consensual pupillary light reflex are sluggish. The pupil slowly constricts to near focus. The syndrome typically occurs in young females after a viral illness. Application of dilute pilocarpine 0.125% (a muscarinic agonist agent) to both eyes has no effect in the normal eye but causes constriction of the Adie's pupil due to denervation hypersensitivity.

27.7. Answer: B.
With age, the vitreous progressively liquefies, a process known as synersis. When a break in the posterior hyaloid face occurs, escaping fluid separates the vitreous from the retina, causing a posterior vitreous detachment (PVD). An impression where the posterior hyaloid face was once attached to the optic nerve becomes visible to the patient as a large central floater and to the clinician on examination as a circular opacity or Weiss ring. PVD occurs earlier in myopia, collagen and connective tissue disorders, and may be triggered by trauma or inflammation. PVD is a risk factor for a retinal tear and subsequent detachment. A thorough examination of the retina is required.

27.8. Answer: B.
Although all of these complications are possible after cataract surgery, this is a presentation of endophthalmitis until proven otherwise and requires specialist review. The worrying features are the initial subjectively good vision, followed by rapid deterioration, new floaters, which may suggest infection in the vitreous, and increasing pain.

27

27.9. Answer: A.

Optic neuritis is an acute inflammatory process affecting the optic nerve. It usually presents with sudden monocular visual loss over hours to days and eye pain in young adults, more commonly in women. The Optic Neuritis Treatment Trial (ONTT) elucidated the typical features of a demyelinating optic neuritis as follows:

- Age 20–50 years
- Unilateral
- Worsens over hours/days
- Recovery starts within 2 weeks
- Retrobulbar pain
- Reduced colour vision
- Relative afferent pupillary defect

In two-thirds of cases, the optic disc itself appears normal because the area of inflammation is deeper within the nerve – this is described as a retrobulbar optic neuritis.

Leber's hereditary optic neuropathy is a rare progressive hereditary optic neuropathy: those affected are usually male and present with painless severe unilateral loss of central vision; the second eye may become affected within weeks to months of the first.

27.10. Answer: D.

The history is convincing of giant cell arteritis. Whilst inflammatory markers are usually raised, these are non-specific. A patient with suspicion of giant cell arteritis with raised inflammatory markers should be commenced on high-dose glucocorticoid without delay. This is due to the serious nature of the condition and risk of ocular involvement. Temporal artery biopsy remains the gold standard investigation. Histopathological features include inflammation of the arterial wall with fragmentation and disruption of the internal elastic lamina. The vessel may be affected in a 'patchy' manner; therefore, obtaining a specimen of at least 1 cm in length is recommended whenever possible.

27.11. Answer: B.

Papilloedema describes bilateral optic disc swelling secondary to raised intracranial pressure. Severity is described by Frisen's scale where:

- stage 1: the optic disc is raised superiorly, nasally and inferiorly, creating a C-shape

- stage 2: the temporal disc head becomes involved, creating a 360° circumferential swelling
- stage 3: vessel obscuration occurs at the disc margin
- stage 4: vessel obscuration occurs at the disc head

In established papilloedema, circumferential retinal folds or Paton lines may form. Haemorrhage and cotton wool spots represent ischaemic damage. In this setting, optic nerve function will be reduced on examination and may not recover. Severe hypertension causes bilateral optic disc swelling in the absence of raised intracranial pressure.

27.12. Answer: C.

The fundus image shows the early changes of dry age-related macular degeneration (AMD). Smoking is associated with a 2- to 3-fold increased risk of developing age-related macular degeneration. Use of the AREDS (Age-Related Eye Disease Study) vitamin formulation was found to reduce the progression to severe AMD by 25% in those with advanced AMD in the fellow eye. There is currently no evidence to suggest that modification of hypertension or glycaemic control has an effect on progression of AMD. Intravitreal anti-VEGF therapy is currently reserved for patients with neovascular AMD.

27.13. Answer: A.

The image shows retinal vein occlusion. Unlike vasculature elsewhere in the body, retinal arteries and veins share their adventitial sheath. This means that arteriosclerotic changes in the artery can directly compromise the lumen of the vein. This is the most common mechanism where hypertension, hypercholesterolaemia, diabetes, smoking and obesity contribute the majority of risk. In younger patients, inflammatory conditions that result in inflammation of the vessel wall must be considered. Less common associations with retinal vein occlusion include hyperviscosity, inherited or acquired thrombophilias. The most common predisposing ocular condition is glaucoma.

27.14. Answer: A.

The earliest feature of diabetic retinopathy on retinal angiography is ischaemia characterised by capillary dropout. Microaneurysms can appear in background diabetic retinopathy, whereas intraretinal microvascular anomalies, venous changes and lipid exudate characterise more advanced disease.

27.15. Answer: D.
Pan-retinal photocoagulation ablates the peripheral ischaemic retina and permanently reduces production of pro-angiogenic factors. Intravitreal anti-VEGF injection can cause temporary regression of neovascularisation. Focal and diffuse macular laser are treatments for diabetic macular oedema, although this is being rapidly succeeded by intravitreal anti-VEGF therapy. Photodynamic therapy with verteporfin is a treatment for other macular disorders, predominantly central serous chorioretinopathy.

27

28

Medical psychiatry

Multiple Choice Questions

28.1. A psychiatric history differs from a general medical history in which of the following key respects?

A. 'Drug history' refers to recreational drugs rather that prescribed medication
B. 'Family history' refers to relationships within the family rather than illnesses affecting first- and second-degree relatives that might indicate genetic risk
C. 'Past medical history' is less important
D. Much of the examination is conducted during the course of history taking
E. The psychiatric history does not include 'history of presenting complaint'

28.2. You are working in an emergency department. A 30 year old man presents with excoriations on both forearms and tells you that he is experiencing a sensation of something crawling under his skin. When documenting this patient's mental state, under which heading would you record his tactile hallucinations?

A. Cognition
B. Insight
C. Mood
D. Perception
E. Thought

28.3. Which of the following psychiatric presentations is rare amongst general medical inpatients?

A. Adjustment reactions
B. Alcohol-related disorders
C. Delirium
D. Depression
E. Schizophrenia

28.4. You are working in an emergency department. An elderly woman who has presented with a pretibial laceration is loudly demanding that she be given priority treatment on the grounds that she is a close personal friend of the Prime Minister. A psychiatric diagnosis of 'persistent delusional disorder' is recorded in her case notes. Which of the following statements best describes a delusion?

A. A recurrent and intrusive thought that enters the patient's mind against their conscious resistance and is recognised by the patient as being a product of their own mind
B. An understandable belief that a patient becomes preoccupied with to an unreasonable extent
C. An unshakeable false belief that is not accepted by other members of the patient's culture
D. A patient's perception and/or belief that thoughts are being implanted into his/her own head by someone or something else
E. When a patient's stream of thought shifts suddenly from one thought to another very loosely or entirely unrelated thought

28.5. When reviewing a patient's neurology case notes, you read that her temporal lobe epilepsy is characterised by a prodrome comprising olfactory hallucinations. Which of the following most accurately describes an hallucination?

A. A belief that has no rational basis
B. A false perception experienced by the patient as arising in his/her own mind
C. A fixed, false belief out of keeping with a patient's cultural background

D. A misperception of real external stimuli

E. A sensory perception occurring without an external stimulus

28.6. When on-call over the weekend in a large general hospital, you are asked to attend the toxicology unit. Which of the following is true of self-harm?

A. Incidence increases with age

B. It is more common in men than women

C. It is the term psychiatrists use for 'attempted suicide'

D. Methods that carry high risk of death are more likely to be associated with mental disorder than are methods that carry low risk of death

E. There is a lower incidence in lower socioeconomic groups

28.7. An 80 year old retired lawyer who lives independently is brought to the emergency department by a neighbour who found him wandering on the street in the early hours of the morning. He has no past psychiatric history. As you attempt to interview him, the man says, 'This is a wonderful party. It is great to see all those young people dancing.' Which is the most likely diagnosis?

A. Delirium

B. Dementia

C. Histrionic personality disorder

D. Mania

E. Schizophrenia

28.8. As a 35 year old man wakes from sleep he briefly sees a lion at the foot of his bed. Which of the following most accurately describes his experience?

A. Autoscopic hallucination

B. Functional hallucination

C. Hypnagogic hallucination

D. Hypnopompic hallucination

E. Kinaesthetic hallucination

28.9. A 48 year old barman is brought to the emergency department by his wife from whom he has recently separated. She is concerned that he is confused and 'talking nonsense'. He has an unsteady gait yet his breath alcohol level is zero. On examination he has ophthalmoplegia and is disorientated in time. His liver function tests are deranged.
  Which is the most likely diagnosis?

A. Alcohol withdrawal

B. Alcoholic dementia

C. Alcoholic hallucinosis

D. Delirium tremens

E. Wernicke–Korsakoff syndrome

28.10. A 28 year old businesswoman presents to the emergency department with chest pain and various other symptoms. She admits to the doctor that she has been taking cocaine and some other recreational drugs. Which of the following combination of features could be attributable to cocaine intoxication?

A. Auditory hallucinations and hypothermia

B. Constricted pupils and sedation

C. Formication and auditory hallucinations

D. Hypothermia and constricted pupils

E. Sedation and formication

28.11. A 46 year old man is brought to the emergency department by emergency ambulance. He says he is unable to breathe, his hands and feet are tingling, he feels that he is about to collapse and possibly die. On examination he has sinus tachycardia. Oxygen saturation is 100%. You notice that this is his fifth attendance at the emergency department in 3 months. Which is the most likely diagnosis?

A. Factitious disorder

B. Generalised anxiety disorder

C. Hypochondriacal disorder

D. Obsessive–compulsive disorder

E. Panic disorder

28.12. A 32 year old man with diabetes mellitus survives an 8-day admission to critical care with overwhelming sepsis and ketoacidosis. On discharge from hospital he appears happy and glad to be alive. You review him at the diabetic clinic 2 months later and he tells you that he is waking in the middle of the night with vivid nightmares. He is now struggling to sleep, he feels anxious and jumpy all of the time and finds himself bursting into tears very easily. His mother has been admitted to hospital but the thought of visiting her on a hospital ward terrifies him. Which is the most likely diagnosis?

A. Acute stress reaction

B. Adjustment disorder

C. Delirium

D. Depression

E. Post-traumatic stress disorder

28

28.13. You review a 55 year old man in the cardiology outpatient clinic. Two months ago he suffered an acute myocardial infarct requiring thrombolysis and subsequent coronary artery stenting. He appears to be making a good physical recovery but he tells you that for the past few weeks he has been unable to experience pleasure from activities that he would ordinarily enjoy (such as watching his favourite football team score a goal). Which of the following terms most accurately describes this symptom?

A. Anhedonia
B. Depression
C. Dysphoria
D. Euthymia
E. Hypomania

28.14. Which one of the following statements about psychiatric treatment is true?

A. Most patients treated with psychiatric medication suffer significant sedation as a side-effect
B. Psychotropic medications can be prescribed by psychiatrists and psychologists
C. The majority of psychiatric patients are given treatment against their will
D. There is considerable randomised controlled trial evidence to support use of cognitive behavioural therapy (CBT) for depression and anxiety disorders
E. There is little randomised controlled trial evidence to support pharmacological interventions in psychiatry

28.15. A 43 year old woman attends your general medical clinic for investigation of severe and persistent fatigue. No abnormalities are evident on examination or investigation. On reviewing her medical record you see that over the past 25 years she has had numerous visits to hospital, including to the ear, nose and throat (ENT) department, where she was diagnosed with temporomandibular joint dysfunction; psychiatry, where she was diagnosed with depression; gynaecology, where a hysterectomy was performed for menorrhagia; and gastroenterology, where she was diagnosed with irritable bowel syndrome. What is the most likely diagnosis?

A. Factitious disorder
B. Fibromyalgia
C. Hypochondriacal disorder
D. Malingering
E. Somatisation disorder

28.16. A 45 year old man presents with dry, broken skin on both hands. He reports a 10-month history of distressing repetitive thoughts with a theme of hygiene. He recognises that these are his own thoughts. He describes a short-lived reduction in distress following hand washing and says that in recent weeks he has been washing his hands more and more. What are the man's thoughts most likely to be?

A. Auditory hallucinations
B. Catastrophisations
C. Compulsions
D. Obsessions
E. Ruminations

28.17. A 19 year old female student is brought to the emergency department at midnight by her friends. They had been out drinking together but when she became so intoxicated that she was unable to walk they became worried about her and took her to hospital. She is admitted overnight for observation (temperature, blood pressure, heart rate and respiratory rate are all normal) and you review her on the ward round the following day.

Her urea and electrolytes, liver function tests, thyroid function tests and full blood count are all normal. On examination she is extremely thin, weight 38 kg (body mass index 16 kg/m^2) with lanugo hair on her arms and back. You tell her you are concerned about her low weight and ask her about her eating. She tearfully tells you that she started dieting 8 months ago but it now dominates her life and she thinks she has developed anorexia nervosa. Unfortunately the hospital has no psychiatric liaison service. What is the most appropriate immediate management?

A. Dietetic review and referral for urgent psychiatric outpatient assessment
B. Mental health act detention and compulsory refeeding
C. Prescribe mirtazapine as an antidepressant and appetite enhancer
D. Transfer to the local psychiatric hospital for specialist inpatient treatment
E. Voluntary refeeding as a medical inpatient

28.18. A 30 year old man brings his 27 year old wife and 10 day old son to the emergency department. He says that over the past 2 days his wife has not been her normal self. Initially she appeared unusually anxious about the baby, unable to put him down for more than a few minutes. Last night she stayed up through the night and this morning she refused to accept any of the food or drink that he offered her and will not let him hold the baby. She will not tell him what is wrong but agreed to come to the hospital as she said she would 'feel safer there'. What is the likely diagnosis?

A. Post-partum blues
B. Post-partum depression
C. Post-traumatic stress disorder
D. Puerperal psychosis
E. Schizophrenia

28.19. Which of the following statements is true about the biological basis of psychiatric disorders?

A. A large number of conditions have an identified single genetic cause
B. Depression is associated with focal reductions in 5-hydroxytryptamine (5-HT, serotonin) receptor binding
C. Most disorders have a discrete underlying abnormality on neuroimaging
D. Schizophrenia is associated with increased post-synaptic dopamine D_2 receptor binding
E. Task-based functional magnetic resonance imaging (MRI) is the technique of choice for analysing the interactions between multiple brain regions

28.20. Which of the following complaints are later (as opposed to earlier) manifestations in the natural history of dementia?

A. Difficulty getting dressed
B. Getting lost in familiar surroundings
C. Personality change
D. Subjective memory problems
E. Disinhibited behaviour

28.21. A 70 year old widowed woman is brought to your clinic with a history of memory impairment and aggressive behaviour for investigation and treatment. Which of the following statements is true of the pathophysiology and management of dementia?

A. Anticholinesterase medication is indicated to treat memory impairment in Pick's disease
B. Anticholinesterases may of some benefit in the late stages of Alzheimer's disease
C. Creutzfeldt–Jakob disease has characteristic electroencephalogram (EEG) abnormalities of generalised slow waves

D. Genetic mutations that cause frontotemporal dementia are also associated with amyotrophic lateral sclerosis
E. The genetic basis of Alzheimer's disease is unknown

28.22. A 50 year old woman with alcohol dependence syndrome is admitted to hospital with cellulitis in her foot. When the nurse gives her lunch, she comments that this is the first meal she has had for weeks as she has been spending all of her money on cider. On examination she is fully orientated and does not appear confused. She has a tremor, is sweating and tachycardic. What would appropriate management comprise?

A. Acamprosate and diazepam
B. Diazepam and parenteral vitamins (Pabrinex)
C. Disulfiram and acamprosate
D. Haloperidol and disulfiram
E. Parenteral vitamins (Pabrinex) and haloperidol

28.23. A 22 year old male is brought into the emergency department. He is agitated, difficult to converse with, smells of alcohol and says that he is being persecuted by secret services; however, he is fully oriented. Which of the following is the most likely diagnosis?

A. Alcohol withdrawal
B. Bipolar affective disorder
C. Drug intoxication
D. Drug-induced psychosis
E. Schizophrenia

28.24. A patient with schizophrenia getting treated with clozapine wants to speak to you about her treatment. Which of the following statements are true of clozapine?

A. Electrocardiogram (ECG) monitoring is mandatory as clozapine commonly causes cardiac arrythmias
B. It can cause dry mouth
C. It is a first-line treatment for schizophrenia
D. It is associated with constipation
E. It is associated with myeloproliferation

28.25. A 30 year old woman with a history of bipolar disorder treated with lithium wants to have a child and wonders if she should stay on the treatment. Which of the following statements are true of lithium salts?

A. Hypopararathyroidism is a potential risk
B. They are contraindicated in pregnancy because of a risk of neural tube defects

28

C. They have a wide therapeutic range
D. They should be reserved for treatment-resistant cases of bipolar disorder
E. Toxic effects include nausea, vomiting, tremor and convulsions

28.26. A 55 year old man with a history of ischaemic heart disease complains of low mood and an inability to derive pleasure from activities he used to enjoy, as well as fatigue, disturbed sleep, poor concentration and reduced appetite. Which of the following

statements relating to depression is true and might guide diagnosis and management?

A. Antidepressants do not work if patients have ongoing medical problems
B. CBT and other psychotherapies are less effective for depression than antidepressants
C. Electroconvulsive therapy (ECT) is the treatment of choice for severe depression
D. Depression has a similar prevalence in people with chronic medical complaints as in the general population
E. Tricyclic antidepressants and SSRIs can cause QTc interval prolongation

Answers

28.1. Answer: D.

'Drug history' refers to both recreational and prescribed medication (and over-the-counter and herbal preparations!). This is true of both a general medical and a psychiatric history. In the psychiatric history, 'family history' refers to both familial conditions and relationships. Much of the mental state examination is conducted during the course of psychiatric history taking, rather than as a separate set of procedures at the end (Box 28.1). 'History of presenting complaint' is as prominent in a psychiatric history as it is in clinical histories taken in other specialties, as is 'past medical history'.

28.2. Answer: D.

A tactile hallucination is the experience of perceiving touch in the absence of a touch stimulus. It is an abnormality of perception.

The mental state examination (MSE) is a systematic examination of the patient's thinking, emotion and behaviour. As with the clinical examination in other areas of medicine, the aim is to elicit objective clinical signs. Whilst many aspects of the patient's mental state may be observed as the history is being taken, specific enquiries about important features should always be made.

28.3. Answer: E.

Adjustment reactions, alcohol-related disorders, delirium and depression are all very common within the general medical inpatient population (Box 28.3). Rates of schizophrenia in the general medical inpatient population are similar to rates in the general population. The lifetime prevalence of schizophrenia is approximately 1%.

i 28.1 How to structure a psychiatric interview
Presenting problem
Reason for referral
Why the patient has been referred and by whom
Presenting complaints
The patient should be asked to describe the main problems for which help is requested and what they want the doctor to do
History of present illness
The patient should be asked to describe the course of the illness from when symptoms were first noticed
The interviewer asks direct questions to determine the nature, duration and severity of symptoms, and any associated factors
Background
Family history
Description of parents and siblings, and a record of any mental illness in relatives
Personal history
Birth and early developmental history, major events in childhood, education, occupational history, relationship(s), marriage, children, current social circumstances
Previous medical and psychiatric history
Previous health, accidents and operations
Use of alcohol, tobacco and other drugs
Direct questions may be needed concerning previous psychiatric history since this may not be volunteered: 'Have you ever been treated for depression or nerves?' or 'Have you ever suffered a nervous breakdown?'
Previous personality
The patterns of behaviour and thinking that characterise a person, including their relationships with other people and reactions to stress (useful information may be obtained from an informant who has known the patient well for many years)

28.3 Prevalence of psychiatric disorders by medical setting

	Medical/surgical			General psychiatric services
	General practice	Outpatients	Inpatients	
Delirium	–	–	+++	–
Alcohol/substance abuse	++	++	+++	+++
Schizophrenia	–	–	–	+++
Bipolar affective disorder	–	–	–	+++
Depression	++	++	+++	+++
Anxiety disorders	++	++	++	+++
Adjustment disorders	++	++	+++	+
Somatoform disorders	+	+++	++	–
Personality disorders	+	+	+	+++

– 'rare' (2%); + 'uncommon' (2–5%); ++ 'common' (5–10%); +++ 'very common' (10%)

28.4. Answer: C.

A delusion is a false belief, out of keeping with a patient's cultural background, which is held with conviction despite evidence to the contrary. It is common to classify delusions on the basis of their content. They may be:

- persecutory – such as a conviction that others are out to harm one
- hypochondriacal – such as an unfounded conviction that one has cancer
- grandiose – such as a belief that one has special powers or status
- nihilistic – such as 'My head is missing', 'I have no body' or 'I am dead'

Option A describes an obsessional thought, B describes an over-valued idea, D describes thought insertion and E describes loosening of associations.

28.5. Answer: E.

A sensory perception arising without an external stimulus is an hallucination. Meanwhile, an external stimulus that is misperceived is an illusion. A false perception that does not have the characteristics of a normal sensory perception (such as a voice heard in one's head rather than in external space) is called a pseudo-hallucination. A belief that has no rational basis is simply a false belief. 'A fixed, false belief out of keeping with a patient's cultural background' is the conventional definition of a delusion.

28.6. Answer: D.

Self-harm (SH) is a common reason for presentation to medical services. 'Self-harm' and 'attempted suicide' are not synonymous. Whilst some patients who self-harm are motivated by a desire to end their life, many have other motivations.

Most cases of SH that come to medical attention involve overdose, but other methods include asphyxiation, drowning, hanging, jumping from a height or in front of a moving vehicle, and firearms. Methods that carry a high chance of being fatal are more likely to be associated with serious psychiatric disorder. Self-cutting is common and often repetitive, but rarely leads to contact with medical services.

SH is more common in women than men, in young adults than the elderly, and in lower socioeconomic groups. In contrast, completed suicide is more common in men and the elderly (Box 28.6).

28.6 Risk factors for suicide

Psychiatric illness (depressive illness, schizophrenia)
Older age
Male sex
Living alone
Unemployment
Recent bereavement, divorce or separation
Chronic physical ill health
Drug or alcohol misuse
Suicide note written
History of previous attempts (especially if a violent method was used)

28.7. Answer: A.

The main differentials in a man of this age with no previous psychiatric history are delirium and dementia. The acute onset, disrupted sleep–wake cycle and visual hallucinations are all suggestive of delirium.

Personality disorders, bipolar affective disorder and schizophrenia typically emerge during adolescence or early adult life; they are unlikely to present for the first time at the age of 80.

28.8. Answer: D.

An autoscopic hallucination is the experience of seeing an image of oneself in external space. A functional hallucination is a false perception that

28

is triggered by a (normal) sensory stimulus: for example, a flash of light causing an olfactory hallucination. A hypnagogic hallucination is a brief hallucination experienced whilst going to sleep, whereas a hypnopompic hallucination is experienced whilst waking from sleep. A kinaesthetic hallucination is a false perception of joint or muscle sense (proprioception): for example, a hypnagogic hallucination of falling through space.

28.9. Answer: E.
Wernicke–Korsakoff syndrome is classically described as a combination of ataxia, delirium and ophthalmoplegia (Wernicke's encephalopathy) with short-term memory loss leading to disorientation and confabulation (Korsakoff's syndrome).

This man is presenting with acute signs suggestive of Wernicke's encephalopathy, which is a medical emergency. Urgent treatment with parenteral thiamin is needed to prevent permanent brain damage.

28.10. Answer: C.
Cocaine intoxication causes heightened arousal (not sedation) and pupillary dilatation (not constriction). At higher doses, the heightened arousal can lead to agitation and to psychotic symptoms such as auditory hallucinations and formication (the sensation of ants crawling under one's skin). Cocaine can also cause hyperthermia (rather than hypothermia).

28.11. Answer: E.
The clinical presentation is highly suggestive of a panic attack. Anxiety leads to hyperventilation and a respiratory alkalosis that triggers the physical symptoms described. These physical symptoms are catastrophically interpreted, thereby generating more anxiety and a vicious cycle is established.

Acute treatment involves helping patients to control their breathing, sometimes even getting them to re-breathe exhaled air (using a paper bag) to correct the respiratory alkalosis. Panic attacks are differentiated from general anxiety disorder by the episodic rather than chronic nature of the anxiety, although the two can coexist.

Factitious disorder is the deliberate feigning of physical symptoms or induction of physical signs for no obvious gain. The core feature of hypochondriacal disorder is a fear of a specific serious disease (such as cancer).

Obsessive–compulsive disorder is characterised by repetitive, intrusive, anxiety-provoking thoughts, images or impulses that give rise to repeated behaviours (compulsions) such as checking, washing or counting, which initially reduce the anxiety but over time become problematic in themselves.

28.12. Answer: E.
Post-traumatic stress disorder (PTSD) is relatively common in patients who recover after being in critical care. It is characterised by a period of latency followed by intrusive flashbacks or nightmares, psychophysiological hyper-arousal and avoidance.

'Acute stress reaction' is the diagnostic term for what is colloquially termed 'shock' – a transient sense of bewilderment or 'daze' arising in the context of a profoundly stressful situation. An adjustment disorder is a state of distress and emotional disturbance (that can include symptoms of depression and/or anxiety) arising during a period of adaptation to a significant life event. Delirium is a state of altered brain function arising from physical illness or other physiological challenge.

28.13. Answer: A.
'Anhedonia' is classically described as the inability to feel pleasure in normally pleasurable activities. The term 'depression' is often used in a non-medical context to mean 'low mood' but in a medical context it is a diagnosis rather than a symptom. This man is not reporting low mood per se but rather an inability to feel pleasure. 'Dysphoria' is a feeling of being ill at ease. 'Euthymia' describes mood that is neither high nor low. 'Hypomania' is a milder form of mania.

28.14. Answer: D.
Psychiatrists are medical practitioners and are therefore licensed to prescribe medication. Psychologists are not medically qualified; therefore, in the majority of jurisdictions, psychologists are not licensed to prescribe. There is a great deal of randomised controlled trial evidence to support both psychotropic medications and psychotherapies such as CBT. A relatively small minority of patients require compulsory treatment (detention under mental health legislation). Sedation can occur with some medications (e.g. high-dose antipsychotics) but most of the commonly prescribed medications (for example, selective

serotonin re-uptake inhibitors; SSRIs) do not cause sedation.

28.15. Answer: E.
Somatisation disorder is the diagnostic term for patients who, over many years, experience (and present to medical services with) somatoform (medically unexplained) symptoms affecting more than one system. Such patients are not faking their symptoms (in contrast to patients with factitious disorder or malingering) and they are not usually worried about a possible serious underlying condition (hypochondriasis). When assessing patients with somatoform symptoms it is important to recognise and acknowledge that their symptoms are real, distressing and disabling and to explain that doctors often see patients whose symptoms cannot be explained by disease.

28.16. Answer: D.
This is a typical description of obsessive–compulsive disorder (OCD), and the thoughts are 'obsessions'. The repetitive hand washing sustained by the temporary relief from anxiety is the 'compulsion'. 'Rumination' refers to the focusing of attention on one's symptoms. Catastrophising is viewing a situation as much worse than it actually is (relatively common in depression and anxiety).

28.17. Answer: A.
Despite her low weight, this woman is not acutely medically unwell: hence neither psychiatric nor ongoing medical admission are indicated. She needs to be supported to gain weight but this is best done collaboratively as an outpatient. Antidepressant medication does not have a major role to play in the management of anorexia nervosa.

28.18. Answer: D.
Puerperal psychosis affects approximately 1 in 500 women, with a peak onset in the first 2 weeks after birth. It usually takes the form of an affective psychosis (manic, depressive or mixed) but can sometimes resemble schizophrenia. The onset is often rapid, with transition from normal mental state to psychosis in a matter of days. Women often conceal their symptoms, which can place both the woman and her baby at significant risk.

Post-partum blues is the term used to describe a transient, self-limiting period of increased emotional reactivity during the first few weeks after delivery. Post-partum depression is depression arising following childbirth. Post-traumatic stress disorder is a delayed reaction to an extremely stressful event. It is characterised by flashbacks, avoidance and hyper-arousal.

28.19. Answer: B.
Very few psychiatric disorders have a single cause of any sort; most are multifactorial and polygenic. Very few conditions have a discrete underlying brain lesion: abnormalities on neuroimaging, even in dementia or schizophrenia, occur in <10% and most disorders are characterised by 'dysconnectivity' (abnormal interactions between brain regions). Schizophrenia is associated with increased *pre*-synaptic dopamine synthesis and turnover. *Resting-state* functional MRI is the technique of choice for analysing the interactions between multiple brain regions.

28.20. Answer: A.
Subjective memory complaints are a common early manifestation of all dementias. Getting lost in familiar surroundings is a common presenting feature of Alzheimer's. Difficulty getting dressed and other dyspraxias are usually more of a problem in the later stages of Alzheimer's disease. Behaviour and personality change are common early manifestations of the frontotemporal dementias.

28.21. Answer: D.
Creutzfeldt–Jakob disease is characterised by a generalised periodic *sharp* wave pattern on EEG. Mutations in several genes have been described in Alzheimer's disease but most are rare and/or of small effect (such as apolipoprotein E epsilon 4; *APOε4*). Anticholinesterases have been shown to be of some benefit at slowing progression of cognitive impairment, but only in the early stages of the disease, while post-synaptic cholinergic receptors are still available. Although Alzheimer's and Pick's (as one of the frontotemporal dementias; FTDs) share certain symptoms, they cannot be treated with the same pharmacological agents because the cholinergic systems are not affected in FTD.

28.22. Answer: B.
This woman is at risk of Wernicke–Korsakoff's syndrome as a consequence of alcohol dependence and poor nutrition. She should be

28

given prophylactic parenteral vitamins (Pabrinex). She is also showing early signs of alcohol withdrawal and should therefore be prescribed an alcohol withdrawal regime (diazepam or similar). Haloperidol is not effective in alcohol withdrawal and may precipitate alcohol withdrawal seizures. Disulfiram and acamprosate are both used to support long-term abstinence in alcohol dependence syndrome. They have no role in acute presentations.

28.23. Answer: E.
Alcohol addiction sufficient to cause a withdrawal syndrome is rare in the young and the patient smells of alcohol, suggesting he still has some in his system. Cannabis, stimulant or hallucinatory drug intoxication or induced psychosis could cause such a presentation, but would usually also be associated with some degree of cognitive impairment and/or disorientation. Bipolar disorder is possible but the content of any delusions present is usually mood-congruent, for example, a patient with mania might report being persecuted because of some special talents or identity.

28.24. Answer: D.
Clozapine is the only treatment licensed for the treatment of schizophrenia that has not responded to antipsychotic drugs. It is not a first-line treatment because of a range of dangerous adverse effects. Hypersalivation is a common adverse effect. White blood cell monitoring is required to monitor for the uncommon adverse effect of agranulocytosis. Constipation is a common adverse effect.

Clozapine is not typically associated with cardiac arrhythmias. ECG monitoring is good medical practice, and myocarditis and circulatory collapse are rare but may arise in the first months of treatment.

28.25. Answer: E.
Lithium is the treatment of choice for bipolar disorder, as it has proven efficacy in both phases of the disorder. Lithium salts are associated with hyperparathyroidism and have a narrow therapeutic range. They may be teratogenic, although this has probably been exaggerated over the years and the risk (if anything) is with Ebstein's anomaly; thus, pregnant mothers with bipolar disorder may be better treated than untreated, although this is a clinical decision that should be made in consultation with a specialist following exploration of the risks and benefits for the patient and her unborn child. Neural tube defects are associated with valproate and carbamazepine, which are therefore contraindicated in pregnancy.

28.26. Answer: E.
Depression affects about 20% of patients with chronic medical complaints, but these patients are still likely to benefit from antidepressant treatment. CBT and other psychotherapies are about as effective as antidepressants for depression in general, although they are probably less effective in severe depression where antidepressants are the first-line treatment. ECT is the treatment of choice for severe depression that has not responded to antidepressants and for psychotic depression.

29

Dermatology

Multiple Choice Questions

29.1. A 23 year old woman presents with a history of an itchy papular rash (see below), which developed on her chest and arms in the evening, after sitting in the sun for 2 hours, earlier that day. The eruption lasts for 3 days before fully resolving. What is the most likely diagnosis?

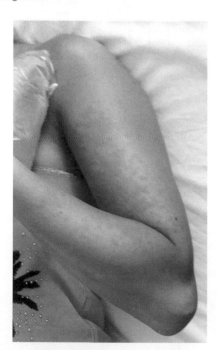

A. Chronic actinic dermatitis
B. Erythema multiforme
C. Lupus erythematosus
D. Polymorphic light eruption
E. Solar urticaria

29.2. A 45 year old farmer is prescribed doxycycline 200 mg orally daily for rosacea. A week later he experiences a severe sunburn reaction after being out one morning on his tractor on a cloudy day (see below). What is the most likely finding on investigation?

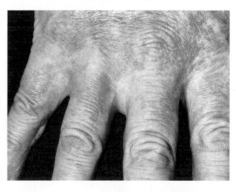

A. Abnormal plasma porphyrin scan
B. Positive antinuclear antibodies (ANA) and antibodies to extractable nuclear antigens (ENA)
C. Positive patch testing to doxycycline
D. Positive ultraviolet B (UVB) sensitivity on monochromator phototesting
E. Ultraviolet A (UVA) sensitivity on monochromator phototesting

29.3. A 22 year old pregnant woman presents to her family physician at 32 weeks' gestation with a 1-week history of intense generalised pruritus, which is preventing her from sleeping. Her family physician examines her and finds no abnormalities.

Which of the following would be the most important investigation to undertake?

A. ANA and complement
B. Full blood count
C. Liver function tests
D. Thyroid function tests
E. Urinalysis

29.4. An 86 year old man is referred to the dermatology clinic with a 2-week history of bilateral lower leg redness, scaling and swelling. He has a history of leg ulcers on both lower legs for the last 2 years and full-layer compression stockings were introduced 6 weeks previously. He is otherwise well and on examination there is sharply defined bilateral erythema and scaling, with associated oedema of the lower legs and a sharp cut-off below the knee. There is also ulceration of both medial lower legs, which is long-standing with surrounding lipodermatosclerosis.

What is the most likely diagnosis?

A. Acute ischaemia
B. Bacterial cellulitis
C. Allergic contact dermatitis
D. Deep venous thrombosis
E. Necrotising fasciitis

29.5. A 35 year old woman presents to the emergency department with a 2-day history of painful erythema, which commenced on the trunk and spread rapidly to the limbs, and a 1-day history of soreness of the mouth and dysuria. She had been commenced on carbamazepine for epilepsy 3 weeks earlier and trimethoprim 3 days ago. On assessment there is extensive erythema, with incipient blistering and denudation of the epidermis affecting about 60% body surface area and a positive Nikolsky sign. She is tachycardic, normotensive and afebrile.

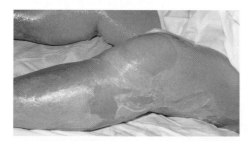

A diagnosis of drug-induced toxic epidermal necrolysis (TEN) is considered most likely. Which of the following statements is true?

A. Antibiotics should be prescribed, given the symptom of dysuria

B. Carbamazepine is the likely cause
C. Full recovery is likely for patients who are under 60 years of age
D. Skin pain suggests a possible viral trigger
E. There is good evidence to support the use intravenous immunoglobulins (IVIg)

29.6. A 75 year old woman presents to clinic with 12-month history of a crusted plaque on her lower leg, which has increased in size despite the use of potent topical corticosteroid. Examination reveals a well-defined crusty plaque 2 cm in diameter that is considered most likely to be a patch of Bowen's disease (see below). The patient also has a history of varicose veins and ankle swelling, which are evident on examination.

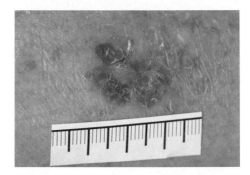

Which of the following would be the most appropriate management plan?

A. Cryotherapy
B. Photodynamic therapy
C. Radiotherapy
D. Refer for excisional surgery
E. Topical ingenol mebutate

29.7. A 33 year old woman presents with a 3-month history of an enlarging pigmented nodule on the forearm. On examination by the naked eye and under a dermatoscope, a diagnosis of melanoma is suspected. What would be the most appropriate next step in management?

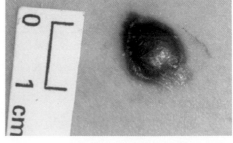

A. Curettage and cautery
B. Excision with a 1 cm margin
C. Excision with a 2 cm margin
D. Excision with a 2 mm margin
E. Initial incisional biopsy

29.8. A 23 year old woman is attending for narrowband UVB phototherapy for the treatment of guttate psoriasis (see below). After the third treatment she reports the development of an itchy papulovesicular rash on the arms, legs and trunk, and a clinical diagnosis of polymorphic light eruption (PLE) is made. Her only medication is the contraceptive pill.

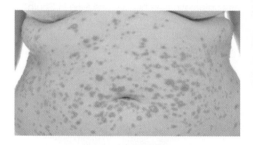

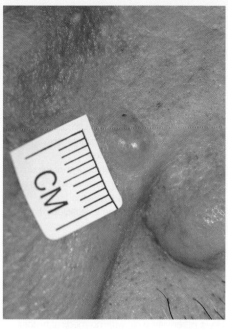

Which of the following statements is correct?

A. Phototherapy should be discontinued
B. PLE is a common cause of photo-aggravation of psoriasis
C. PLE is more common in patients on the contraceptive pill
D. PLE is more common in patients with psoriasis
E. Systemic prednisolone should be prescribed

29.9. A 68 year old man presents with a 2-year history of a nodular lesion on the right cheek, which has gradually increased in size but otherwise does not trouble him. He is well, although he is on warfarin as he has a history of transient ischemic attacks. Examination reveals a translucent nodule on the right nasolabial fold region, with telangiectatic vessels (see below). What is the most appropriate management approach?

A. Mohs' micrographic surgery
B. Photodynamic therapy
C. Standard excisional surgery
D. Topical imiquimod
E. Topical ingenol mebutate

29.10. A 16 year old girl presents with a history of persistent papulopustular inflammatory acne, which has not responded to topical antibiotics or benzoyl peroxide preparations (see below). She is otherwise well but is very troubled by her acne and it is stopping her from socialising. What is the most appropriate next management step?

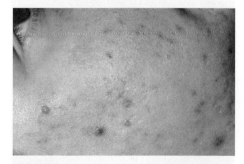

A. Combined oestrogen/anti-androgen orally for 3 months
B. Erythromycin 250 mg orally daily for 3 months
C. Isotretinoin 0.5 mg/kg orally daily for 4 months
D. Lymecycline 408 mg daily for 3 months
E. Minocycline 100 mg daily for 3 months

29.11. A 12 year old girl complains of itching of the scalp and has recently returned from a residential school camp. Her mother thought her daughter had more dandruff than usual and tried her with an over-the-counter anti-dandruff shampoo, which did not help. She then asked the advice of her family physician, who thought the daughter may have 'nits'.

Which of the following statements is correct?

A. 'Nits' are the active head louse *Pediculus humanus capitis* and are easily seen on the scalp and often confused with dandruff
B. All cases of head lice need intensive treatment with insecticides
C. Head lice infestation is highly contagious and all members of the family and all classmates should be treated at the same time
D. Malathion would be the insecticide of choice for active treatment
E. Thorough combing of wet, conditioned hair may be effective

29.12. A 10 year old boy presents with a patch of inflammation and hair loss in the scalp, which was noticed when he went for a haircut. He is otherwise well, with no medical history and lives at home with his mother, brother and pets. They have just returned home from a holiday on a farm. On examination, there is a boggy area of inflammation in the scalp, with overlying pustules and hair loss (see below). This is thought most likely to be tinea capitis.

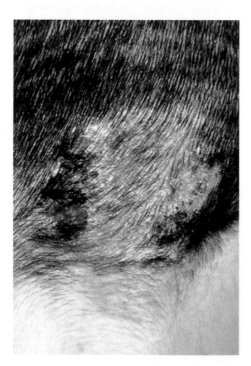

Which of the following statements is correct?

A. Examination with Wood's light will show areas of fluorescence if the endothrix is involved
B. If the diagnosis is confirmed he should be treated with topical terbinafine
C. Oral griseofulvin is the antifungal agent of choice for children in the UK
D. Systemic glucocorticoids will prevent any further hair loss
E. Tinea capitis is a dermatophyte fungal infection of the scalp hair bulb

29.13. A 62 year old woman presents with a 6-week history of a rapidly enlarging lesion on the right cheek, which is otherwise asymptomatic (see below). She lived in South Africa until the age of 20 years and has previously had three BCCs excised. What would be the most appropriate course of action?

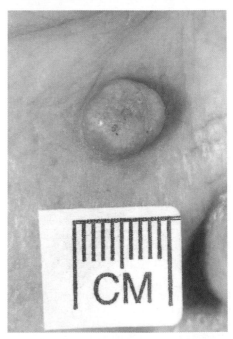

A. Biopsy and photodynamic therapy
B. Biopsy and topical imiquimod
C. Excisional surgery
D. Mohs' micrographic surgery
E. Observation

29.14. A 65 year old man presents with an enlarging, darkening patch of brown pigmentation adjacent to the eye, and biopsy confirms lentigo maligna. The patient is otherwise fit and well.

Which statement is correct?

A. Excisional surgery is usually curative
B. Histological disease often persists despite clinical clearance
C. Lentigo maligna is best treated non-surgically by topical imiquimod
D. Lentigo maligna should be treated by photodynamic therapy
E. There is high risk of invasive SCC if left untreated

29.15. A 65 year old female presents with a 2-year history of recurrent crops of pustules on the palms and soles (see below). There is no past history of dermatological disease. She has diabetes and is hypertensive but is otherwise well and has recently been trying to stop smoking. She is informed that the diagnosis is palmoplantar pustulosis.

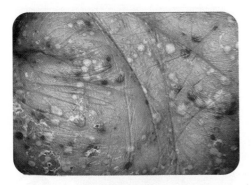

Which of the following is correct?

A. Bacterial swabs from pustules usually grow *Staphylococcus aureus*
B. Palmoplantar pustulosis is usually associated with chronic plaque psoriasis
C. PUVA (psoralen and ultraviolet A) treatment is usually effective
D. Smoking cessation is likely to result in disease improvement
E. Topical glucocorticoids should be avoided due to potential flaring of psoriasis

29.16. A 32 year old woman presents with a painful, well-demarcated erythematous plaque on the buttock, which occurs most months pre-menstrually. She is otherwise well and has recently started the oral contraceptive for menorrhagia. On close inspection, there is a well-defined plaque on the right buttock with clustered vesicles evident.

What is the most likely diagnosis?

A. Contact allergy
B. Fixed drug eruption
C. Herpes simplex virus
D. Molluscum contagiosum
E. Tinea corporis

29.17. A 64 year old man presents with three episodes of angioedema occurring over 6 weeks. He has a complex medical history with hypertension, diabetes mellitus and ischaemic heart disease, but has not previously had any dermatological disease. His medications include ramipril, insulin, bendroflumethiazide, clopidogrel and warfarin.
Which of the following statements is correct?

A. It is unusual that he does not also have urticaria
B. Patch testing would be the investigation of choice
C. Ramipril-induced angioedema is the most likely diagnosis
D. There is an increased incidence of angioedema in patients with diabetes
E. Bendroflumethiazide-induced angioedema is the most likely diagnosis

29.18. Which cells in the skin are primarily involved in antigen presentation?

A. B lymphocytes
B. Keratinocytes
C. Langerhans' cells
D. Merkel cells
E. T lymphocytes

29.19. The basement membrane serves as an anchor for the epidermis and allows movement of cells and nutrients between the dermis and the epidermis. Which of the following statements is correct?

A. The anchoring fibrils consist of type IV collagen
B. The lamina densa contains mainly type VII collagen
C. The lamina lucida lies above the basal cell membrane
D. The main hemidesmosomal collagen is type XIV
E. The tonofilaments mainly consist of keratin 5 and 14

29.20. The parents of a child with xeroderma pigmentosum, a rare genetic disease associated with severe photosensitivity, have

29

found out through the internet that vitamin D deficiency can lead to impaired bone health, rickets and osteomalacia. Which of the following statements is correct?

A. Dietary vitamin D intake is effective for vitamin D deficiency

B. Skin fibroblasts are the main source of vitamin D synthesis

C. UVA exposure is required for cutaneous vitamin D synthesis

D. UVB exposure is required for cutaneous vitamin D synthesis

E. Vitamin D toxicity is a risk for patients with increased photosensitivity

29.21. A 54 year old woman with chronic urticaria, without obvious history of trigger, is referred to dermatology for investigation and management (see below). With the exception of hay fever and long-standing vitiligo, she is otherwise well and is taking no medications.

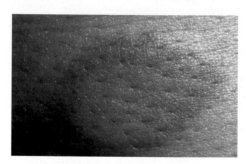

Which would be the most appropriate investigation?

A. Patch testing

B. Prick tests

C. Specific immunoglobulin E (IgE)

D. Thyroid function tests

E. Total IgE

29.22. A 28 year old woman, 32 weeks into her first pregnancy, presents with an itchy erythematous papular eruption that she first noticed in the stretch marks on her abdomen and thighs 2 weeks earlier. A diagnosis of pruritic urticarial papules and plaques of pregnancy (polymorphic eruption of pregnancy) is made and she is offered advice and treatment.

Which of the following statements is correct?

A. Abnormalities in liver function tests commonly occur

B. Non-sedating antihistamines are usually effective

C. She is advised that she should be delivered early because of fetal risk

D. She is advised that this is unlikely to be a problem in subsequent pregnancies

E. Topical glucocorticoids should be avoided due to potential adverse fetal effects

29.23. A 63 year old woman presents with a pigmented lesion on the anterior chest noted by her family physician during Well Woman screening. She had been aware of the lesion for 10 years and did not think it had significantly changed, although on closer questioning, she said it had enlarged over the last year. Excisional surgery confirms a diagnosis of invasive superficial spreading malignant melanoma (Breslow thickness 0.8 mm).

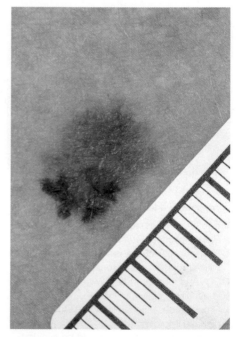

Which of the following statements is correct?

A. Breslow thickness is the most important prognostic factor

B. Five-year disease-free survival is about 85%

C. The patient will need indefinite follow-up

D. Total body computed tomography (CT) scan is recommended

E. Wide local excision with a 0.5-cm margin is advised

29.24. A 62 year old man presents with a 2-month history of blistering and fragility on the back of his hands (see below). He is otherwise well and enjoys socialising with his friends.

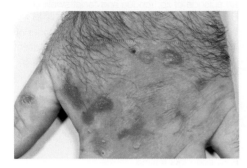

Which of the following investigations would be most useful?

A. Lupus serology
B. Patch testing
C. Porphyrin plasma scan
D. Skin biopsy and direct immunofluorescence
E. Urinalysis

29.25. A 39 year old woman with psoriasis, which is controlled by acitretin, wishes to become pregnant. What advice would you give her with regard to her plans to conceive?

A. Acitretin is not as teratogenic as isotretinoin so she can conceive on drug
B. She can try to conceive once she has been off acitretin for 1 year
C. She can try to conceive once she has been off acitretin for 6 months
D. She can try to conceive once she has been off acitretin for 3 years
E. She can try to conceive once she has been off acitretin for 2 months

29.26. A 64 year old man with recalcitrant psoriasis, despite UVB, PUVA and methotrexate, is being considered for biological therapy. He has extensive chronic plaque psoriasis, nail and scalp involvement and troublesome psoriatic arthritis. On assessing the Psoriasis Area and Severity Index (PASI), which of the following is included in the assessment?

A. Area of involvement
B. Degree of lichenification
C. Severity of joint involvement

D. Severity of nail involvement
E. Type of psoriasis

29.27. Which of the following conditions would be likely to flare if treated with PUVA photochemotherapy?

A. Atopic dermatitis
B. Bullous pemphigoid
C. Chronic urticaria
D. Lichen planus
E. Pustular psoriasis

29.28. A 56 year old man presents with an ill-defined nodular lesion on the nasal bridge abutting the medial canthus (see below). What would be the most appropriate management approach?

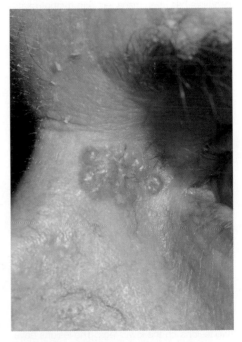

A. Curettage and cautery
B. Mohs' surgery
C. Photodynamic therapy
D. Radiotherapy
E. Topical imiquimod

29.29. Which of the following is a normal variant of nail growth?

A. Longitudinal ridging
B. Nail furrowing
C. Onycholysis
D. Pitting
E. Transverse ridging

29

29.30. A 35 year old woman presents with a 6-month history of sudden onset of hair loss. On examination there is complete loss of scalp hair, eyebrows, eyelashes and hair at all other body sites. There is no evidence of scalp inflammation, scarring or regrowth. She is otherwise well, although she has a history of vitiligo and treated hypothyroidism.

Which of the following management approaches would be most appropriate?

A. Discuss consideration of a wig
B. Finasteride
C. Intralesional corticosteroids
D. Topical minoxidil
E. UVB phototherapy

29.31. A 42 year old man with chronic plaque psoriasis has been managed with methotrexate, with partial control of his skin disease, for the last 5 years. He had previously failed to respond to UVB and PUVA. He is otherwise well, although he has a history of hypertension and is a smoker. He has increasingly had problems with pain and swelling of joints in the hands and feet and in the sacroiliac joints. On examination he has extensive plaque psoriasis and evidence of synovitis and dactylitis in fingers and toes. The PASI is 15 and Dermatology Life Quality Index (DLQI) 25, despite methotrexate 25 mg/week subcutaneously.

What would be the most appropriate next treatment approach?

A. Switch to adalimumab
B. Switch to apremilast
C. Switch to ciclosporin
D. Switch to fumaric acid esters
E. Switch to PUVA plus acitretin

29.32. A 93 year old woman is noted to have two lesions on the lower legs. The lesions have been unchanged and asymptomatic for 2 years and don't trouble her. Her daughter brought her to clinic for an opinion. On examination she has two well-defined erythematous scaly plaques on the lower legs, with dermatoscopic features consistent with Bowen's disease. She additionally has pitting ankle oedema, varicose veins and absent foot pulses. Her daughter asks for advice as to what would be the most appropriate treatment option.

Which of the following is most appropriate?

A. Cryotherapy
B. Excision

C. Imiquimod
D. Ingenol mebutate
E. No treatment

29.33. A 21 year old woman presents following an episode of lip, tongue and facial swelling, occurring within minutes of blowing up a balloon. The episode resolved within an hour of taking a non-sedating antihistamine. The patient asks whether this can be related to the rubber balloon and is keen to know what the most useful method of investigation would be?

A. Oral challenge
B. Patch testing
C. Prick testing
D. Specific IgE testing
E. Specific IgG testing

29.34. The skin changes as people age and there are many important differences between young and old skin. Which of the following statements relating to the skin of the elderly is correct?

A. Absorption and clearance of topical medications is reduced
B. Photo-ageing is accelerated intrinsic ageing due to sunlight exposure
C. Skin cancer is more common because of increased immune reactions in the skin
D. The skin thickens as it ages
E. There is less risk of developing irritant dermatitis

29.35. A 62 year old man presents with a 6-week history of itchy blistering rash occurring on the trunk and limbs (see below). He is otherwise in good health apart from controlled hypertension. His medications are ramipril and aspirin. On examination he has several tense, clear and haemorrhagic-fluid filled blisters arising on erythematous plaques on the trunk and limbs. A diagnosis of bullous pemphigoid is suspected.

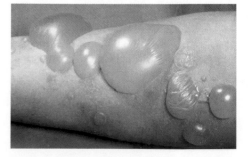

Which of the following would you expect to find?

A. Mucosal involvement
B. Neutrophilia
C. Positive circulating anti-epidermal antibodies
D. Positive Nikolsky sign
E. Subcorneal blister on histology

29.36. An 85 year old woman presents with a 6-month history of generalised itch, but no rash. Investigations do not identify a cause and symptomatic management is offered. Which is likely to be the most effective management option?

A. High-dose tricyclic antidepressants
B. High-dose antihistamines
C. Topical capsaicin
D. UVB phototherapy
E. Very potent topical glucocorticoids

29.37. A 45 year old man attends clinic for topical photodynamic therapy (PDT) for a superficial BCC on his leg (see below). He is keen to ask about how the treatment works. PDT is increasingly used to treat superficial non-melanoma skin cancer. Which of the following statements is correct?

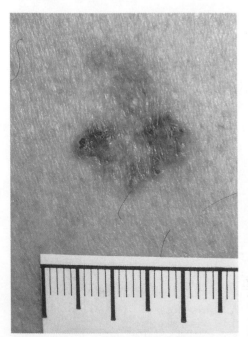

A. A cream containing a photosensitiser is applied

B. Oxygen is required for the photodynamic reaction
C. PDT should not be used for nodular BCC
D. PDT should not be used in elderly frail patients
E. Red laser light is required for irradiation during PDT

29.38. There has been a rising epidemic of skin cancer in white-skinned populations. Which of the following statements is correct?

A. Malignant melanoma usually arises on sites of chronic sun exposure
B. Most patients with sporadic BCC carry a germline mutation in the *PTCH1* gene
C. There is a greatly increased risk of BCC in immunosuppressed patients
D. There is convincing evidence that sunscreen use lowers risk of BCC development
E. There is marked genetic heterogeneity in SCC

29.39. Actinic keratoses are extremely common in white-skinned populations and occur as scaly erythematous lesions on chronically sun-exposed sites (see below). Histological evidence of dysplasia is the hallmark and progression to Bowen's disease and/or invasive SCC may occur. Which of the following statements is correct?

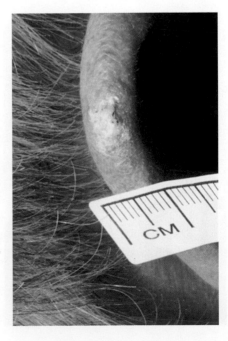

29

A. Approximately 3% of actinic keratosis transform into invasive SCC
B. Field-directed treatment is typically required
C. Hyperkeratotic actinic keratosis usually responds to cryotherapy
D. Invasive SCC invariably arises from actinic keratosis
E. Spontaneous resolution of actinic keratosis may occur

29.40. Which of the following statements is correct with respect to malignant melanoma?

A. Acral melanoma is less common in dark-skinned populations
B. Lentigo maligna melanoma usually occurs in younger patients
C. Most patients with melanoma have a positive family history of melanoma
D. Nodular melanoma is most common in men
E. The majority of melanomas arise from a pre-existing naevus

29.41. A 3 year old boy presents with a 2-day history of tense blisters and superficial erosions arising on a background of erythema affecting the trunk and face (see below). He has been off his food and is febrile. On examination, extensive superficial erosions are evident in the groins and affected large areas on the trunk. There is no mucosal involvement.

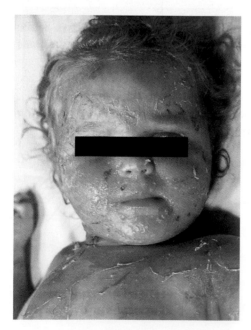

What is the most likely diagnosis?

A. Epidermolysis bullosa
B. Impetigo
C. Staphylococcal scalded skin syndrome (SSSS)
D. Stevens–Johnson syndrome
E. Toxic epidermal necrolysis

29.42. A 32 year old man with chronic plaque psoriasis has been attending for UVB phototherapy. He was starting to respond to treatment but in the second week commented that he had developed a new asymptomatic rash on the back and chest. On examination, in addition to chronic plaque psoriasis affecting extensor surfaces, sacral area and buttocks, a rash is evident on the upper trunk, consisting of oval scaly macules and hypopigmentation (see image). What is the most likely diagnosis?

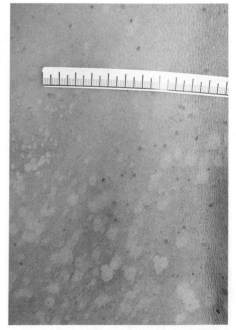

A. Pityriasis rosea
B. Pityriasis versicolor
C. Polymorphic light eruption
D. Psoriasis
E. Secondary syphilis

29.43. A 35 year old woman returns to clinic for management of chronic atopic eczema (see image). She has a life-long history of eczema with whole-body and facial activity over the last 5 years, despite topical emollients, glucocorticoids, phototherapy and PUVA. She is otherwise in good health, works in an office and does not smoke or drink. She needs a considerable amount of time off work because of her skin, which is adversely impacting on her life, with a DLQI score of 24. What would be the next most appropriate management step to consider?

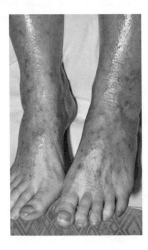

A. Acitretin
B. Apremilast
C. Ciclosporin
D. Dupilumab
E. Methotrexate

29.44. Early clinical trial data on biological agents for severe recalcitrant atopic dermatitis look promising. Which of the following pathways is implicated for therapeutic response to biological agents in atopic dermatitis?

A. IL-12 inhibition
B. IL-13 inhibition
C. IL-17 inhibition
D. IL-23 inhibition
E. TNF-α inhibition

29.45. A 28 year old mother of 6 month old twins presents with a rash on the back of hands and between the fingers. Examination reveals erythema and scaling at these sites, with bilateral involvement and a relatively sharp cut-off at the wrists. There is no previous history of relevance and she is not known to be atopic. What is the most likely diagnosis?

A. Allergic contact dermatitis
B. Dermatophyte fungal infection
C. Irritant contact dermatitis
D. Late-onset atopic dermatitis
E. Progesterone dermatitis

29.46. A 14 year old boy attends the paediatric dermatology clinic with his mother who is seeking a second opinion for treatment of long-standing chronic atopic eczema. On examination he has extensive eczema affecting the trunk and flexor and extensor surfaces of the limbs, with chronic inflammation and lichenification (see below). He is using Eumovate ointment daily, approximately 100 g per fortnight to the trunk and limbs, emulsifying ointment as emollient and fexofenadine at night to help with itch. Which of the following changes to his management is likely to be most effective?

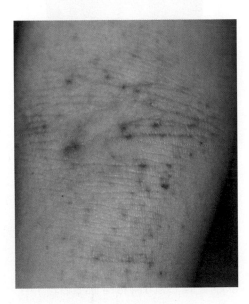

A. Changing from emulsifying ointment to aqueous cream
B. Changing vehicle formulation to Eumovate cream
C. Increasing the amount of topical glucocorticoid use
D. Increasing the dose of fexofenadine
E. Increasing the potency of topical glucocorticoid, e.g. to Betnovate ointment

29

29.47. A 72 year old man with previously stable chronic plaque psoriasis presents with extensive erythroderma and sheets of pustules affecting the trunk, limbs and flexures (see below). He has a history of chronic obstructive pulmonary disease and has recently completed a course of prednisolone for a respiratory exacerbation. Topical treatment with a vitamin D agonist to the skin has been ineffective. Which of the following statements is correct?

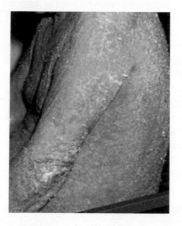

A. Coal tar and UVB phototherapy should be commenced
B. He should be admitted and treated with topical dithranol
C. Methotrexate would be the systemic immunosuppressant of choice because of rapid onset of action
D. The flare of pustular psoriasis may be related to prednisolone use
E. Vitamin D analogues are the topical treatment of choice for pustular psoriasis

29.48. A 49 year old man presents with an itchy violaceous papular rash affecting the flexural surfaces of forearms and shins. Skin biopsy shows a lichenoid reaction pattern and a drug cause is considered. Which of the following drugs is the most likely to be the culprit?

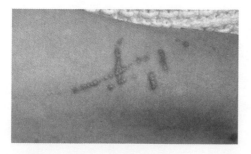

A. Aspirin
B. Bendroflumethiazide
C. Doxycycline
D. Furosemide
E. Ranitidine

29.49. A 29 year old man attends a consultation for advice with respect to further management of chronic urticaria that has troubled him for 6 months. There are no known triggers and investigations are normal. He has not responded well to H_1 antihistamines. Which of the following treatment options has been shown to be effective in this setting?

A. Montelukast
B. Narrowband UVB phototherapy
C. Oral prednisolone
D. PUVA photochemotherapy
E. Ranitidine

29.50. An 85 year old woman presents with a 6-week history of severe oral ulceration. On examination it is also noted that she has an extensive erythematous rash on the neck and upper trunk, with erosions evident and Nikolsky sign positive. Skin biopsy is undertaken and shows intra-epidermal blistering, acantholysis and IgG and C_3 deposition within the epidermis on immunofluorescence. Which of the following statements is correct?

A. Long-term treatment is often required
B. Low-dose systemic glucocorticoids are usually effective
C. Positive Nikolsky sign usually indicates a drug-induced cause
D. The disease can be treated with penicillamine
E. Underlying malignancy is found in most cases

29.51. A 27 year old woman presents with progressive symmetrical depigmentation affecting the face, hands and feet (see below). There is no history of preceding inflammation and no altered sensation within the areas of hypopigmentation. A diagnosis of vitiligo is established. Which of the following is associated with an improved prognosis for repigmentation in vitiligo?

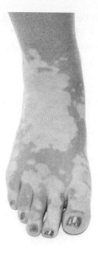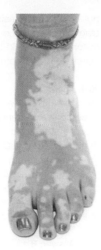

she has multiple erythematous annular targetoid lesions. She is otherwise well, with no preceding medical history. A diagnosis of erythema multiforme is suspected. Which of the following is most likely to have provoked this?

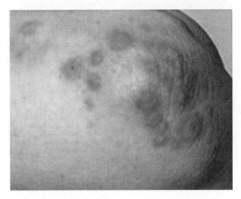

A. Associated hypothyroidism
B. Facial involvement
C. Involvement of the distal limbs
D. The presence of a trichrome pattern
E. The presence of leucotrichia

A. Adenovirus
B. Herpes simplex virus
C. Ibuprofen
D. Paracetamol
E. Oral contraceptive

29.52. A 53 year old woman with a known diagnosis of hepatitis C attends a general medical clinic for routine review. On enquiry she comments that she has been aware of blistering occurring on the backs of her hands, in particular when she had minor trauma to the skin. On examination there is nothing much to see other than mild scarring and milia. What would be the most appropriate course of action?

A. Check renal function, as this may indicate renal failure
B. Patch testing, as this may be allergic contact dermatitis
C. Porphyrin investigations, as this may be a cutaneous porphyria
D. Reassurance that this is likely due to the hepatitis C infection
E. Skin biopsy and direct immunofluorescence to exclude immunobullous disease

29.53. A 25 year old woman presents to her family physician with a 2-day history of a rash on her hands and forearms. On examination

29.54. A 66 year old woman was commenced on carbamazepine and co-codamol 10 days previously for trigeminal neuralgia. She was otherwise well, having just returned from a holiday in the Caribbean. She presents to out-of-hours primary care with an acute onset of extensive rash, systemic malaise and high fever. Examination reveals a widespread erythematous maculopapular and purpuric rash, with prominent facial involvement and facial oedema. She has generalised lymphadenopathy and a temperature of 40°C. Initial investigations show an eosinophilia and marked elevation of liver function tests. She is admitted to an infectious disease department. What would be the most likely diagnosis?

A. Carbamazepine-induced drug reaction
B. Co-codamol-induced drug reaction
C. Hepatitis
D. Leptospirosis
E. Meningococcal sepsis

29

Answers

29.1. Answer: D.
This immunological photodermatosis occurs in 18% of the population in Northern Europe. It presents as a delayed-onset papulovesicular eruption, typically occurring a few hours after sun exposure and lasting a few days before resolving. In contrast, solar urticaria will almost invariably occur within 15 minutes of sun exposure and will last only a few hours before resolving. Chronic actinic dermatitis can occur

at any age but typically presents in elderly males and the morphology of rash is a dermatitis. It usually takes a few hours to days of sun exposure to develop and it persists until treated. Lupus erythematosus is a photo-aggravated autoimmune disorder and the skin features more typically develop a day, or so, after sun exposure and persist for weeks. Erythema multiforme is a photo-aggravated disease often triggered by herpes simplex virus infection and can be most prominent on sun-exposed sites although usually affects sun-protected sites as well. The rash is usually more targetoid and less papular.

29.2. Answer: E.

Most drugs, including doxycycline, photosensitise maximally in the UVA region and this would usually be detected on monochromator phototesting. Patch testing is not the investigation of choice for suspected systemic drug-induced photosensitivity. Both false-positive and false-negative results mean that patch testing using topical delivery of a drug that has been used systemically is an unreliable investigation. It is usually not indicated nor of clinical relevance. Positive ANA and ENA autoantibodies can be seen with some systemic drug photosensitisers: for example, thiazides or proton pump inhibitors. However, this is not typically the case with doxycycline and, indeed, the most common presentation of drug-induced photosensitivity is through a phototoxic non-immunological mechanism. UVB provocation testing may be positive in drug-induced photosensitivity but is much less likely to be abnormal than UVA phototesting, which is the main part of the ultraviolet spectrum implicated in drug-induced photosensitivity. Whilst some drugs can cause minor derangements of porphyrins, this is not the case with doxycycline and one would not expect abnormal porphyrins in doxycycline-induced photosensitivity.

29.3. Answer: C.

Acute cholestasis of pregnancy is uncommon but usually presents in the third trimester of pregnancy. It is essential to diagnose this promptly as there is increased fetal and maternal risk; urgent diagnosis and treatment, which may include early delivery, are required. The other investigations of full blood count, urinalysis and thyroid function tests would all be important to undertake in this clinical setting but liver function tests would be most important diagnostically. In the absence of other relevant history, there would be no specific indication to check ANA and complement.

29.4. Answer: C.

The scenario of the relatively recent introduction of compression bandaging a few weeks earlier raises the possibility of allergic contact dermatitis. Specifically, rubber additives or preservatives in any of the topical preparations could be culprits. All of the other diagnoses should, of course, be considered and excluded but a bilateral symmetrical presentation of each of these diagnoses would be extremely unlikely.

29.5. Answer: B.

The Nikolsky sign is when gentle lateral pressure on stroking the skin results in epidermal detachment. Carbamazepine is a drug that is associated with many cutaneous adverse effects and is one of the most common culprits in TEN. Evidence relating to the use of IVIg in TEN is controversial at best and overall not advised (see British Association of Dermatology guidelines). The symptom of dysuria is much more likely to be due to inflammation and desquamation of the uroepithelial tract due to involvement in the TEN process. Catheterisation should be avoided unless necessary, such as for monitoring fluid balance – and in that instance should be performed with caution. A mid-stream urine should be undertaken, but antibiotics should not be prescribed empirically. Skin pain is a characteristic feature of TEN and the prognosis is better for patients who are less than 40 years of age, although other prognostic indicators need to be taken into account when assessing the disease severity score (SCORTEN), which is predictive of risk of mortality (Box 29.5).

29.6. Answer: B.

Photodynamic therapy is approved for use in Bowen's disease. Given its relative specificity of treatment and improved healing compared with other treatments such as cryotherapy and 5-fluorouracil, this would be the treatment of choice on a lower leg site where there is coexistent oedema and vascular insufficiency, either venous and/or arterial. Definitive surgical excision would be an option but in this instance a non-surgical approach would usually be advised in order to reduce morbidity, given the

i	29.5 Disease severity score for toxic epidermal necrolysis: SCORTEN
Factor	
Age > 40 years	
Heart rate > 120 beats/min	
Cancer or haematological malignancy	
Involved body surface area > 10%	
Blood urea > 10 mmol/L (28 mg/dL)	
Serum bicarbonate < 20 mmol/L (20 mEq/L)	
Blood glucose ≥ 14 mmol/L (252 mg/dL)	
Mortality rates	
0–1 factor present = 3%	
2 factors = 12%	
3 factors = 35%	
4 factors = 58%	
≥5 factors = 90%	

From Bastuji-Garin S, Fouchard N, Bertocchi M, et al. SCORTEN: a severity-of-illness score for toxic epidermal necrolysis. J Invest Dermatol 2000; 115:149–153.

very low risk of malignant transformation. Cryosurgery to a lesion of this size, on an oedematous lower leg site with venous insufficiency, would be associated with a higher risk of poor healing and ulceration. Radiotherapy would not usually be used on a lower leg site with these coexistent morbidities as the risk of radionecrosis, scarring and ulceration are relatively high. Ingenol mebutate is not licensed or approved for use in Bowen's disease.

29.7. Answer: D.

The first step in this situation would be an initial excision with a narrow margin in order to establish the diagnosis. Thereafter, the next step would be to re-excise with wider margins (1–2 cm) once the diagnosis of melanoma was confirmed, and dependent on the Breslow thickness. An initial wide excision would not usually be advocated in case the clinical diagnosis was incorrect. Incisional biopsy is not advised when melanoma is suspected if it can be readily excised. Curettage would also not be recommended if melanoma was suspected.

29.8. Answer: B.

There is no evidence that PLE is more common either in patients taking the contraceptive pill or in psoriasis. The prevalence of PLE is approximately 18% in Northern Europe and, as it most commonly occurs in young females of child-bearing age, the contraceptive pill and PLE are commonly associated but there is no evidence to indicate a causal relationship. PLE does commonly occur during a course of phototherapy and, if this is the case, there is concern that Köbnerisation of psoriasis

may occur. Indeed, most cases of photo-aggravation of psoriasis are through the mechanism of induced PLE. If PLE develops during a course of phototherapy, then it is advisable to stop treatment until the rash has settled and then to restart at a lower dose, with reduced dose increments and, if necessary, a topical corticosteroid application after treatment. Systemic corticosteroids are uncommonly required for PLE occurring during a course of phototherapy and might cause a rebound flare of psoriasis on cessation.

29.9. Answer: C.

The image shows a well–defined, nodular basal cell carcinoma (BCC). If he is agreeable to surgery, then the most appropriate approach would be excision of the lesion. Mohs' micrographic surgery would only be required if the lesion is poorly defined, in order to ensure complete excision and preservation of normal tissue.

Warfarin does not preclude a surgical approach as long as the international normalised ratio (INR) is checked 48 hours before the procedure in order to ensure the patient is not over-anticoagulated and as long as additional precautionary measures are taken at the time of surgery in order to ensure haemostasis. Medical treatments, including photodynamic therapy, imiquimod and ingenol mebutate, would be unlikely to be effective with this prominently nodular BCC. Medical treatments are best reserved for either superficial BCC or thin, nodular BCC, and would only be considered for a lesion such as this if surgery was contraindicated or the patient refused to consider a surgical approach.

29.10. Answer: D.

In the first instance, as a trial, lymecycline would be an appropriate next step. Erythromycin would be an alternative but the dose of 250 mg daily is sub-therapeutic and would be unlikely to be effective. Minocycline is not the first antibiotic of choice given the risk of skin pigmentation and of drug-induced lupus. Antibiotics will need to be continued for several months, and a trial of at least 3 months is required. Combined oestrogen/anti-androgen contraceptives, such as those including cyproterone acetate, may be appropriate but would usually only be considered or added in if there was an inadequate response to a trial of systemic antibiotics. Isotretinoin would not be

29

considered at this early stage in management of a patient with papulopustular acne. The hope would be that this case would respond well to systemic antibiotics; systemic retinoids would only be required if there was a failure to respond to 3–6 months of antibiotic treatment.

29.11. Answer: E.

Scalp infestation with the head louse *Pediculus humanus capitis* is very common. A diagnosis is confirmed by identifying a living louse or nymph. However, the 'nits' are actually empty egg cases, not the head lice themselves, and are signs of there having been an infestation. 'Nits' are yellowish in colour and can be confused with dandruff. Not all cases require treatment with insecticide, as regular wet combing of conditioned hair may be effective in physical removal of lice. Malathion would not be the insecticide of choice as resistance is fairly common; alternatives such as dimeticone may be used. Whilst the infestation is highly contagious, treatment is only recommended for the affected individual and close contacts, such as family members or close school class members where there has been direct head-to-head contact. Treatment of all classmates is not required.

29.12. Answer: C.

Fluorescence with Wood's light is only seen with some species of dermatophyte infection and not with those involving the endothrix (within the hair shaft). Dermatophyte infection of the scalp hair affects the shaft as opposed to the bulb. Topical treatment will not be sufficient for clearance of inflammatory active fungal infection within the hair-bearing scalp. Griseofulvin is the only systemic antifungal agent licensed for use in children in the UK. There is no convincing evidence that systemic glucocorticoids reduce hair loss associated with tinea capitis.

29.13. Answer: C.

From the history, this lesion is most likely a benign keratoacanthoma, but it is impossible to distinguish this from a rapidly growing squamous cell carcinoma (SCC). Given her history of significant sun exposure and previous BCC, it would be important to excise in order to exclude invasive SCC. Mohs' micrographic surgery would not usually be required for this well-defined tumour and is most commonly used, in particular, for poorly defined BCC. Observation is an option, because if this is a benign keratoacanthoma, then it should

regress. However, given that spontaneous resolution of keratoacanthoma often leaves cosmetically unacceptable scars and that it is impossible to distinguish from invasive SCC, active intervention and removal is important. An incisional biopsy may not clearly distinguish between keratoacanthoma and invasive SCC: the distinction often remains difficult; thus, usually these lesions are definitively excised. A nodular lesion such as this would be unlikely to respond to treatment with either topical imiquimod or photodynamic therapy.

29.14. Answer: B.

Lentigo maligna may be very difficult to treat and to achieve clinical and histological clearance. It is not unusual for clinical response to occur but abnormal cells to remain histologically. Treatment of choice would be definitive surgical excision although this can be difficult as dysplastic cells often persist at the margins, arising as part of field change carcinogenesis. Imiquimod may be used if surgery is not appropriate but the risk of recurrence is higher. Left untreated, there is a significant risk of invasive melanoma developing into lentigo maligna. Pigmented lesions with metastatic potential would not be appropriately treated by photodynamic therapy, and melanin absorbs red light; thus efficacy would not be expected.

29.15. Answer: C.

Whilst some consider palmoplantar pustulosis to be a variant of psoriasis, most patients with this condition do not have other features of chronic plaque psoriasis and there is increasing evidence to suggest that the two conditions are distinct. Palmoplantar pustulosis is almost invariably associated with smoking but there is no convincing evidence that stopping smoking results in disease improvement. Topical glucocorticoids are usually a mainstay treatment in palmoplantar pustulosis. Bacterial swabs from the pustules are usually sterile. PUVA may be effective for disease suppression in this condition.

29.16. Answer: C.

Clustered painful vesicles recurring at the same site in association with the pre-menstrual period are most likely to be extra-labial herpes simplex virus infection. Pain and clustered vesicles would not be expected in fixed drug eruption, although this should certainly be something to be considered, particularly if the patient is taking paracetamol or non-steroidal anti-inflammatory medication in the pre-menstrual phase. In tinea corporis or dermatophyte fungal infection, the most likely presentation would be a raised edge with pustules and scaling and central clearing, and it would be unlikely to clear and recur at the same site each month or be painful. In molluscum contagiosum, whilst these are due to a pox virus infection, the lesions are not vesicular but are usually solid umbilicated papules and they are not usually painful or intermittent. Whilst an acute vesicular eczema can occur in association with contact allergy, the intermittent and isolated nature of this would make this diagnosis unlikely.

29.17. Answer: C.
A relatively common side-effect of angiotensin-converting enzyme (ACE) inhibitors is angioedema and this usually occurs without associated urticaria. Thiazide diuretics do not typically cause angioedema. Patch testing is used to investigate type IV delayed hypersensitivity and not type I immunological reactions. There is no evidence that angioedema is increased in patients with diabetes.

29.18. Answer: C.
Langerhans' cells have the primary function of antigen presentation to lymphocytes.

29.19. Answer: E.
The tonofilaments mainly consist of keratins 5 and 14. The lamina lucida lies immediately below the basal cell membrane. The lamina densa is made up mainly of type IV collagen. The main hemi-desmosomal collagen is type XVII. The anchoring fibrils consist of type VII collagen.

29.20. Answer: D.
The main cell type involved in vitamin D photosynthesis in skin is the keratinocyte. UVB is required for this. UVA exposure does not result in adequate cutaneous vitamin D production. Dietary absorption of vitamin D is poor and vitamin D and calcium supplements are required in vitamin D deficiency. Vitamin D deficiency is a potential concern for patients with photosensitivity diseases.

29.21. Answer: D.
This patient is atopic and has autoimmune disease. Urticaria may be a manifestation of autoimmune hypo- or hyperthyroidism. Patch testing is the investigation of choice for delayed type IV cell-mediated hypersensitivity but not type I antibody-mediated allergy. Most patients

with chronic urticaria do not have an obvious trigger and total IgE and specific IgE testing are unlikely to be helpful in the absence of a history suggestive of trigger factors. Prick testing would, again, be unlikely to be contributory unless there was a specific trigger identified in the history.

29.22. Answer: D.
The condition is usually treated with topical glucocorticoids, which can be safely prescribed in pregnancy. The condition is not known to be associated with any adverse effects to the fetus and early delivery is not generally required. Abnormal liver function tests are not associated with polymorphic eruption of pregnancy. Sedating antihistamines, such as chlorphenamine, may be required but as this is not primarily a histamine-mediated disease, non-sedating antihistamines are not advised as their safety in pregnancy is unproven. Polymorphic eruption of pregnancy usually persists until delivery and may even continue for some time into the post-partum period before spontaneous resolution. It does not usually occur in subsequent pregnancies.

29.23. Answer: A.
Breslow thickness is the most important prognostic factor. For a tumour less than 1 mm in histological thickness, routine CT scanning and sentinel node biopsy would not be indicated. Prognosis should be around 95% disease-free survival at 5 years. Wide local excision with a 1-cm margin is advised. For a good prognosis in melanoma such as this, long-term follow-up is not required.

29.24. Answer: C.
This history is very suggestive of a diagnosis of porphyria cutanea tarda, and this would be an easy screening test. If this proved positive, then more detailed investigations would be required including urine porphyrins and investigating for an underlying cause of iron overload and liver disease. In this case it may be due to alcohol-induced liver disease. Skin biopsy and immunofluorescence may show characteristic changes of subepidermal blistering and periodic acid–Schiff (PAS) staining but would not be the investigation of choice. Patch testing, urinalysis and lupus serology would not be specifically indicated.

29.25. Answer: D.
Acitretin has a long half-life and high lipid bioavailability; pregnancy should be avoided for

29

3 years after the drug has been stopped, which is why it is not often used in women of child-bearing age. Acitretin is at least as teratogenic as isotretinoin and the effect is of longer duration.

29.26. Answer: A.
The body is divided into four areas and each is scored individually based on area involved and the redness, thickness and scaling of psoriatic plaques. Joint and nail involvement are not assessed and neither is the type of psoriasis. Lichenification is taken into account in eczema severity scores.

29.27. Answer: B.
The autoimmune bullous diseases are usually exacerbated by light-based therapies and should be avoided. All of the other diseases may respond therapeutically to PUVA.

29.28. Answer: B.
The image is of a BCC. Mohs' surgery, if available, would be preferred to excisional surgery at this site given the need for preservation of normal tissue and structures. Curettage and cautery may lead to unacceptable scarring at this site and is less likely to result in tumour clearance. Topical imiquimod may cause significant inflammation, blepharitis and conjunctivitis at this site. Photodynamic therapy, given the nodular nature of the tumour, would be unlikely to result in complete clearance. Radiotherapy would be likely to result in poorer cosmetic outcome and risk damage to the medial canthus and lacrimal duct.

29.29. Answer: A.
Longitudinal ridging can be a normal part of the ageing process. Pitting, onycholysis, transverse ridging and nail furrowing are associated with pathological processes.

29.30. Answer: A.
Intralesional corticosteroids are unlikely to be effective in sudden-onset alopecia universalis and is mainly indicated for patchy alopecia areata. There is no evidence for efficacy of topical minoxidil, finasteride or UVB phototherapy in the treatment of alopecia areata. The most appropriate option is psychological support and discussion of realistic expectations for hair regrowth, which may include whether she wishes to consider use of a wig, given the complete alopecia.

29.31. Answer: A.
As tumour necrosis factor alpha (TNF-α) antagonists have efficacy both in psoriasis and psoriatic arthritis, adalimumab would be the most appropriate next treatment approach to consider. Ciclosporin could only be used short-term and other treatment options would not be effective for psoriatic arthritis.

29.32. Answer: E.
Given that this patient is 93 years old and has other comorbidities, active treatment may result in ulceration and poor healing. Given that these lesions have not significantly changed and are asymptomatic and not bothering her, the most appropriate treatment option would likely be to leave these untreated, as the risk of significant change and development of invasive SCC is very low (approximately 3%). This case demonstrates how every patient must be individually assessed in order to ascertain what is most appropriate in any clinical scenario.

29.33. Answer: D.
Specific IgE testing is also known as the radioallergosorbent test (RAST) and could be helpful in this situation, which is most likely to have been caused by type I latex rubber allergy. Patch testing is used to investigate delayed type IV cell-mediated hypersensitivity. Prick testing may be positive and helpful in type I allergy but is risky to undertake in a patient who has already experienced angioedema as this may trigger anaphylaxis and should not be undertaken without anaesthetic support available. Thus, the specific IgE test would be a safe initial investigation. It is important to be aware that both specific IgE and prick testing can be falsely positive or falsely negative. If specific IgE testing is negative but clinical suspicion is high, further investigations with prick testing in a controlled situation could be indicated in order to try and clarify the diagnosis. IgG antibodies are not elevated in type I hypersensitivity reactions as the mechanism is mediated via IgE immediate antibody reactions. Oral challenge would not be appropriate and would, again, carry an unnecessary risk of anaphylaxis.

29.34. Answer: A.
As people get older there is reduced absorption and clearance of topical medications. Skin immune reactions are reduced with ageing. Photo-ageing is a different process to intrinsic

ageing but is superimposed on intrinsic ageing. There is increased susceptibility to irritants and irritant dermatitis. The skin becomes thin and atrophic with ageing.

29.35. Answer: C.
Circulating anti-epidermal antibodies may be present in bullous pemphigoid. In this condition, the split is below the basement membrane and therefore the subepidermal blisters are tense and intact. Nikolsky sign is thus negative. Mucous membrane involvement is uncommon in bullous pemphigoid. Eosinophilia is usually evident.

29.36. Answer: D.
Great caution needs to be taken with high doses of antihistamines in elderly patients because of the risk of over-sedation, delirium and falls. Likewise, low-dose tricyclic antidepressants may be considered but a high-dose approach would not be advisable. In the absence of rash, very potent topical glucocorticoids would be unlikely to be of therapeutic benefit and, in the elderly, adverse effects of striae and purpura may occur. Topical capsaicin would be unlikely to be of benefit for generalised pruritus as it can only be applied to localised areas.

29.37. Answer: B.
Oxygen is required for the photodynamic therapy effect. The cream contains a photosensitiser prodrug and not the photosensitiser itself as the prodrug needs to be taken up and converted to the photosensitiser in the skin cells. Laser light is not required for irradiation and most dermatological PDT is undertaken using broadband and light-emitting diode (LED) light sources. Nodular BCC can be treated with PDT, particularly if surgery is contraindicated. However, recurrence rates at 5 years are higher following PDT for nodular BCC than for surgical excision. PDT is often the most appropriate treatment choice for elderly frail patients. It can be used to treat large areas, on an outpatient basis, without the need for surgery and with improved healing.

29.38. Answer: E.
Malignant melanoma usually occurs on intermittently sun-exposed sites. The immunosuppressed patient population is most at risk of SCC, with only a slight increased risk of BCC. There is good epidemiological evidence to suggest that regular sunscreen use reduces the risk of actinic keratosis (AK) and SCC, although whilst assumed that it will reduce BCC risk, there is no good evidence to support this. In most BCCs, the PTCH1 gene mutations are somatic and not germline. SCC is a highly genetically heterogeneous tumour.

29.39. Answer: E.
Invasive SCC may arise de novo or from the background of AK. The risk of transformation of AK into invasive SCC is <1%. A field-directed approach, such as with 5-fluorouracil, PDT or imiquimod, is required for multiple AK and field-change carcinogenesis. Isolated lesions may be treated with a lesion-directed approach such as cryotherapy. Hyperkeratotic AK usually does not respond well to cryotherapy, and curettage and cautery and preparations containing salicylic acid in combination with 5-fluorourcil are usually required. Spontaneous resolution of AK may occur.

29.40. Answer: D.
Most patients with melanoma do not have a positive family history for melanoma and approximately 50% of melanomas arise from pre-existing naevus. Lentigo maligna melanoma tends to occur in the elderly, and acral melanoma is more common in dark-skinned populations. Nodular melanoma is more common in men.

29.41. Answer: C.
The description of the rash, the age of onset, associated systemic features of irritability, fever, extensive areas of rash with erosions and blistering, and systemic upset are most in keeping with staphylococcal scalded skin syndrome. Toxic epidermal necrolysis is much less likely in this age group and usually occurs in association with drug ingestion. Stevens–Johnson syndrome typically has mucosal involvement, lesions are more targetoid and often there is a precipitant of herpes simplex virus infection. Epidermolysis bullosa is a genetically inherited blistering disease, which does occur in children but is not associated with systemic upset. Impetigo is a localised form of superficial bacterial infection, usually due to Staphylococcus aureus.

29.42. Answer: B.
The description of the rash and its distribution are consistent with pityriasis versicolor and it is

29

likely that, as the patient has started to tan with phototherapy, the areas of hypopigmentation have become more obvious, making him aware of this second diagnosis. Pityriasis rosea would usually be more widespread, not just restricted to the central trunk, and would usually be associated with a herald patch. In addition, lesions would be erythematous and not hypopigmented. Polymorphic light eruption commonly occurs during phototherapy but is a papulovesicular eruption. This is unlikely to be psoriasis because it is hypopigmented and also other sites of psoriasis are improving with phototherapy. Secondary syphilis should always be considered with new development of erythematous scaly rash, but lesions do not tend to be hypopigmented and are usually more prominently found on distal sites, including palms and soles.

29.43. Answer: E.
Methotrexate can be very effective for chronic management of eczema, including atopic eczema. It would not be sensible to move to the newer drugs – apremilast or the biological agent dupilumab – without having a therapeutic trial of more conventional immunosuppressants such as methotrexate. Ciclosporin can be very effective for clearing eczema; however, for chronic disease activity without acute flare, the use of a drug that can only be continued in the short term would not be ideal. Acitretin would not usually be used in a woman of child-bearing age unless she had definitely completed her family, as there is a requirement for her to abstain from pregnancy for 3 years after cessation of drug because of teratogenicity.

29.44. Answer: B.
Biological agents blocking and inhibiting interleukin (IL)-4R and IL-13 are being trialled for use in atopic dermatitis. TNF-α inhibition and inhibition of IL-12, IL-23 and IL-17 pathways by biological agents have been shown to be effective in psoriasis.

29.45. Answer: C.
In the absence of a history of atopic dermatitis, bilateral dermatitis developing on the backs of hands and between the fingers in a young woman on maternity leave and likely to have a lot of exposure to water and detergents is most likely to be irritant contact dermatitis. Allergic contact dermatitis is a possibility and if irritant avoidance does not suffice then patch testing should be considered. Late-onset atopic

dermatitis would be unusual, although not impossible at this age. The distribution, however, is more suggestive of external causes. The distribution would be unusual for dermatophyte fungal infection as this is usually unilateral. Progesterone dermatitis is thought to be due to autoimmune sensitisation to progesterone and occurs cyclically with the menstrual cycle but this distribution would be unusual.

29.46. Answer: E.
Moderate-strength topical glucocorticoid such as Eumovate would usually not be sufficient to gain adequate control of significant eczema activity on the trunk and limbs, and increasing the potency of glucocorticoid to a potent agent such as betamethasone 17-valerate (Betnovate) would be likely to be more effective. Increasing the amount but not the potency would be unlikely to suffice. For chronic lichenified eczema, ointments are the preferred vehicle. Emulsifying ointment is a very good emollient and barrier for chronic lichenified eczema. Changing to aqueous cream, which can be irritant, would not be advisable. Increasing the dose of fexofenadine would be unlikely to be beneficial, as fexofenadine is a non-sedating antihistamine and, as atopic eczema is not primarily a histamine-mediated disease, the beneficial effect of antihistamines would usually be via sedating antihistamines, in order to break the itch/scratch cycle at night.

29.47. Answer: D.
Pustular psoriasis can often be triggered as a rebound secondary to commencement and sudden cessation of systemic glucocorticoids. It can also be triggered by topical use of glucocorticoids and other irritants, which include dithranol, coal tar and vitamin D analogues. These should all be avoided in pustular psoriasis. Whilst PUVA light therapy can often be effectively used in pustular psoriasis, UVB, although highly effective for chronic plaque psoriasis, often causes further flaring of unstable pustular disease. The effects of methotrexate may take several weeks to become established as it does not have a rapid onset of action.

29.48. Answer: B.
There are many common culprits for drug-induced lichenoid reactions, which include gold, penicillamine, thiazides, β-adrenoceptor antagonists (β-blockers), ACE inhibitors, proton pump inhibitors, non-steroidal anti-

inflammatories, antituberculous drugs, sulphonamides, lithium and antimalarials. The other drugs listed are not common culprits.

29.49. Answer: B.

With narrowband UVB phototherapy there is randomised controlled trial evidence to show efficacy in recalcitrant chronic urticaria. There is no conclusive evidence for the use of H_2 blockers, such as ranitidine, nor of montelukast, although both are widely used. There is no randomised controlled trial evidence showing efficacy with PUVA.

29.50. Answer: A.

Long-term treatment is often required as this condition, pemphigus, is an autoimmune blistering disorder that tends to last for many months or years; it requires long-term treatment to prevent disease relapse. The condition is more difficult to treat than bullous pemphigoid and higher doses of systemic glucocorticoids are required. There may be underlying malignancy but not in most cases. Investigations should be with this in mind. Penicillamine may actually trigger pemphigus and a positive Nikolsky sign indicates that there is superficial intra-epidermal blistering but does not necessarily indicate a drug-induced cause.

29.51. Answer: D.

The presence of a trichrome pattern, where normal skin colour, hypopigmentation and depigmentation are present, is a good prognostic factor. All of the others are poorer prognostic factors.

29.52. Answer: C.

The description of tense blistering, scarring and milia on photo-exposed sites of back of hands in a patient with underlying liver disease should strongly raise the suspicion of a diagnosis of porphyria cutanea tarda, which is almost invariably associated with chronic liver disease and iron overload. Examination findings are often not striking if the disease is relatively quiescent but the presence of scarring and milia should raise suspicions. The screening investigation of choice would be porphyrin plasma scan as a first step. The abnormal porphyrins in porphyria cutanea tarda are water soluble and thus biochemical analysis of urine will also show raised porphyrins in urine. Hepatitis C, per se, does not cause blistering and most patients with hepatitis C will not have porphyria cutanea tarda. Skin biopsy to exclude immunobullous disease such as bullous pemphigoid would not be the investigation of choice in this clinical setting as porphyria cutanea tarda should be suspected. There are characteristic changes of porphyria cutanea tarda on histology but, if the porphyrin investigations are abnormal, then skin biopsy would not necessarily be indicated, although it would be confirmatory. Blistering can occur in allergic contact dermatitis but blisters are usually multilocular and milia and scarring are uncommon. Thus, patch testing would not be the investigation of choice. In chronic renal failure, patients can present with a porphyria cutanea tarda-like presentation due to uraemia and this may be associated with some elevation of porphyrins due to impaired elimination. However, in a patient with known underlying chronic liver disease, the most likely diagnosis would be porphyria cutanea tarda.

29.53. Answer: B.

Erythema multiforme may have multiple triggers, which include infections and drugs. However, in many cases, a trigger is not identified. Where there is an evident provoking factor, this is most usually herpes simplex virus infection.

29.54. Answer: A.

The description of her presentation is very much consistent with drug reaction and eosinophilia with systemic symptoms (DRESS). This diagnosis is often confused with an infectious cause and patients are not uncommonly admitted to infectious diseases units for investigation. High fever can occur due to drug hypersensitivity and can be misleading. Facial oedema and lymphadenopathy, with eosinophilia and systemic involvement such as hepatitis, are classical features of DRESS. Carbamazepine is one of the most common culprits for DRESS. Co-codamol is not a typical culprit. Patients are usually investigated for underlying infection, including meningococcal infection given the purpura, and other causes of hepatitis. Overseas travel should always raise the possibility of an infectious cause. However, these patients are often extensively investigated for underlying infection because of high fever. The diagnosis of DRESS is often not reached until a dermatological consultation is requested or infection screening is negative, so this is a diagnosis to be aware of.

29

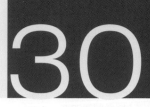

Maternal medicine

Multiple Choice Questions

30.1. A 25 year old woman with a 5-year history of rheumatoid arthritis is planning her first pregnancy. Which of the following drugs should be avoided in pregnancy?

A. Azathioprine
B. Hydroxychloroquine
C. Methotrexate
D. Prednisolone
E. Sulfasalazine

30.2. A 40 year old woman is 6 weeks pregnant. She has a diagnosis of epilepsy. Which of the following pieces of advice is correct?

A. Drug doses should routinely be doubled in the second trimester
B. Pregnancy reduces the frequency of seizures
C. She should start high-dose folic acid
D. She should stop anticonvulsant therapy
E. Sodium valproate is the antiepileptic drug of choice in pregnancy

30.3. An 18 year old woman is admitted to the gynaecology ward at 8 weeks' gestation in her first pregnancy. She has a known diagnosis of epilepsy and takes levetiracetam. Her epilepsy is usually well controlled but she has had three seizures in the last 2 days. Four of the answers below need to be considered as possible contributing factors; however, one is unlikely. Which of the following factors is LEAST likely to have contributed to the increasing frequency of seizures?

A. Serum drug levels have reduced due to increased renal clearance and increased plasma volume
B. She has nausea and vomiting of pregnancy and cannot keep her tablets down

C. She has stopped her medication for fear of teratogenicity
D. She is anxious about the pregnancy and is having pseudoseizures
E. Sleep deprivation has caused a worsening of her epilepsy

30.4. A 35 year old primiparous woman attends the antenatal day unit at 18 weeks' gestation with a history of vomiting, dysuria, left loin pain and rigors for 24 hours. A urine dipstick is positive for leucocytes and nitrites. Her C-reactive protein is 140 mg/L. Which of the following findings on examination and investigation would require urgent attention?

A. A decrease in urea and creatinine values from her pre-pregnancy levels
B. A mild respiratory alkalosis on the arterial blood gas
C. A raised alkaline phosphatase result
D. A respiratory rate of 24 breaths/min
E. The presence of a systolic murmur

30.5. A 22 year old woman is 9 weeks into her first pregnancy, and presents with vomiting. Which of the following is a feature of hyperemesis gravidarum?

A. Abdominal pain
B. Hyper-reflexia
C. Lactate >2 mmol/L (18.0 mg/dL)
D. Vomiting intermittently
E. Weight loss >5%

30.6. A 34 year old primiparous woman is admitted to hospital at 32 weeks' gestation with central crushing chest pain, ST segment elevation on her electrocardiogram (ECG) and a troponin T of 840 ng/L. She has a background of smoking a pack of cigarettes daily for 18 years, essential hypertension and a family history of ischaemic heart disease. Which of the following is the appropriate management?

A. Aspirin 300 mg
B. Aspirin, clopidogrel and fondaparinux
C. Primary percutaneous coronary intervention (PPCI)
D. Therapeutic low-molecular-weight heparin
E. Thrombolysis with alteplase

30.7. A 19 year old woman is contemplating her first pregnancy. She has lupus nephritis, which is stable and takes azathioprine and tacrolimus. Which of the following pieces of advice should she be given?

A. She is at increased risk of fetal growth restriction
B. She is likely to be infertile
C. She should be warned that dialysis is contraindicated in pregnancy
D. She should start antihypertensive therapy prior to conception
E. She should stop her tacrolimus

30.8. A 30 year old woman, who is normally well, is 22 weeks into her second pregnancy and is seen on the acute medical unit with cough with green sputum for the last 3 days. Her respiratory rate is 12 breaths/min, oxygen saturations 98% on air, blood pressure 110/76 mmHg, heart rate 90 beats/min and temperature 38.4°C. Her chest X-ray shows right middle lobe consolidation.

Which of the following is the most appropriate treatment?

A. Amoxicillin 500 mg 3 times daily and clarithromycin 500 mg twice daily
B. Doxycycline 200 mg immediately, then 100 mg daily thereafter
C. Oseltamivir 75 mg twice daily for 5 days
D. Piperacillin/tazobactam (Tazocin) 4.5 g intravenously (IV) 3 times daily
E. Trimethoprim 200 mg twice daily

30.9. A 17 year old woman who is 30 weeks into her first pregnancy is admitted to hospital with acute severe asthma. Which of the following statements is TRUE?

A. Chest X-ray is generally avoided in this situation
B. Inhalers should be stopped in pregnancy

C. Intravenous magnesium sulphate is contraindicated
D. Nebulised salbutamol can be given safely
E. Peak flow measurement is not helpful in pregnancy

30.10. A 36 year old woman with type 2 diabetes is planning her first pregnancy. She takes metformin 500 mg 3 times daily and her HbA$_{1c}$ is 45 mmol/mol (6.3%). Which of the following pieces of advice should she be given regarding medication?

A. Double her metformin dose before she conceives
B. Start aspirin 75 mg daily at 12 weeks' gestation
C. Start gliclazide 40 mg daily after she has conceived
D. Start subcutaneous insulin at 12 weeks' gestation
E. Stop metformin after she has conceived

30.11. A 40 year old woman is examined at 32 weeks' gestation in the antenatal clinic. She has upper abdominal pain and pruritus. Which of the following physical signs can be part of normal pregnancy?

A. Ascites
B. Palmar pigmentation
C. Spider naevi
D. Upper abdominal tenderness
E. Yellow sclerae

30.12. An 18 year old woman presents at 36 weeks' gestation with 24 hours of vomiting. The differential diagnosis includes viral gastroenteritis, pre-eclampsia/haemolysis, elevated liver enzymes, and low platelets (HELLP) and acute fatty liver of pregnancy. Which of the following would be in keeping with a diagnosis of acute fatty liver of pregnancy?

A. Blood glucose 3.2 mmol/L (58 mg/dL)
B. Creatinine 100 μmol/L (1.13 mg/dL)
C. Oliguria
D. Platelets 85 × 10^9/L
E. Temperature 39°C

30.13. A 25 year old woman with ulcerative colitis is planning her first pregnancy, and attends clinic for pre-pregnancy counselling. Which of the following pieces of advice is TRUE?

A. She should be advised against pregnancy
B. She should stop taking sulfasalazine during the first trimester

30

C. She should deliver by caesarean section

D. She should stop infliximab once she has conceived

E. She should stop taking methotrexate 3 months prior to conception

30.14. A 42 year old woman presents at 12 weeks post-partum with palpitations and irritability. On examination she has a fine tremor. What is the most likely diagnosis?

A. Anxiety

B. Graves' disease

C. Hashimotos's thyroiditis

D. Post-partum depression

E. Post-partum thyroiditis

Answers

30.1. Answer: C.
Methotrexate should be stopped 3 months before pregnancy and throughout pregnancy and breastfeeding. All other medications can be taken during pregnancy and breastfeeding. Women taking sulfasalazine should also receive high-dose (5 mg daily) folic acid from pre-conception until at least 12 weeks' gestation.

30.2. Answer: C.
Women with epilepsy should take high-dose folic acid prior to conception and throughout the pregnancy. This is because women with epilepsy who take antiepileptic drugs (AEDs) that induce cytochrome P450 (for example phenytoin, carbamazepine) are at risk of low levels of folic acid. Anticonvulsant therapy should be reviewed prior to conception, and should not be stopped. Sodium valproate is associated with a higher risk of major congenital malformations compared to other AEDs and there should be a discussion between the woman and her epilepsy specialist about switching to another AED prior to pregnancy. Pregnancy does not reduce the frequency of seizures. Women with well-controlled epilepsy are not more likely to have increased seizures in pregnancy, but those with poorly controlled epilepsy may find their condition deteriorates. There is no rationale for routinely doubling drug doses in the second trimester, although some AEDs, for example lamotrigine, may need a dose increase during pregnancy.

30.3. Answer: D.
Profound physiological changes in pregnancy can cause a significant reduction in serum concentrations of some drugs – this is particularly true for lamotrigine and levetiracetam. Non-adherence is common due to concerns over teratogencity and non-reassurance or reticence to prescribe by health-care professionals. Nausea and vomiting is very common in early pregnancy and antiemetics may be used safely to allow regular medication to be given. All these factors need to be thought about and addressed to ensure women feel confident and comfortable in their decisions and their chronic condition can be optimally managed in pregnancy. Pseudoseizures in this scenario would be very uncommon.

30.4. Answer: D.
Pregnancy does not cause a significant increase in respiratory rate. A respiratory rate >20 breaths/min is abnormal in pregnancy. All of the others are part of normal physiological changes of pregnancy.

30.5. Answer: E.
Hyperemesis gravidarum (HG) can be diagnosed in the first trimester of pregnancy, when other causes of persistent nausea and vomiting have been excluded. It is associated with >5% pre-pregnancy weight loss, electrolyte imbalance and dehydration. Nausea and vomiting in pregnancy (NVP) is common, but not all of these women have HG.

30.6. Answer: C.
Myocardial infarction is more common in pregnancy compared to age-matched controls. PPCI is not contraindicated in pregnancy, and should be carried out where benefits outweigh risks. Both chest X-rays and ECGs are useful investigations for chest pain in pregnancy. Management of chest pain where an acute coronary syndrome is suspected should be the same as in a non-pregnant woman.

30.7. Answer: A.

Many women with chronic kidney disease (CKD) have successful pregnancies. However, there are increased risks of pre-eclampsia, fetal growth restriction, miscarriage, pre-term delivery and fetal death for these women. Women with CKD are more likely to require antihypertensives, but they do not need to be started routinely. Women who are already taking angiotensin-converting enzyme inhibitors should stop this drug at conception and switch to an alternative therapy, such as labetalol, methyldopa or nifedipine.

30.8. Answer: A.

The diagnosis is community-acquired pneumonia. Doxycycline is a tetracycline and is associated with discolouration of infant teeth when used in the second and third trimesters. Intravenous Tazocin is unnecessary, and oral therapy is more appropriate for this woman. Oseltamivir is not indicated for community-acquired pneumonia. Trimethoprim is not an appropriate antibiotic for community-acquired pneumonia: it is avoided in the first trimester due to its anti-folate effects. Amoxicillin and clarithromycin are the most appropriate choice of antibiotic for community-acquired pneumonia, and both are safe in pregnancy.

30.9. Answer: D.

Chest X-ray should be carried out for the same reasons as outside of pregnancy, and is safe. Nebulised salbutamol and ipratropium, steroids, magnesium sulphate and aminophylline can all be given safely in pregnancy. Peak flow measurement is valid in pregnancy, and should be carried out. Women should be advised to continue their inhalers in pregnancy, and aim for freedom from symptoms.

30.10. Answer: B.

Women with type 2 diabetes should take aspirin 75 mg once daily from 12 weeks' gestation to delivery to reduce the risk of developing pre-eclampsia. Insulin and metformin are both used to manage women with type 2 diabetes in pregnancy. Tight glycaemic control is advocated prior to pregnancy to reduce the risk of major congenital malformations and miscarriage but the decision to alter medication is based on blood glucose levels (BGs); therefore the first step would be to start monitoring BGs before deciding on treatment.

30.11. Answer: C.

Spider naevi and palmar erythema (not pigmentation) can be part of normal pregnancy, and are also signs of chronic liver disease. The other physical signs are not seen in normal pregnancy. Ascites is observed in chronic liver disease, and yellow sclerae indicate raised bilirubin, which is not part of normal pregnancy.

30.12. Answer: A.

Oliguria could be associated with viral gastroenteritis if there was an associated acute kidney injury (AKI). Creatinine of 100 μmol/L (1.13 mg/dL) could be seen in pre-eclampsia/HELLP and gastroenteritis with an AKI. A blood glucose of <4 mmol/L (72 mg/dL) is a feature of acute fatty liver of pregnancy (AFLP), and is one of the 'Swansea Criteria' for diagnosis of AFLP. This condition is associated with polydipsia/polyuria. Creatinine >150 μmol/L (>1.70 mg/dL) is a feature of AFLP. It is associated with hypoglycaemia, but not typically thrombocytopenia or a fever. Thrombocytopenia is more commonly associated with pre-eclampsia/HELLP.

30.13. Answer: E.

Some women with complex ulcerative colitis will require a caesarean section, but this mode of delivery is usually reserved for obstetric indications. Methotrexate is teratogenic and should be stopped 3 months prior to conception. Most women with well-controlled ulcerative colitis will have uneventful pregnancies. Sulfasalazine can be taken safely throughout pregnancy. Infliximab can be taken safely in the first and second trimesters.

30.14. Answer: E.

Post-partum thyroiditis commonly presents at 3–4 months post-delivery, although it can present up to 6 months post-delivery. It can present with a transient hyperthyroidism, hypothyroidism, or a biphasic pattern, with a period of hyperthyroidism followed by hypothyroidism. Graves' disease is possible, but post-partum thyroiditis is more likely at 12 weeks post-partum. Hashimoto's thyroiditis leads to symptoms of fatigue, weight gain, cold intolerance, constipation and depression (in association with biochemical hypothyroidism). Post-partum depression and anxiety can only be diagnosed once organic causes of symptoms and signs have been excluded.

30

31

Adolescent and transition medicine

Multiple Choice Questions

31.1. Adolescence is a complex developmental stage characterised by physical, biochemical and emotional changes that see a child or young person transition to adulthood. Which of the following statements is true about male pubertal physiology?

A. Follicle-stimulating hormone (FSH) production ultimately stimulates the growth of pubic, facial and axillary hair

B. Gonadatrophin-releasing hormone (GnRH) produced in the pituitary stimulates luteinising hormone (LH) and FSH release from the hypothalamus

C. Growth hormone increases skeletal growth and promotes development of the male genital organs

D. Leydig cells in the testis produce testosterone

E. Puberty is initiated by pulsatile release of testosterone in the testis

31.2. In relation to the normal adolescent female, which of the following statements is most correct?

A. A fall in growth hormone levels is associated with a climb in insulin-like growth factors 1 and 2 (IGF-1 and IGF-2)

B. Breast bud development and the development of pubic hair are seen around the time of menarche

C. Insulin levels fall by around 30%, coinciding with an increased risk of type 2 diabetes

D. Investigation should be considered if she has not started menstruating by the age of 18 years

E. The ovary produces both oestrogen and testosterone and there is a rise in adrenal androgen production

31.3. Adolescence is a period of time when adherence with medications and treatment regimes can fall significantly. Which factors might predict that a young person is at particular risk of low adherence?

A. Acceptance of the seriousness of their health problems

B. Female gender

C. High self-esteem and high levels of self-confidence and motivation

D. Patients treated with complex medicines

E. Use of treatments with good short-term symptom relief

31.4. On a global basis, what is the commonest cause of death in adolescents?

A. Complications of pregnancy

B. Infective gastroenteritis

C. Late effects of childhood cancer treatment

D. Malaria

E. Road injury

31.5. Which of the following characteristics are particularly associated with risk-taking behaviours in teenagers?

A. Female gender

B. Having good health and high levels of physical well-being

C. Higher educational status

D. Maturation of the prefontal cortex, resulting in development of frontal lobe control

E. Maturity of the frontostriatal reward circuits, encouraging novel and adult-like activities

31.6. Which of the following is a key component of a successful transition programme?

A. A dedicated transition nurse to support patient education throughout adolescence

B. A range of detailed patient information leaflets about the patient's medical condition and treatment and prognosis

C. A well-developed website/online support service with up-to-date information about the service and transition arrangements

D. A written transition policy, developed in conjunction with young patients and implemented with a staff training package

E. Access to a patient support group

31.7. At your first appointment with a 17 year old female kidney transplant recipient, she discloses that she is pregnant. The pregnancy is unplanned. Her current treatment comprises alternate-day prednisolone, mycophenolate mofetil, enalapril, amlodipine and azathioprine. Which of the following statements is most correct in relation to the pregnancy?

A. Mycophenolate is the immunosuppressant of choice in pregnancy

B. Prednisolone easily crosses the placenta and causes a risk of impaired fetal growth

C. Stable blood pressure control is essential and enalapril should be continued

D. The patient needs to be aware that pregnancy adversely affects long-term renal allograft survival so close monitoring is necessary

E. There is an increased risk of pre-eclampsia in women who have received a renal transplant

31.8. You have just completed a consultation with a 17 year old male with epilepsy. He is about to leave college and asks for advice about employment and driving. He is seeking further information about other lifestyle choices. Which of the following statements is true?

A. Illicit drugs can affect seizure threshold, as well as affect adherence to antiepileptic drugs (AEDs)

B. In the UK he will not be able to drive unless he is seizure-free for 2 years

C. Sodium valproate can affect spermatogenesis and is teratogenic when taken by men

D. There is no evidence that alcohol independently affects seizure control, so he does not need to be concerned about his alcohol intake

E. There are no restrictions on application for jobs in the armed forces

31.9. A 17 year old male with a diagnosis of ulcerative colitis has been referred to your clinic. He is currently well and completely asymptomatic on mesalazine. The only relevant history is that his healthy brother has recently been investigated for a raised bilirubin. Routine liver function tests are as detailed:

Alkaline phosphatase 420 U/L, alanine aminotransferase 36 U/L, bilirubin 34 µmol/L (1.99 mg/dL), albumin 48 g/L, γ-glutamyl transferase (GGT) 25 U/L.
Which of the following is true?

A. Gilbert's syndrome is a common cause of hyperbilirubinaemia and is the most likely explanation of these liver function tests

B. It is important to check hepatitis serology

C. It is important to undertake alkaline phosphatase isoenzymes to exclude bone or liver disease

D. The albumin suggests active inflammatory bowel disease

E. The alkaline phosphatase result suggests vitamin D deficiency

31.10. A 20 year old woman with learning difficulties and epilepsy is attending your clinic for the first time. She is accompanied by her new boyfriend who she has just started living with. She is currently taking high-dose sodium valproate and has generalised seizures every few weeks. What is your highest priority to clarify or assess during your consultation?

A. Assess her sodium valproate levels as you are concerned about adherence

B. Find out whether she is taking any recreational drugs

C. Procure a detailed family history, particularly regarding epilepsy risk

D. Request an up-to-date electroencephalo-gram report

E. Review the patient's and her partner's understanding of teratogenicity of sodium valproate, their plans for having children and/or whether they are using contraception

31

31.11. You are taking over the care of a 18 year old male with severe spastic quadriplegic cerebral palsy. Which of the following statements is true?

A. A common cause of mortality is renal failure related to recurrent urinary tract infections
B. Formal assessment of respiratory function such as spirometery and peak flows will help assess respiratory risks
C. Gastro-oesophageal reflux is an important comorbidity that needs to be assessed and treated if necessary
D. Now that he is 18 years old he automatically assumes the capacity to consent to treatment and decisions about his care
E. Nutritional support is unlikely to be necessary now growth has been completed

31.12. An 18 year old male with Duchenne muscular dystrophy is admitted in end-stage respiratory failure. After treatment with antibiotics and stabilisation on non-invasive respiratory support, he is ready for discharge with ongoing respiratory support and careful long-term follow-up. At his next clinic appointment, he asks for a discussion about the genetics of his condition and how it might involve his wider family – his younger brother is also a Duchenne sufferer. He has a 10 year old sister.
Which of the following statements are true?

A. He will be infertile
B. His father must be a carrier of the Duchenne gene
C. His sister could be affected
D. His sister should be referred for genetic testing for carrier status
E. There are no genetic implications for second-generation family members

31.13. A 17 year old female with cystic fibrosis (CF) is referred to your adolescent respiratory clinic. She has good nutritional status and is generally well, attending full-time school. Which of the following are true regarding her current status?

A. As she has good nutritional status and growth, her bone mineral density is likely to be normal and treatment with vitamin D is not necessary
B. Clarithromycin will affect oral contraceptive pill (OCP) effectiveness
C. Most patients gain benefit from newer treatments that rectify defects in the CF

transmembrane conductance regulator (CFTR) protein
D. She is likely to be infertile, and the chances of pregnancy are low
E. The OCP seems to be safe and effective for most patients with CF

31.14. An 18 year old female has been referred to your late-effects clinic, after treatment for acute lymphoblastic leukaemia (ALL) in childhood, ultimately requiring treatment with total body irradiation and bone marrow transplantation at 15 years of age. She is currently treated with thyroxine but her general health seems good. Which of the following statements is true?

A. As her periods are regular she can be reassured of normal fertility in the future
B. Her risk of future malignancy is no higher than the normal population
C. She has previously been treated with high-dose doxorubicin and therefore is at risk of cardiomyopathy
D. She needs 7 years more follow-up before discharge, as 10-year disease-free survival equates to cure in ALL
E. When plotted on a centile chart, her growth is 50th centile for height and weight, suggesting she has normal growth hormone levels

31.15. A 16 year old girl has undergone liver transplant following a Kasai procedure for biliary atresia in the newborn period. She has been well for 8 years post-transplant. She had a viral illness characterised by lymphadenopathy, malaise and hepatosplenomegaly 6 months ago and now has persistent palpable cervical lymphadenopathy. Which of these statements is most correct?

A. If her lymphadenopathy persists you need to consider blood tests, including a full blood count, liver function tests, Epstein–Barr virus (EBV) and cytomegalovirus (CMV) PCR and serology
B. She is at increased risk of chronic fatigue syndrome
C. T-cell activation and proliferation is the likely underlying pathological process in post-transplant lymphoproliferative disorder (PTLD), often triggered by EBV infection
D. The most likely cause of her infection was hepatitis B infection
E. There is a 10% chance of this being a PTLD

31.16. A 16 year old boy presents with an 8-week history of diarrhoea, weight loss and raised inflammatory markers. A biopsy is consistent with Crohn's disease. Which of the following is the most correct statement in relation to this case?

A. Anti-tumour necrosis factor (TNF) therapy, for example infliximab, is more commonly needed for adolescents, and he has about a 50% chance of needing treatment with a biological agent.
B. First-line treatment is with steroid therapy, most commonly oral prednisolone or pulsed intravenous methylprednisolone
C. Methotrexate is a helpful first-line maintenance therapy
D. There is a 50% chance of him requiring surgery in the next 5 years
E. When offering lifestyle advice, particular emphasis should be given to reducing smoking, as smoking increases disease activity and reduces effectiveness of biological agents

31.17. Adherence with treatment is a particular challenge for teenagers and young adults with long-term medical conditions such as diabetes. Which of the following statements is most correct in relation to studies in adolescents with diabetes?

A. About 15% of adolescents do not check blood glucose levels regularly and fabricate results for the medical team looking after them

B. Eighty per cent of adolescents follow their diet reasonably well
C. In females, concern about body image, including the desire for weight loss, can be a significant factor in non-adherence to insulin therapy
D. Microvascular complications can begin from 20 years after diagnosis, and so can already be emerging in patients in their 20s and 30s
E. The majority of patients do not take their insulin injections reliably and this results in an increased admission rate with diabetic ketoacidosis (DKA)

31.18. When planning adult services for a young person with juvenile idiopathic arthritis (JIA), which one of the following statements is most accurate?

A. All children with oligoarticular juvenile arthritis will require long-term follow-up into adulthood
B. Antinuclear antibody (ANA)-positive patients need ophthalmic screening for eye involvement
C. Methotrexate is a first-line treatment if multiple joints are affected, and it should be used early, particularly in polyarticular JIA
D. Systemic JIA can often be treated with a combination of long-term NSAIDs and systemic glucocorticoids
E. When offering lifestyle advice, particular emphasis should be given to reducing alcohol intake as it increases disease activity and reduces effectiveness of biological agents

Answers

31.1. Answer: D.
Puberty is initiated by pulsatile GnRH production, which stimulates FSH and LH production in the pituitary gland. LH stimulates Leydig cells in the testis to produce testosterone, which causes androgenisation and skeletal growth. FSH acts on Sertoli cells to stimulate spermatogenesis and not to increase androgenisation.

31.2. Answer: E.
Adolescent females have a increase in testosterone and androgen production (manifest as the development of pubic hair, increased sweating, acne) from the ovaries and the adrenal glands. The earliest pubertal

changes are breast bud development and early pubic hair growth, which can be seen from around 10 years of age. Menarche arises relatively late in puberty, but an adolescent who has not started her periods by 16 years of age should be investigated for delayed puberty. Growth hormone levels, IGF-1 and IGF-2 levels climb steadily during puberty, as do insulin levels by about 30%.

31.3. Answer: D.
Complex medicine and treatment regimes make it harder for young people to adhere strictly to their treatment. The other factors are all associated with better patient adherence with medication and treatment regimes, and in

31

many conditions have been associated with a better long-term outlook. Younger patients find it harder to adhere to medicines where the long-term health benefits are considerable if there is no short-term improvement in symptoms.

31.4. Answer: E.
Road injury/fatal road traffic accidents account for a significant proportion of adolescent deaths on a worldwide basis. Death from road injury is independently associated with alcohol and drug ingestion. Whilst malaria and infective gastroenteritis are important causes of death in younger children, teenagers have better immune responses and these conditions are a common cause of morbidity but have a lower mortality rate than in younger children. Lower respiratory tract infections and suicide are also important global causes of adolescent mortality.

31.5. Answer: E.
The highest-risk adolescents, in terms of risk-taking and self-harming behaviour such as heavy alcohol intake, illicit drug ingestion and non-adherence to treatment regimes, are males, older adolescents and those with serious long-term health conditions. It is thought that maturation of the frontostriatal reward circuits in early/mid-adolescence drives individuals towards impulsive and pleasure-seeking behaviours that place the adolescent at risk. With time, frontal lobe control of impulsivity improves and more stable and safe behaviour patterns develop.

31.6. Answer: D.
The starting point in the development of an effective transition policy is the local development of a programme that meets the medical, social and cultural needs of your local population. The other measures may support the implementation of your transition programme, but often services overly focus upon a series of information-giving interventions rather than developing an ethos of patient autonomy and control.

31.7. Answer: E.
There is an increased risk of hypertension during pregnancy in all women with renal disease, so they require close monitoring throughout – the pre-eclampsia rate is around 30%. Prednisolone crosses the placenta poorly and is not a particular risk to the fetus. Neither mycophenolate nor azathioprine are safe during pregnancy. When pregnancy is diagnosed, angiotensin-converting enzyme (ACE) inhibitors should be stopped immediately, and alternative therapy commenced, due to human fetotoxicity. With careful monitoring, transplant survival rates are good.

31.8. Answer: A.
Illicit drugs have an adverse affect on seizure control through both lowering seizure threshold and adversely affecting adherence. Alcohol does not seem to independently increase seizure activity, but binge drinking can be associated with significant sleep disturbance and reduced AED compliance. In the UK, drivers are not permitted to drive unless they have had no daytime seizures for 1 year, but if seizures only occur during sleep then driving can be considered. There is no evidence of teratogenicity in men taking sodium valproate but it reduces sperm count in some. In most parts of the world there are restrictions on entry to the armed forces, driving heavy goods vehicles and driving emergency vehicles.

31.9. Answer: A.
The liver function tests (including raised alkaline phosphatase) are normal for a male of this age, with the exception of the isolated raised bilirubin. Hypoalbuminaemia can be a marker of inflammatory bowel disease, but this albumin is normal. There is no need to check alkaline phosphatase isoenzymes as the GGT is normal. Gilbert's syndrome affects 5–10% of the Western European population, and is one of the commonest causes of isolated elevation in bilirubin. It is autosomally recessively inherited and so his brother's jaundice is likely to also be due to Gilbert's syndrome.

31.10. Answer: E.
All these issues may be important. However, in a young person who has recently started a sexual relationship, establishing his/her understanding of the reproductive implications of his/her condition and treatment is of vital importance – particularly with an agent as teratogenic as sodium valproate.

31.11. Answer: C.
Gastro-oesophageal reflux is common in patients with severe neurodisability. It places patients at significant risk of aspiration as they may not have adequate airway-protective

reflexes. Most patients with four-limb cerebral palsy are also intellectually impaired, and many do not have the capacity to give informed consent. They are unlikely to be able to comply with formal lung function tests, although respiratory disease, often complicated by recurrent chest infections or aspiration and scoliois, is a common cause of death. Many do not manage to ingest their full nutritional requirements and need additional/supportive feeding, often by gastrostomy.

31.12. Answer: C.

Female carriers of Duchenne muscular dystrophy are at risk of cardiomyopathy and around 10% also experience muscle weakness and fatigue. They should be referred for genetic testing when they are able to understand the implications of the diagnosis, possibly in the mid-teens. This patient's mother must be a carrier of the Duchenne muscular dystrophy gene, not his father, and his sister has a 50% risk of also being a carrier. Fertility is normal in males. There are potentially risks for the wider family, with his mother's sisters having a 50% chance of being carriers of the Duchenne genetic mutation.

31.13. Answer: E.

The OCP is contraindicated in patients with pulmonary hypertension but is safe and effective in most patients with CF. There is increasing evidence of effectiveness of CFTR modification in patients with specified (G551D) CFTR gene mutations, but these affect a very small proportion of CF sufferers. Females with CF usually have normal fertility if their general nutrition and health are good; males have obstructive azoospermia. All patients are at significant risk of osteoporosis.

31.14. Answer: C.

There is a well-recognised risk of cardiomyopathy in patients exposed to high-dose anthracyclines such as doxorubicin, so long-term follow-up is recommended. There is also an increased risk of second malignancy. Many female survivors of childhood cancer have reduced long-term fertility due to reduced ovarian reserves, and total-body irradiation makes this patient at risk of pituitary dysfunction, including growth hormone deficiency. The hypothyroidism might be central or peripheral in aetiology.

31.15. Answer: E.

PTLD is a well-recognised complication occurring in more than 10% of solid organ recipients – particularly those who receive a solid organ in childhood when they are commonly EBV seronegative. It is often triggered by EBV infection leading to uncontrolled B-cell proliferation and tumour proliferation, including development of lymphoma. Blood tests need to be undertaken immediately in this high-risk patient and further investigation for possible lymphoma is necessary.

31.16. Answer: E.

Smoking is a particular risk factor for exacerbation and reduces effectiveness of many immunosuppressant therapies, as well as increasing the risk of steroid and other therapy. Adolescents/teenagers do have more aggressive disease than older patients, and about 20% will require surgery or treatment with biological agents. First-line therapy is a 6- to 8-week trial of elemental diet; methotrexate is used as maintenance therapy but is not a first-line agent.

31.17. Answer: C.

A few adolescents present with repeated episodes of DKA because of non-adherence with insulin therapy. In females it is thought that motivating factors might include weight loss/concerns about body image. The extent of non-adherence amongst adolescents is high, with 25% not taking their insulin as prescribed, 80% not following their diet and around 30% not checking blood glucose and/or submitting fabricated results. Microvascular complications can develop within 10 years of diagnosis, so may already be present in later teenage years.

31.18. Answer: C.

Methotrexate and earlier use of anti-TNF agents such as etanercept have significantly improved outcome in the 30% of patients with polyarticular JIA. All patients, even those who are not ANA positive, need screening for uveitis, which can be silent and persist into adulthood (Box 31.18). As many as 50% of children with oligoarticular JIA go into remission, so long-term follow-up into adulthood may not be required.

31

i 31.18 Juvenile idiopathic arthritis in adolescence

Uveitis: may be clinically silent and persist into adulthood. All (not just those who are ANA positive) need ophthalmic screening for eye involvement.

Persistence into adulthood: occurs in 50% of cases, especially in systemic disease. Specific supportive management through transition from adolescence to adulthood should be planned.

Reduced peak bone mass: common in polyarthritis and systemic juvenile idiopathic arthritis but there are few data on fracture risk and the evidence base for treatment is poor.

Therapy: methotrexate is standard treatment, used after NSAIDs alone are insufficient. Anti-TNF therapy is effective in all forms of juvenile idiopathic arthritis but long-term safety remains unclear.

(ANA = antinuclear antibody; NSAIDs = non-steroidal anti-inflammatory drugs; TNF = tumour necrosis factor)

32

Ageing and disease

Multiple Choice Questions

32.1. A 79 year old man who lives in his own home presents with several recent falls, all of which have taken place whilst walking in town. Witnesses report no loss of consciousness. He takes thyroxine and paracetamol but no other medications. Which of the following interventions is most likely to reduce his risk of falls?

A. Calcium and vitamin D supplementation
B. Cardiac pacemaker
C. Hip protectors
D. Home environment modification
E. Strength and balance training

32.2. An 86 year old woman complains of incontinence for the last 2 years. She describes wanting to pass urine 10–12 times a day, has to rush to the toilet, and if she does not get there in time, urine is passed in a flood. Which of the following would be the most useful treatment for her symptoms?

A. Antimuscarinic medication
B. Long-term prophylactic antibiotics
C. Long-term urinary catheter
D. Pelvic floor muscle training
E. Tension-free vaginal tape surgery

32.3. A 68 year old woman presents complaining of dizziness. She says that this started 2 days ago, and that she cannot walk in a straight line. She feels sick and the room is spinning. What is the most likely cause?

A. Fast atrial fibrillation
B. Lumbar nerve root entrapment
C. Orthostatic hypotension

D. Transient ischaemic attack
E. Vestibular neuronitis

32.4. An 84 year old man presents with falls and ankle swelling. He was started on amlodipine 3 months ago for hypertension, and started furosemide 2 weeks ago for the ankle swelling. He complains of feeling lightheaded when standing, and thinks he might have lost consciousness before the last fall. His blood pressure is 165/97 mmHg lying, 142/88 mmHg standing.

What changes to his medication are most appropriate?

A. Add an angiotensin-converting enzyme (ACE) inhibitor, continue the amlodipine and furosemide
B. Add an ACE inhibitor and stop the amlodipine
C. Stop the furosemide and amlodipine
D. Stop the furosemide and amlodipine and add an α-adrenoceptor antagonist (α-blocker)
E. Stop the furosemide and continue the amlodipine

32.5. Which of the following is an essential component of a successful rehabilitation programme?

A. A dedicated rehabilitation ward
B. Clearly defined diagnoses
C. Goal setting
D. Medical leadership
E. The Barthel Index

32.6. Which of the following outcomes does Comprehensive Geriatric Assessment (CGA) improve?

A. Chance of living independently at 6 months
B. Mortality at 3 years
C. Speed of recovery from surgery
D. Time to onset of dementia
E. Time to onset of frailty

32.7. A 76 year old man is admitted to hospital with a urinary tract infection. As the admitting doctor, you are concerned that he is frail. Which of the following measurements would most assist you in assessing whether he is frail?

A. Blood pressure
B. Body mass index
C. Hand grip strength
D. Number of medications
E. Six-minute walk distance

32.8. You see an 87 year old woman in your clinic, newly diagnosed with heart failure with preserved systolic function. She is sceptical that her condition is real, and would prefer to attribute it to old age. Which one of the following cardiovascular changes is attributable to normal ageing?

A. Development of left ventricular hypertrophy
B. Fatty infiltration of the myocardium
C. Increased left ventricular end diastolic volume
D. Reduced left ventricular ejection fraction
E. Reduced maximum heart rate

32.9. You are assessing a 78 year old woman as part of Comprehensive Geriatric Assessment. Which one of the following measurements would best allow you to predict her falls risk?

A. Abbreviated Mental Test score
B. Barthel Index
C. Hand grip strength
D. Six-minute walk test
E. Timed 'get up and go' test

32.10. You are assessing a 91 year old man who recently fractured his hip in a fall. Which one of the following components of examination is most likely to influence your immediate management of his falls risk?

A. Cardiac auscultation
B. Geriatric Depression Scale
C. Hallpike manoeuvre

D. Hip extension range
E. Supine blood pressure

32.11. An 82 year old man presents with delirium, which has been gradually worsening for 6 weeks. His niece thinks that it started after his last hospital stay, when he was treated for pneumonia. His blood tests show a sodium of 122 mmol/L. What is the most likely cause for his hyponatraemia and delirium?

A. Addison's disease
B. Bendroflumethiazide
C. Carcinoma of the lung
D. Ibuprofen
E. Inadequate salt intake

32.12. A 92 year old woman presents with urinary incontinence, which the nursing home staff are finding difficult to manage. She has severe dementia, and the incontinence has been gradually worsening for several years. She often declines to wear incontinence pads, appears to be unaware that she needs to pass urine, and consequently is found by the staff to have been incontinent sitting in her chair. Which management strategy is most likely to improve her continence?

A. A course of antibiotics
B. Intermittent self-catheterisation
C. Long-term urinary catheter
D. Pelvic floor exercises
E. Regular prompted toileting

32.13. You are assessing an 83 year old woman, who wishes to undergo a hip replacement. She has not lost any weight in the last 12 months, her grip strength is 15 kg, and her 5 m walk time is 6 seconds. She admits to feeling tired a lot of the time, but still manages to do her own shopping, a little gardening, and goes out to play cards 3 evenings a week. Which description best fits her current functional status?

A. Disabled
B. Frail
C. Functionally impaired
D. Not frail
E. Pre-frail

32.14. A 77 year old woman complains of unsteadiness on her feet, which started a few months ago and has gradually worsened. She finds it difficult to walk in a straight line, and often overbalances when she turns. On examination, she has no nystagmus or past pointing, tone and power are normal, but Romberg's test is positive. What is the most likely cause for her unsteadiness?

A. Benign positional vertigo
B. Cerebellar infarction
C. Parkinson's disease
D. Peripheral neuropathy
E. Vestibular neuronitis

32.15. A 93 year old man presents having fallen three times in the last week. He has significant bruising over the side of his face from the last fall. His wife saw the last fall; she is sure that her husband lost consciousness for a few seconds, but came round after 2–3 minutes on the ground. Lying and standing blood pressure are 155/92 mmHg and 148/90 mmHg, respectively, and cardiac auscultation is normal. Which course of action would be most appropriate for this man?

A. 24-Hour electrocardiogram (ECG) monitoring
B. Echocardiography
C. Referral to physiotherapist for strength and balance training
D. Start calcium and vitamin D supplementation
E. Tilt table testing

32.16. An 85 year old woman presents with diarrhoea and vomiting. Her blood tests show acute kidney injury. Which one of the following changes in kidney structure is attributable to ageing, rather than to an underlying disease process?

A. Glomerulosclerosis
B. Porosity of the glomerular filtration barrier
C. Reduction in nephron numbers
D. Renal arteriolar hyaline deposition
E. Stenosis of the renal arteries

32.17. A 94 year old man presents with three falls over a 2-day period. On assessment, he is disoriented and dehydrated. His chest is clear to auscultation, temperature is 35.2°C, pulse 90 beats/min, blood pressure 110/50 mmHg. His respiratory rate is 18 breaths/min and his oxygen saturations are 89% on air. What is the most likely cause for his falls?

A. Cerebral infarction
B. Pneumonia
C. Poor fluid intake
D. Spinal cord compression
E. Subdural haematoma

32.18. An 82 year old woman with advanced dementia is noticed by the nursing home staff to look rather pale. She does not complain of breathlessness or tiredness; she had a severe stroke 3 years ago and has been unable to walk since; she sits in a wheelchair during the day and is helped into bed by two helpers at night. Her bowels are open normally and she does not complain of indigestion. She has been in hospital twice in the last 3 months and during her last admission stated a wish to be allowed to die. What is the most appropriate investigation for this woman?

A. Abdominal ultrasonography
B. Full blood count
C. No investigation
D. Upper and lower gastrointestinal endoscopy
E. Upper gastrointestinal endoscopy

32.19. An 86 year old woman presents having taken to her bed for the last 2 days. She is normally mobile around the house using a walking frame, but does not usually leave the house. Carers come to help her wash and dress twice a day. On examination, her pulse is 110 beats/min, blood pressure 90/50 mmHg, respiratory rate 24 breaths/min, oxygen saturations 96% on air. Her temperature is 37.0°C. Her chest is clear, she has a gallop rhythm on cardiac auscultation, and her jugular venous pressure is not elevated. She is disoriented, drowsy, but able to move all her limbs. She opens her eyes when you raise your voice. Her ECG shows deep T-wave inversion across the anterior leads. What is the most likely diagnosis?

A. Depression
B. Myocardial infarction
C. Parkinson's disease
D. Pneumonia
E. Pulmonary embolism

32.20. A 77 year old man complains of difficulty walking. On inspection of his gait, he struggles to start walking, but then accelerates into a series of small steps, and fails to lift his feet very far from the floor. He does not swing his arms when walking, and has difficulty turning at the end of the walk. What is the most likely explanation for his gait?

A. Bilateral parietal lobe stroke disease
B. Cerebellar stroke
C. Hip osteoarthritis
D. Parkinson's disease
E. Peripheral neuropathy

32

Answers

32.1. Answer: E.
His falls do not occur at home: thus, home modification is unlikely to help in this case. Calcium and vitamin D is effective only in patients in institutional care, who are those with the lowest vitamin D levels. Hip protectors do not reduce falls, and current evidence suggests that they do not reduce fractures either. A pacemaker would help only if cardioinhibitory carotid sinus hypersensitivity was demonstrated.

32.2. Answer: A.
She is describing urge incontinence. Antimuscarinic medication can be helpful but carries a high burden of side-effects. Her symptoms have been continuous for 2 years; they are not therefore due to infection and antibiotic therapy is inappropriate. For most people, long-term catheters bring as much harm as benefit. Tension-free vaginal tape and pelvic floor training are useful interventions for stress incontinence but not for urge incontinence.

32.3. Answer: E.
She is describing vertigo, which may be due to either labyrinth or brainstem disease. As her symptoms have persisted for 2 days, a transient ischaemic brainstem attack is less likely than vestibular neuronitis – although note that a completed stroke involving the brainstem might produce similar symptoms.

32.4. Answer: C.
This is a classic case of treating drug side-effects with further drugs. The amlodipine has caused ankle oedema; the furosemide has then caused intravascular volume depletion and orthostatic hypotension. The safest course of action is to stop both agents, then reassess the blood pressure (perhaps using a 24-hour blood pressure monitor). If the blood pressure is still high, an alternative agent (such as an ACE inhibitor) could be considered. α-Blockers are particularly likely to worsen orthostatic hypotension.

32.5. Answer: C.
Goal setting (and regular review of goals) is an essential component of successful rehabilitation. The other components are not.

Leadership is necessary, but does not have to be medical or doctor leadership. Assessment of needs is necessary, but this does not have to be via the Barthel score. Rehabilitation can take place in many settings, including the patient's home; a ward is not necessary. It is essential to define the patient's disabilities and functional capabilities; this is more important than the precise underlying diagnoses.

32.6. Answer: A.
CGA reduces short-term mortality or adverse outcomes, but not these outcomes at 12 months. CGA can improve cognition in the medium term, but there is no evidence as to whether it delays the onset of dementia or not. CGA might improve the speed of recovery from surgery, but there is no trial evidence to prove this. It is a key component, however, in maximising function in older people recovering from surgery. CGA is usually offered to those patients who are already frail or pre-frail; thus it is unlikely to affect time to onset of frailty.

32.7. Answer: C.
Hand grip strength forms part of the Fried frailty phenotype, and is a powerful independent predictor of frailty-related outcomes in older people. Blood pressure is not part of frailty syndromes. Although weight loss is part of frailty measurements, current body mass index is not. Similarly, walk speed over a short distance (4 or 5 m) is part of frailty assessment, but 6-minute walk distance is not commonly used; this is a measure of endurance exercise capacity and is more useful in assessing disease severity of cardiorespiratory illnesses such as heart failure and chronic obstructive pulmonary disease. Number of medications is related to multimorbidity, not to frailty.

32.8. Answer: E.
All of the other changes are due to cardiovascular pathology; all are more common with age, but can be attributed to disease processes such as atherosclerosis, hypertension, obesity and myocardial dysfunction.

32.9. Answer: E.
Timed 'get up and go' test is a good predictor of future falls risk, and also allows observation

of the gait for unsteadiness. Six-minute walk test measures endurance rather than 'fast-twitch' lower limb function (which is more closely correlated with balance and falls risk). The Barthel Index measures dependency in activities of daily living, and although hand grip is a good measure of overall physical status (and forms part of the criteria for frailty), it is less directly relevant to falls risk.

32.10. Answer: C.

Benign positional vertigo is common and amenable to treatment with simple positional manoeuvres. Supine blood pressure alone will tell you little; postural blood pressure is more important. Finding a reduced hip extension range would be unsurprising after recent hip surgery. Whilst depression is important, finding it will not directly influence your plans for reducing his falls risk. Cardiac auscultation may uncover a murmur of aortic stenosis – a cause of syncopal episodes potentially amenable to intervention – but this is less likely than option C, and even if you find severe aortic stenosis, comorbid disease and frailty might prevent you from intervening successfully.

32.11. Answer: B.

Drugs are the most common cause of hyponatraemia in older people – and thiazide diuretics are one of the commonest drug causes. Ibuprofen is a less likely cause, unless acute kidney injury has been precipitated by its use. Both carcinoma of the lung and Addison's disease can cause hyponatraemia, but are both much less common causes than drugs. Inadequate salt intake is very unlikely to lead to low serum sodium levels.

32.12. Answer: E.

Her dementia is likely to be severe enough that she is unaware of needing to pass urine; the normal inhibitory signals preventing bladder emptying are lost and the signals indicating that the bladder is full are either not processed or not acted on. Regular toilet visits (e.g. every 2–3 hours) can be helpful in ensuring that voiding occurs before the bladder is full. Pelvic floor exercises are useful in stress incontinence, but require active participation and understanding by the patient. Catheterisation is not the first choice for any continence problem, and this woman is unlikely to have sufficient cognitive function to self-catheterise. The long-standing nature of the problem makes it

very unlikely that urinary infection is playing any part in her symptoms.

32.13. Answer: E.

She has 2 of the 5 Fried Frailty criteria – low grip strength and self-reported exhaustion. Three criteria are required to diagnose frailty, but the presence of 1 or 2 criteria is sometimes categorised as 'pre-frail'. You are not given any information to suggest that she has functional impairment – she continues to undertake activities of daily living. Similarly, you are not told anything that suggests the presence of a specific disability.

i	**32.13 How to assess a Fried Frailty score**
Hand grip strength in bottom 20% of healthy elderly distribution*
Walking speed in bottom 20% of healthy elderly distribution*
Self-reported exhaustion
Physical inactivity
At least 4.5 kg weight loss within 1 year
Patient is defined as frail if 3 or more factors are present; 1–2 factors indicate a 'pre-frail' state.
*Varies between populations. Grip cut-off is 30 kg for men and 18 kg for women in US adults; 5 m walk time cut-off is 7 seconds in US adults for both sexes.

32.14. Answer: D.

The lack of nystagmus or past pointing argues against this being due to middle ear, brainstem or cerebellar disease. The normal tone makes Parkinsonian syndromes less likely, although you are not given specific information about bradykinesia. A peripheral neuropathy or dorsal column spinal cord disease would explain the unsteadiness and positive Romberg's test.

32.15. Answer: A.

The witness account suggests that this was a syncopal episode; this requires investigation. 24-Hour ECG monitoring is a reasonable first investigation; if this does not uncover a reason, then further investigation (e.g. tilt table testing) may be required. Echocardiography is likely to be less useful, especially given that no murmur is audible.

32.16. Answer: C.

The other structural changes are due to disease, not ageing. Glomerulosclerosis may be caused by a range of diseases, including diabetes mellitus and infections; diabetes may similarly cause porosity of the filtration barrier, leading to proteinuria. Hypertension leads to

32

arteriolar hyaline deposition, and renal artery stenosis may be caused by atherosclerosis or fibromuscular dysplasia.

32.17. Answer: B.
Onset of falls, particularly several falls in quick succession, should suggest intercurrent illness. Acute illness in older people may present atypically, as here – but there are still clues that this is pneumonia. He has a low temperature (equivalent to a fever of 38.8°C), a raised pulse rate and low oxygen saturations. The other options do not explain all of these features; in particular, they do not explain his hypoxia.

32.18. Answer: C.
It is unlikely that performing any of the listed investigations will improve the quality of this woman's life. She is asymptomatic: therefore even if anaemia was discovered on a full blood count, it is debatable as to whether transfusion would improve her quality of life. Clearly if she were to become symptomatic, this would change. Endoscopy would, in addition, be burdensome given her frailty, and you have some indication from her last illness that she might not want further medical intervention. Even if you did decide to investigate anaemia, ultrasonography is unlikely to find the cause. In real life, the decision-making process would, of course, need to be informed by the wishes of the patient, and of those deputed to make decisions on her behalf should she lack capacity to make decisions about her medical care.

32.19. Answer: B.
The ECG is suggestive of myocardial infarction – perhaps 2–3 days ago, this would also explain her gallop rhythm. Myocardial infarction may present without chest pain in older people – especially older women – and atypical symptoms such as tiredness and delirium are common, as in this case, where she suffers from hypoactive delirium. The problem is acute, making depression or Parkinson's disease unlikely; the normal oxygen saturations make pneumonia and pulmonary embolism less likely diagnoses.

32.20. Answer: D
The gait described is festinant (slow start, then accelerating), and shuffling (not lifting the feet). The lack of arm swing and difficulty turning are also consistent with a Parkinsonian gait. Cerebellar lesions cause ataxia; bilateral parietal lobe stroke disease may cause apraxia (e.g. difficulties starting to walk) or *marche à petits pas* and peripheral neuropathy can cause a stamping gait, which may be high stepping if foot drop is present. Hip osteoarthritis would typically cause an antalgic gait, where the weight-bearing phase is shortened for the affected leg (a 'limp').

GG Dark

33

Oncology

Multiple Choice Questions

33.1. A 52 year old woman presents to her family physician concerned about her risk of cancer from her smoking. She has smoked 20 cigarettes per day for the last 35 years and several of her family members have died of cancer. She is in good health.

What site of cancer is most likely to be caused by inhaled carcinogens from cigarette smoke?

A. Bladder
B. Breast
C. Central nervous system
D. Colon
E. Ovary

33.2. A 44 year old man presents to the urology clinic for assessment. He is suspected of having a bladder tumour in the renal tract and the consultant requests a urine cytology specimen.

What is the best sample for cytological assessment?

A. 24-Hour urine collection
B. First urine sample of the morning
C. Fresh, full voided sample
D. Mid-stream urine
E. Urine that is frozen immediately

33.3. A research student is studying the effects of a new chemotherapy agent on cell cycle and cellular division. What phase of the cell cycle is most likely to correspond with nuclear division followed by cytokinesis?

A. G_0
B. G_1
C. G_2

D. M
E. S

33.4. A 23 year old woman presents to her family physician. She is 8 weeks pregnant and the family physician advises her to take folic acid daily. She asks if it is safe to take other vitamin supplements.

Which vitamin in large doses can be teratogenic and so should be avoided?

A. Vitamin A
B. Vitamin B_{12}
C. Vitamin C
D. Vitamin D
E. Vitamin E

33.5. A 71 year old man presents to the dermatology clinic with an ulcer over his left temple. It has been growing slowly over the previous 3 years. He worked as a farmer and spent most of the working day outdoors.

On clinical examination the lesion appears as a non-healing, indolent, punched-out, clean-looking 2-cm ulcer over the left temple. There are no enlarged lymph nodes in the head and neck.

What is the most appropriate next step in the patient care?

A. Perform a full-thickness biopsy of the centre of this lesion
B. Perform a full-thickness biopsy of the edge of the lesion
C. Perform scrapings and culture from the ulcer base

D. Refer for radiotherapy treatment to this lesion

E. Resection of the whole lesion with a 1-cm clear margin

33.6. A 52 year old man presents to the emergency department complaining of lightheadedness. He has a past medical history of lung cancer, which was diagnosed a month previously and found to be metastatic, involving the bone and pericardium.

On clinical examination, his blood pressure is 70/40 mmHg and his pulse is 100 beats/min. His heart sounds are distant and soft. His electrocardiogram shows low-voltage complexes and electrical alternans is present. A chest X-ray film shows that the cardiac silhouette is enlarged.

What is the most appropriate next step in this patient's care?

A. Intravenous dexamethasone
B. Intravenous fluid challenge
C. Intravenous furosemide
D. Oral ibuprofen
E. Pericardiocentesis

33.7. A 66 year old woman presents to the emergency department holding her right arm with a deformity that signifies an obvious fracture. She described that she was shopping and picked up a bag out of the trolley to place it in her car. She then felt a sharp, sudden pain in the middle of her arm and her humerus suddenly gave way.

What is the most likely reason for the fracture?

A. Bone metastasis in the humerus from breast cancer
B. Osteitis fibrosa cystica from parathyroid disease
C. Osteomalacia from nutritional deficiency
D. Osteoporosis
E. Primary malignant bone tumour of the humerus

33.8. A 51 year old woman presents to the endocrinology clinic for investigation of weight gain. She is found to have an elevated 24-hour urinary free cortisol, elevated serum adrenocorticotrophic hormone (ACTH) and elevated serum cortisol. The serum cortisol does not fall when she is given high-dose dexamethasone.

What serum investigation is most likely to be elevated in this patient?

A. Adrenaline (epinephrine)
B. Lactate dehydrogenase
C. Plasma osmolality
D. Prolactin
E. Renin

33.9. A 65 year old man presents to the emergency department complaining of gradual loss of sensation in his right hand, weakness of the left lower leg and visual disturbance. He has smoked two packs of cigarettes daily for 40 years. His past medical history includes asthma and emphysema.

On clinical examination, he is afebrile, pulse 86 beats/min, blood pressure 137/86 mmHg and respiration rate 24 breaths/min. Eye fundoscopy is normal.

A magnetic resonance imaging (MRI) scan of the brain shows five different intracerebral lesions, ranging from 1 to 3 cm in diameter and located at the gray–white matter junction in both cerebral hemispheres. The lesions are sharply demarcated and contrast enhancement after gadolinium administration is present in all of them.

What is the most likely diagnosis?

A. Arteriovenous malformations
B. Embolic infarcts
C. Multifocal glioblastoma multiforme
D. Multiple abscesses
E. Multiple metastases

33.10. A 65 year old woman presents to the emergency department with constant, severe abdominal pain that has worsened over the previous week. She has no other associated symptoms but has noticed that her daily urine output had decreased significantly. She has had a constant desire to urinate, but when she tries, only a small amount of bloody urine is discharged. She is a long-time smoker, having smoked three packs per day for more than 45 years.

On clinical examination she has a suprapubic mass arising from the bladder and appears to be in urinary retention.

What is most likely to be detected upon imaging the patient's genitourinary system?

A. Bilateral hydronephrosis
B. Bladder dilation
C. Bladder dyskinesis
D. Unilateral hydronephrosis
E. Urethral dilation

33.11. A 54 year old woman presents to the emergency department complaining of severe lower abdominal pain and distension over a 24-hour period. Her bowels had not moved over the same time period and her abdomen has become visibly swollen with associated nausea and vomiting. Over the previous 4 months, she has lost 9 kg in weight and has noted progressive symptoms of constipation. She reports that on several occasions she has passed blood mixed in with her bowel movements, which have become thinner in calibre. She denies any recent travel, use of antibiotics, or fevers.

On clinical examination, she appears acutely uncomfortable and has a temperature of 38.3°C. Her abdomen is diffusely distended and tender to palpation in the left lower quadrant. There are hyperactive rushing bowel sounds. On rectal examination, her stool is brown and tests positive for blood. A plain abdominal X-ray film shows multiple small bowel air fluid levels and a dilated colon proximal to the sigmoid colon.

What is the most likely diagnosis?

A. Amoebic abscess
B. Colonic polyp
C. Diverticulitis
D. Diverticulosis
E. Sigmoid carcinoma

33.12. A 39 year old woman completed her last course of adjuvant chemotherapy for breast cancer 2 years earlier. She presents to the oncology clinic complaining of constant back pain for 3 weeks. On clinical examination she is tender to palpation over two well-circumscribed areas in the thoracic and lumbar spine. There is no neurological deficit.

What is the most appropriate next step in investigation, assuming rapid availability of all?

A. Computed tomography (CT) scan of whole spine
B. Isotope bone scan
C. Needle biopsy of the affected areas
D. Plain film X-rays of the affected areas
E. Ultrasound of the affected areas

33.13. A 62 year old woman has noticed a lesion on her face that has persisted for more than a month. It appears as an ulcerated lesion with a raised, rolled edge (see figure).

What factor is the most likely cause of this problem in the UK?

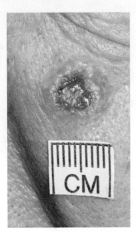

A. Arsenic
B. Benzene
C. Human papilloma virus (HPV)
D. Ultraviolet (UV) radiation
E. Vinyl chloride

33.14. A 42 year old man previously worked at the Fukushima Daiichi Nuclear Power Plant and received radiation exposure as a result of the damage to the reactor caused by an earthquake and the subsequent leakage of nuclear material. He has concerns about his future cancer risk as a direct result of his exposure.

What statement in relation to radiation exposure is the most accurate?

A. Large exposure is required to develop the most serious malignancies
B. Leukaemia has the shortest latency period of all malignancies
C. Malignancies always occur within 10 years of exposure
D. Malignancy risk increases with advancing age at the time of exposure
E. Therapeutic radiation therapy given without chemotherapy does not increase the risk of a second malignancy

33.15. A 22 year old man presents to his family physician complaining of breathlessness worsening over the previous 7 days. He has no cough and denies smoking. A chest X-ray is performed, shown below.

What is the most likely histological type of malignancy?

33

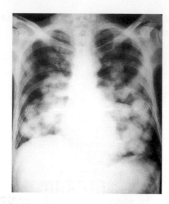

A. Adenocarcinoma
B. Carcinosarcoma
C. Immature teratoma
D. Papillary serous carcinoma
E. Squamous cell cancer

33.16. A 28 year old woman presents to her family physician after finding a breast lump on self-examination. She found the lump 2 months previously, and although she was not initially concerned, has laterly become worried about the possibility of cancer. On further questioning, she reports that the lump had neither increased nor decreased in size since she first noticed it and that she had no family history of breast cancer.

On clinical examination there was a 2×2 cm firm, non-tender, mobile lump in the left breast.

What is the most appropriate next action for the family physician to take?

A. Perform a fine needle aspiration of the lump himself for cytological assessment
B. Reassure the patient that the lump is probably benign and arrange a 1-month follow-up
C. Refer the patient to a breast cancer multidisciplinary team
D. Request a mammogram
E. Request an ultrasound of the breast

33.17. A 64 year old man with known lung cancer presents with a history of progressive leg weakness and numbness, which began in his buttocks and gradually spread down the back of his legs into the soles of his feet. He has recently become impotent and incontinent of both faeces and urine.

On examination there is wasting of the buttocks and calf muscles with bilateral weakness of hip extension, ankle dorsiflexion and plantar flexion. A sensory deficit is demonstrated, extending from the buttocks down the back of the legs and onto the soles of the feet.

What is the most likely site of the lesion?

A. A dorsal column of the spinal cord
B. Cauda equina
C. Distal spinal cord
D. Proximal spinal cord
E. Sciatic nerves

33.18. A 49 year old man presents with a 1-week history of increasing nausea, vomiting and lethargy. He has an extensive smoking history of 30 pack years and was recently diagnosed with lung cancer. He is not taking any medications and has not yet initiated chemotherapy.

On clinical examination, he is afebrile and somnolent. His lungs are clear to auscultation and his heart is regular in rate and rhythm. His skin demonstrates loss of elasticity. Laboratory results indicate a serum calcium level of 2.95 mmol/L (11.8 mg/dL).

What is the most appropriate initial step in management?

A. Calcitonin
B. Hydrochlorothiazide
C. Intravenous normal saline
D. Prednisolone
E. Zoledronic acid

33.19. A 37 year old accountant presents to his family physician to ask for advice regarding the future management of his ulcerative colitis. He has had pancolitis for the past 19 years and has been told that he is at an increased risk for developing colorectal cancer. He asks for recommendation regarding appropriate surveillance.

What is the most appropriate investigation for regular surveillance?

A. Barium enema
B. Colonoscopy
C. Colonoscopy and multiple biopsies
D. Faecal occult blood testing
E. Flexible sigmoidoscopy with multiple biopsies

33.20. A 72 year old woman presents with abdominal distension, feeling bloated and getting full quickly when eating. Her past medical history includes hypertension and she is prescribed an angiotensin-converting enzyme (ACE) inhibitor.

Clinical examination reveals abdominal distension with shifting dullness. Pelvic examination reveals a large, non-tender right adnexal mass.

Abdominal CT scan shows masses arising on both ovaries, ascites and omental thickening. Serum cancer antigen 125 (CA-125) level is 2000 U/mL. Serum alpha-fetoprotein (AFP) and human chorionic gonadotrophin (hCG) are normal.

What is the most likely diagnosis?

A. Choriocarcinoma
B. Dermoid cyst (cystic teratoma)
C. Epithelial ovarian cancer
D. Ovarian sarcoma
E. Sertoli stromal cell tumour

33.21. A 25 year old woman, gravida 2, para 2 presents to her family physician to discuss contraception. She has no medical problems, is on no medications and has no family history of cancer. All clinical examinations are normal. After a discussion with the family physician, she chooses to take the oral contraceptive pill (OCP) and stays on the pill for the following 5 years.

What cancer has the greatest reduction in risk as a result of this medication?

A. Bone sarcoma
B. Breast cancer
C. Cervical cancer
D. Endometrial cancer
E. Hepatocellular carcinoma

33.22. A 73 year old man presents to his family physician complaining of a drooping right eye lid. He has a 70-pack year history and his family physician has been seeing him for more than 10 years for management of his symptoms of chronic obstructive pulmonary disease (COPD). On clinical examination, he has ptosis of the right eye with a constricted right pupil. The remainder of the eye and cranial nerve examination is normal.

What is the most likely finding on a chest X-ray of this patient?

A. A calcified granuloma in the left mid-lung field
B. A left-sided pleural effusion
C. A right upper lobe pneumonia
D. An irregularly shaped mass at the apex of the left lung
E. An irregularly shaped mass at the apex of the right lung

33.23. A 44 year old woman presents to her family physician complaining of a severe headache that had been present for several weeks and had not responded to the usual over-the-counter headache remedies. She locates the headache to the centre of her head and describes it as constant but worse in the mornings. She has no other neurological signs or symptoms. She has had 'tension headaches' previously but those were located in the back of her head and felt different from the present pain. She has a past history of breast cancer 2 years previously, which was treated with surgery followed by adjuvant chemotherapy.

What is the most appropriate next step in diagnosis?

A. Carotid arteriogram
B. CT scan of the head
C. Lumbar puncture
D. Psychiatric evaluation
E. Skull X-rays

33.24. A 43 year old woman presents to the specialist breast clinic with a breast lump that she noticed on self-examination. She has a 2-cm, firm, non-tender mass in the left breast, which is movable from the chest wall, but not movable within the breast. She has no prior history of breast disease.

What is the most appropriate initial step?

A. Arrange a mammogram to find any other lesions that might also need to be addressed
B. Arrange an ultrasound scan and advise the patient she is unlikely to need a biopsy
C. Discuss the surgical options in case cancer is found
D. Obtain a fine needle aspirate and discharge the patient if no malignant cells are found
E. Wait for two menstrual cycles to see whether there is spontaneous resolution

33.25. A 70 year old man presents to his family physician with an episode of visible haematuria. He denies prior episodes and had been previously healthy. He is not on any medication. Urinalysis confirms gross haematuria without proteinuria or casts. The patient denies any pain and all physical examination is normal.

What is the most appropriate next step?

A. CT scan of the pelvis
B. Cystoscopy
C. Renal angiogram
D. Transrectal prostatic biopsy
E. Trimethoprim–sulfamethoxazole

33

33.26. A 73 year old man presents to the chest clinic for annual review for asbestosis. He has a long smoking history and was diagnosed with asbestosis on biopsy 4 years previously. He has no change in his symptoms but continues to smoke cigarettes and denies any cough or shortness of breath. His chest X-ray shows left lower lobe pleural thickening with calcifications at the level of the diaphragm.

He has many questions about his disease and wants to discuss his risk for malignancy and long-term prognosis. What explanation is most appropriate?

A. Asbestosis itself (without smoking) is unlikely to progress to cancer

B. His risk of cancer is greater than 70 times that of the normal population

C. Mesothelioma is the most common cancer associated with asbestosis and smoking

D. Small cell lung cancer is the most common cancer associated with asbestosis and smoking

E. Steroids may slow progression of his disease

33.27. A 42 year old woman presents to the clinic to discuss her concerns regarding breast cancer. She has no symptoms at review, but previously she had noted bilateral breast tenderness prior to her menses, which has since abated. She has had two caesarean deliveries but no other operations. She is taking a low-dose OCP and has no known drug allergies. She does not smoke and has no family history of cancer. All clinical examinations are normal.

She wants to know whether *BRCA1* and *BRCA2* screening would be appropriate for her in addition to routine screening starting at age 50. What is the most appropriate response?

A. *BRCA1* and *BRCA2* screening is not recommended

B. *BRCA1* and *BRCA2* screening should be performed after age 50

C. *BRCA1* and *BRCA2* screening should be performed if breast pain recurs

D. *BRCA1* screening is recommended

E. *BRCA2* screening is recommended

33.28. A 26 year old woman presents to her family physician complaining of facial hair on her upper lip. This has been present for many years and has not bothered her before. She has been trying to conceive for some time without success and previously has taken the OCP for irregular periods.

On clinical examination, her body mass index (BMI) is 32 kg/m^2. Her blood pressure is 135/88 mmHg, pulse is 72 beats/min and skin examination reveals acanthosis nigricans, mild acne and scattered plucked chin with facial hair on the upper lip. Abdominal examination is normal.

This woman is at greatest risk for what condition?

A. Diabetes mellitus

B. Gastric cancer

C. Ovarian cancer

D. Ovarian torsion

E. Uterine cancer

33.29. A 59 year old man presents to his family physician with a 3-week history of dyspnoea, particularly on exertion, and had an occasional cough, which is dry and unproductive. He describes some chest tightness and discomfort, which was mostly dull in nature.

On clinical examination there is nicotine staining of the left index and second fingers. There is no peripheral lymphadenopathy, no evidence of heart failure, the jugulovenous pressure is not raised and heart sounds are normal. On chest examination there is reduced expansion on the right, with decreased tactile vocal fremitus, dullness to percussion and diminished breath sounds. Examination of the left hemithorax is unremarkable. Peak flow rate is 450 L/min. Abdominal examination is normal.

What is the most likely diagnosis?

A. Collapse of the right lung

B. Consolidation of the right lung

C. Interstitial fibrosis throughout right lung field

D. Left tension pneumothorax

E. Right pleural effusion

Answers

33.1. Answer: A.

Inhaled carcinogens are absorbed across the bronchial mucosa and enter the blood stream and are then processed in the liver to become more water-soluble. The metabolised carcinogens are then filtered by the kidney and sit in the bladder for hours. After more than 10 years, the risk of bladder cancer is significantly elevated. The same is true for breast cancer, as carcinogens are secreted into the breast ducts, but the incidence of breast cancer caused by this aetiology is not as great as that for bladder cancer.

Ovarian cancer is not affected by smoking but the risk of endometrial cancer is lower in smokers than non-smokers. Options C and D have no significant linkage to smoking. The best answer is option A.

33.2. Answer: C.
Options A and E would allow the cells to die and therefore be unsuitable for cytological assessment. Option B results in cells sitting in the bladder overnight with some also dying off. This is, however, the best option for suspected *Mycobacterium* infection. Option D is the best sample for culture as it minimises contamination at the start and end of stream. Option C gives the best yield for cytological assessment.

33.3. Answer: D.
The second growth phase precedes nuclear division, which is in mitosis (M), and is followed by cytokinesis, which is still in mitosis (M).

33.4. Answer: A.
It is important to understand which drugs are safe in pregnancy, and vitamin A taken in large doses can cause fetal abnormalities. Other vitamins mentioned are not thought to have any teratogenic effect.

33.5. Answer: B.
This patient is likely to have a basal cell carcinoma from the description.

Options D and E relate to management but identification is required first, particularly before delivering invasive treatment. Option C would be used for a fungal lesion. Option A would biopsy the central necrotic portion and may not yield a diagnosis, whereas option B would sample the proliferative edge and therefore is best for histological diagnosis.

33.6. Answer: E.
The clinical presentation of this patient describes a pericardial effusion resulting from his malignancy: hence the increased cardiac silhouette. His blood pressure is low as he is developing cardiac tamponade. This requires

aspiration, usually under echocardiogram guidance.

33.7. Answer: A.
This patient has no prior history of illness and the fracture has occurred spontaneously, i.e. without any trauma. In view of her gender and age, of the options listed, this is most likely to be due to breast cancer (1 in 8 lifetime risk).

33.8. Answer: B.
The clinical indicators suggest that this patient has Cushing's syndrome. There are four possible causes of Cushing's. These are: exogenous steroids, adrenal adenoma, ectopic ACTH and a pituitary adenoma. Only the latter two give a high ACTH and only ectopic production does not fall on a high-dose suppression test. Therefore, the clinical scenario is describing Cushing's syndrome with ectopic ACTH production. The most likely cause of that is small cell lung cancer (SCLC). LDH is an intracellular enzyme that is released during necrosis as a pathological process; therefore, in rapidly growing tumours (like SCLC), this can be elevated in a serum sample.

Patients with SCLC can develop the syndrome of inappropriate antidiuretic hormone (vasopressin) secretion, but that would decrease plasma osmolality. Renin may be increased in some tumours but not lung. Adrenaline is increased in neuroendocrine tumours of the adrenal gland (phaeochromocytoma) but not neuroendocrine tumours of the lung (SCLC). Prolactin can be produced as a result of an ACTH-producing pituitary tumour causing loss of prolactin inhibitory factor (due to pituitary stalk compression), but ACTH would fall with high-dose dexamethasone in that scenario.

33.9. Answer: E.
The clinical features do not suggest infection (option D) and option A would be more likely to cause a subarachnoid haemorrhage. Option B is more likely to have sudden onset. Option B, C and E are possible from the clinical history but the radiological description is more in keeping with option E.

33.10. Answer: A.
A long smoking history increases the exposure of the urological epithelium to inflammatory mediators such as carcinogens in tobacco. After more than 10 years, this increases the

33

risk of developing a bladder cancer, which in turn is causing urinary retention. Given the time course, it is most likely that bilateral hydronephrosis will be present.

33.11. Answer: E.
This patient is in bowel obstruction and the clinical history suggests many features to locate this to the sigmoid colon. Option A is unlikely in the absence of foreign travel and the symptoms would be right upper quadrant pain. Option B is unlikely to cause thin stools and obstruction. Option C (-itis) has inflammation and could result in abscess formation, even perforation, but would not fully explain the stool history (thin calibre). Option D may explain the increasing constipation over time but not the acute presentation. Option E is the best answer for all symptoms and progression into an emergency presentation to hospital in bowel obstruction. A high temperature can be seen in malignancy or when secondary infection is present.

33.12. Answer: B.
This patient is likely to be pre-menopausal and therefore osteoporosis is less likely. She has a diagnosis of breast cancer and could have progressive recurrent disease and therefore the onset of back pain requires investigation. The first step in investigation is to assess the whole skeleton to see if this is isolated or widespread and that is best done with a radioisotope bone scan. This will be followed with plain film imaging of any hot spots and, if suspicious, thereafter consider a biopsy of the abnormalities.

CT imaging can show bone detail but would be less sensitive than a bone scan. Ultrasound would not be helpful. MRI would be best if there was also a neurological deficit, to look for cord compression or to distinguish osteoporotic collapse from metastatic involvement.

33.13. Answer: D.
Each of these substances is associated with malignancy but UV exposure is most associated with a basal cell carcinoma. These tumours are therefore more common in individuals that work outdoors. Although arsenic is associated with skin cancer, it is most likely to be squamous cell carcinoma. HPV is associated with head and neck cancer and cervical cancer. Benzene is associated with leukaemia, particularly acute myeloid leukaemia but also non-Hodgkin lymphoma and

myeloma. Vinyl chloride is hepatotoxic and has been associated with hepatic angiosarcoma.

33.14. Answer: B.
The carcinogenic effect of radiation exposure is related to the exposure rate. When we consider this in relation to therapeutic radiation, larger doses can be given in lots of small fractions over more time to lessen the effect (55 Gy over 5 weeks on average for radiotherapy treatment, whereas 8 Gy to the whole body over 30 seconds could prove fatal). Second malignancies induced by radiotherapy usually take more than 10 years to manifest. Patients that are young (<18 years) have tissues that are still developing and are therefore at highest risk of transformation. Chemotherapy is administered with radiotherapy to enhance the biologically effective dose, i.e. it produces a greater effect on tissue than the dose of radiation on its own. This acts as a sensitiser for the tissue and would therefore increase the risk of malignant transformation. Leukaemia has the shortest latency period.

33.15. Answer: C.
This question is about understanding the natural history of malignancy. Papillary serous carcinoma is most commonly associated with gynaecological cancers and is therefore unlikely in a male patient, although it can arise in the pancreas in older patients. Carcinosarcoma contains malignant elements from epithelial tissue (carcinoma) and connective tissue (sarcoma) and is most commonly found in the gynaecological system, although rarely it is found as a component of de-differentiated carcinoma of the lung, but not at this age. Adenocarcinoma can develop from many primary sites, including the lung, where it can arise in the periphery or hilar region and is not associated with tobacco products. This, too, is less likely at this age. Testicular immature teratoma is most likely to cause a large-volume lung metastases in a young male.

33.16. Answer: C.
According to the National Institute for Health and Care Excellence (NICE) guidance, the lump requires follow-up and investigation, not reassessment in a month's time by the same doctor. However, whilst one of the listed investigations is the most appropriate (option A), it should be performed and interpreted by specialists and not in the primary care setting.

33.17. Answer: B.
This patient has clinical signs that suggest lower motor neuron weakness and as the spinal cord ends at L1–L2, this abnormality is at a lower level than L2. Lung cancer will commonly metastasise to bone and although it can cause spinal cord compression, the neurology in this presentation infers that this is at a level where it results in compression of the cauda equina.

33.18. Answer: C.
This patient is presenting with hypercalcaemia and the immediate management should be to rehydrate the patient (option C). Bisphosphonate therapy (option E) is indicated once his hydration state improves. Loop diuretics can be used if fully rehydrated but not a thiazide diuretic (option B) as it could increase the serum calcium. In patients with lung cancer, hypercalcaemia is most commonly associated with squamous cell carcinoma.

33.19. Answer: C.
Patients with ulcerative colitis have an increased risk of developing a colonic carcinoma due to the chronic inflammation. It often will have a lead time of 10 years and is more likely in those with more significant inflammation. In order to assess the whole colon and biopsy for histology, option C is the best investigation. Option E will not assess the whole colon and the remaining options (without biopsy) do not allow histological assessment.

33.20. Answer: C.
Epithelial ovarian cancer is most likely to cause a rise in CA-125 and although this tumour marker is rarely diagnostic it can assist in disease activity monitoring. The remaining tumours do not normally cause a rise in CA-125 unless it is a false positive due to inflammatory changes arising from the tumour. Choriocarcinoma would cause a rise in serum hCG.

33.21. Answer: D.
The risk of breast cancer and bone sarcoma remains the same in patients taking the OCP. The risk of cervical cancer is slightly increased, not by the medication but due to the increased sexual activity of this population of patients. The risk of endometrial cancer is reduced due to the reduced stimulation of this tissue. The use of a steroid-based drug such as oestrogen may slightly increase the risk of hepatocellular carcinoma.

33.22. Answer: E.
The clinical features are that of Horner's syndrome and the clinical signs will be ipsilateral, therefore suggesting an invasive lesion in the apex of the right lung (option E). The remaining options are non-invasive or in the wrong location and therefore should not cause impairment of the sympathetic innervation on the right side. The presence of Horner's syndrome in a patient with a chest infection is suggestive of an underlying cancer.

33.23. Answer: B.
The past history of breast cancer should raise an index of suspicion for metastasis and the new headache is different to her previous episodes. This should be investigated as brain metastasis and the best initial investigation of those listed is CT scan (option B). The other options would not enable this diagnosis to be made.

33.24. Answer: A.
The first step is to look for other lesions and to examine for calcification and spiculation (option A). There is no need to wait for the menstrual cycle as the patient has not presented with cyclical changes in the breast. A fine needle aspiration will be required but a negative result does not exclude malignancy. A biopsy will be required, whether a mammogram is performed or not. In practice, patients attending a one-stop specialist breast clinic will have a mammogram or ultrasound, clinical examination and a fine needle biopsy at the same visit.

33.25. Answer: B.
A single episode of frank haematuria requires investigation and is unlikely to be a simple urinary infection (option E). CT imaging may not detect small mucosal lesions (option A) and without stream impairment it is unlikely that this is related to prostatic enlargement (option D). The most likely diagnosis is a bladder lesion or cancer and that requires cystoscopy for inspection and biopsy.

33.26. Answer: B.
Non-small cell cancer is the most likely malignancy that occurs in patients with asbestosis. Although asbestosis is due to previous asbestos exposure, only a small

33

percentage of patients subsequently develop mesothelioma and the continued smoking will increase the risk of lung cancer. Moreover, smoking cessation will not negate the risk of malignancy. Steroid therapy may improve the symptoms but does not alter the natural history of asbestosis.

33.27. Answer: A.

Screening of patients for breast and ovarian susceptibility genes is indicated in individuals that have a personal history of both cancers, or that have a personal diagnosis of either breast or ovarian cancer and a first-degree relative with either breast or ovarian cancer. Routine screening of BRCA genes in a patient with no history would not be indicated.

33.28. Answer: A.

Acanthosis nigricans is a paraneoplastic phenomenon associated with gastric cancer in middle-aged patients and males more than females. However, in younger patients it is more associated with insulin resistance and thus an increased risk of diabetes mellitus and polycystic ovary syndrome, which may explain some of the other signs and symptomatology. Her BMI will increase her risk of uterine cancer but only after she has become post-menopausal.

33.29. Answer: E.

The clinical features at presentation are those of a pleural effusion: reduced expansion, diminished tactile vocal fremitus (vocal resonance), dullness to percussion and diminished breath sounds. Tracheal deviation may be away from the side of the lesion in massive effusion but shift of the lower mediastinum (apex beat) is also likely to be away from the side of the effusion.

34

Pain and palliative care

Multiple Choice Questions

34.1. Which of the following is normally involved in peripheral pain processing?

A. Aβ fibres
B. Calcitonin gene-related peptide (CGRP)-containing C fibres
C. Interneurons
D. Meissner's corpuscles
E. Pacinian corpuscles

34.2. The pain system can change in response to tissue injury. Which of the following neurotransmitters plays a key role in the process of central sensitisation?

A. Galanin
B. Glutamate
C. Glycine
D. β-Endorphin
E. γ-Aminobutyric acid (GABA)

34.3. A previously fit 72 year old man presents with severe pain affecting his right chest wall, such that he is struggling to remain living independently. From his history you discover that his clothes touching his skin is excruciatingly painful. His family physician has started him on tramadol 50 mg twice daily, without significant benefit. What symptom is he describing?

A. Breakthrough pain
B. Formication
C. Hyperalgesia
D. Mechanical allodynia
E. Spontaneous pain

34.4. A 64 year old man with type 2 diabetes mellitus is complaining of numbness, paraesthesia and pain in both feet, spreading into his legs. On examination, light touch is painful, and he has reduced sensation to pin-prick testing in a stocking distribution, typical of peripheral diabetic neuropathy. His blood glucose control is not good, his renal function is impaired and he is overweight. He is reluctant to walk because of the pain, and lives alone, becoming increasingly socially isolated. What factor may make pharmacological management more difficult?

A. Impaired renal function
B. Obesity
C. Pin-prick hypoalgesia
D. Reduced mobility
E. Social isolation

34.5. A range of patient-reported outcome measures have been validated for use in patients with chronic pain. Which one of the following assessment tools is likely to be most helpful in making the diagnosis of neuropathic pain?

A. Beck Depression Inventory
B. Brief Pain Inventory
C. Pain Catastrophising Scale
D. Pain Detect
E. Tampa Scale of Kinesiophobia

34.6. A 79 year old woman has osteoporosis with vertebral collapse at T10, demonstrated on plain X-ray. She is now struggling with washing and dressing herself because of severe pain. She lives alone, although she has a daughter who visits her every day, who has been giving her two co-codamol 30/500 (30 mg codeine and 500 mg of paracetamol), morning and evening. Her daughter is concerned that her mother's memory is not as good as it used to be. What is the likeliest cause of the memory impairment?

A. Borderline cognitive impairment exacerbated by opioid medication
B. Depression
C. Lack of sleep due to pain
D. New onset of Alzheimer's disease
E. Undiagnosed malignant disease, with brain metastases

34.7. A 27 year old man had a severe injury to his left arm in a motorcycle accident 4 years ago. He had extensive surgery, complicated by post-operative infection, and required a high dose of opioids to manage it at that time. He has had persistent pain since then, being unable to return to his job as a builder. When assessed in the pain clinic he has very limited movement, mechanical allodynia and intermittent swelling (below). The affected limb is noticeably colder than the other arm, with increased sweating in his hand.

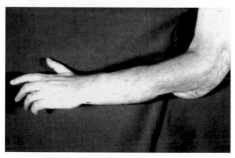

What is the likeliest diagnosis?

A. Chronic osteomyelitis
B. Complex regional pain syndrome (CRPS) type 1
C. CRPS type 2
D. Secondary osteoarthritis
E. Ulnar neuropathy

34.8. A 24 year old woman with long-standing Crohn's disease, currently quiescent, has chronic abdominal pain. She is on modified-release oxycodone 30 mg twice daily, plus immediate-release (IR) oxycodone 5–10 mg as required for pain, up to 6 times a day. She is regularly admitted with a flare-up in her pain, despite no evidence of active disease, although she is often very constipated. What is the best long-term management option for her?

A. Add in tramadol 100 mg 4 times daily for additional short-acting analgesia

B. Develop a management plan with the patient to support her in using self-management strategies
C. Ensure she has a thorough assessment by a dietician and advice on diet
D. Increase oxycodone IR to 15 mg with an increase in frequency, as required for the pain, up to 8 times a day.
E. Stop her strong opioids, as they may be causing the constipation

34.9. A 49 year old man with an advanced oropharyngeal tumour has severe pain in his mouth and jaw, and is also struggling to eat. He is taking soluble co-codamol, which helped initially but is not really working now. He has a past history of peptic ulcer disease. What type of analgesic would you choose next?

A. A strong opioid should be considered, with appropriate formulation or route of administration (e.g. suspension or liquid; transdermal)
B. Diazepam should be given to help with any anxiety
C. Diclofenac should be started at maximum dose to reduce any inflammation
D. Low-dose amitriptyline, or other tricyclic antidepressant, should be started in case there is any neuropathic pain
E. Paracetamol should be added in

34.10. A 65 year old man with inoperable lung cancer has increasing breathlessness. He is struggling to climb the stairs to his bedroom and more recently has found holding a conversation difficult. What would the first step be in managing his symptoms?

A. A comprehensive assessment to determine if there is a reversible cause
B. Breathing retraining should be used to improve mechanical effectiveness of the respiratory system
C. Use of a hand-held fan to cool the air flowing over nasal receptors
D. Referral for physical therapy to reduce disability and strengthen muscles
E. Reassurance and involvement of a psychologist to manage anxiety

34.11. A 72 year old man with metastatic prostate cancer is admitted with severe nausea and some delirium. He is on morphine for pain control, for bony metastases. What investigations should you do initially?

A. Blood test, including full blood count, urea and electrolytes, calcium and albumin
B. Computed tomography (CT) scan of abdomen and pelvis
C. CT scan of head
D. Electrocardiogram (ECG) and echocardiogram
E. Endoscopy

34.12. A 68 year old patient with chronic obstructive pulmonary disease (COPD) attends your outpatient clinic after a recent admission to the high dependency unit. He remains short of breath on minimal exertion. His daughter asks whether he might be referred to the local palliative care team. Which of the following statements applies?

A. He should be judged to be in the last 6 months of his life in order to benefit from specialist palliative care team input
B. He should have a diagnosis of cancer to be suitable for referral
C. He should have up-to-date pulmonary function tests before referral
D. He would benefit from advice on anticipatory planning for future exacerbations of his disease
E. Opiate medication is the likely treatment of choice for this patient

34.13. A 79 year old man is in the ward. He has presented with right flank pain and a sense of abdominal fullness. His liver function tests are abnormal and an ultrasound shows multiple lesions in the liver. He is tender over the right upper quadrant and tells the medical team that his pain is not helped by paracetamol.

He has a past medical history of ischaemic heart disease, gout, total hip replacement and a resection of a colonic cancer 2 years ago.

Which of the following would be a reasonable strategy if his pain persists?

A. A glucocorticoid such as prednisolone or dexamethasone
B. An NSAID
C. Antispasmodic medication such as hyoscine butylbromide
D. Gabapentin
E. Oral morphine solution

34.14. A 52 year old woman has metastatic cancer with bony metastases throughout her pelvis. She is requiring increasing doses of her opiate medication, and is concerned about the

side-effects associated with the medication. Which of the following pieces of advice is true?

A. Drowsiness after a dose increase is common and may improve within a few days
B. Morphine is the opiate of choice regardless of renal function
C. Once established on the right dose, further adjustments will not usually be necessary
D. The dry mouth associated with her morphine prescription will improve within a week of starting the drug
E. The nausea and vomiting are likely to persist and she should take long-term antiemetic medication in addition

34.15. A 71 year old woman with lung cancer and end-stage COPD is becoming increasingly distressed by dyspnoea and is referred to the respiratory team for assessment. She is tachypnoeic and anxious. Her symptoms are no longer relieved by inhaled bronchodilators. She has a cough productive of grey phlegm, which is unchanged from her normal situation. Her husband supports her at home; both of them continue to smoke.

Her chest X-ray shows hyperinflation of both lungs and the known tumour at the left apex. Observations are unremarkable other than oxygen saturations of 89%.

Which of the following might play a role in helping to manage her current condition?

A. An oxygen concentrator, for use as required at home
B. Antibiotic therapy
C. Initiation of citalopram medication
D. Oral diuretic therapy to treat any coexisting cardiac failure
E. Sublingual lorazepam, to be taken as required

34.16. A 76 year old woman is an inpatient in the general medical unit. She is known to have multiple myeloma with bony metastases and has presented with vomiting. Her bowels have not moved for 8 days. She is delirious and looks as though she may be dying.

Her initial blood results are as follows: haemoglobin 79 g/L, white cell count 6.7×10^9/L, platelets 314×10^9/L; urea 18.3 mmol/L (110 mg/dL), sodium 143 mmol/L, potassium 4.2 mmol/L, creatinine 213 μmol/L (2.4 mg/dL), calcium 2.94 mmol/L (11.8 mg/dL), albumin 23 g/L, adjusted calcium 3.28 mmol/L (13.1 mg/dL).

34

Which of the following initial treatments would be most helpful to this patient?

A. A subcutaneous infusion of haloperidol for her delirium and nausea

B. Blood transfusion to bring haemoglobin above 100 g/L and addition of a proton pump inhibitor

C. Intramuscular cyclizine

D. Intravenous fluids and bisphosphonate therapy

E. Intravenous fluids and laxatives to address the constipation

34.17. You are asked by hospital colleagues to undertake a palliative care review of a 77 year old man who is dying of end-stage cardiac failure in one of the general hospital wards. He is no longer able to eat or drink and is completely bed bound. He is now unconscious and is now unable to communicate his needs to his family or the nursing team caring for him. He is currently undistressed.

Which of the following statements applies to his ongoing management?

A. As he is unconscious, there is now no need for religious or spiritual support in this situation

B. He should have his urea and electrolytes checked at least twice weekly to check for worsening of his renal function

C. If he is unable to swallow medication, then he should receive his usual dose of diuretics by an intravenous route

D. Parenteral medication should be available as required for any symptoms that might arise

E. The family can be advised that he is likely to die within the next 2–3 days

Answers

34.1. Answer: B.
Normally, light touch and pressure cause activation of specialised mechanoreceptors such as Pacinian and Meissner's corpuscles, with transmission of sensation such as light touch being via large myelinated Aβ fibres. Painful stimuli activate high-threshold nociceptors, found on small unmyelinated C fibres. C fibres may contain a range of neuropeptides involved in pain processing, such as CGRP. Spinal interneurons modulate input from peripheral nerves.

34.2. Answer: B.
A wide range of neurotransmitters are involved in pain processing (Box 34.2), with changes occurring in response to tissue injury. Glutamate, acting via the N-methyl-D-aspartate (NMDA) receptor plays a key role in central sensitisation (Fig. 34.2), with increased neuronal

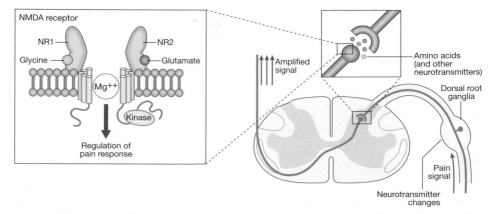

Fig. 34.2 Mechanisms of central sensitisation. Post-synaptic activation of the *N*-methyl-*D*-aspartate (NMDA) receptor by the amino acids glycine and glutamate, which bind to the NR1 and NR2 subunits, respectively, amplify pain signals at the level of the spinal cord. In contrast, magnesium ions block receptor activation.

34.2 Neurotransmitters and receptors involved in pain processing in the spinal cord			
Neurotransmitter	Receptor(s)	Receptor type	Comments*
Amino acids			
Glutamate	AMPA	Ion channel	Excitatory; permeable to cations: can be Ca^{2+}, Na^+ or K^+, depending on subunit structure
	NMDA	Ion channel	Excitatory; blocked by Mg^{2+} at resting state; block can be altered if membrane potential changes; permeable to Ca^{2+}, Na^+ and K^+
	Kainate	Ion channel	Post synaptic – excitatory
	Gp I	GPCR	Pre-synaptic – inhibitory through GABA release; permeable to Na^+ and K^+
	Gp II	GPCR	Activates a range of signalling pathways; long-term effects on synaptic excitability
	Gp III	GPCR	Probably inhibitory; can decrease cAMP production; pre-synaptic; decreases glutamate release
Glycine	GlyR	Ion channel	Mainly inhibitory; permeable to Cl^- blocked by caffeine
γ-aminobutyric acid	$GABA_A$	Ion channel	Mainly inhibitory in spinal cord; permeable to Cl^-; indirectly modulated by benzodiazepines (increased ion channel opening); not specifically involved in nociception, generally depressant effect on spinal cord activity
	$GABA_B$	GPCR	Predominantly inhibitory; activated by baclofen
Neuropeptides			
Substance P	Neurokinin receptors	GPCR	Mainly excitatory; increased in inflammation, decreased in neuropathic pain
Cholecystokinin	CCKRs1–8	GPCR	Excitatory; clinical trials of antagonists in progress
Calcitonin gene-related peptide	CALCRL	GPCR	Excitatory; slows degradation of substance P; implicated in migraine
Opioids			
Dynorphin	OP1 (kappa)	GPCR	Excitatory??; may be pro-nociceptive
β-endorphin	OP3 (mu)	GPCR	Inhibitory
Nociceptin	ORL-1	GPCR	Inhibitory; also expressed by immune cells

*Excitatory = increased pain; inhibitory = reduced pain.
(AMPA = α-amino-3-hydroxy-5-methyl-4-isoxazolepropionic acid; CALCRL = calcitonin receptor-like receptor; cAMP = cyclic adenosine monophosphate; GABA = γ-aminobutyric acid; Gp = group; GPCR = G-protein-coupled receptor; NMDA = N-methyl-D-aspartate; OP = opioid; ORL-1 = opioid receptor-like I)

activity at the spinal cord level. Inhibitory amino acid neurotransmitters include glycine and GABA, with neuropeptides such as β-endorphin and galanin having inhibitory actions, although these may be altered in some chronic pain states.

34.3. Answer: D.
When normally non-painful stimuli become painful (either thermal or mechanical), the term 'allodynia' is used. This can occur in neuropathic pain, and may be associated with other sensory changes, resulting in other symptoms such as formication – the sensation of insects crawling over the skin. Breakthrough pain tends to occur when the usual pain is controlled by analgesia and something (such as movement) precipitates an increase in pain that

is not controlled by the background analgesia. Hyperalgesia occurs in a painful area when the pain experienced is much greater than would be expected from the painful stimulus. Pain can also occur spontaneously without any precipitating stimulus, and may be related to spontaneously occurring electrical discharges in injured nerves.

34.4. Answer: A.
Assessment has shown features typical of diabetic neuropathy: stocking distribution, reduced sensation to pin-prick and mechanical allodynia. This man needs multidisciplinary management to address the range of issues that are affecting him. Psychosocial factors need to be considered with support in active rehabilitation, and use of non-pharmacological

34

techniques to self-manage his pain. Support in managing his diabetes better will reduce the risk of worsening symptoms, and lifestyle/dietary advice is needed to increase what he is able to do. The renal impairment means that anti-neuropathic drugs such as pregabalin and duloxetine need to be used with care, as toxicity may result on lower doses than expected.

34.5. Answer: D.
The Brief Pain Inventory was originally designed for use in cancer patients and measures pain intensity and its interference with different aspects of life. It does not assess the character of the pain, which is necessary to make a diagnosis of neuropathic pain. Pain Detect does do this, and has been validated in a range of neuropathic pain types. The other measures

assess physical and psychological effects of chronic pain in general (Box 34.5).

34.6. Answer: A.
While all of the above may impact on memory, the likeliest cause is borderline opioid toxicity. Elderly patients with limited reserve in terms of cognitive function are much more sensitive to even low doses of opioids (Box 34.6).

34.7. Answer: B.
The diagnosis of CRPS type 1 requires a combination of sensory, vasomotor, sudomotor and motor changes to be present. It can occur after an injury such as a fracture, without definite peripheral nerve lesion. CRPS type 2 occurs if there is a defined peripheral nerve lesion. CRPS is commoner in females between the ages of 35 and 50, occurring in about 20

i 34.5 Instruments used in the assessment of pain and its impact	
Instrument	Comments
Brief Pain Inventory	Developed for use in cancer pain, validated and widely employed for chronic pain; based on 0–10 ratings of pain intensity and the impact of pain on a range of domains, including sleep, work and enjoyment of life
Pain Detect, s-LANSS, DN-4	A number of screening questionnaires to aid diagnosis of neuropathic pain
Pain Catastrophising Scale	Developed to assess individual levels of catastrophising, encompassing three different domains: helplessness, rumination and magnification
Tampa Scale of Kinesiophobia	Measures how much an individual is fearful of movement
Pain Self-efficacy Questionnaire	Assesses individual beliefs about self-efficacy in the context of chronic pain, and how this impacts on function
Visual analogue scale (VAS)	Patient marks pain intensity on a horizontal line
Localisation of pain	Body chart, allowing the patient to indicate where pain is situated
Beck Depression Inventory	Assesses emotional function
SF-36/EQ-5D	Assesses health-related quality of life

(DN-4 = Douleur Neuropathique questionnaire; EQ-5D = EuroQol 5-Domain questionnaire; SF-36 = Short Form 36; s-LANSS = Leeds Assessment of Neuropathic Signs and Symptoms)

i 34.6 Challenges in pain assessment in particular patient populations		
Patient population	Challenges	Comments
Paediatric	Assessment needs to be appropriate to developmental stage	Consider visual tools to aid pain assessment
Elderly	May have impaired cognitive function Cultural factors may reduce self-reporting of pain Risk of adverse effects of medication increased	Consider formal assessment of cognitive function Consider non-verbal assessment Consider visual tools to assess pain Employ a number of tools assessing pain behaviours
Cognitive impairment	Reporting and expression of pain may change Increased sensitivity to central nervous system effects of analgesics	Perform formal assessment of cognitive function Use non-verbal assessment: facial expressions, vocalisations, body movements, changes in social interactions
Substance misuse	Response to analgesics altered Increased tolerance Increased risk of addiction Substance misuse may affect reporting of pain	Seek specialist support early Ensure prescribing is safe

per 100 000 individuals. Active rehabilitation with early physiotherapy is important in management.

34.8. Answer: B.
This is a challenging pain syndrome to manage, with very limited evidence for efficacy of long-term opioids, and growing evidence of possible harms. While opioids may be required for short-term use, regular use of short-acting strong opioids should be avoided if possible. Support in developing pain management strategies, maintaining function, ensuring adequate nutrition and reducing opioids should be the goal. Strong opioids should not be stopped abruptly unless the patient is at risk of overdose.

34.9. Answer: A.
The pain has responded to a weak opioid, but either some tolerance has developed or there is disease progression. He is, therefore, likely to get better analgesia from a strong opioid. Diazepam is not an analgesic, although it can be used for short-term anxiolysis. While there may be neuropathic features, a strong opioid should be started first. Non-steroidal anti-inflammatory drugs (NSAIDs) should be avoided if there is a history of peptic ulcer disease. Adding in paracetamol is unlikely to be effective, as he is already taking paracetamol in the compound preparation (co-codamol) and may result in exceeding safe dosing limits.

34.10. Answer: A.
While all of the options given can be used in the management of breathlessness, it is important to assess for treatable causes first, such as pleural effusion, cardiac failure or bronchospasm, even though the patient is being managed palliatively. Options B–E can all be useful in the management of breathlessness, but it is important to diagnose and start to treat any potentially reversible underlying cause first.

34.11. Answer: A.
There are many potential causes for confusion and nausea, including raised intracranial pressure and hypoxaemia due to a cardiovascular problem. While many of these tests may be appropriate, rapid checking of blood results allows exclusion of correctable causes such as electrolyte imbalance and, particularly, hypercalcaemia.

34.12. Answer: D.
Palliative care is the active total care for patients with incurable disease. A palliative care approach is likely to be suitable where symptom management becomes more important than aggressive treatment of the underlying disease, although the two goals of treatment can exist side by side. Although initially targeted at patients with malignant disease, patients with other life-limiting conditions such as COPD are now often suitable for palliative care input. There are usually no stringent guidelines regarding physiological parameters. Prognosis is often difficult to judge, but key events such as an admission to higher-level care are good opportunities to consider the future and make anticipatory care plans for the next exacerbation. Opiate medication is a possibility, but in the first instance he may benefit from non-pharmacological treatments and an assessment as to whether his inhaled medication is optimised.

34.13. Answer: A.
It is likely that this patient has liver capsule pain as a result of metastases from his previous colonic carcinoma. This type of pain responds poorly to opiates and is best treated by glucocorticoids. An antispasmodic will not relieve the stretch of the liver capsule. An NSAID is better suited to ischaemic or bone pain and gabapentin to neuropathic pain (Box 34.13).

34.14. Answer: A.
Nausea and vomiting can occur initially with opiate therapy but usually settle after a few days. Dry mouth and constipation are long-term effects, however, and will need ongoing treatment. Tolerance usually develops to drowsiness, so this problem is often transient after an increase in dose. Opiate toxicity is an ongoing concern for any patient on this medication and so follow-up review is advisable. This patient may need adjustments to her medication over time depending on increasing pain, changes in renal function or development of toxicity, if it arises.

Patients who develop renal failure are at particular risk of opiate toxicity and consideration should be given to swapping from morphine to an alternative opiate such as alfentanil.

34

i	34.13 Common types of pain in cancer	
Type of pain	Features	Management options
Bone pain	Tender area over bone Possible pain on movement	NSAIDs Bisphosphonates Radiotherapy
Increased intracranial pressure	Headache, worse in the morning, associated with vomiting and occasionally confusion	Glucocorticoids Radiotherapy Codeine
Abdominal colic	Intermittent, severe, spasmodic, associated with nausea or vomiting	Antispasmodics Hyoscine butylbromide
Liver capsule pain	Right upper quadrant abdominal pain, often associated with tender enlarged liver Responds poorly to opioids	Glucocorticoids

Neuropathic pain	Spontaneous pain
	Light touch, pressure and temperature changes are painful; increased pain on pin-prick
	Numbness, tingling or loss of temperature sensation
	Skin feels abnormal
		Anticonvulsants:
		  Gabapentin
		  Pregabalin
		Antidepressants
		  Amitriptyline
		  Duloxetine
		  Ketamine

Ischaemic pain	Diffuse, severe, aching pain associated with evidence of poor perfusion Responds poorly to opioids	NSAIDs Ketamine
Incident pain	Episodic pain usually related to movement or bowel spasm	Intermittent short-acting opioids Nerve block

(NSAIDs = non-steroidal anti-inflammatory drugs)

34.15. Answer: E.

Breathlessness is one of the most common symptoms in palliative care and is distressing for both patients and carers. Patients with breathlessness should be fully assessed to determine whether there is a reversible cause, such as a pleural effusion, heart failure or bronchospasm; if so, this should be managed in the normal way. There is no suggestion in the scenario here of fluid overload or new infection to justify antibiotics or diuretics.

There are many potential causes of dyspnoea in cancer patients and in other chronic diseases; apart from direct involvement of the lungs, muscle loss secondary to cachexia, anxiety and fear can all contribute. A cycle of panic and breathlessness, often associated with fear of dying, can be dominant. Exploration of precipitating factors is important and patient education about breathlessness and effective breathing has been shown to be effective. Non-pharmacological approaches that include using a hand-held fan, pacing, and following a tailored exercise programme can help. There is no evidence to suggest that oxygen therapy reduces the sensation of breathlessness in advanced cancer any better than cool air flow, and oxygen is indicated only if there is significant hypoxia. In this case, oxygen is also likely to be precluded by both the husband and wife continuing to smoke in the house.

Opioids, through both their central and their peripheral action, can palliate breathlessness and might be an alternative in this scenario. If anxiety is considered to be playing a significant role, a quick-acting benzodiazepine, such as lorazepam (used sublingually for rapid absorption), may also be useful. Citalopram would be useful for longer-term treatment of established anxiety or depression, but would not give instant relief in the short term in the way that lorazepam would.

34.16. Answer: D.

Although this patient is very unwell, her hypercalcaemia may be amenable to treatment. Even if it is not life saving, it will make her feel more comfortable and reducing her calcium level will be the most effective way to help her vomiting. The other treatments may have a role

i 34.17 How to manage a patient who is dying	
Patient and family awareness	**Support for family**
Assess patient's and family's awareness of the situation Ensure family understands plan of care	Make sure you have contact details for family, that you know when they want to be contacted and that they are aware of facilities available to them
Medical interventions	
Stop non-essential medications that do not contribute to symptom control Stop inappropriate investigations and interventions, including routine observations	**Religious and spiritual needs**
	Make sure any particular wishes are identified and followed
	Ongoing assessment
Resuscitation	Family's awareness of condition Management of symptoms Need for parenteral hydration
Complete Do Not Attempt Cardiopulmonary Resuscitation (DNACPR) form Deactivate implantable defibrillator	
	Care after death
Symptom control	Make sure family know what they have to do Notify other appropriate health professionals
Ensure availability of parenteral medication for symptom relief	

in due course, but would be of lower priority than addressing her hypercalcaemia.

34.17. Answer: D.

When patients with any advanced condition become comatose and unable to take medication or oral intake with no reversible cause, they are likely to be dying. Although many will die within 2–3 days, this stage of life is often unpredictable and doctors should be cautious in any prognosis they give to families.

Once the conclusion has been reached that a patient is dying, there is a significant change in management (Box 34.17). Symptom control, relief of distress and care for the family become the most important elements of care. Medication and investigation are only justifiable

if they contribute to these ends. In the case of this patient, he has no oral intake and is undistressed; therefore diuretics are unlikely to help and intravenous treatment will be unnecessarily burdensome. Religious and spiritual support are very important in this situation, for the family as much as the patient. Priority should be given to checking the understanding of family members regarding the situation and their wishes regarding care, visiting and how they wish to be contacted.

Although the patient does not currently have any symptoms at present, it is possible that he may develop them at some point in future. It is important to ensure availability of parenteral medication for symptom relief so that it can be given without delay should the need arise.

34

35

Laboratory reference ranges

Notes on the International System of Units (SI Units)

Système International (SI) d'Unités are a specific subset of the metre–kilogram–second system of units and were agreed on as the everyday currency for commercial and scientific work in 1960, following a series of international conferences organised by the International Bureau of Weights and Measures. SI units have been adopted widely in clinical laboratories but non-SI units are still used in many countries. For that reason, values in both units are given for common measurements throughout this textbook and commonly used non-SI units are shown in this chapter. The SI unit system is, however, recommended.

Examples of basic SI units

Length	metre (m)
Mass	kilogram (kg)
Amount of substance	mole (mol)
Energy	joule (J)
Pressure	pascal (Pa)
Volume	The basic SI unit of volume is the cubic metre (1000 litres). For convenience, however, the litre (L) is used as the unit of volume in laboratory work.

Examples of decimal multiples and submultiples of SI units

Factor	Name	Prefix
10^6	mega-	M
10^3	kilo-	k
10^{-1}	deci-	d
10^{-2}	centi-	c
10^{-3}	milli-	m
10^{-6}	micro-	μ
10^{-9}	nano-	n
10^{-12}	pico-	p
10^{-15}	femto-	f

Exceptions to the use of SI units

By convention, blood pressure is excluded from the SI unit system and is measured in mmHg (millimetres of mercury) rather than pascals.

Mass concentrations such as g/L and μg/L are used in preference to molar concentrations for all protein measurements and for substances that do not have a sufficiently well-defined composition.

Some enzymes and hormones are measured by 'bioassay', in which the activity in the sample is compared with the activity (rather than the mass) of a standard sample that is provided from a central source. For these assays, results are given in standardised 'units' (U/L), or 'international units' (IU/L), which depend on the activity in the standard sample and may not be readily converted to mass units.

Laboratory reference ranges in adults

35

Reference ranges are largely those used in the Departments of Clinical Biochemistry and Haematology, Lothian Health University Hospitals Division, Edinburgh, UK. Values are shown in both SI units and, where appropriate, non-SI units. Many reference ranges vary between laboratories, depending on the assay method used and on other factors; this is especially the case for enzyme assays. Reference ranges and the definition of 'abnormal' results are based on distributions in the population of interest and may differ between settings. No details are given here of the collection requirements, which may be critical to obtaining a meaningful result. Unless otherwise stated, reference ranges shown apply to adults; values in children may be different.

Many analytes can be measured in either serum (the supernatant of clotted blood) or plasma (the supernatant of anticoagulated blood). A specific requirement for one or the other may depend on a kit manufacturer's recommendations. In other instances, the distinction is critical. An example is fibrinogen, where plasma is required, since fibrinogen is largely absent from serum. In contrast, serum is required for electrophoresis to detect paraproteins because fibrinogen migrates as a discrete band in the zone of interest.

i 35.1 Urea and electrolytes in venous blood

Analysis	Reference range SI units	Non-SI units
Sodium	135–145 mmol/L	135–145 mEq/L
Potassium*	3.6–5.0 mmol/L	3.6–5.0 mEq/L
Chloride	95–107 mmol/L	95–107 mEq/L
Urea	2.5–6.6 mmol/L	15–40 mg/dL
Creatinine		
Male	64–111 µmol/L	0.72–1.26 mg/dL
Female	50–98 µmol/L	0.57–1.11 mg/dL

Serum values are, on average, 0.3 mmol/L higher than plasma values.

i 35.2 Analytes in arterial blood

Analysis	Reference range SI units	Non-SI units
Bicarbonate	21–29 mmol/L	21–29 mEq/L
Hydrogen ion	37–45 nmol/L	pH 7.35–7.43
$PaCO_2$	4.5–6.0 kPa	34–45 mmHg
PaO_2	12–15 kPa	90–113 mmHg
Oxygen saturation	>97%	

i 35.3 Hormones in venous blood

Hormone	Reference range SI units	Non-SI units
Adrenocorticotrophic hormone (ACTH) (plasma)	1.5–13.9 pmol/L (0700–1000 hrs)	63 ng/L
Aldosterone		
Supine (at least 30 mins)	30–440 pmol/L	1.09–15.9 ng/dL
Erect (at least 1 hr)	110–860 pmol/L	3.97–31.0 ng/dL
Cortisol	Dynamic tests are required Plasma cortisol > 500 nmol/L (approximately 18 µg/dL)* either at baseline or at 30 mins post 250 µg ACTH$_{1-24}$ (Synacthen) by IM injection	
Follicle-stimulating hormone (FSH)		
Male	1.0–10.0 IU/L	0.2–2.2 ng/mL
Female	3.0–10.0 IU/L (early follicular) >30 IU/L (post-menopausal)	0.7–2.2 ng/mL >6.7 ng/mL

Continued

i	35.3 Hormones in venous blood – cont'd	
Hormone	Reference range SI units	Non-SI units
Gastrin (plasma, fasting)	<40 pmol/L	<83 pg/mL
Growth hormone (GH)	Dynamic tests are usually required – see Ch. 18 <0.5 µg/L excludes acromegaly (if insulin-like growth factor 1 (IGF-1) in reference range) >6 µg/L excludes GH deficiency >18 mIU/L	< 2 mIU/L
Insulin	Highly variable and interpretable only in relation to plasma glucose and body habitus	
C-peptide	Highly variable and interpretable only in relation to plasma glucose and body habitus. However very low levels are found in conditions of insulin deficiency e.g. type 1 diabetes	
Luteinising hormone (LH)		
Male	1.0–9.0 IU/L	0.1–1.0 µg/L
Female	2.0–9.0 IU/L (early follicular) >20 IU/L (post-menopausal)	0.2–1.0 µg/L > 2.2 µg/L
17β-Oestradiol		
Male	<160 pmol/L	<43 pg/mL
Female: early follicular	75–140 pmol/L	20–38 pg/mL
mid-follicular	100–453 pmol/L	27–123 pg/mL
post-menopausal	<150 pmol/L	<41 pg/mL
Parathyroid hormone (PTH)	1.6–6.9 pmol/L	16–69 pg/mL
Progesterone (in luteal phase in women)		
Consistent with ovulation	>30 nmol/L	>9.3 ng/mL
Probable ovulatory cycle	15–30 nmol/L	4.7–9.3 ng/mL
Anovulatory cycle	<10 nmol/L	<3 ng/mL
Prolactin (PRL)	60–500 mIU/L	–
Renin concentration		
Supine (at least 30 mins)	5–40 mIU/L	–
Sitting (at least 15 mins)	5–45 mIU/L	–
Erect (at least 1 hr)	16–63 mIU/L	–
Testosterone		
Male	10–38 nmol/L	2.9–10.9 ng/mL
Female	0.3–1.9 nmol/L	0.1–0.9 ng/mL
Thyroid-stimulating hormone (TSH)	0.2–4.5 mIU/L	–
Thyroxine (free), (free T$_4$)	9–21 pmol/L	700–1632 pg/dL
Triiodothyronine (free), (free T$_3$)	2.6–6.2 pmol/L	160–400 pg/dL

Notes

1. A number of hormones are unstable and collection details are critical to obtaining a meaningful result. Refer to local laboratory handbook.

2. Values in the table are only a guideline; hormone levels can often be meaningfully understood only in relation to factors such as gender (e.g. testosterone), age (e.g. FSH in women), pregnancy (e.g. thyroid function tests, prolactin), time of day (e.g. cortisol) or regulatory hormones (e.g. insulin and glucose, PTH and [Ca^{2+}]).

3. Reference ranges are usually dependent on the method used for analysis.

35

i **35.4 Other common analytes in venous blood**

Analyte	Reference range SI units	Non-SI units
α$_1$-Antitrypsin	1.1–2.1 g/L	110–210 mg/dL
Alanine aminotransferase (ALT)	10–50 U/L	–
Albumin	35–50 g/L	3.5–5.0 g/dL
Alpha-fetoprotein	<10 ng/mL	1000 ng/ dL
Alkaline phosphatase	40–125 U/L	–
Amylase	<100 U/L	–
Aspartate aminotransferase (AST)	10–45 U/L	–
Bilirubin (total)	3–16 μmol/L	0.18–0.94 mg/dL
Calcium (total)	2.1–2.6 mmol/L	4.2–5.2 mEq/L or 8.5–10.5 mg/dL
Carboxyhaemoglobin	0.1–3.0% Levels of up to 8% may be found in heavy smokers	–
Caeruloplasmin	0.16–0.47 g/L	16–47 mg/dL
Cholesterol	Target cholesterol levels will vary according to individual cardiovascular risk, with stricter goals for those most at risk. Normal ranges are misleading as they cover both a healthy and unhealthy population. A rough guide to treatment targets is given below, but further guidance, e.g. National Cholesterol Education Programme Adult Treatment Panel III (ATPIII) guidelines, should be used for individual case management. See Box 35.15 for treatment guidelines in diabetes	
Approx Treatment Targets:		
Cholesterol (total) (see also Fig. 35.1)	<5–5.2 mmol/l	<200 mg/dL
LDL-cholesterol	<2–2.5 mmol/l	<100 mg/dL
HDL-cholesterol		
Low	<1.0 mmol/L	<40 mg/dL
High (desirable)	≥1.5 mmol/L	≥60 mg/dL
Complement		
C3	0.81–1.57 g/L	–
C4	0.13–1.39 g/L	–
Total haemolytic complement	0.086–0.410 g/L	–
CA-125	<35 U/mL	
CEA	<3 ng/mL	
Copper	10–22 μmol/L	64–140 μg/dL
C-reactive protein (CRP)	<5 mg/L Highly sensitive CRP assays also exist that measure lower values and may be useful in estimating cardiovascular risk	
Creatine kinase (CK; total)		
Male	55–170 U/L	–
Female	30–135 U/L	–
Creatine kinase MB isoenzyme	<6% of total CK	–
Ethanol	Not normally detectable	
Marked intoxication	65–87 mmol/L	300–400 mg/dL
Stupor	87–109 mmol/L	400–500 mg/dL
Coma	>109 mmol/L	>500 mg/dL
γ-glutamyl transferase (GGT)	Male 10–55 U/L Female 5–35 U/L	–
Glucose (fasting)	3.6–5.8 mmol/L See Box 35.15 for definitions of impaired glucose tolerance and diabetes mellitus. Hypoglycaemia is defined as a blood glucose of less than 3.9 mmol/L (70 mg/dL)	65–104 mg/dL
Glycated haemoglobin (HbA$_{1c}$)	4.0–6.0% 20–42 mmol/mol Hb See Box 35.15 for diagnosis of diabetes mellitus	–
Ketones	<1 mg/dL Note: levels can be mildly physiologically elevated during periods of starvation	

Continued

i 35.4 Other common analytes in venous blood – cont'd

Analyte	Reference range SI units	Non-SI units
Lactate	0.6–2.4 mmol/L	5.40–21.6 mg/dL
Lactate dehydrogenase (LDH; total)	125–220 U/L	–
Lead	<0.5 µmol/L	<10 µg/dL
Magnesium	0.75–1.0 mmol/L	1.5–2.0 mEq/L or 1.82–2.43 mg/dL
Osmolality	280–296 mOsmol/kg	–
Osmolarity	280–296 mOsmol/L	–
Phosphate (fasting)	0.8–1.4 mmol/L	2.48–4.34 mg/dL
Protein (total)	60–80 g/L	6–8 g/dL
Sex hormone-binding globulin (SHBG)	18.4–75.6 nmol/L	175–718 µg/dL
Triglycerides (fasting)	0.6–1.7 mmol/L	53–150 mg/dL
Troponins	Values consistent with myocardial infarction are crucially dependent on which troponin is measured (I or T) and on the method employed. Interpret in context of clinical presentation. Troponin I and troponin T are structural cardiac muscle proteins that are released during myocyte damage and necrosis, and represent the cornerstone of the diagnosis of acute myocardial infarction. Modern assays are extremely sensitive, however, and can detect minor degrees of myocardial damage, so that elevated plasma troponin concentrations may be observed in conditions other than acute MI, such as pulmonary embolus, septic shock and pulmonary oedema.	
Tryptase	0–135 mg/L	–
Urate		
Male	0.12–0.42 mmol/L	2.0–7.0 mg/dL
Female	0.12–0.36 mmol/L	2.0–6.0 mg/dL
Vitamin D (25(OH)D)		
Normal	>50 nmol/L	>20 ng/mL
Insufficiency	25–50 nmol/L	10–20 ng/ml
Deficiency	<25 nmol/L	<10 ng/mL
Zinc	10–18 µmol/L	65–118 µg/dL

Calculated blood values

Anion gap

The **anion gap** is the difference between the primary measured cations (sodium Na+ and potassium K+) and the primary measured **anions** (chloride Cl− and bicarbonate HCO_3^-) in serum

A normal anion gap using ion selective electrodes is 3–11 mEq/L

Previous measures of anion gap using colorimetry gave a normal range of **8–16** mEq/L

when not including K+ and 10–20 mEq/L when including K+

eGFR

The estimated glomeral filtration rate (eGFR) is calculated from age, sex and blood creatinine level. An adjustment is needed for certain ethnic groups. eGFR levels have been used to categorise degrees of renal impairment

eGFR (mL/min/1.73 m²)	Stage of chronic kidney disease (CKD)	Description
>90	Stage 1	Normal
60–89	Stage 2	Mild reduction (not considered CKD)
45–59	CKD stage 3A	Moderately reduced function
30–44	CKD stage 3B	Moderately reduced function
15–29	CKD stage 4	Severely reduced function
<15	CKD stage 5	Very severely reduced function/end-stage kidney failure

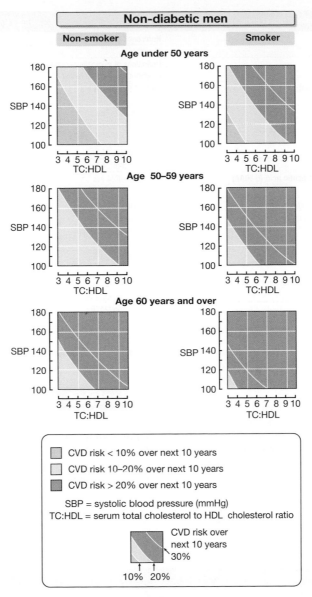

Fig. 35.1

Serum osmolality

The **serum** or plasma **osmolality** is a measurement of the different solutes in plasma. It is primarily determined by sodium, chloride, bicarbonate, glucose and urea. Osmoles per kilogram of water defines **osmolality**. Normal range is 280–**296 mOsm**/kg.

i 35.5 Common analytes in urine

Analyte	Reference range SI units	Non-SI units
Albumin	Definitions of microalbuminuria are given in Box 35.6 Proteinuria is defined below	
Calcium (normal diet)	Up to 7.5 mmol/24 hrs	Up to 15 mEq/24 hrs or 300 mg/24 hrs
Copper	<0.6 μmol/24 hrs	<38 μg/24 hrs
Cortisol	20–180 nmol/24 hrs	7.2–65 μg/24 hrs
Creatinine		
Male	6.3–23 mmol/24 hrs	712–2600 mg/24 hrs
Female	4.1–15 mmol/24 hrs	463–1695 mg/24 hrs
5-hydroxyindole-3-acetic acid (5-HIAA)	10–42 μmol/24 hrs	1.9–8.1 mg/24 hrs
Metadrenalines		
Normetadrenaline (normetanephrine)	0.4–3.4 μmol/24 hrs	73–620 μg/24 hrs
Metadrenaline (metanephrine)	0.3–1.7 μmol/24 hrs	59–335 μg/24 hrs
Oxalate	0.04–0.49 mmol/24 hrs	3.6–44 mg/24 hrs
Phosphate	15–50 mmol/24 hrs	465–1548 mg/24 hrs
Potassium*	25–100 mmol/24 hrs	25–100 mEq/24 hrs
Protein	<0.3 g/L	<0.03 g/dL
Sodium* (random sample)	40–220 mmol/L	40–220 mEq/L
Sodium*	100–200 mmol/24 hrs	100–200 mEq/24 hrs
Urate	1.2–3.0 mmol/24 hrs	202–504 mg/24 hrs
Urea	170–600 mmol/24 hrs	10.2–36.0 g/24 hrs
Zinc	3–21 μmol/24 hrs	195–1365 μg/24 hrs

*The urinary output of electrolytes such as sodium and potassium is normally a reflection of dietary intake. This can vary widely. The values quoted are appropriate to a 'Western' diet.

Urinalysis

Urinalysis is a point of care test normally assessing the pH (normal range pH 4.6 to pH 8.0), specific gravity (normal range 1.005–1.030) and the prescence of components such as blood, protein, glucose, ketones, nitrites, leukocyte esterase, bilirubin and urobilirubin. A normal result is negative for all parameters. If present, a scale of + to ++++ is used to describe the degree of positivity.

Calculated urine values

Urine Osmolality

Urine osmolality is a **measure** of the concentration of osmotically active particles, principally **sodium**, chloride, potassium and urea; glucose can contribute significantly to the **osmolality** when present in substantial amounts in **urine**

i 35.6 Albumin : Creatinine Ratio (ACR)

ACR[1]	Category	PCR[2]	Typical dipstick results[3]	Significance
<2.5 mg/mmol (males) <3.5 mg/mmol (females)	A1 Normal	< 25	–	Normal
2.5–30 mg/mmol (males) 3.5–30 mg/mmol (females)	A2 Mildly raised	25–50	–	Moderately elevated albuminuria Known as 'Microalbuminuria'
30–70	A3 Moderately raised	50–100	+ to ++	Dipstick positive Known as 'Proteinuria'
70–300		100–350	++ to +++	Glomerular disease more likely; equivalent to > 1 g/24 hrs Known as 'Heavy Proteinuria'
> 300		> 350	+++ to ++++	Nephrotic range: almost always glomerular disease, equivalent to > 3.5 g/24 hrs

[1]Urinary albumin (mg/L)/urine creatinine (mmol/L). [2]Urine protein (mg/L)/urine creatinine (mmol/L). (If urine creatinine is measured in mg/dL, reference values for PCR and ACR can be derived by dividing by 11.31.) [3]Dipstick results are affected by urine concentration and are occasionally weakly positive on normal samples.

Random urine osmolality should average **300–900** mOsm/kg of water

Calcium clearance: creatinine clearance ratio

This test is generally done in the context of hypercalcaemia in association with a normal or raised plasma PTH level.

The ratio is calculated using the following formula:

urine calcium (mmol/L) × [serum creatinine (μmol/L) /1000]

serum calcium (mmol) × urine creatinine (mmol/L)

Interpretation

- Calcium creatinine clearance ratio > 0.01 is suggestive of primary hyperparathyroidism (PHPT).
- Calcium creatinine clearance ratio < 0.01 is suggestive of familial hypocalciuric hypocalcaemia (FHH) but may also be seen in PHPT with vitamin D deficiency.
- Urine calcium is also usually <200 mg/24 hrs (50 mmol/24 hrs) in FHH.

35

ℹ 35.7 Analytes in cerebrospinal fluid (CSF)

Analysis	Reference range SI units	Non-SI units
Cells	<5×10⁶ cells/L (all mononuclear)	<5 cells/mm³
Glucose[1]	2.3–4.5 mmol/L	41–81 mg/dL
IgG index[2]	<0.65	–
Total protein	0.14–0.45 g/L	0.014–0.045 g/dL

[1]Interpret in relation to plasma glucose. Values in CSF are typically approximately two-thirds of plasma levels.
[2]A crude index of increase in immunoglobulin G (IgG) attributable to intrathecal synthesis.

ℹ 35.8 Analytes in faeces

Analyte	Reference range SI units	Non-SI units
Calprotectin	<50 μg/g	–
Elastase	>200 μg/g	–

ℹ 35.9 Analytes in pleural fluid

Analyte	Reference range SI units	Non-SI units
Lactate dehydrogenase	125–220 U/L	–

ℹ 35.10 Haematological values

Analysis	Reference range SI units	Non-SI units
Activated partial thromboplastin time (APTT)	24–34 secs	–
Bleeding time (Ivy)	<8 mins	–
Blood volume		
Male	65–85 mL/kg	–
Female	60–80 mL/kg	–
CD4 count	>500 cells/mm³	–
Coagulation screen		
Prothrombin time (PT)	10.5–13.5 secs	–
Activated partial thromboplastin time (APTT)	26–36 secs	–
D-dimers		
Interpret in relation to clinical presentation	<200 ng/mL	–
Erythrocyte sedimentation rate (ESR)	Higher values in older patients are not necessarily abnormal	
Adult male	0–10 mm/hr	–
Adult female	3–15 mm/hr	–
Erythropoietin (EPO) (adults)	4.1–19.5 mU/mL	
Factor VIII	RR is 50–150% of normal	
Ferritin		
Male (and post-menopausal female)	20–300 μg/L	20–300 ng/mL
Female (pre-menopausal)	15–200 μg/L	15–200 ng/mL
Fibrinogen	1.5–4.0 g/L	0.15–0.4 g/dL
Folate		
Serum	2.8–20 μg/L	2.8–20 ng/mL
Red cell	120–500 μg/L	120–500 ng/mL
Haemoglobin		
Male	130–180 g/L	13–18 g/dL
Female	115–165 g/L	11.5–16.5 g/dL
Haptoglobin	0.4–2.4 g/L	0.04–0.24 g/dL

Continued

i 35.10 Haematological values – cont'd

Analysis	Reference range SI units	Non-SI units
Iron		
Male	14–32 μmol/L	78–178 μg/dL
Female	10–28 μmol/L	56–157 μg/dL
Leucocytes (adults)	4.0–11.0×10⁹/L	4.0–11.0×10³/mm³
Differential white cell count		
Neutrophil granulocytes	2.0–7.5×10⁹/L	2.0–7.5×10³/mm³
Lymphocytes	1.5–4.0×10⁹/L	1.5–4.0×10³/mm³
Monocytes	0.2–0.8×10⁹/L	0.2–0.8×10³/mm³
Eosinophil granulocytes	0.04–0.4×10⁹/L	0.04–0.4×10³/mm³
Basophil granulocytes	0.01–0.1×10⁹/L	0.01–0.1×10³/mm³
Mean cell haemoglobin (MCH)	27–32 pg	–
Mean cell volume (MCV)	78–98 fl	–
Packed cell volume (PCV) or haematocrit		
Male	0.40–0.54	–
Female	0.37–0.47	–
Platelets	150–350×10⁹/L	150–350×10³/mm³
Prothrombin time (PT)	10–13.5 secs	–
Red cell count		
Male	4.5–6.5×10¹²/L	4.5–6.5×10⁶/mm³
Female	3.8–5.8×10¹²/L	3.8–5.8×10⁶/mm³
Red cell lifespan		
Mean	120 days	–
Half-life (⁵¹Cr)	25–35 days	–
Reticulocytes (adults)	25–85×10⁹/L	25–85×10³/mm³
Total iron-binding capacity	43–81 μmol/L	240–453 μg/dL
Transferrin	2.0–4.0 g/L	0.2–0.4 g/dL
Transferrin saturation		
Male	25–50%	–
Female	14–50%	–
Vitamin B₁₂		
Normal	>210 ng/L	–
Intermediatev	180–200 ng/L	–
Low	<180 ng/L	–
von Willebrand factor activity (ristocetin co-factor)	RR is 50–200%	

i 35.11 Immunological reference ranges

Anti-tissue transglutaminase antibody (anti-tTG)	Negative <20 U, positive >75 U
Anti-citrullinated peptide antibodies (ACPA)	Normal <4.5 U
Anti-DNA antibody titre	0–5 IU/L
TSH receptor antibodies (TRAbs)	0–1.6 IU/L
Serum allergen testing (Specific IgE)	Interpretation <0.35 kU/L – no specific IgE antibody detected 0.35–0.70 kU/L – low level 0.70–3.50 kU/L – moderate level 3.50–17.5 kU/L – high level 17.5–100 kU/L – very high level >100.0 kU/L – extremely high level
Immunoglobulins (Ig)	
IgA	0.8–4.5 g/L
IgE	0–250 kU/L
IgG	6.0–15.0 g/L
IgM	0.35–2.90 g/L

Laboratory reference ranges in pregnancy

The levels of many analytes in blood vary during pregnancy, when many hormonal and metabolic changes occur. The standard adult reference ranges may therefore not be appropriate and it is important for the clinician reviewing the results to be aware of this to enable appropriate interpretation and patient management.

i 35.12 Analytes that may be significantly affected by pregnancy*

Analyte	Reference range First trimester	Second trimester	Third trimester
Alkaline phosphatase	17–88 U/L	25–126 U/L	38–229 U/L
Packed cell volume (PCV) or haematocrit	0.31–0.41	0.30–0.39	0.28–0.40
Haemoglobin	116–139 g/L	97–148 g/L	95–150 g/L
Human chorionic gonadotrophin	4 weeks: 16–156 IU/L 4–9 weeks: 101–233 000 IU/L 9–13 weeks: 20 900–291 000 IU/L	4270–103 000 IU/L	2700–78 300 IU/L
17β-Oestradiol	690–9166 pmol/L (188–2497 pg/mL)	4691–26 401 pmol/L (1278–7192 pg/mL)	12 701–22 528 pmol/L (3460–6137 pg/mL)
Progesterone	25–153 nmol/L (8–48 ng/mL)	Not available	314–1088 nmol/L (99–342 ng/mL)
Prolactin	765–4532 mIU/L	2340–7021 mIU/L	2914–7914 mIU/L
Thyroid-stimulating hormone (TSH)	0.60–3.40 mIU/L	0.37–3.60 mIU/L	0.38–4.04 mIU/L
Thyroxine (free), (free T$_4$)	10–18 pmol/L (777–1399 pg/dL)	9–16 pmol/L (699–1243 pg/dL)	8–14 pmol/L (621–1088 pg/dL)

*Non-SI equivalents are given in brackets where appropriate.

Laboratory reference ranges in childhood and adolescence

The levels of many analytes in blood vary due to the physiological changes that occur during growth and adolescence. Hospital laboratories may provide reference ranges that are age-adjusted or based on pubertal stage but this is not always the case. It is therefore important for the doctor requesting these tests to understand the impact of age and puberty on interpretation of the results. For example, a creatinine of 70 μmol/L (0.79 mg/dL) is perfectly normal for the majority of adults but may indicate significant renal impairment in a child. Reference ranges for hormone results are described according to the Tanner stages of puberty (see Fig. 35.2).

i 35.13 Analytes that may be significantly affected by growth and puberty*

Analyte	Age/pubertal stage	Gender	Reference range
Alkaline phosphatase (ALP)	<1 year	M, F	80–580 U/L
	1–16 years	M, F	100–400 U/L
	16–20 years	M	50–250 U/L
		F	40–200 U/L
Creatinine	<1 year	M, F	12–39 μmol/L (0.14–0.44 mg/dL)
	1–4 years	M, F	13–42 μmol/L (0.15–0.48 mg/dL)
	4–12 years	M, F	20–57 μmol/L (0.23–0.64 mg/dL)
	12–15 years	M, F	31–67 μmol/L (0.35–0.76 mg/dL)

Continued

	35.13 Analytes that may be significantly affected by growth and puberty* – cont'd		
Analyte	Age/pubertal stage	Gender	Reference range
	15–18 years	M	39–92 µmol/L (0.44–1.04 mg/dL)
		F	34–72 µmol/L (0.38–0.81 mg/dL)
Follicle-stimulating hormone	Prepubertal	M	<3.0 IU/L (<0.6 ng/mL)
		F	<3.2 IU/L (<0.64 ng/mL)
	Pubertal stage 2	M	<6.6 IU/L (<1.32 ng/mL)
		F	<4.1 IU/L (<0.82 ng/mL)
	Pubertal stage 3	M	0.7–5.0 IU/L (0.14–1 ng/mL)
	Pubertal stages 4–5	M	1.5–6.0 IU/L (0.3–1.2 ng/mL)
	Pubertal stages 3–5	F	2.5–13.5 IU/L (0.5–2.7 ng/mL)
Insulin-like growth factor 1	<7 years	M	15–349 µg/L
		F	17–272 µg/L
	8–16 years	M	67–510 µg/L
		F	59–502 µg/L
Luteinising hormone	Prepubertal	M	<1.0 IU/L (<0.1 µg/L)
	Pubertal stage 2	M	<3.0 IU/L (<0.3 µg/L)
	Prepubertal and pubertal stage 2	F	<1.0 IU/L (<0.1 µg/L)
	Pubertal stage 3	M	1.0–4.0 IU/L (0.1–0.4 µg/L)
	Pubertal stages 4–5	M	1.0–5.0 IU/L (0.1–0.6 µg/L)
	Pubertal stages 3–5	F	1.0–8.0 IU/L (0.1–0.9 µg/L)
17β-Oestradiol	Prepubertal and pubertal stages 2–3	M	<75 pmol/L (<20 pg/mL)
	Prepubertal and pubertal stage 2	F	<100 pmol/L (<27 pg/mL)
	Pubertal stages 4–5	M	<130 pmol/L (<35 pg/mL)
	Pubertal stages 3–5	F	<150 pmol/L (<41 pg/mL)
Testosterone	Prepubertal	M	<0.5 nmol/L (<0.1 ng/mL)
		F	<0.6 nmol/L (<0.2 ng/mL)
	Pubertal stage 2	M	<10.6 nmol/L (<3.1 ng/mL)
		F	<1.4 nmol/L (<0.4 ng/mL)
	Pubertal stage 3	M	0.4–30 nmol/L (0.1–8.7 ng/mL)
	Pubertal stage 4	M	5.6–30 nmol/L (1.6–8.7 ng/mL)
	Pubertal stage 5	M	10–30 nmol/L (2.9–8.7 ng/mL)
	Pubertal stages 3–5	F	0.4–1.9 nmol/L (0.1–0.5 ng/mL)

*Non-SI equivalents are given in brackets where appropriate.

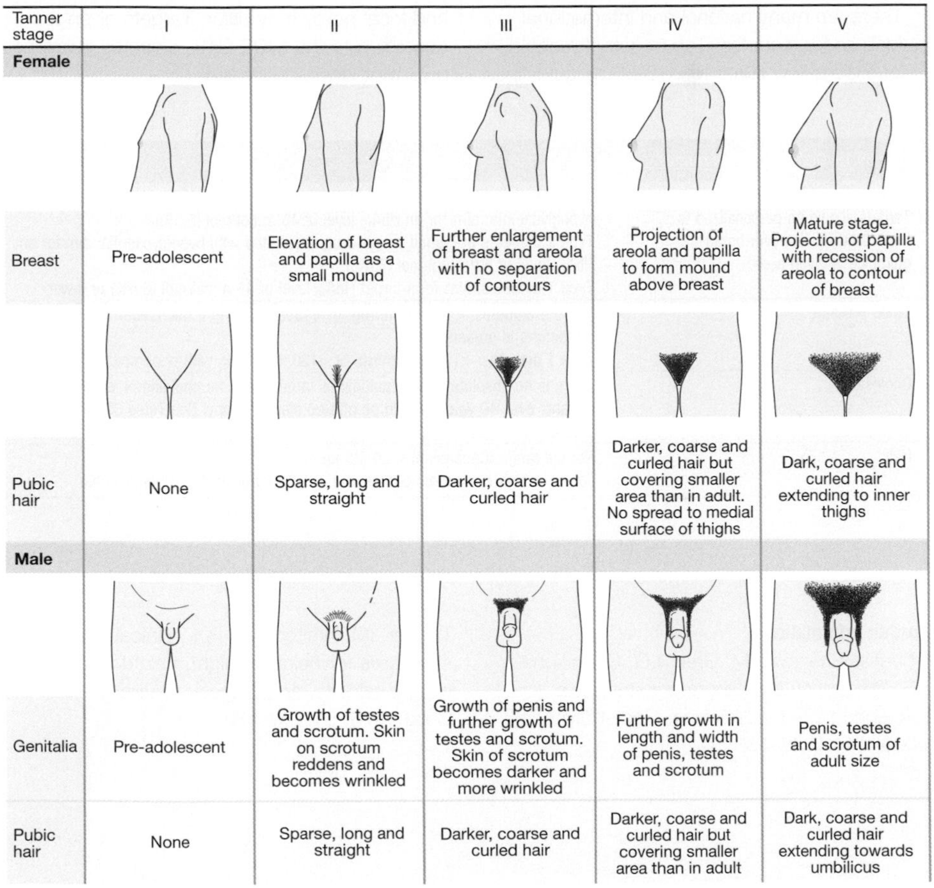

35

Tanner stage	I	II	III	IV	V
Female					
Breast	Pre-adolescent	Elevation of breast and papilla as a small mound	Further enlargement of breast and areola with no separation of contours	Projection of areola and papilla to form mound above breast	Mature stage. Projection of papilla with recession of areola to contour of breast
Pubic hair	None	Sparse, long and straight	Darker, coarse and curled hair	Darker, coarse and curled hair but covering smaller area than in adult. No spread to medial surface of thighs	Dark, coarse and curled hair extending to inner thighs
Male					
Genitalia	Pre-adolescent	Growth of testes and scrotum. Skin on scrotum reddens and becomes wrinkled	Growth of penis and further growth of testes and scrotum. Skin of scrotum becomes darker and more wrinkled	Further growth in length and width of penis, testes and scrotum	Penis, testes and scrotum of adult size
Pubic hair	None	Sparse, long and straight	Darker, coarse and curled hair	Darker, coarse and curled hair but covering smaller area than in adult	Dark, coarse and curled hair extending towards umbilicus

Fig. 35.2

---

i 35.14 Diagnostic cut-offs in diabetes and other glucose–related disorders

Diabetes is confirmed by:
- *either* plasma glucose in random sample or 2 hrs after a 75 g glucose load ≥11.1 mmol/L (200 mg/dL) *or*
- fasting plasma glucose ≥ 7.0 mmol/L (126 mg/dL) *or*
- HbA$_{1c}$ ≥ 48 mmol/mol

In asymptomatic patients, two diagnostic tests are required to confirm diabetes; the second test should be the same as the first test to avoid confusion

'Pre-diabetes' is classified as:
- impaired fasting glucose = fasting plasma glucose ≥ 6.1 mmol/L (110 mg/dL) and < 7.0 mmol/L (126 mg/dL)
- impaired glucose tolerance = fasting plasma glucose < 7.0 mmol/L (126 mg/dL) *and* 2-hr glucose after 75 g oral glucose drink 7.8–11.1 mmol/L (140–200 mg/dL)

HbA$_{1c}$ criteria for pre-diabetes vary. The National Institute for Health and Care Excellence (NICE) guidelines (UK) recommend considering an HbA$_{1c}$ range of 42–47 mmol/mol to be indicative of pre-diabetes; the American Diabetes Association (ADA) guidelines suggest a range of 39–47 mmol/mol. The ADA also suggests a lower fasting plasma glucose limit of ≥ 5.6 mmol/L (100 mg/dL) for impaired fasting glucose.

Gestational diabetes is classified by:
Plasma glucose ≥5.6 mmol/L (100 mg/dL) (fasting) ≥7.8 mmol/L (140 mg/dL) 120 mins post 75 g OGTT, according to NICE 2015 guidelines, but other regions may differ

There are many national and international guidelines for diabetes. The targets/threshold discussed below relate to current UK guidelines and local policy may differ. Targets given are according to the NICE 2015 diabetes guidelines unless otherwise specified

i	35.15 Diabetes target ranges
HbA$_{1c}$ Targets should be personalized to the individual. However broad guidance is given here	Type 2 diabetes managed by lifestyle/ diet +/- a single drug not associated with hypoglycaemia: aim for an HbA$_{1c}$ level of 48 mmol/mol (6.5%) Type 2 diabetes managed with a drug associated with hypoglycaemia: aim for an HbA$_{1c}$ level of 53 mmol/mol (7.0%) Type 1 diabetes: aim for a target HbA$_{1c}$ level of 48 mmol/mol (6.5%) or lower
Blood pressure	*Type 2 diabetes: <140/80 mmHg, or <135/75 mmHg if microalbuminuria or proteinuria is present Type 1 diabetes: <135/85 mmHg, or <130/80 mmHg with nephropathy
Cholesterol	There is no absolute agreed guidelines target levels for cholesterol levels but all patients over 40 years should be offered statin therapy. See Table 35.4 for cholesterol targets
BMI	Normal range (Caucasian) = 20–25 kg/m^2 (lower in high-risk ethnic groups: e.g. 20–23 kg/m^2 in Asian populations)

Further information

Abbassi-Ghanavati M, Greer LG, Cunningham FG. Pregnancy and laboratory studies: a reference table for clinicians. Obstet Gynecol 2009; 114:1326–1331.

Tanner JM, Whitehouse RH. Clinical longitudinal standards for height, weight, height velocity, weight velocity, and stages of puberty. Arch Dis Child 1976; 51:170–179.

Colour illustrations

These illustrations are shown here in colour. They are also reproduced in black and white alongside their associated questions.

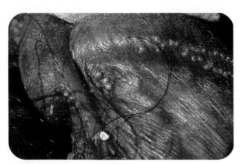

Fig. 13.5

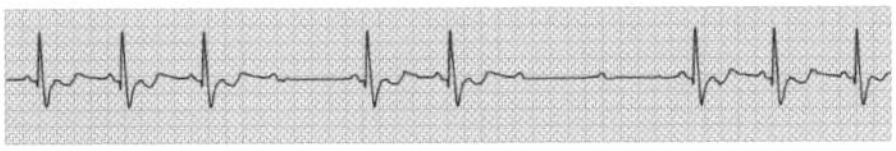

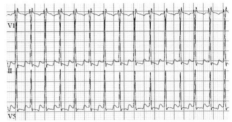

Fig. 16.21

Fig. 16.25

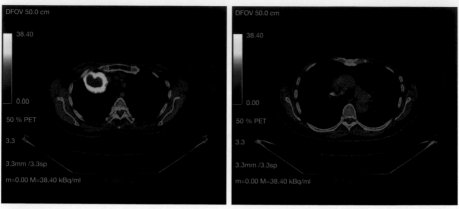

Fig. 17.15a

Fig. 17.15b

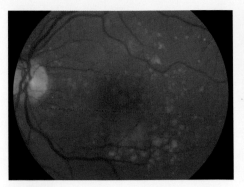

Fig. 27.12

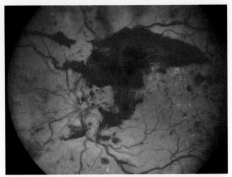

Fig. 27.15

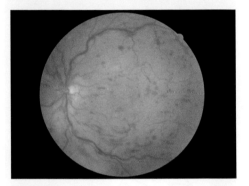

Fig. 27.13

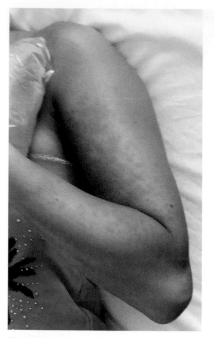

Fig. 29.1

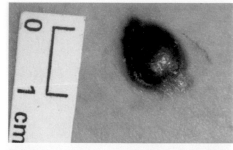

Fig. 29.7

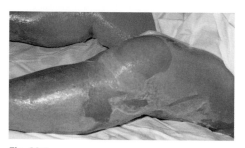

Fig. 29.5

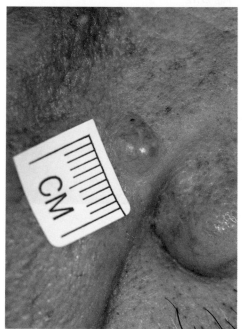

Fig. 29.9

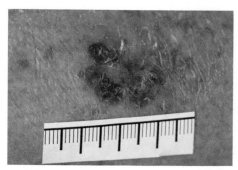

Fig. 29.6

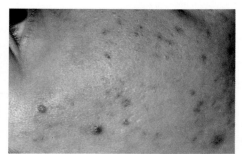

Fig. 29.10

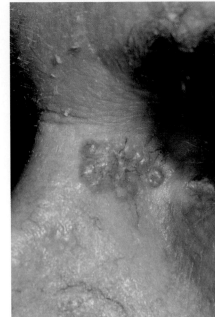

Fig. 29.13

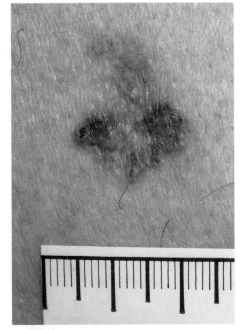

Fig. 29.28

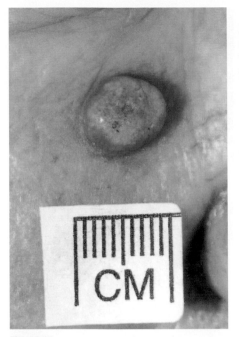

Fig. 29.23

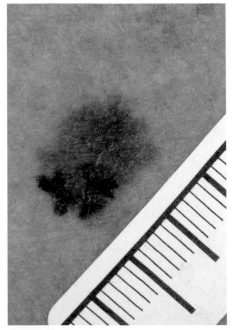

Fig. 29.37

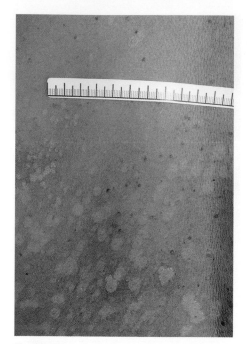

Fig. 29.42

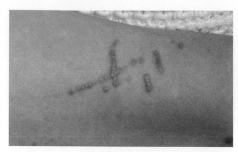

Fig. 29.48

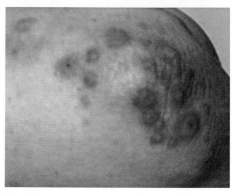

Fig. 29.53

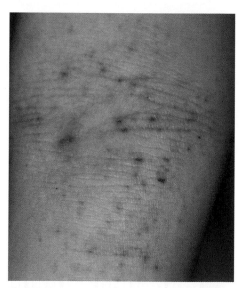

Fig. 29.46

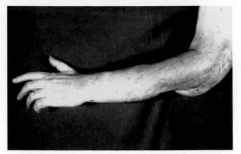

Fig. 34.7

Fig. 34.7

Index

Page numbers followed by "*f*" indicate figures, "*t*" indicate tables, and "*b*" indicate boxes.